Thieme

Musculoskeletal Imaging

A Concise Multimodality Approach

Klaus Bohndorf, M. D.
Professor and Chair
Klinik für Diagnostische Radiologie
und Neuroradiologie
Zentralklinikum Augsburg
Augsburg, Germany

Herwig Imhof, M. D.
Professor
Universitätsklinik für Radiodiagnostik
Allgemeines Krankenhaus der Stadt Wien
Vienna, Austria

Thomas Lee Pope, Jr., M. D., FACR
Professor and Chair
Department of Radiology
Medical University of South Carolina
Charleston, South Carolina, USA

With contributions by

W. Fischer, M. Breitenseher, J. Demharter,
J. Haller, H. Häuser, J. Hodler, J. Hofmann,
F. M. Kainberger, E. Knöpfle, W. Michl,
Th. Rand, G. Seidl, S. Trattnig, K. Turetschek,
S. Youssefzadeh

Translated by Peter Winter, M. D.

1300 illustrations

Thieme
Stuttgart · New York

Library of Congress Cataloging-in-Publication Data

Bohndorf, Klaus.
[Radiologische Diagnostik der Knochen und Gelenke, English]
Radiologic diagnosis of the bones and joints/Klaus Bohndorf, Herwig Imhof, Thomas Lee Pope, Jr.; with contributions by W. Fischer … [et al.]; translated by Peter Winter. p.; cm.
Includes bibliographical references and index.
ISBN 3131274417 (GTV) –
ISBN 1-58890-060-6 (TNY)
1. Bones–Radiography. 2. Joints–Radiography.
3. Bones–Diseases–Diagnosis. 4. Joints–Diseases–Diagnosis. I. Imhof, H. (Herwig).
II. Pope, Thomas Lee. III. Title.
[DNLM: 1. Bone Diseases–radiography.
2. Arthrography. 3. Bone and Bones–radiography.
WE 141 B677r2001a]
RC930.5.B5813 2001
616.7'107572–dc21 2001027188

This book is an authorized translation of the German edition published and copyrighted 1998 by Georg Thieme Verlag, Stuttgart, Germany. Title of the German edition: Radiologische Diagnostik der Knochen und Gelenke.

Translated by
Peter Winter, M. D.
Clinical Assistant Professor
University of Illinois
College of Medicine at Peoria
Peoria, IL, USA

Rüdigerstraße 14, D-70469 Stuttgart, Germany
Thieme New York, 333 Seventh Avenue,
New York, N. Y. 10001 U. S. A.

Cover design: Martina Berge, Erbach-Ernsbach
Typesetting by Ziegler + Müller, Kirchentellinsfurt
Printed in Germany by Appl, Wemding
ISBN 3-13-127441-7 (GTV)
ISBN 1-58890-060-6 (TNY) 1 2 3 4 5

Preface

This book makes the somewhat daring claim of offering a new approach to diagnostic imaging of bones and joints by redesigning the very concept of the book, the classic vehicle of relating knowledge. The authors composed most of the pages themselves with the help of personal computers, scanners, and appropriate software. The format chosen was to present the material in units of two opposing pages, with the left-hand page for reading and the right-hand page for viewing, thereby integrating text, tables, diagrams, and carefully selected images. Like radiology, the presentation is heavily image oriented. Whenever necessary, the images have been annotated for easier comprehension of the radiologic findings. Text and figures have to be seen as a unit, so not every figure is annotated in the text.

This is not a conventional multi-authored book since every chapter was thoroughly revised and edited to harmonize style and content and to create a coherent whole. Colleagues from the disciplines of orthopedics, rheumatology, traumatology, internal medicine, and nuclear medicine have reviewed the chapters and made useful suggestions.

This book attempts to define what a board-certified radiologist should know, or at one time should have known. Looking things up is legitimate and even intended. The point is to know where to look, and finding out should be made easy by the lucid presentation and systematic outline.

According to Shakespeare, brevity is the soul of wit ("Hamlet," Act II, Sc 2, Polonius) – but does this also apply to a textbook? The process of selecting, deleting, and emphasizing is one grounded on experience in and mastery of the subject. This book does not describe all there is, but rather, it is hoped, all that is deemed relevant. For good reason, traumatology (Chapter 1) and arthrology (Chapter 9) are the supporting pillars of the book. Conventional radiology of the bones and joints continues to take first place in describing the features that can be extracted from the images and used for interpretation. At the same time, the book follows a multi-modality approach. MRI, CT, nuclear medicine, and ultrasound are presented in depth when they supplement, replace, or add information that cannot be inferred from radiography. The modalities are integrated wherever they belong together. This takes into consideration that training in radiology generally involves working with one modality at a time, though diagnosing diseases by imaging requires a profound understanding of various modalities. This book is not meant to be used with one particular modality.

Who can benefit from this book? Above all, residents who want to learn more about musculoskeletal radiology. The structure and outline of the book make it especially suitable for review in preparation for the board examination. Furthermore, it is hoped that this book might be a useful reference text for practicing radiologists and other specialists to solve problems encountered in day-to-day practice.

The authors' text was edited into the final version by our technical editor Wolfgang Fischer, M.D., who made this project possible through his commitment, ideas, and hard work. Cliff Bergman, M.D., Gert Krueger and their team eagerly took on the last hurdle by formatting the files into printable book pages. Donna Garrison did a great job in editing the English text. Last but not least, the English version was made possible through the translation by our good friend Peter Winter, M.D.

Augsburg, Vienna, Charleston
Spring 2001

Klaus Bohndorf
Herwig Imhof
Thomas Lee Pope

Acknowledgements

With thanks to those who have contributed images:

V. Cassar-Pullicino, M.D., Oswestry

S. Ehara, M.D., Morioha

Prof. Dr. J. Freyschmidt, Bremen

G. Greenway, M.D., Dallas

Prof. Dr. M. Heller, Kiel

R. Kerr, M.D., Los Angeles

P. Kindynis, M.D., Geneva

Doz. Th. Leitha, Vienna

Dr. Mathson, Riad

Priv.-Doz. Dr. A. Prescher, Aachen

D. Resnick, M.D., San Diego

Scanco Medical, Bassersdorf

K. Tallroth, M.D., Helsinki

Yung Chan Wang, M.D., Taipeh

Contributors

Martin Breitenseher, M.D.
Professor
Universitätsklinik für Radiodiagnostik
Allgemeines Krankenhaus der Stadt Wien
Vienna, Austria

Johannes Demharter, M.D.
Klinik für Diagnostische Radiologie
und Neuroradiologie
Zentralklinikum Augsburg
Augsburg, Germany

Wolfgang Fischer, M.D.
Klinik für Diagnostische Radiologie
und Neuroradiologie
Zentralklinikum Augsburg
Augsburg, Germany

Jörg Haller, M.D.
Zentralröntgeninstitut
Hanusch-Krankenhaus
Vienna, Austria

Hannes Häuser, M.D.
Klinik für Diagnostische Radiologie
und Neuroradiologie
Zentralklinikum Augsburg
Augsburg, Germany

Juerg Hodler, M.D.
Abteilung Radiologie
Klinik Balgrist
Zurich, Switzerland

Johannes Hofmann, M.D.
Zentralröntgeninstitut
Hanusch-Krankenhaus
Vienna, Austria

Franz M. Kainberger, M.D.
Professor
Universitätsklinik für Radiodiagnostik
Allgemeines Krankenhaus der Stadt Wien
Vienna, Austria

Egbert Knöpfle, M.D.
Klinik für Diagnostische Radiologie
und Neuroradiologie
Zentralklinikum Augsburg
Augsburg, Germany

Wolfgang Michl, M.D.
Klinik für Diagnostische Radiologie
und Neuroradiologie
Zentralklinikum Augsburg
Augsburg, Germany

Thomas Rand, M.D.
Professor
Universitätsklinik für Radiodiagnostik
Allgemeines Krankenhaus der Stadt Wien
Vienna, Austria

Gerald Seidl, M.D.
Universitätsklinik für Radiodiagnostik
Allgemeines Krankenhaus der Stadt Wien
Vienna, Austria

Siegfried Trattnig, M.D.
Professor
Universitätsklinik für Radiodiagnostik
Allgemeines Krankenhaus der Stadt Wien
Vienna, Austria

Karl Turetschek, M.D.
Universitätsklinik für Radiodiagnostik
Allgemeines Krankenhaus der Stadt Wien
Vienna, Austria

Soraya Youssefzadeh, M.D.
Universitätsklinik für Radiodiagnostik
Allgemeines Krankenhaus der Stadt Wien
Vienna, Austria

Contents

1 Trauma

Definitions . . . 2
- Fracture . . . 2
- Joint Injury . . . 2
- Muscle Injury . . . 2
- Tendon Injury . . . 2

Role of Imaging in Trauma to the Musculoskeletal System . . . 2
K. Bohndorf
- Conventional Radiology . . . 4
  - Digital Radiology . . . 4
- Computed Tomography . . . 4
  - Spiral CT, 2-D and 3-D Reconstruction . . . 6
- Arthrography . . . 6
- Sonography . . . 8
- Magnetic Resonance Imaging . . . 8
- Scintigraphy . . . 10

Practical Suggestions for Imaging in the Trauma Setting . . . 11
K. Bohndorf

Fracture Classifications and Types . . . 12
K. Bohndorf
- Fracture Types . . . 12
- Special Considerations in the Pediatric Age Group . . . 14
- Fractures of the Articular Surfaces (Chondral and Osteochondral Fractures) . . . 16
- Stress and Insufficiency Fractures . . . 18
- Pathologic Fracture . . . 22

Fracture Healing . . . 24
K. Bohndorf
- Primary Fracture Healing . . . 24
- Secondary Fracture Healing . . . 24
- Radiographic Signs of Osseous Consolidation . . . 24
- Basic Principles of Fracture Treatment . . . 24
- Delayed Fracture Healing . . . 26
- Pseudarthrosis . . . 26

Complications after Fractures . . . 26
M. Breitenseher
- Reflex Sympathetic Dystrophy (RSD) . . . 30

Trauma-Induced Soft-Tissue Changes . . . 32
K. Bohndorf
- Tendon Injuries . . . 32
- Ligamentous Injuries . . . 32
- Muscle Injuries . . . 32
- Rhabdomyolysis . . . 34
- Myositis Ossificans . . . 34
- Compartment Syndrome . . . 34

Radiologic Reporting of Fractures . . . 36
K. Bohndorf

Special Traumatology . . . 38
- Skull and Spine . . . 38
  K. Turetschek
  - Fractures of the Cranial Vault . . . 38
  - Fractures of the Cranial Base . . . 38
  - Fractures of the Temporal Bone . . . 38
  - Fractures of the Facial Bones . . . 40
  - Spine . . . 44
- Pelvis . . . 54
  J. Demharter
  - Pelvic Injuries . . . 54
  - Acetabular Fractures . . . 58
  - Hip Dislocation without Acetabular Fracture . . . 60
  - Hip Dislocations with Fracture of the Femoral Heads (Pipkin Fractures) . . . 60
- Shoulder Girdle . . . 62
  J. Hodler
  - Sternoclavicular Dislocation . . . 62
  - Clavicular Fracture . . . 62
  - Acromioclavicular Separation . . . 64
  - Impingement and Rotator Cuff Rupture . . . 65
  - Shoulder Dislocation, Shoulder Instability . 70
- Upper Extremity . . . 74
  H. Häuser
  - Humeral Fractures . . . 74
  - Dislocation of the Elbow . . . 78
  - Subluxation of the Radial Head (Chassaignac) . . . 78
  - Tennis Elbow . . . 78
  - Fractures of the Proximal Forearm . . . 80
  - Forearm Fractures . . . 82
  - Distal Forearm Fractures . . . 84
  - Dislocation of the Distal Forearm . . . 88
  - Injuries of the Triangular Fibrocartilage Complex (TFCC) . . . 88
  - Fractures of the Carpal Bones . . . 90
  - Carpal Derangements . . . 92
  - Carpometacarpal Injuries . . . 96
- Lower Extremity . . . 98
  - Femur and Patella . . . 98
  S. Trattnig, W. Fischer

The Post-Surgical Hip 102
E. Knöpfle
Internal Lesions of the Knee 108
S. Trattnig
Tibia/Fibula 114
J. Demharter
Fractures of the Ankle 120
J. Demharter
Tarsal and Metatarsal Bones 122
J. Demharter
Ligamentous Injuries of the Ankle 126
M. Breitenseher
Special Problems Encountered in Children 128
W. Michl
The Normal Development of the Epiphyseal Growth Zone, Developmental Variations, and Transition to Pathologic Cases 128
Battered Child Syndrome 132

2 Bone and Soft-Tissue Infections

Osteomyelitis 136
K. Bohndorf
Acute Hematogenous Osteomyelitis 136
Newborn Osteomyelitis 136
Juvenile Hematogenous Osteomyelitis .. 138
Acute Hematogenous Osteomyelitis in the Adult 138
Imaging Features of Acute Hematogenous Osteomyelitis (All Ages) 138
Evidence of Healing of Acute Osteomyelitis 140
Complications of Acute Hematogenous Osteomyelitis (All Age Groups) 140
Chronic Hematogenous Osteomyelitis 142
Brodie Abscess 144
Chronic Recurrent Multifocal Osteomyelitis 144
Post-traumatic Osteomyelitis 146
Tuberculosis 150
Soft-Tissue Infections 152
K. Bohndorf

3 Tumors and Tumorlike Lesions of the Skeleton and Soft Tissues

General Considerations in Diagnosing Skeletal Tumors 154
K. Bohndorf
The Role of the Radiologist in Evaluating Skeletal Lesions Suspicious for Tumors .. 155
The Role of Diagnostic Imaging 155
Ten Rules for Classifying Skeletal Lesions Suspicious for Tumors 156
Staging (Determining the Extent of the Lesion) 157
Relative Values of the Different Imaging Modalities for Tissue Diagnosis, Biologic Activity, and Staging 157
Conventional Radiography 157
Scintigraphy 157
CT 157
Sonography 157
Angiography 158
MRI 158
Staging and MRI 159
Therapeutic Strategies of Bone and Soft-Tissue Tumors 159
Primary Bone Tumors 160
K. Bohndorf
Bone-Producing Tumors 160
Osteoid Osteoma 160
Osteoblastoma 160
Osteosarcoma 162
"Conventional" Osteosarcoma 162
Cartilage-Producing Tumors 164
Osteochondroma 164
Enchondroma 166
Chondroblastoma 166
Chondromyxoid Fibroma 168
Chondrosarcoma 168
Giant Cell Tumor 170
Tumors Arising from Bone Marrow 172
Ewing Sarcoma 172
Vascular Tumors 174
Hemangiomas 174
Tumors Arising From Connective Tissue 177
Lipoma 177
Other Tumors 180
Chordoma 180
Adamantinoma of the Long Tubular Bones 180
Tumorlike Lesions 182
K. Bohndorf
Osteoma, Bone Islands, Osteopoikilosis 182
Fibrous Cortical Defect/Nonossifying Fibroma 184

Simple (Juvenile) Bone Cyst 186
Aneurysmal Bone Cyst 188
Eosinophilic Granuloma and Histiocytosis X . 190
Fibrous Dysplasia 192
Metastases 196
K. Bohndorf
Soft-Tissue Tumors 200
K. Bohndorf

4 Hematologic Disorders

Plasmocytoma 204
Th. Rand
Leukemias 208
Th. Rand
Acute Leukemia in Children 208
Chronic Leukemia in Adulthood 208
Malignant Lymphoma 210
Th. Rand
Anemias 212
Th. Rand
Sickle Cell Anemia 212
Thalassemias 214
Myelofibrosis 216
Th. Rand
Lipidoses 216
Th. Rand

5 Ischemic Bone Disease

Osteonecrosis 218
M. Breitenseher
Osteonecrosis of the Hip 218
Osteonecrosis in other Locations 224
Osteonecrosis of the Lunate 224
Osteonecrosis of the Scaphoid 226
Osteonecrosis of the Metatarsal Heads ... 226
Osteonecrosis of the Distal Femur 226
Bone Infarct 228
M. Breitenseher
Bone Marrow Edema Syndrome 230
M. Breitenseher
Legg-Calvé-Perthes Disease 232
Osteochondritis Dissecans (OCD) 234
K. Bohndorf

6 Metabolic, Hormonal, and Toxic Osteopathies

Osteoporosis 236
G. Seidl
X-Ray Absorptiometry and Osteoporosis 240
Rickets and Osteomalacia 242
S. Youssefzadeh
Hyperparathyroidism 244
S. Youssefzadeh
Renal Osteodystrophy 248
S. Youssefzadeh
Hypoparathyroidism 250
S. Youssefzadeh
Toxic Osteopathies 250
S. Youssefzadeh
Metal Poisoning (Lead, Bismuth, Phosph.) .. 250
Aluminum Bone Disease 250
Fluorosis 250
Corticosteroids 252
Other Medications 252
Amyloidosis 254
S. Youssefzadeh, K. Bohndorf
Acromegaly 254
W. Fischer

7 Constitutional Disorders of Bone Growth

Skeletal Dysplasias 256
W. Michl
Early Onset Types 258
Thanatophoric Dysplasia 258
Achondroplasia 258
Chondrodysplasia Punctata 260
Asphyxiating Thoracic Dysplasia 260
Dyschondrosteosis 260
Cleidocranial Dysplasia 262
Late-Onset Types 262
Predominantly Epiphyseal Dysplasias 262
Predominantly Metaphyseal Dysplasias .. 262
Predominantly Spondyloepiphyseal
or Metaphyseal Dysplasias 264
Skeletal Dysplasia with Disorganized
Development of Cartilage
and Fibrous Components 266
Enchondromatosis 266
Polyostotic Fibrous Dysplasia 266
Congenital Generalized Fibromatosis 266
Skeletal Dysplasias with Abnormal
Density of Osseous Structures 266

Increased Bone Density 270
Dysostosis Multiplex 272
W. Michl
Mucopolysaccharidoses 272
Mucolipidoses and Gangliosidoses 272
Dysostoses 274
W. Michl

8 Various Bone and Soft-Tissue Disorders

Paget Disease 276
W. Fischer
Sarcoidosis 280
W. Fischer
Hypertrophic Osteoarthropathy 282
W. Fischer
Melorheostosis 282
W. Fischer
Calcifications and Ossifications of the Soft Tissues 284
W. Fischer, K. Bohndorf
Soft-Tissue Calcification Secondary to Imbalanced Calcium-Phosphate Metabolism 284
Soft-Tissue Calcifications with Normal Calcium-Phosphate Metabolism 284
Dystrophic Calcifications 284
Myositis Ossificans 286
Chronic Venous Stasis 286
Pustulotic Arthro-osteitis 288
K. Bohndorf
Congenital Hip Dysplasia 290
W. Fischer

9 Joints

Introduction and Synopsis 292
Anatomy of the Synovial Joints 292
W. Fischer
Signs of Joint Diseases on Radiography and CT 293
F. Kainberger, W. Fischer, K. Bohndorf
Radiographic Signs of the Peripheral Joints and Their Role in the Differential Diagnosis 294
Radiographic Signs at Specific Joints 298
Sonography 300
F. Kainberger
Scintigraphy 300
F. Kainberger
MRI 301
F. Kainberger
Arthritis versus Osteoarthritis (Overview) 302
W. Fischer
Enthesopathies (Fibro-ostosis and Fibro-ostitis) 306
K. Bohndorf
Fibro-ostosis 306
Fibro-ostitis 306
Degenerative Joint Diseases 308
H. Imhof
Osteoarthritis of the Peripheral Joints 308
Osteoarthritis of Specific Joints 312
Osteoarthritis of the Hip 312
Osteoarthritis of the Shoulder 314
Osteoarthritis of the Finger and Carpal Bones 314
Osteoarthritis of the Toes 314
Disk Degeneration (Chondrosis, Osteochondrosis) 320
Degeneration of the Intervertebral Articulations (Facet Joint Osteoarthritis) 326
Advantages and Disadvantages of the Different Imaging Modalities in Degenerative Disease of the Spine with Neurologic Findings (Radiculopathy) 326
Comments on Interpreting MRI, CT, and CT Myelography in Disk Diseases 326
Diffuse Idiopathic Skeletal Hyperostosis (DISH, Forestier Disease) 328
Inflammatory Joint Diseases 331
Classification of the Arthritides 331
W. Fischer
Special Problems 331
Infectious Arthritis, Spondylitis and Spondylodiskitis 332
W. Fischer, K. Bohndorf
Bacterial Arthritis 332
Infectious Spondylitis and Spondylodiskitis 334
Rheumatoid Arthritis 338
J. Haller, J. Hofmann
Juvenile Rheumatoid Arthritis (Juvenile Chronic Arthritis) 344
J. Haller, J. Hofmann
Ankylosing Spondylitis 346
J. Haller, J. Hofmann

Reactive Arthritis 350
J. Haller, J. Hofmann
Reiter Syndrome 350
Psoriatic Arthropathy 352
J. Haller, J. Hofmann
Enteropathic Arthropathies 354
J. Haller, J. Hofmann
Articular Changes in Inflammatory Systemic Connective Tissue Diseases 354
J. Haller, J. Hofmann
Systemic Lupus Erythematosus (SLE) 355
Progressive Systemic Scleroderma (PSS) .. 355
Polymyositis, Dermatomyositis 355
Polyarteritis Nodosa 356
Mixed Collagenosis 356
HIV-Associated Articular Disease 356
J. Haller, J. Hofmann
Differential Diagnosis of Arthritis 358
W. Fischer
Neurogenic, Metabolic, and Hematologic Joint Diseases 360
Neurogenic Osteoarthropathy (Charcot Joint) 360
F. Kainberger
The Diabetic Foot 362
Corticosteroid-Induced Neuropathic-Like Alterations (Pseudo-Charcot Joint) 362
Crystal-Induced Arthropathies and Periarthropathies 364
Gout (Gouty Arthritis) 364
G. Seidl, W. Fischer
Pyrophosphate Arthropathy 368
F. Kainberger
Hydroxyapatite Disease 370
F. Kainberger
Arthropathy in Hemophilia 372
F. Kainberger
Tumors and Tumorlike Lesions of the Joints 374
K. Bohndorf
Intraosseous Ganglion 374
Synovial Chondromatosis 374
Pigmented Villonodular Synovitis (PVNS) 376

Index 378

Dedicated to Susanne, Katharina, Ilse, Klaus, and Andrea.

Klaus Bohndorf, Herwig Imhof

Dedicated to Lou, David, Jason, my Mom, my Dad, and my brother Robin.

Thomas Lee Pope

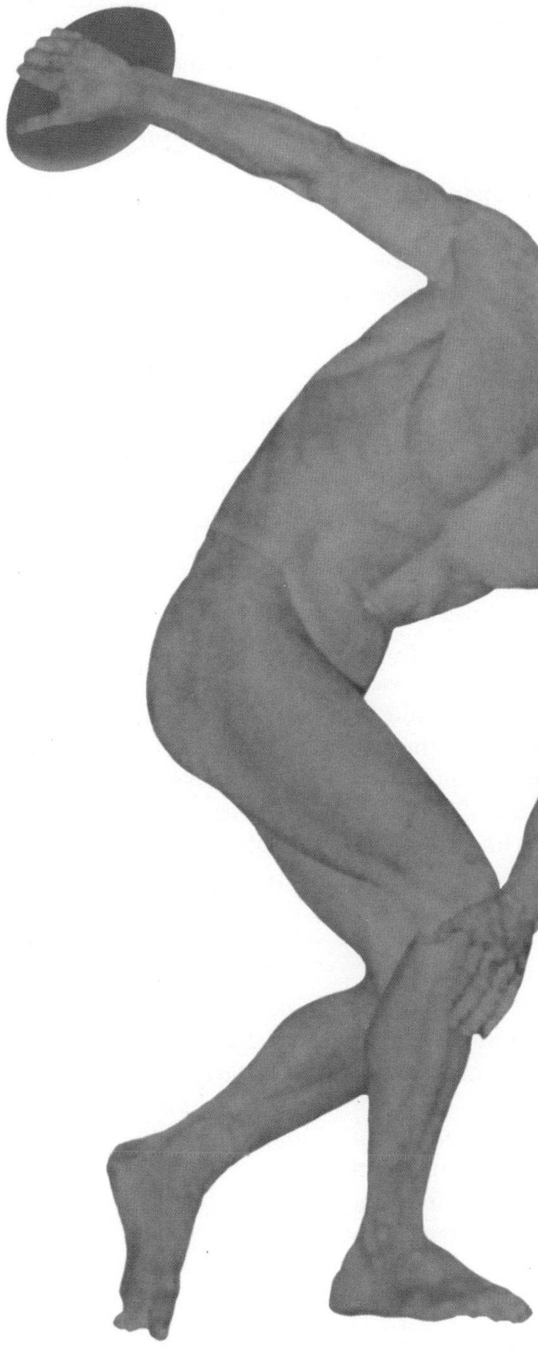

1 Trauma

In the broadest sense of its meaning, traumatology can be described as the medical specialty that studies damage to the human body, especially to the cell. The traumatic agent can be physical (e.g., mechanical trauma, temperature changes, radiation), chemical, or biologic (e.g., bacteria, viruses, etc.). Regardless of the etiology, the body can be expected to exhibit two effects: a local effect at the site of the trauma, and a systemic effect on the body (e.g., shock, fever, and others).

In a narrower sense, traumatology deals with mechanically induced injuries of the musculoskeletal tissue. For practical reasons, other physical etiologies, such as thermal injuries, are included in this chapter.

Definitions

Fracture

A fracture is a break in the continuity of bone. Where the bone is not completely separated, a break is called a fissure.

Etiologically, fractures can be classified as direct fractures (a fracture at the site of the causative force, Fig. 1.**1**) or indirect fractures (a fracture at a site remote from the causative force). Furthermore, the degree and extent of the injury differentiate complete from incomplete fractures. Typical incomplete fractures are greenstick fractures, buckle fractures, and fissures.

Joint Injury

Joint injury refers to any damage to the capsuloligamentous system, cartilaginous structures, and osseous articular surfaces following contusions, subluxations, and dislocations.

Since the ligaments that connect the joints are more or less incorporated in the joint capsule, the term 'capsuloligamentous injury' is frequently used. Such an injury can be an elastic strain, a plastic sprain, or a complete rupture.

Joint injuries of particular interest are fractures and avulsions of cartilage (chondral fractures) with or without attached osseous fragments (osteochondral fractures, 'flake fractures', Fig. 1.**2**).

Subluxation and dislocation result from forcefully displaced articular surfaces that have failed to return to their normal position.

Muscle Injury

Muscles can suffer closed or open tears and crush injuries. Furthermore, indirect injuries can cause elastic strains, plastic sprains, or tears (Figs. 1.**3**–1.**5**).

Tendon Injury

Direct mechanical trauma (e.g., lacerations) and indirect trauma that triggers maximum muscular contraction can tear a tendon. The tear frequently occurs where the tendon shows signs of degeneration.

Role of Imaging in Trauma to the Musculoskeletal System

Roentgen's discovery of X-rays at the end of the 19th century not only revolutionized the diagnostic evaluation of trauma, but also transformed the treatment of injuries to the skeleton, joints, and soft tissues. The dominant role of conventional radiology now must be reassessed at increasingly shorter intervals in view of the continuing emergence of new imaging modalities. Some of the recently introduced techniques use X-rays, such as digital radiography or CT, while others are based on completely different physical principles, such as sonography or MRI.

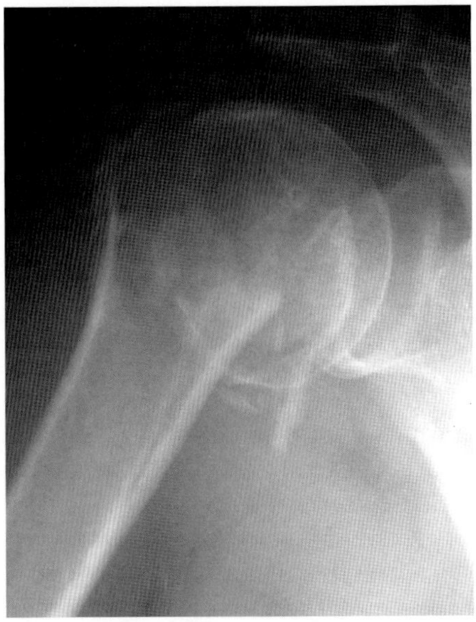

Fig. 1.1 Fractures. Subcapital fracture of the humerus with avulsion of the greater and lesser tuberosity and varus position of the humeral shaft.

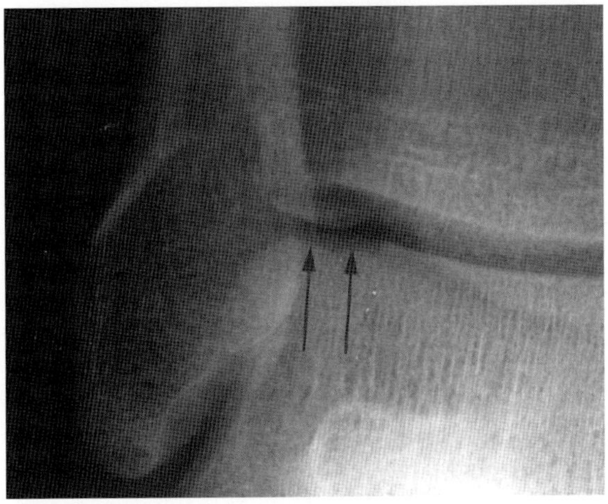

Fig. 1.2 Joint injury. Osteochondral fracture of the lateral talus.

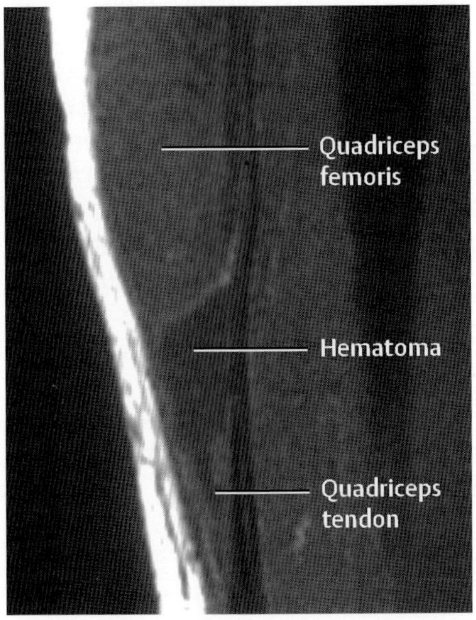

Fig. 1.3 Tendon injury. Acute hematoma at the transition of the quadriceps femoris muscle with the quadriceps tendon on sagittal T1-weighted spin echo image.

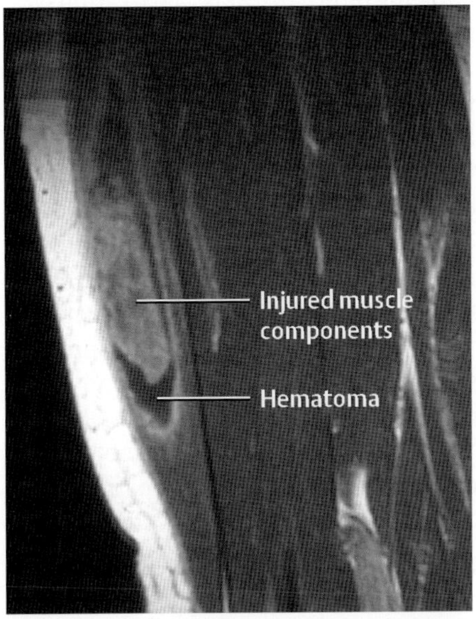

Fig. 1.4 Tendon injury. Large subacute hematoma in the femoris muscle on enhanced T1-weighted spin echo image.

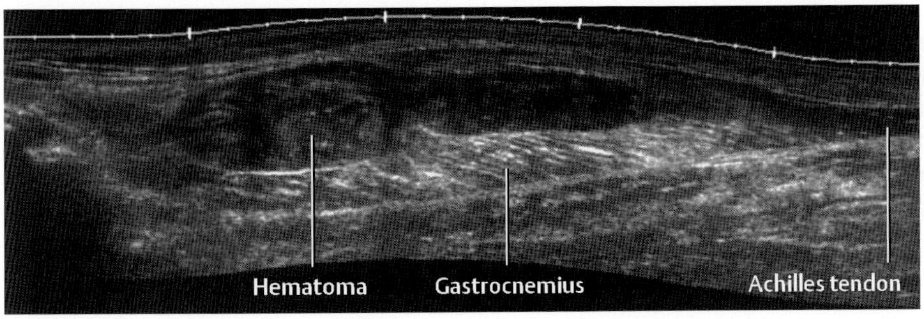

Fig. 1.5 Sonographic visualization of a muscle injury. Large hematoma in the gastrocnemius muscle secondary to torn muscle fibers. The tear itself is not discernible.

Conventional Radiology

Radiographs in two projections perpendicular to each other, preceded only by the clinical assessment, are generally the first and often the only diagnostic images needed for the evaluation of trauma. Some fractures, such as fractures of the radial head or femoral condyles, are only visible on additional oblique views (Fig. 1.**6**). Special views designed to eliminate superimposed structures are used to display complicated anatomic structures such as those encountered in the facial and carpal bones, in the shoulder and hip joint, and in the mid foot. In general, conventional radiography promptly diagnoses fractures and provides relevant information as to whether the adjacent joint is involved and how the fracture fragments are positioned. Conventional radiographs can almost always be obtained under the difficult circumstances encountered in the acute setting of severe trauma. Even with the availability of more advanced methods, such as MRI, surgical planning is still guided primarily by the clinical and radiographic findings. Following internal or external fixation with reduction of dislocations and alignment of displaced fracture fragments, radiographs are mandatory to confirm the results of these therapeutic measures. Radiographs, however, cannot always monitor the progress of healing adequately. Complications of the healing process, such as infections, reflex osteodystrophy or inadequate internal fixation, are still diagnosed clinically, and radiographs are only confirmative. Radiographs play a limited role in skeletal regions that have complex anatomy or are superimposed by soft tissues and bowel loops, and in the evaluation of soft-tissue injuries. On the other hand, radiographically demonstrated soft-tissue changes can be used as indirect signs of osseous pathology.

Digital Radiology

Diagnostic imaging and image-guided therapy are inconceivable today without digital manipulation. Computed tomography (CT), digital subtraction angiography (DSA), and magnetic resonance imaging (MRI) rely on digital image acquisition and processing.

Two digital methods are used for projection radiography today: **digital image enhancement** and **digital luminescence radiography.** Both methods store the intensity distribution of the transmitted X-rays as a set of binary data, instead of analog data as with the film-screen system.

Digital enhancement radiography is a fluoroscopic method that can be implemented as digital cardiography, digital subtraction angiography, and digital spot films. Their numerous advantages have led to the acceptance of digital methods in diagnostic and therapeutic cardiology and angiography. Because of digital enhancement radiography's limited spatial resolution, it is rarely used as a substitute for X-rays, except for intra- and postoperative assessment of the position of fracture fragments.

Currently, digital luminescence radiography or storage phosphor radiography is the most commonly used digital method for obtaining radiographs (Figs. 1.**7**, 1.**8**), using the established projections of the film-screen technique. It can also be used with existing conventional tomographic equipment. The conventional film-screen cassette is replaced with a reusable storage phosphor imaging plate which captures the incoming X-rays as a latent image. The reader scans the plate with a laser beam and releases the stored energy as light. This stimulated light emission is measured by a photomultiplier tube interfaced to the image processor. The quality of digital luminescence radiography is adequate for diagnosing traumatic changes in all parts of the skeleton. The inferior spatial resolution of digital luminescence radiography is compensated for by its superior contrast resolution, i.e., the superior detection of small contrast differences. The linear response curve (gradient type) of the storage phosphor and the capability of display processing give this method a high tolerance for variations in exposure, reducing the number of films that have to be repeated because of inadequate exposure and ultimately decreasing the radiation dose to the patient.

Radiography of the bones and joints with **flat panel detectors**, an emerging new technique, is still work in progress.

Computed Tomography

CT generates images without superimposed structures, usually along the axial plane. While the patient is in a resting supine position, even anatomically difficult body regions can readily be evaluated noninvasively. A single section can be imaged in seconds and, with the addition of spiral technique (see below), an entire body region obtained during a single breath-hold. CT provides information about the bones and soft tissues and, while the resolution is slightly inferior compared to conventional radiography, is fully adequate to evaluate skeletal trauma.

CT may often show post-traumatic changes not shown by radiography (Fig. 1.**9**). The established in-

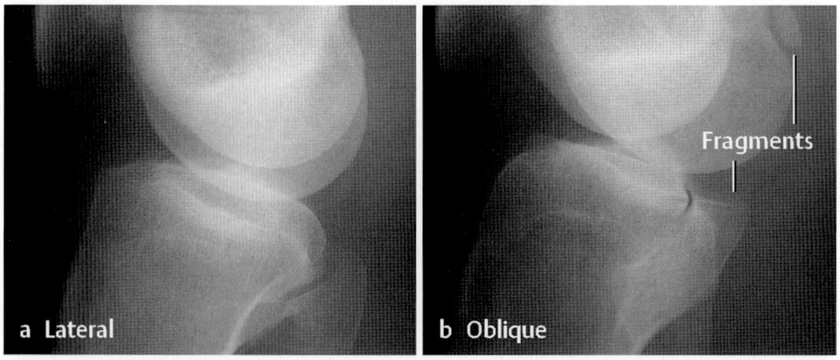

Fig. 1.**6** Dorsal avulsion of the tibial plateau and femoral condyles. The fractures are seen *only* in the *oblique* projection (**b**).

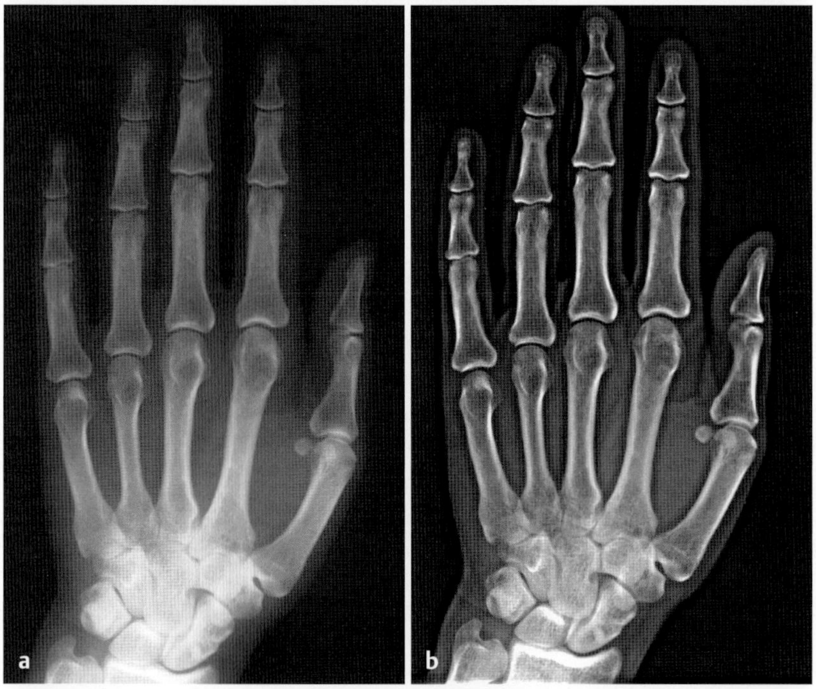

Fig. 1.**7** Different displays of a digital radiograph with:
a contrast scaling adjusted to that of a normal radiograph,
b frequency processing with edge enhancement.

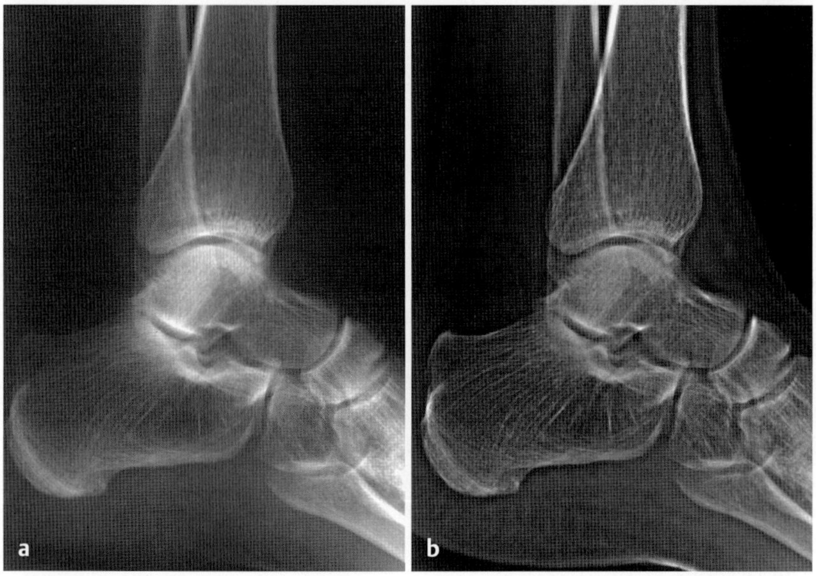

Fig. 1.**8** Further examples of various displays of digital images:
a contrast scaling adjusted to that of a normal radiograph,
b edge enhancement.

dications of CT in trauma are summarized in Table 1.1. It has been reported that up to 18% of fractures not seen on conventional radiographs may be detected by CT in the occipitocervical transition when CT is routinely performed on severely injured patients.

Any standard CT unit can easily demonstrate rotational anomalies, length discrepancies of the long bones of the extremities, and anteversion of the femoral neck with high accuracy and reproducibility. No complicated patient positioning or dedicated software is needed. In view of its excellent results and lower radiation dose, CT should replace the conventional methods of measuring the antetorsion angle, such as the Ripstein method.

Spiral CT, 2-D and 3-D Reconstruction

Spiral CT acquires a three-dimensional data set by continuous rotation of the X-ray tube around the moving examination table. The selected parameters for section thickness and table motion determine the volume of the body region and the resultant spatial resolution. From the three-dimensional data set, axial images are reconstructed as needed to address the clinical questions. Furthermore, the three-dimensional data set can be used to reformat images in other planes (2-D technique) and to render volume images (3-D technique) (Fig. 1.**10**). The tremendous improvements in processing speed over the last few years have made volume rendering feasible in daily clinical work. Reconstruction of isotropic voxels generated by the new generation of multi slice spiral CTs also has improved 3-D volume imaging.

The 2-D reformatting of sagittal and coronal images from axial images can highlight longitudinal fracture lines and can make it easier to evaluate horizontal interfaces, such as the acetabular roof or orbital floor (Fig. 1.**10 a**).

The 3-D rendering allows different displays of the volume data. Surface rendering by thresholding is the most widely used technique. The relatively rapid surface-rendering algorithms dismiss attenuation values below the user-selected threshold of bone attenuation. The soft tissues are computationally removed and the surface of the underlying osseous structure is displayed (Fig. 1.**11**). The surface rendering for the display of bone has the drawback of including other high-attenuation structures, such as atheromatous plaques, contrast agents, and internal fixation devices. The osseous structures depicted can be manipulated by semiautomatic subtraction of superimposed and potentially interfering anatomic structures. For instance, acetabular fractures can be displayed without the femoral head, or calcaneal fractures without the talus, essentially enacting an 'electronic disarticulation'. By adding a virtual light source, a shaded surface display (SSD) can be achieved, which enhances the 3-D understanding of the image.

Volume rendering requires more computer manipulation. It classifies each voxel of the volume data set and incorporates it into the displayed image. It can provide a transparent 3-D display of any apparent surface from any point of view and allows the comprehensive visualization of fractures. Powerful computers are required to achieve volume rendering at a reasonable speed in clinical applications.

All reconstruction methods offer a more effective display of complex anatomic and pathologic structures. Three-dimensional imaging improves the assessment of fractures. Location and extent of the fracture, shape and position of the fracture fragments and the condition of articular surfaces can be better appreciated, making it easier to assess comminuted fractures. Surface rendering, which, in contrast to volume rendering, incorporates only a portion of the data into the 3-D image, provides an inadequate display of undisplaced and intra-articular fragments and fails to show any soft-tissue changes. In comparison to sectional imaging, surface rendering does not increase the detection rate of fractures and should only be supplementary to plain films and axial CT sections in the evaluation of comminuted fractures.

Arthrography

The role of arthrography has declined because of the excellent visualization of the intra-articular structures by MRI. However, arthrography still has a role for certain clinical questions, such as adhesive capsulitis, and is still considered to be the 'gold standard' for the evaluation of ligamentous injuries of the hand (Fig. 1.**12**). Moreover, arthrography remains part of CT- or MRI-arthrography and is superior to imaging without intra-articular contrast medium for the evaluation of shoulder instability because of the detailed arthrographic visualization of anatomic structures and pathologic changes. This feature is especially helpful for conditions involving the glenoid labrum and joint capsule.

Table 1.1 Established indications for CT in skeletal traumatology

Indication	Clinical question
Facial bone injuries	Exact determination of the fracture sites and position of the fracture fragments
Vertebral injuries	Stability, intraspinal fragment, paravertebral/intraspinal hemorrhage, traumatic disk extrusion, fractures of the occipitocervical transition
Pelvic and hip fractures	Fractures of the posterior pelvic ring, acetabular fracture, intra-articular fragment, degree and type of fragment displacement
Wrist injuries	Unclear extent of trauma, radioulnar/carpal dislocation, rotational deformity
Calcaneal fractures	Fragment displacement, articular involvement
Biometric views	Determination of malrotation, length discrepancy, angulation (antetorsion angle of the femoral neck)

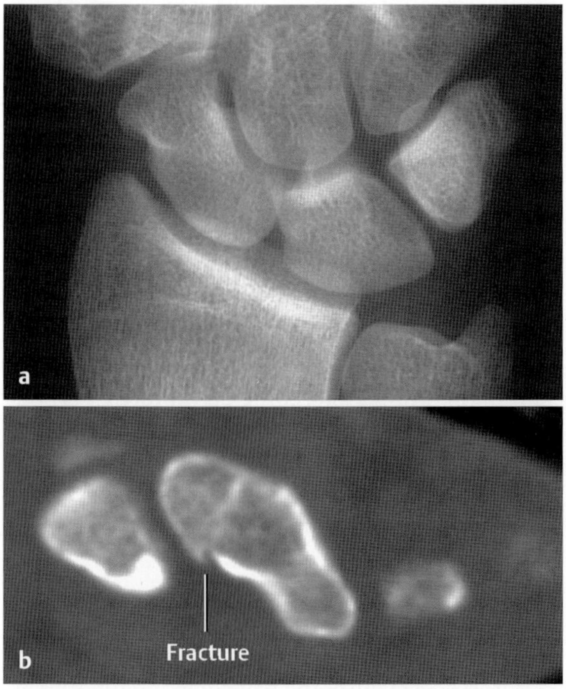

Fig. 1.9 Scaphoid fracture. **a** The AP radiograph is normal. **b** The fracture line is clearly delineated by CT.

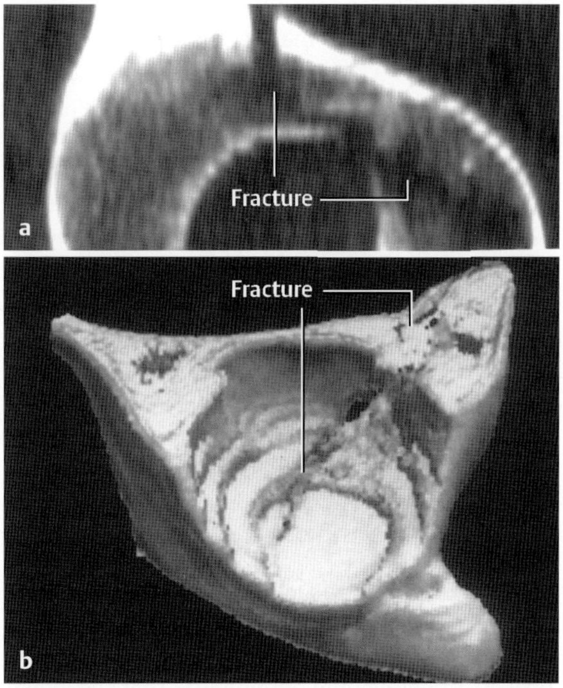

Fig. 1.10 2-D (**a**) and 3-D (**b**) reconstruction of an acetabular fracture. The 3-D reconstruction displays the joint as seen from the patient's feet.

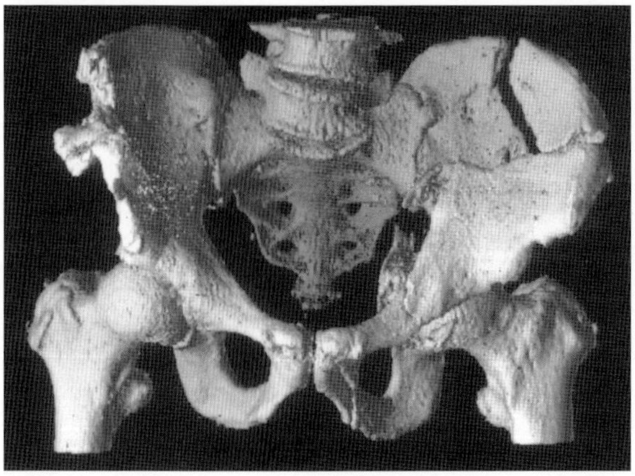

Fig. 1.11 3-D visualization of fractures of left iliac wing and acetabulum.

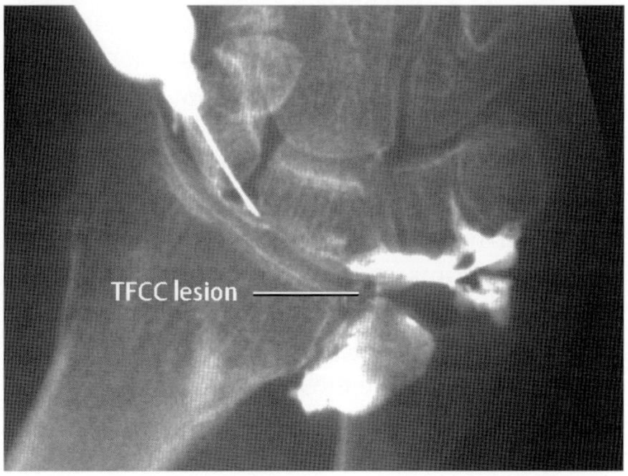

Fig. 1.12 Arthrography showing a tear of the triangular fibrocartilage complex (TFCC).

Sonography

Sonography is beginning to play an increasingly important role in trauma. Among its advantages are availability, low cost, patient acceptance, and lack of radiation exposure. Its disadvantages are operator dependence, long examination times, selective and often incomprehensible documentation, and the inability to penetrate osseous structures. Reasonable indications for sonography in trauma are outlined in Table 1.**2.** Ruptures of the Achilles and patellar tendons can be diagnosed instantly with great accuracy. Sonography cannot always differentiate between partial and complete rotator cuff tear, and MRI must be added in these cases.

Intrafascial hematomas in the musculature of the extremities can be visualized by sonography and, if necessary, drained under sonographic guidance. Sonography should also be the primary method for evaluation of a suspected sternal fracture. Sternal fractures, which have become a frequent seat belt injury, are seen as breaks in the normal contour of bone surrounded by a hematoma, with inducible relative motion of the fracture fragments (Fig. 1.**13**). Radiographic visualization of sternal fractures is often inadequate because of superimposed ribs and soft tissues and inherent low bone contrast. Finally, sonography can be superior to radiography in demonstrating rib fractures.

Magnetic Resonance Imaging

MRI can effectively visualize traumatic changes of the skeleton and peripheral soft tissues, such as intramuscular hematomas and ligamentous tears. Initially, the prevailing opinion was that the signal void of cortical bone would preclude the evaluation of skeletal injuries, but this theory has been disproved. In fact, the opposite is true; the lack of any signal from cortical bone augments the signal from adjacent tissues. In particular, visualization of bone marrow has opened entirely new perspectives (Table 1.**3**).

Stress and insufficiency fractures can present as radiographically unexplained pain. If radiographic changes are present, they might be mistaken for neoplasms or infection, particularly in the absence of periosteal reaction. A space-occupying process can be excluded invariably by MRI. These advantages of MRI are most valuable for evaluating skeletal regions with a complex internal architecture.

Before the availability of MRI, radiologically **occult fractures** often posed a diagnostic dilemma. MRI can detect not only these fractures, but also other conditions, such as osteonecrosis, degenerative subchondral cysts, and metastases, which might be the cause of the patient's symptoms (Fig. 1.**16**).

MRI has its major impact on diagnosing traumatic **joint** injury. Traumatic injury to the joints was once the domain of arthroscopy, but this has now changed with the introduction of MRI and has led to a better understanding of the immediate and delayed effects of trauma on the joints. Although hyaline cartilage, subchondral lamellar and trabecular bone can be considered separately, they are now increasingly seen as a functional unit. The most frequently encountered and characteristic constellation is the subchondral trabecular fracture with underlying marrow edema. The therapeutic ramification of the bone marrow edema, the so-called 'bone bruise', is still not fully understood.

Because of its complex anatomy, the **wrist** was one of the first anatomic regions to be investigated by MRI, and special surface coils allow high-resolution visualization of the carpal bones. For imaging with conventional MRI, patients must place their hands over their heads, putting them in a relatively uncomfortable position that is rarely tolerated for examination times exceeding 20 minutes. This has been overcome by open MRI systems, which allow the patient to sit outside the unit. The inferior spatial resolution of the open systems, however, can be a problem for those clinical questions that require the evaluation of the triangular fibrocartilage complex or ligaments. Established MRI indications in the wrist include the search for occult fractures of the carpal bones as well as the assessment of osteonecroses, especially of the navicular and lunate. Numerous publications have addressed the role of MRI in the evaluation of injuries of the triangular fibrocartilage complex (TFCC). Like arthrography, MRI visualizes a variety of changes in the TFCC in asymptomatic patients, and it is difficult to determine whether the particular change seen after trauma is traumatic or degenerative in origin.

The evaluation of **knee pain** undiagnosed by physical examination in the patient with normal radiographs has become the domain of MRI. This technique can demonstrate intraosseous microfractures and has increased our understanding of post-traumatic pain. These trabecular fractures, which are radiographically occult but often scintigraphically positive, can be clearly identified by location and configuration of the abnormal signal pattern. These otherwise unidentifiable microfractures must be considered the most frequent cause

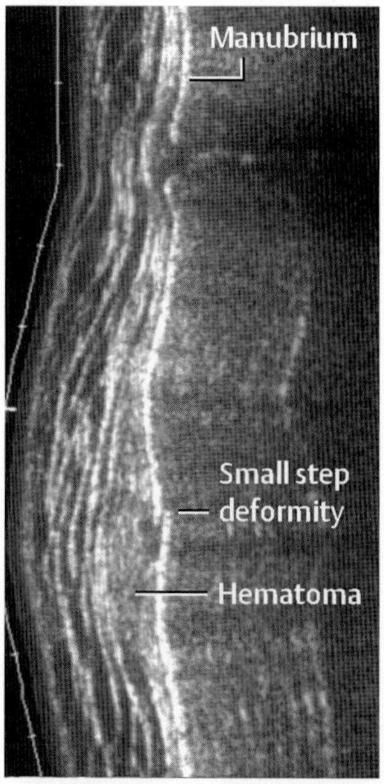

Fig. 1.**13** Sonographic visualization of a sternal fracture. The sonographically visualized hematoma makes it easy to find nondisplaced fractures, making sonography more sensitive than radiography.

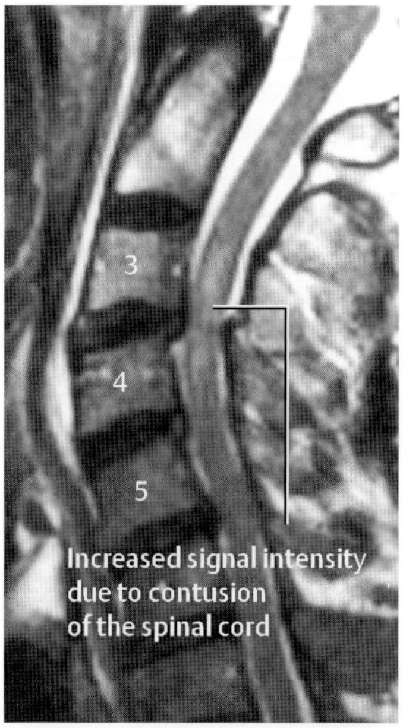

Fig. 1.**14** Contusion of the spinal cord and posterior subluxation of C3 on C4 in a trauma patient with neurologic findings (T2-weighted SE images).

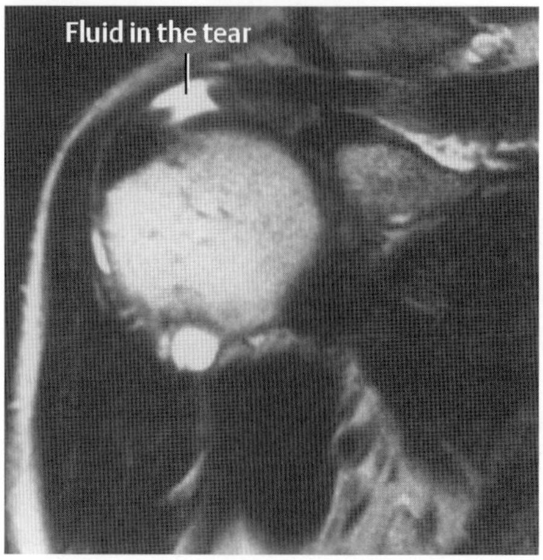

Fig. 1.**15** Full-thickness tear of the supraspinatus tendon on T2-weighted SE image.

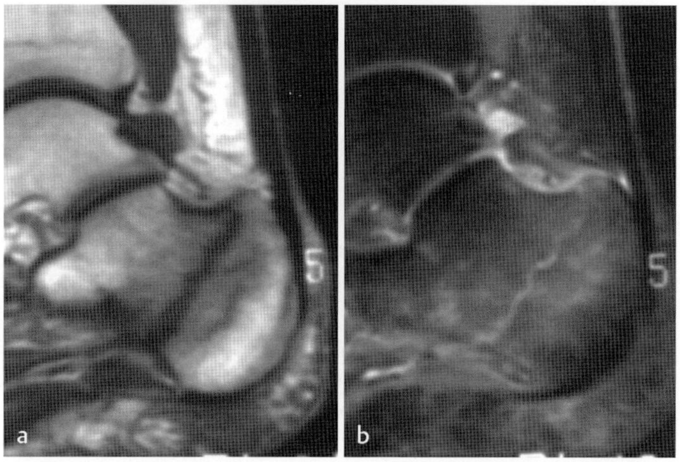

Fig. 1.**16** Occult calcaneal fracture with associated bone marrow edema following minor trauma 6 weeks previously and with persistent pain. The radiograph was normal. **a** T1-weighted SE sequence showing the fracture line as low signal intensity, **b** STIR sequence showing the fracture line as high signal intensity surrounded by bone marrow edema.

Table 1.**2** Established indications for sonography in the diagnostic evaluation of osseous, articular, and soft-tissue injuries

Body region	Indications
Shoulder	Rotator cuff tear, biceps tendon tear and dislocation, Hill-Sachs lesion, avulsion fracture, joint effusion, AC joint separation
Elbow, hand, foot	Achilles tendon tear, joint effusion, rupture of the distal triceps and biceps tendon, avulsion fracture
Hip	Joint effusion, avulsion fracture, slipped capital femoral epiphysis (epiphyseolysis of the femoral head)
Knee	Rupture of quadriceps and patellar tendons, rupture of collateral ligament, joint effusion, Baker cyst
Soft tissues	Muscle tear, hematoma, foreign body
Ribs, sternum	Radiographically occult fractures

of acute post-traumatic pain. Generally MRI findings resolve within 5 to 15 days, although no satisfactory prospective studies have been reported.

MRI detects **meniscal tears** with an accuracy of 80 – 90%, but it is still uncertain whether degenerative and traumatic tears can be distinguished by MRI. Not every meniscal lesion identified by MRI is symptomatic, and all those identified do not need surgical intervention. Obliquely oriented horizontal tears, which are commonly found on the undersurface of the meniscus, are invariably degenerative in nature, whereas vertical tears usually are traumatic in origin.

Complete tears of the anterior cruciate ligament (ACL) are detected with an average accuracy of 90%. Partial tears or distortions of the anterior cruciate ligament, which are characterized by partially intact fibers and severe intra- and periligamentous edema, are not always distinguishable from complete tears. Injuries of the posterior cruciate ligament are less common than ACL tears but are easily detected by MRI.

Even after numerous technical refinements, evaluation of the hyaline cartilage by MRI remains inferior to direct visualization by arthroscopy. This superiority of arthroscopy applies only to chondromalacia and superficial lesions of questionable therapeutic relevance. However, in many instances, osteochondral injuries are easily identified by MRI as the cause of hemarthrosis.

MRI is the most sensitive imaging test for identifying lesions of the **rotator cuff** of the shoulder joint (Fig. 1.**15**). Evaluating shoulder instability by MRI remains a controversial issue, as CT-arthrography represents a competing imaging method for this indication. But MRI-arthrography, analogous to CT-arthrography, can be viewed as the 'gold standard' for evaluating complex labrocapsular and ligamentous anatomy and pathology. MRI-arthrography can visualize anterior, posterior, or inferior labral injuries and Hill-Sachs defects, as well as injuries of the superior labral-biceps tendon junction.

Scintigraphy

Bone scans are performed with Tc 99 m–labeled diphosphonate and can be obtained as a static study or a dynamic study using the three-phase technique. Other scintigraphic techniques, such as In111- or Tc 99 m–labeled white blood cell scans, or Tc 99 m – labeled monoclonal antibody scans do not play a significant role in the evaluation of trauma.

Bone scans are established for the detection of radiologically occult fractures, but MRI has replaced this technique in most centers.

The bone scan is well suited for surveying the patient with multiple trauma for the extent of skeletal involvement. It should be kept in mind that reparative changes in juxta-articular appendicular bone might be visible only after the third day. In the diaphyses of the long bones and in the central skeleton, the bone scan might even become positive as late as one week after the trauma. Because of the known low specificity of increased bone activity on bone scan, a positive finding should be correlated with the radiographs.

In pediatrics, bone scanning plays a major role in screening for battered child syndrome (see pp. 132 ff).

Another indication for bone scanning is the search for stress fractures, including stress-induced spondylolysis of the lower lumbar spine. Focally increased osseous activity is often seen well before radiographic changes are detected.

Stress fractures should be differentiated from traumatic or degenerative irritation of tendon insertions (enthesopathy) and traumatic periosteal reaction along diaphyseal bone. Periosteal reaction along the tibia is referred to as 'shin splints'. In comparison to stress fractures, shin splints show no increased blood flow on the blood pool images.

Post-traumatic complications of the healing process, such as pseudarthrosis and reflex osteodystrophy, can also be demonstrated by bone scanning.

Practical Suggestions for Imaging in the Trauma Setting

1. Any traumatized bone must be visualized in at least two projections. It is difficult to meet this requirement for certain anatomic locations, such as the hip or shoulder. Special projections have been proposed for these anatomic regions. (Refer to other texts dedicated to radiographic positioning.)
2. For any fracture visualized next to a joint, any articular extension must be searched for. Special views must often be added to the two standard views. If conventional imaging is inconclusive, MRI should be considered.
3. If one of two parallel long bones (such as the ulna and radius or the tibia and fibula) is fractured, a fracture of the companion bone must be excluded.
4. Any long bone must be visualized in its **entire length.** In other words, the proximal and distal joint bearing ends have to be included.
5. In patients with multiple fractures, subtle findings may be missed if other major injuries are present. A second look at a less busy time or a second reading can be beneficial in detecting findings which might be overlooked. This is particularly applicable to films of patients with multiple trauma.
6. Whenever possible, the referring physician should state the traumatic forces and the expected **pattern** of the traumatic changes. This allows a focused search with the expected injuries kept in mind.
   Example: The supination-adduction trauma to the ankle causes a transverse fracture of the lateral malleolus below the syndesmosis, or a rupture of the lateral collateral ligament. Furthermore, this can lead to a vertical osteochondral fracture of the medial talar articulating surface. An awareness of the mechanism of injury will help direct the search pattern. This follows the adage 'you will find what you look for'.
7. It is mandatory to correlate clinical and radiological findings. If no exact or reliable clinical information is supplied, the radiologist or technologist must obtain it directly from the patient.
8. While many direct signs of fracture are easily appreciated, indirect signs such as soft-tissue changes are often overlooked. It is important for all images to include indirect signs in the diagnostic process (refer to special traumatology).
9. Equivocal radiographic findings should be further evaluated by additional views in other projections, such as oblique views. Other imaging modalities, such as sonography and CT, should be incorporated early in the diagnostic process.
10. Fracture lines are not invariably radiolucent. They can be radiodense if fracture fragments
    a) overlap,
    b) are impacted,
    c) are rotated relative to each other, with the radiodense line often sharply delineated, in contrast to a) and b).

Table 1.**3** Established indications for MRI in the diagnostic evaluation of osseous, articular, and soft-tissue injuries

Indications	Clinical question
Skeletal trauma	Trabecular fractures, occult fractures, stress fractures, vertebral fractures, suspected spinal cord involvement, posttraumatic osteonecroses, post-traumatic chronic osteomyelitis
Joint trauma	Osteochondral fractures, intra-articular ligamentous lesions (cruciate ligaments, collateral ligaments), meniscus injuries (especially in the knee)
Trauma of the peripheral soft tissues	Tendon and muscle injuries (hematoma, rupture, ligamentous injury [e.g., shoulder]), tendosynovitis in chronic repetitive microtrauma

Fracture Classifications and Types

Classification of fractures by their causative mechanisms:

1. **Traumatic Fractures**
   These fractures are caused by excessive mechanical loading, which can be sustained by deforming forces that act directly on bone such as tapping, crushing, or penetration, or indirectly from a distance, as occurs with traction, angulation, shearing, or compression. If the loading of bone exceeds a certain point, the bone will fail and fracture.
2. **Stress and Insufficiency Fractures**
   Stress fractures are caused by fatigue failure of otherwise normal bone induced by repeated or cyclical stresses. Insufficiency fractures are caused by normal forces or microtrauma and occur in bones of reduced internal strength, such those bones weakened by osteoporosis.
3. **Pathologic Fractures**
   These fractures occur in bone weakened by a preexisting condition and are caused by a force that would not break normal bone. They can be considered a local manifestation of an insufficiency fracture. The most common preexisting conditions are bone cysts, osteolytic metastases, and plasmocytoma.

Fracture Types

The morphology of the fracture reflects the direction and level of the traumatic forces. A practical classification of fracture types is illustrated in Fig. 1.**20.**

A special type of fracture is the compression fracture of the spine (Fig. 1.**17**).

The classification can be slightly modified by determining whether the fracture is associated with a dislocation (Fig. 1.**18**), or whether the fracture lines extend to the articular surface (Fig. 1.**19**).

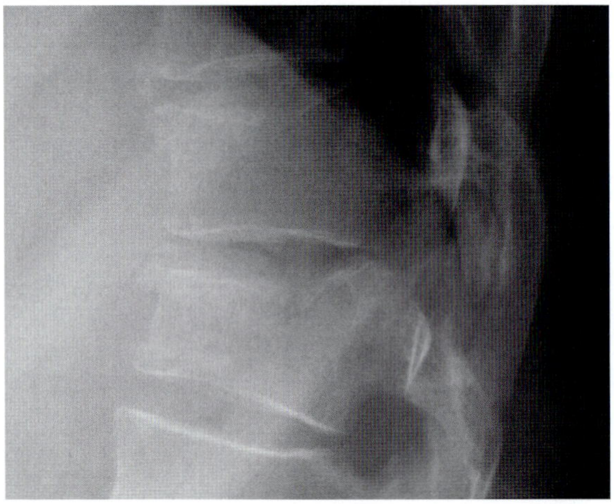

Fig. 1.**17** Compression fracture of the T9 and T10 vertebral bodies. There is increased density in the impacted anterior components of the vertebral bodies.

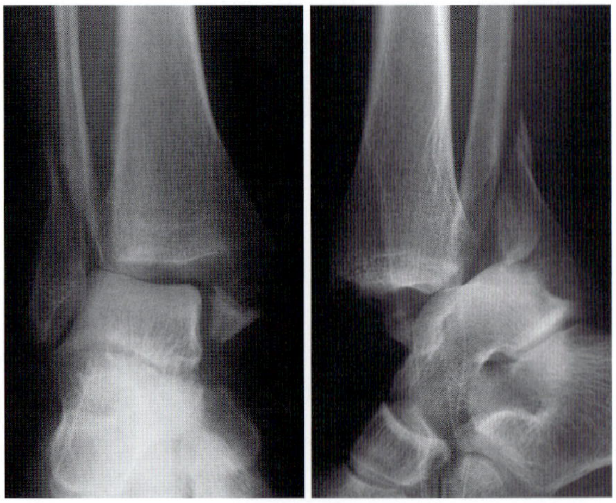

Fig. 1.**18** Bimalleolar fracture-dislocation of the ankle. Only the lateral view shows the full extent of the injury.

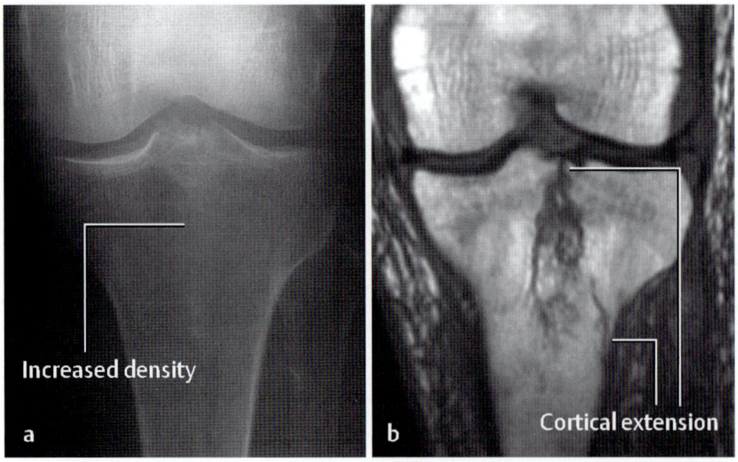

Fig. 1.**19** Longitudinal fracture of the tibial plateau seen as indistinct increased density on the conventional radiograph (**a**). MRI (T1-weighted SE sequence) shows the full extent of the fracture and the cortical involvement (**b**).

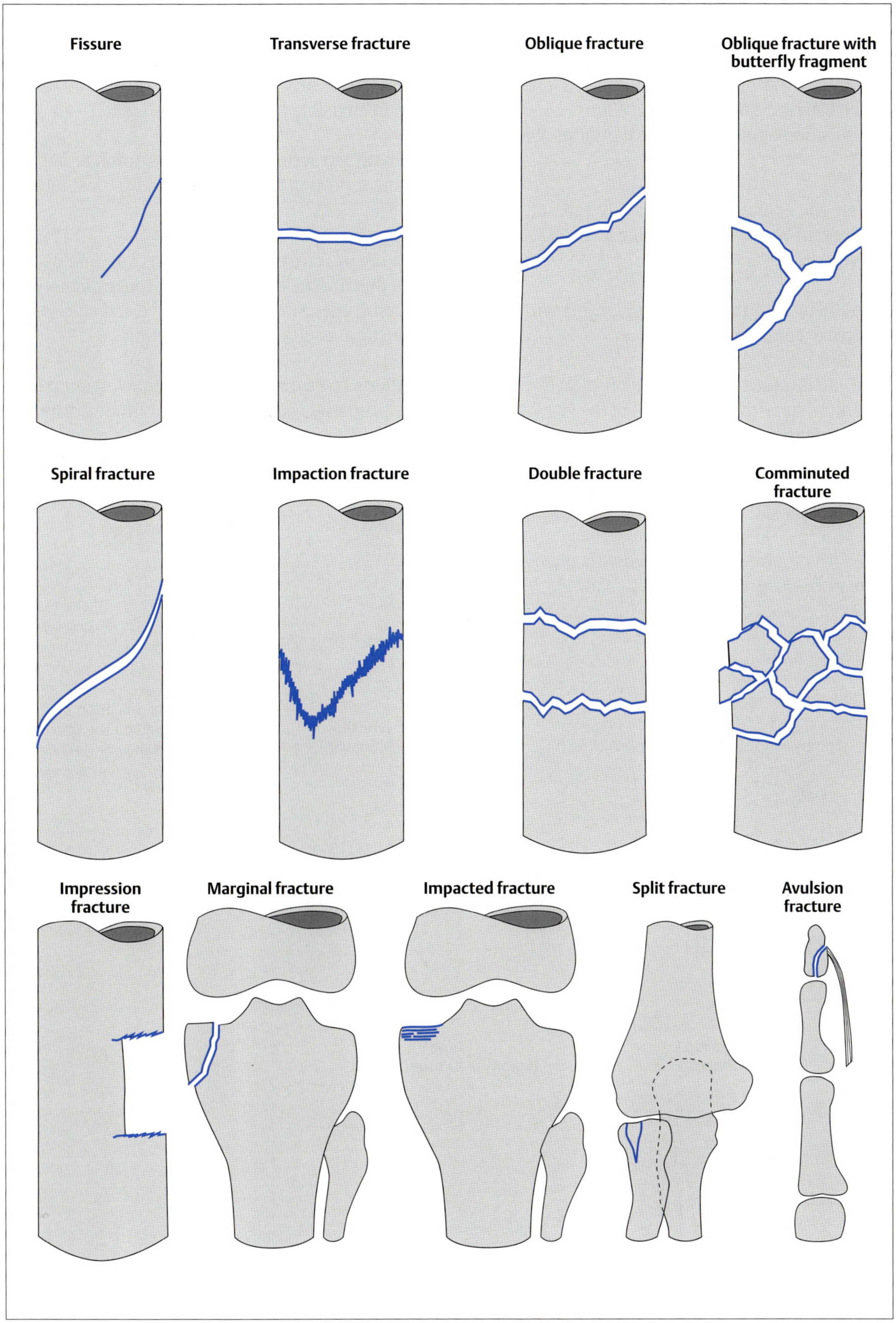

Fig. 1.**20** Summary of the most important fracture types.

Special Considerations in the Pediatric Age Group

Trauma to the epiphysis and growth plate: The **Salter-Harris** classification is the most widely used classification applied to physeal injuries (Figs. 1.**21**, 1.**24**).

Type I: The epiphysis is completely separated from the metaphysis without evidence of osseous involvement.

Type II: Fracture through the epiphysis with a metaphyseal 'corner' fragment.

Type III: Intra-articular extension of a fracture of the epiphysis with involvement of the growth plate. The epiphyseal fragment can be displaced.

Type IV: Vertical fracture that crosses epiphysis, growth plate and metaphysis.

Type V: Compression of the growth plate (risk of premature closure of the growth plate).

Buckle or **torus fracture:** This is an impaction injury of the metaphysis, causing the cortex to buckle. It is frequently asymmetric with one side of the cortex more involved than the other and might even be invisible on one side (Fig. 1.**22**).

Greenstick fracture: This is an incomplete fracture leaving a portion of the cortex and periosteum intact (Fig. 1.**23**).

Growing fracture: Skull fractures in infants can grow due to development of a 'leptomeningeal cyst' that protrudes into the fracture line and causes it to widen as a result of marginal erosion.

Toddler's fracture: This is an oblique or spiral fracture, primarily seen in the tibia, without displacement of the fracture fragments. It is a torsional injury found in children who are just beginning to walk.

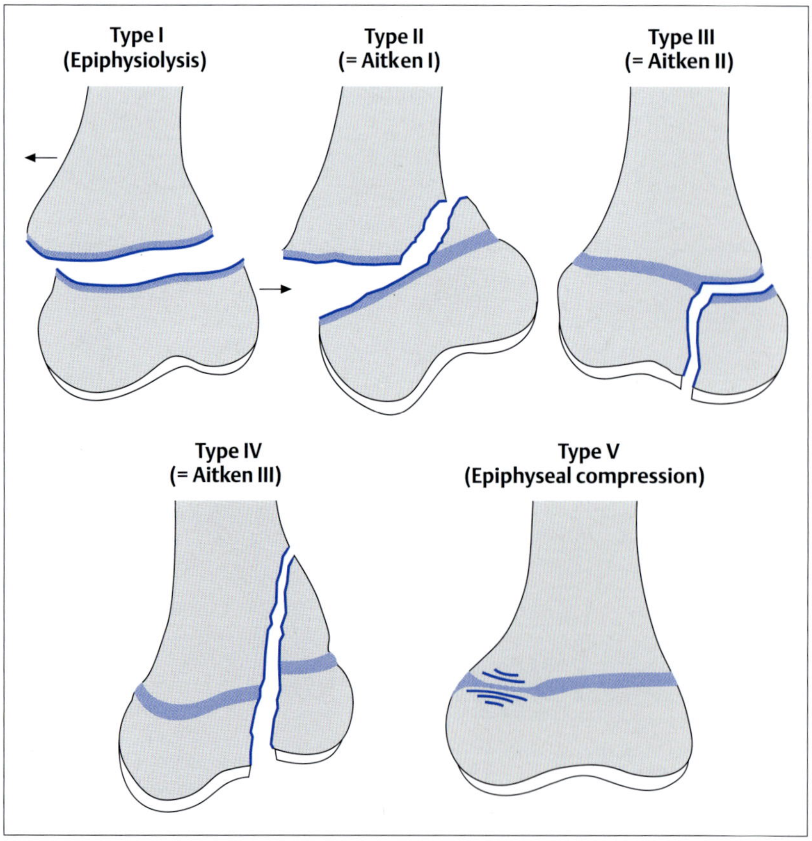

Fig. 1.**21** Classification of the fractures involving the growth plates after **Salter** and **Harris.** Aitken's classification is shown in brackets.

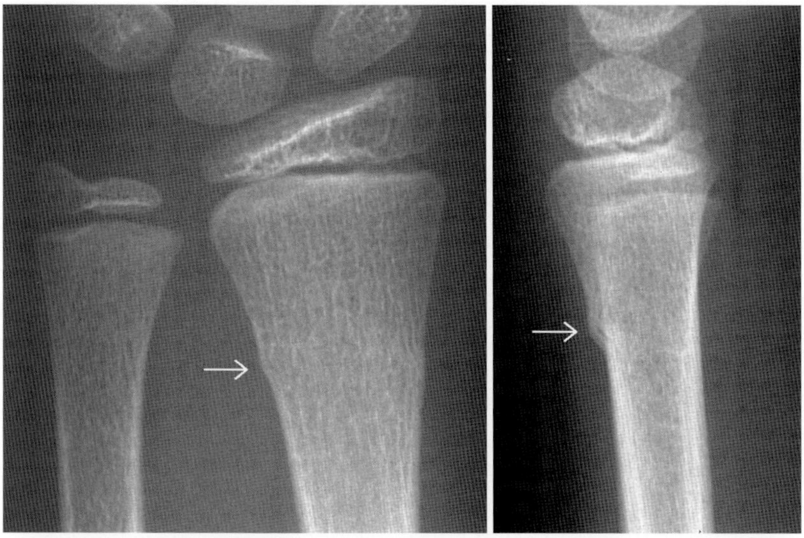

Fig. 1.**22** Buckle fracture in a 9-year-old girl.

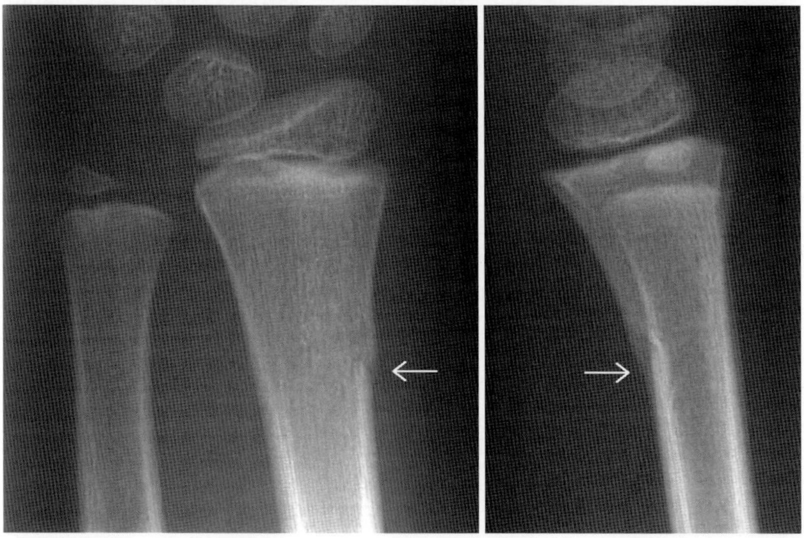

Fig. 1.**23** Greenstick fracture in a 7-year-old girl. Only one side of the cortex is fractured.

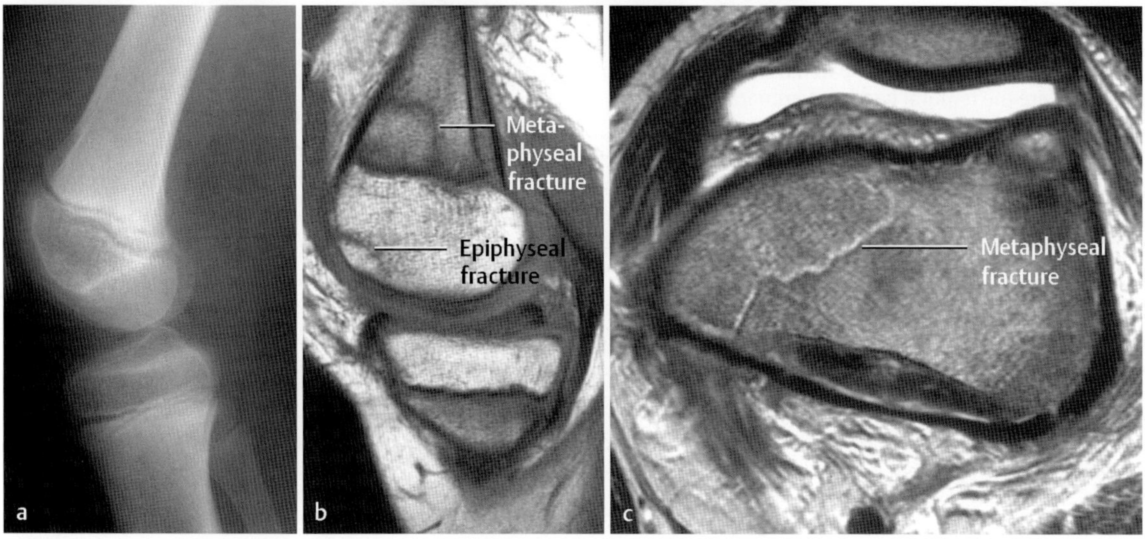

Fig. 1.**24** Unusual fracture in the pediatric age group. Fracture across the metaphysis (corresponds to the **Salter-Harris** type II fracture), together with a subchondral fracture of the epiphysis (cartilage intact). **a** Unremarkable radiograph, **b** sagittal T1-weighted SE sequence, **c** axial T2-weighted sequence at the level of the femoral metaphyses.

Fractures of the articular surfaces (chondral and osteochondral fractures)

PATH The most important biomechanical properties of hyaline cartilage are protection against excessive strain and providing a smooth surface for the joint. These properties are determined by the chemical composition and the complex spatial interaction of the extracellular matrix of the cartilage. The matrix is primarily composed of water and macromolecules (collagen, proteoglycan, and other proteins). Hyaline cartilage consists of several layers, and the deep calcified zone and the subchondral bone are closely intertwined. An avulsion of the cartilage (traumatic separation) occurs primarily between the deep calcified and the juxta-articular noncalcified cartilage.

It is known from experimental studies that compression and trabecular fractures of the subchondral bone can occur without injury to the cartilage. This can be attributed to the greater elasticity of the cartilage in comparison to the subchondral trabecular osseous structure.

Fractures of the joints can be divided into typical skeletal fractures with articular involvement and specific fractures confined to the cartilage and subchondral bone. The latter fractures are caused primarily by pressure directly transmitted onto the cartilage by a vertical load. Concurrent shearing and rotatory load can not only increase the pressure on the articular surface but can also avulse cartilaginous fragments (with or without attached bone) from the articular surface.

CLINIC Frequent causes of articular surface fractures are torsion or supination/pronation injuries and these are often associated with ligamentous injuries.

The clinical findings are nonspecific, but a hemorrhagic joint effusion is invariably present. This finding can also be associated with any trauma involving the intra-articular structures.

Dislodged chondral or osteochondral fragments must be surgically reattached, but shallow articular compression deformities can be treated conservatively.

Location: The principal sites of involvement are the ankle and knee, including the patella. Other less common locations are the femoral head and humeral head.

> **!** Chondral fractures occur primarily in children and adolescents, and osteochondral fractures occur primarily in adults.

X-RAY **Technical considerations:** If an osteochrondral fracture of the ankle is suspected, a radiographic examination in three projections is indicated: AP, lateral, and AP oblique in slight internal rotation. The oblique view projects the articular surface of the talar trochlea without superimposition.

Ankle: The lateral osteochondral fractures of the talus are horizontally oriented and have a thin, small fragment (Fig. 1.**28**). The medial fractures are generally deeper and produce a crater-like defect.

Patella: The diagnostic evaluation rests on axial views, possibly obtained at different angles. Small contour defects are seen along the articular surface (Fig. 1.**27**).

Femoral condyles: The fracture line is invariably parallel to the articular surface. The following specific findings can occur alone or in any combination:

- linear densities in the subchondral bone (caused by superimposed fragments on the summation view),
- irregularity of the osseous contour (undulated, serrated; Figs. 1.**25**, 1.**29**),
- large avulsion with complete or partial separation of the fragments (Fig. 1.**30**),
- loose fragment in the joint capsule (Fig. 1.**26**).

When the epiphyses are unfused, chondral/osteochondral fractures can be mistaken for variants of the epiphyseal ossification. This will be addressed further (see pp. 128 ff).

> **!** Conventional radiography has a high rate of false negative findings. For example, up to 30% of ankle fractures are overlooked.

MRI MRI is the imaging method of choice for the definitive evaluation of altered articular surfaces.

Technical considerations: The examination protocol offers several sequences. The recommended sequences are STIR, T1-weighted, and T2-weighted (turbo) spin echo and, for more comprehensive evaluation of cartilage, gradient echo sequences. The selection of section planes depends on the anatomy and the expected site of the injury. Images should be obtained in at least two planes.

With a properly selected examination technique, MRI should disclose the findings needed for the clinically relevant differentiation between injuries **with** cartilaginous defects and those with intact cartilage.

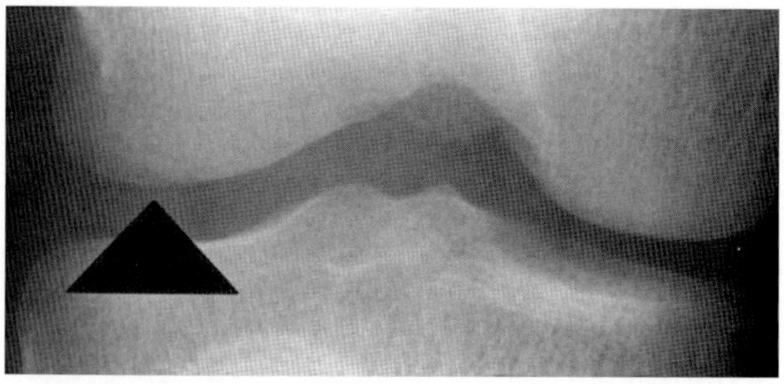

Fig. 1.25 Osteochondral fracture, seen only as irregular contour of the femoral condyle.

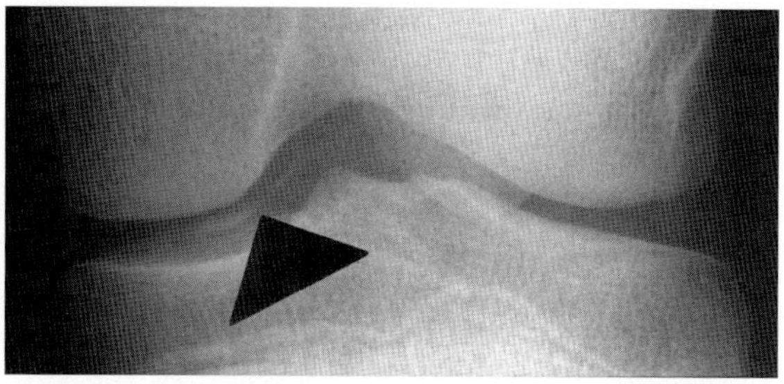

Fig. 1.26 Osteochondral fracture with loose fragment.

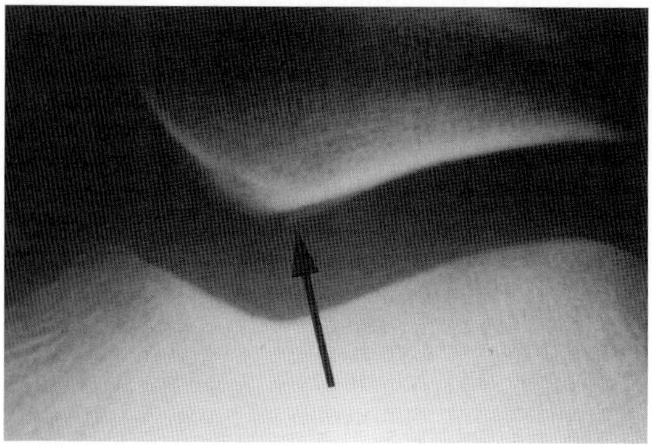

Fig. 1.27 Osteochondral fracture of the retropatellar articular surface.

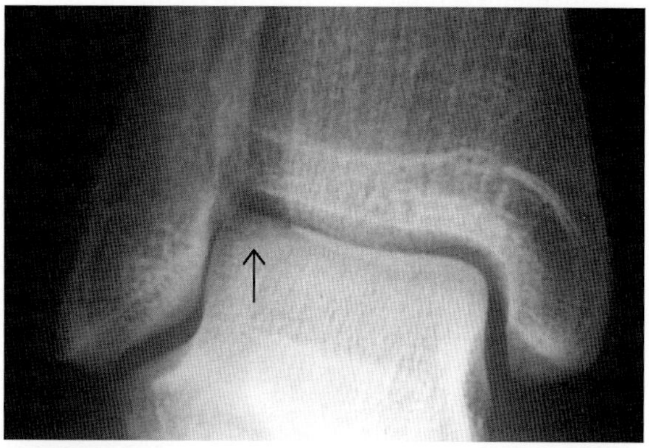

Fig. 1.28 Osteochondral fracture of the lateral aspect of the talar trochlea.

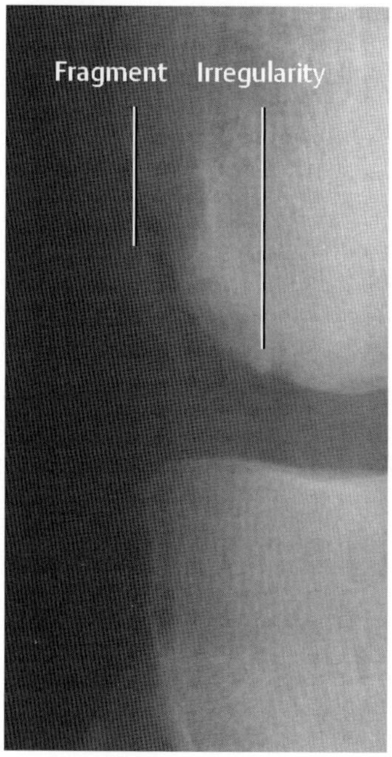

Fig. 1.29 Osteochondral fracture of the lateral femoral condyle. Shell-like osseous fragment and irregular condylar contour.

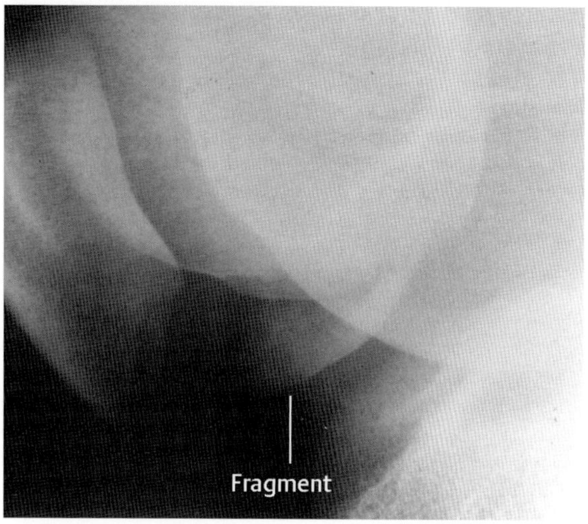

Fig. 1.30 Large osseous fragment of osteochondral fracture of the femoral condyle.

Injuries with cartilage defects: The major discriminating feature distinguishing strictly chondral lesions from osteochondral fractures is contour irregularity (Figs. 1.**32**, 1.**33**).

Injuries of the articular surface with intact cartilage: The following distinctions have to be made

- subchondral impaction (Fig. 1.**31**):
  This produces a subtle depression of the subchondral bone parallel to the articular surface. Occasionally, scalloped signal changes and fracture lines are observed.
- subchondral trabecular fracture (bone bruise):
  This represents bone marrow edema detectable by MRI without subchondral impaction.

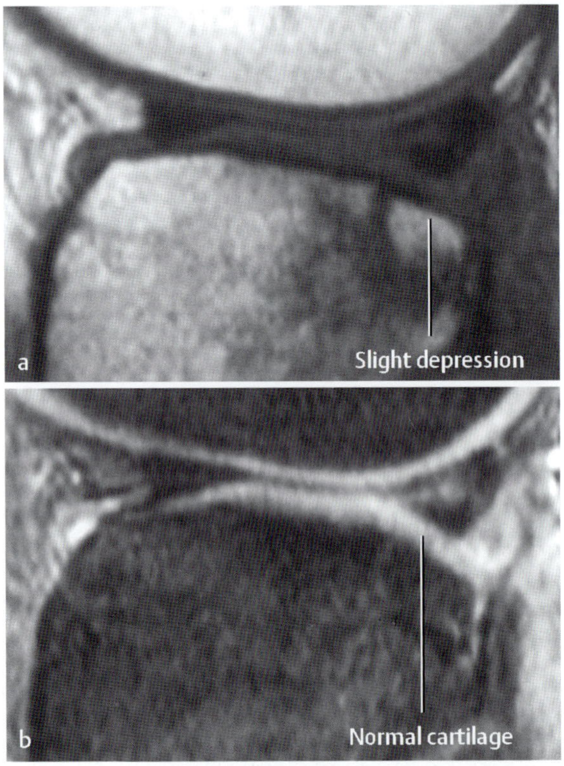

Fig. 1.**31** Subchondral impaction with normal overlying cartilage. **a** T1-weighted SE image, **b** GRE image.

Stress and Insufficiency Fractures

Stress can be defined as the load sustained by bone. Bone is a dynamic tissue and needs stress for its normal development. The mechanical response to stress determines the osseous texture. Absence of normal stress induces rapid osteoclastic resorption of cancellous and cortical bone as well as cessation of the osteoblastic activity, leading to disuse osteoporosis.

Stress is also placed on bone from muscular activity and body weight.

It is not entirely understood how stress shapes the mechanical function of bone, but evidence suggests that the adaptive process is mediated by microfractures. Bone subjected to more than normal stress responds with osteoclastic resorption. The osteoclastic cavities are subsequently filled with lamellated bone. The formation of new bone is a slow process (weeks to months), and stress in excess of the normal levels results in an imbalance between bone resorption and bone formation for the first few weeks. Therefore, new periosteal and endosteal bone formation represents a passing reparative mechanism needed to support the transiently weakened bone, especially the critical cortex. This process is basically the same in cortical and cancellous bone.

This normal physiologic adaptive process to micro damage (stress) becomes pathologic whenever there is an imbalance between the damage and repair. Continued and repetitive imbalance causes fatigue fractures of the cortical and cancellous bone. If the excessive stress abates (e.g., joggers curtail their activity because of the pain induced by the disproportionally high stress of running), a fracture line may not become visible despite radiographically apparent **periosteal** reaction as an adaptation to the stress. This phenomenon is referred to as **stress reaction** rather than stress fracture (Fig. 1.**34**).

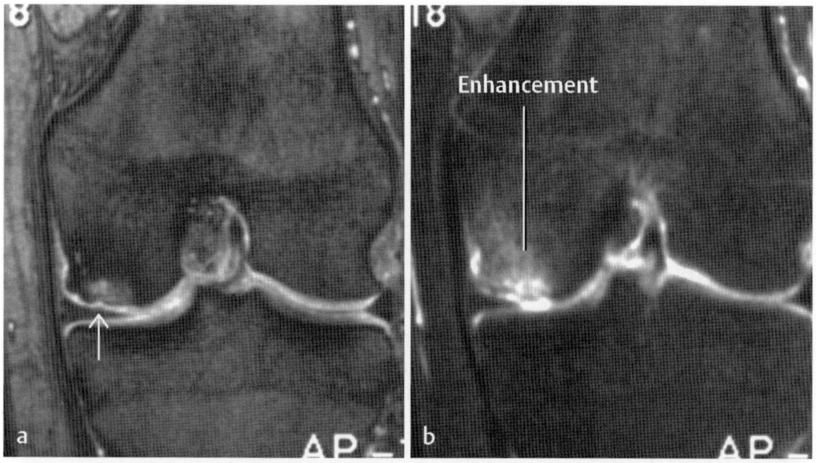

Fig. 1.32 One-year-old osteochondral fracture without intact cartilage. Enhancement of the subchondral bone indicates reactive changes.
a T1-weighted GRE sequence after intravenous injection of contrast medium (indirect arthrography),
b T1-weighted SE sequence with frequency selective fat suppression following administration of contrast medium.

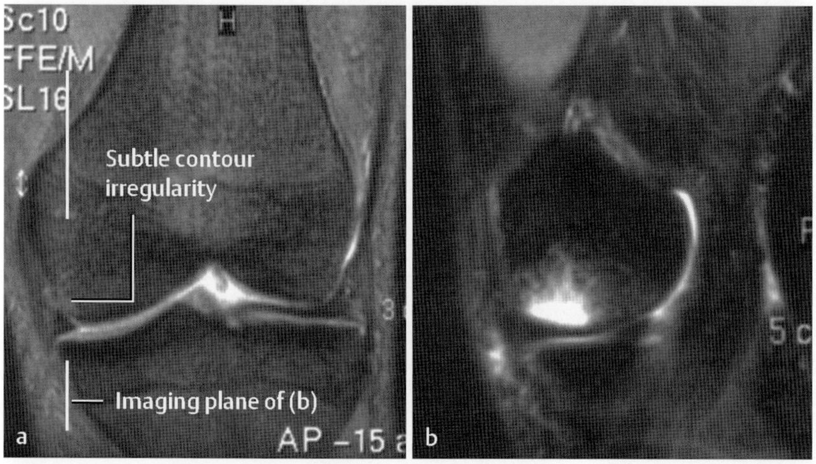

Fig. 1.33 Acute osteochondral fracture with surrounding edema laterally.
a Coronal T2-weighted GRE sequence with fat suppression,
b sagittal STIR sequence.

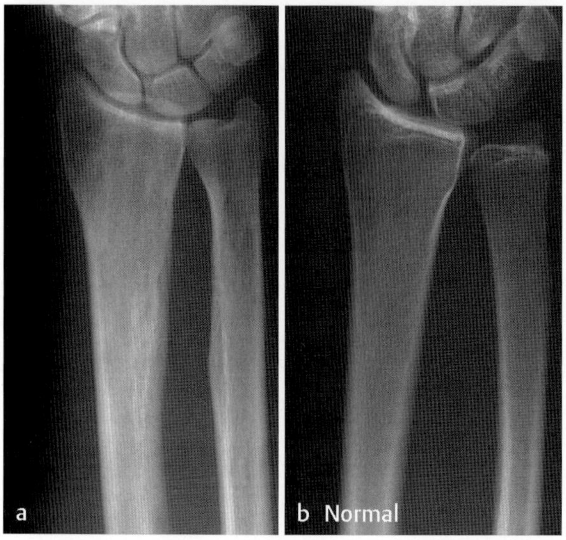

Fig. 1.34 **a** Stress reaction with periosteal and endosteal adaptation. The patient played volleyball for 30 years but was asymptomatic. The radiographic examination was obtained because of acute trauma. **b** Normal radiograph for comparison.

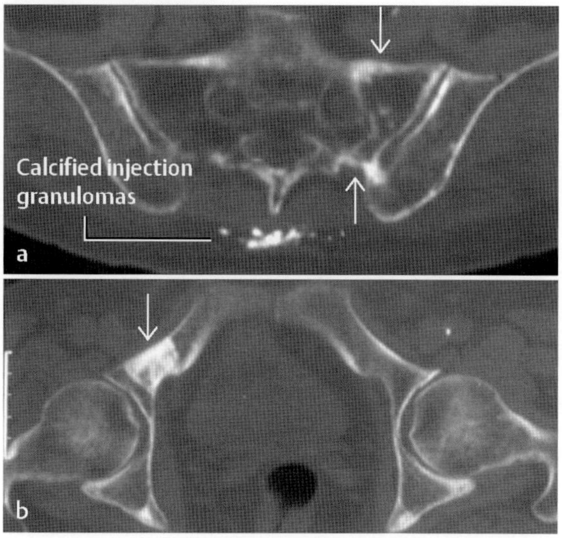

Fig. 1.35 Elderly female patient with pain for two years. **a** Remote insufficiency fracture of the right sacral ala. **b** The diagnosis of an insufficiency fracture is supported by a remote insufficiency fracture in the left superior ischial ramus (axial CT).

Fatigue fractures are divided into two categories, depending upon the underlying conditions of bone:

Stress fractures: The density and structure of bone are normal. Only the stressed portion of the bone is (reversibly) weakened according to the mechanism described above.

Insufficiency fractures: Normal or slightly above normal stress acts on a bone of abnormal density or structure. The pathologic fracture is a special case of insufficiency fracture. While the pathologic fracture occurs at a site of local bone loss, such as that caused by tumor destruction for instance, the insufficiency fracture generally affects bone of diffusely reduced bone mineral density (BMD) (Figs. 1.**35**, 1.**37**, 1.**45**).

Risk factors:
1. Excessive mechanical strain, especially during walking.
2. Estrogen deficiency in women.
3. Elderly (osteoporotic bone).
4. Reduced bone density from other causes (e.g., steroids).

CLINIC **Location:** The tubular bones of the appendicular skeleton as well as the axial skeleton can be affected. Insufficiency fractures primarily involve the femoral neck, distal forearm, spine, and sacrum, whereas stress fractures have a tendency to occur in the tarsal bones, tibia, and femur.

The clinical findings of insufficiency lesions consist of localized pain and soft-tissue swelling with overlying warmth. The stress fracture of the femoral neck can remain asymptomatic for a long time.

X-RAY It is important to remember that conventional radiography might show no abnormality for several weeks. Within the first few weeks, the radiographic sensitivity approaches 15–50%.
- A lamellated periosteal reaction is frequently the first radiographic sign.
- In selected cases, a subtle radiolucency and an indistinctly outlined cortex may be seen early.
- Endosteal thickening becomes discernible at a later stage of the process.
- The fracture line is usually apparent only after the periosteal reaction has appeared.
- An indistinctly outlined sclerotic zone is seen across the cancellous bone and the cortex (late stage, Fig. 1.**38**).

NUC Bone scintigraphy with Tc 99 m diphosphonate is well suited for the detection of stress and insufficiency fractures. A false negative finding is extremely rare.

A direct correlation exists between the intensity of tracer uptake and the extent of the stress fracture. Stress fractures appear as ill-defined focal areas of increased uptake, primarily in the cortex (Fig. 1.**36**).

Bone scintigraphy also reveals clinically asymptomatic lesions. Though the nature of these lesions cannot always be established, they are often attributed to stress reactions that have not yet become clinically apparent and have not yet induced any radiographic abnormalities.

Above all, bone scintigraphy contributes to the evaluation of anatomically complex osseous structures. Sacral insufficiency fractures present as linear or H-shaped radionuclide accumulation (the so-called 'Honda sign'); this latter pattern is essentially pathognomonic of stress injury and not malignancy.

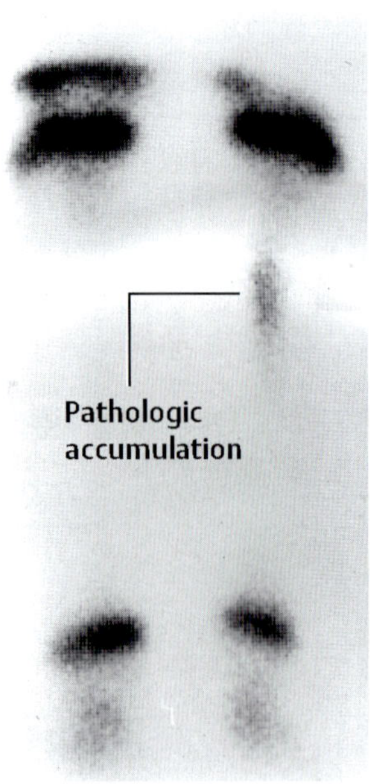

Fig. 1.**36** Stress fracture of the tibia in a 6-year-old boy, with only minimally increased osseous uptake.

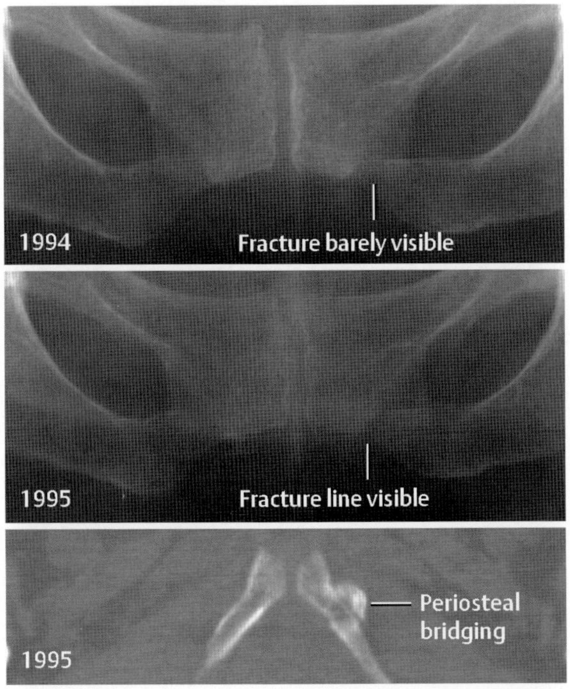

Fig. 1.**37** Insufficiency fracture in the presence of severe osteoporosis.

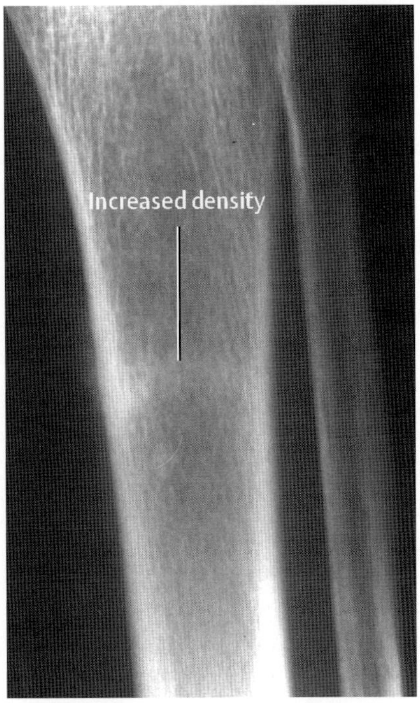

Fig. 1.**38** Remote stress fracture in a marathon runner, seen as a subtle band of increased density.

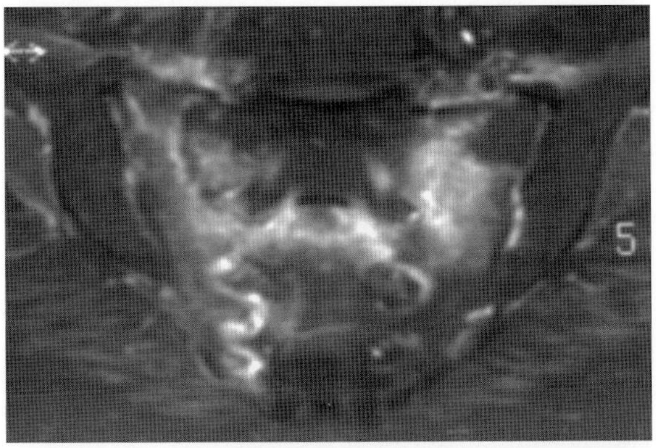

Fig. 1.**39** Bilateral insufficiency fractures of the sacrum. Enhanced T1-weighted MR sequence with fat suppression showing the 'H' configuration ('Honda sign').

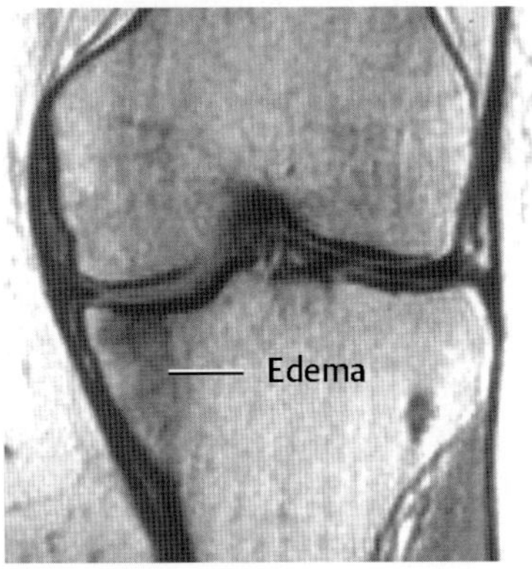

Fig. 1.**40** Insufficiency fracture of the tibial plateau in an overweight osteoporotic woman with pain for three weeks.

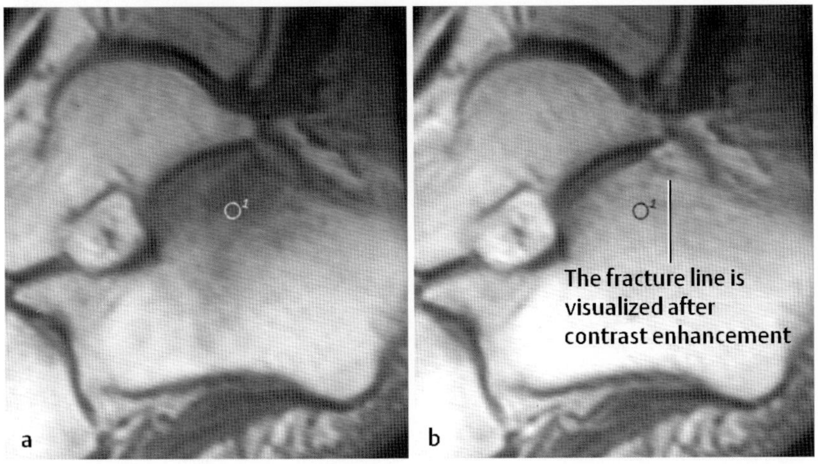

Fig. 1.**41** Insufficiency fracture of the calcaneus, T1-weighted spin echo sequence before (**a**) and after (**b**) administration of contrast medium. After enhancement, the fracture line is seen as a band of decreased signal intensity.

CT CT is a good method for delineating fracture lines, especially those in the sacrum, tarsal bones, and tubular bones. A definitive diagnosis can usually be made if the fracture line is surrounded by reactive sclerosis (Figs. 1.**35**, 1.**37**, 1.**44**).

MRI MRI is an extremely sensitive method for the detection of stress and insufficiency fractures since both conditions are associated with a bone marrow edema and can be used as an alternative to bone scintigraphy (Figs. 1.**39**, 1.**40**, 1.**41**, 1.**43**). The most helpful sequences are STIR images and T1-weighted and T2-weighted images. A fracture line is not always visualized, and in cases where the MR findings are nonspecific, osteomyelitis should be included in the differential diagnosis. In selected cases, enhancement with Gd-based contrast medium might help delineate the fracture line, which remains of low signal intensity relative to the enhancing edematous bone marrow (Fig. 1.**41**).

DD **Osteoid osteoma:** The radiographic findings of this lesion are a round radiolucency surrounded by an irregularly outlined sclerotic rim without evidence of a linear component perpendicular to or at an acute angle with the cortex found in stress fractures.

Chronic osteomyelitis, another cause of diffuse cortical thickening usually involves the entire cortical circumference. Linear radiolucencies are not seen in this condition.

On MRI, the differential diagnosis includes an acute **bone infarct,** especially after radiotherapy to the pelvic region. In this setting differentiation of infarct from stress fracture can be difficult. Bone infarcts show a diffuse enhancement of bone marrow edema, and CT can be helpful in certain cases to search for fracture lines.

Pathologic Fracture

This condition represents a special case of insufficiency fracture. It is a fracture that develops in an osseous structure weakened by tumor or tumor-like conditions. These injuries are usually caused by inadequate stress or minor trauma (Figs. 1.**42**, 1.**46**).

The commonest pathologic fracture is one occurring through a juvenile bone cyst or a nonossifying fibroma. Any osseous tumor, especially metastases, can be the underlying cause of a pathologic fracture. However, the notable exception to this rule is primary or secondary bone-forming tumors, such as osteosarcoma and osteoblastic metastases, which rarely result in a pathologic fracture.

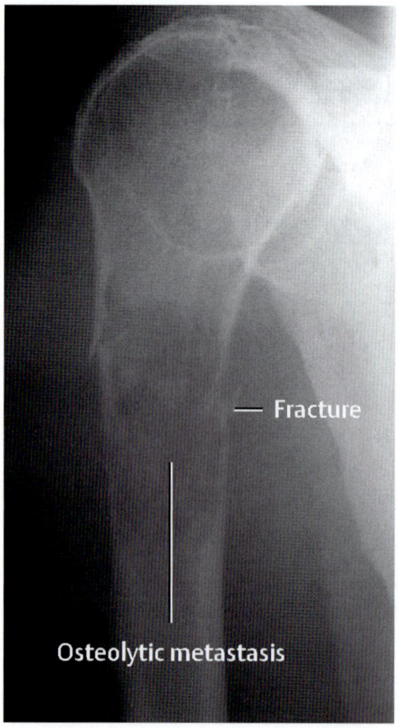

Fig. 1.**42** Pathologic fracture of the proximal humerus through an osteolytic metastasis from thyroid carcinoma.

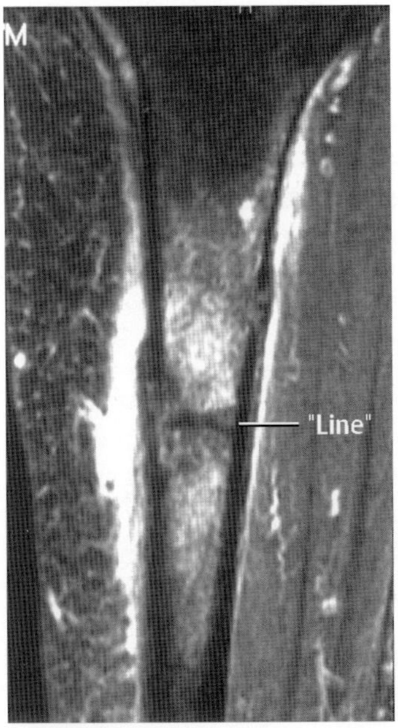

Fig. 1.43 Insufficiency fracture (STIR sequence). The clinical findings consisted of pain and tenderness, as well as swelling. The linear decrease in signal intensity distinguishes this finding from chronic osteomyelitis.

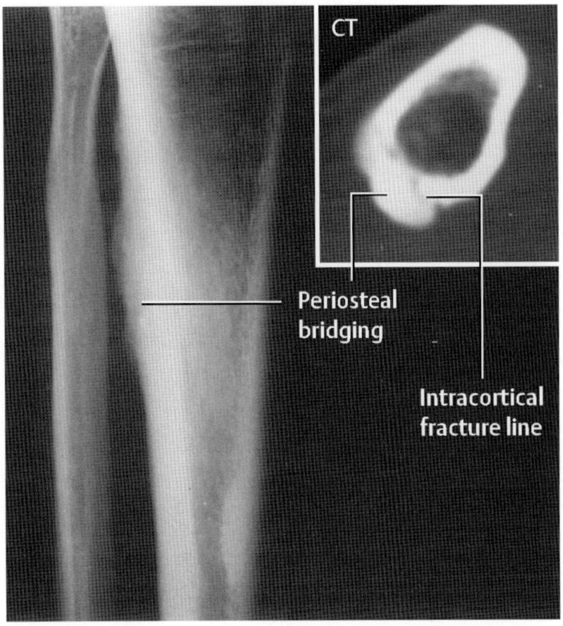

Fig. 1.44 Pain for three months, no discernible fracture line: Stress fracture with periosteal new bone formation.

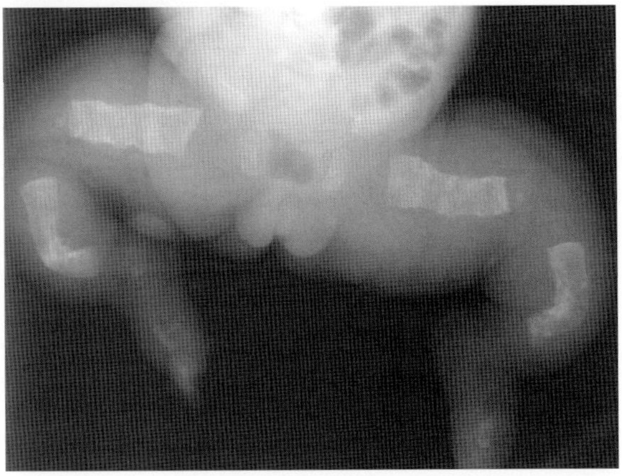

Fig. 1.45 Insufficiency fracture in osteogenesis imperfecta.

Below:

Fig. 1.46 Pathologic fracture in fibrous dysplasia (**a**). The patient suffered minor trauma. **b** Control radiography after internal fixation. The fibrous dysplasia was initially overlooked and only recognized after removal of the internal fixation device. **c** Conventional tomography.

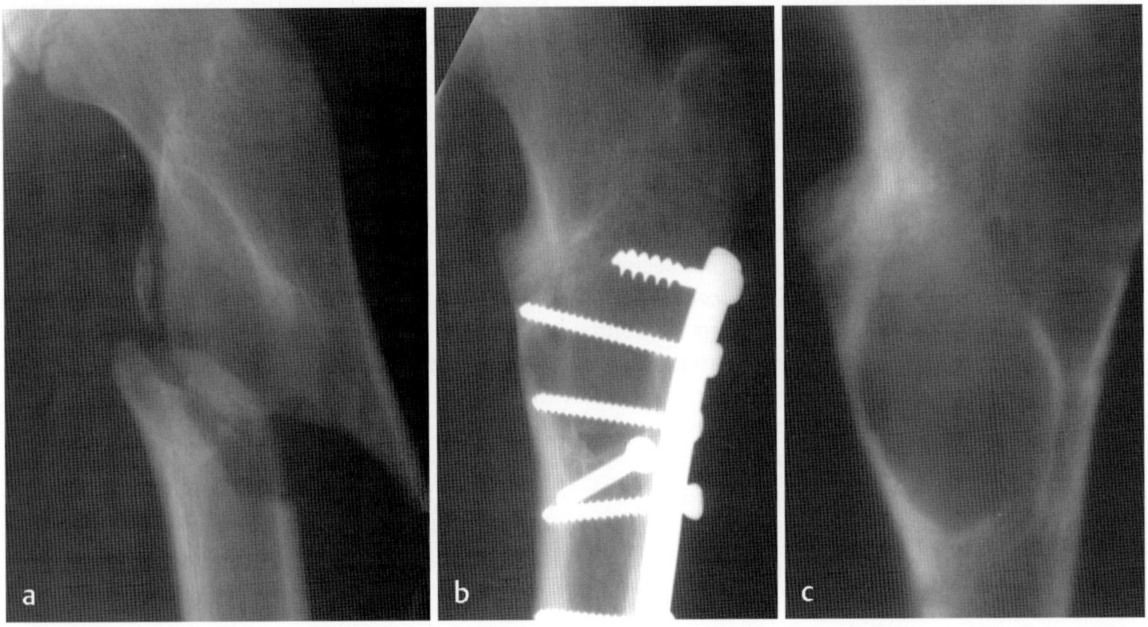

Fracture Healing

■ Primary (direct) and secondary (indirect) healing of the fractures returns osseous stability by restoring the original tissue. ■

Primary Fracture Healing

Definition: Primary healing is characterized by the absence of callus formation and requires:
- Contact between fragments with a maximum fracture gap of 0.5 mm. Internal compression fixation of the fragments increases the chance of a primary fracture healing.
- Immobilization of the fracture fragments (e.g., internal fixation).
- Adequate blood supply and viability of the fragments.

The fracture fragments unite by direct extension of the Haversian canals from one fragment to the other ('contact healing'), or by the formation of lamellar bone, which is later replaced by longitudinally oriented osteons ('gap healing'). The periosteal or endosteal mesenchymal cells are **not** activated in this setting.

X-RAY
- Indistinct cortical structures,
- invisible or faint fracture line.

Visualized interosseous or periosteal callous formation indicates the formation of 'restless' callus, followed by fixation callus. Furthermore, widening of the fracture line or the appearance of a 'new' fracture line reflects osseous resorption of the fracture fragments and indicates an impaired primary fracture healing.

Secondary Fracture Healing

A widened fracture line or inadequate mechanical fixation of the fracture fragments results in secondary fracture healing, consisting of the formation of a 'periosteal cuff' around the fracture gap. This cuff arises from connective tissue and represents mesenchymal new bone formation. In addition to connective tissue proliferation, cartilage is usually formed by metaplasia and ultimately transformed into osseous tissue. Thus, the original structure is restored via a detour (lamellar osseous tissue, osteons).

Secondary osseous healing passes through characteristic stages and their corresponding radiographic findings are shown in Table 1.**4.**

! Trabecular fractures initially show increased density. Within weeks, the increased density resolves and is replaced by normal trabecular texture. A periosteal reaction always indicates cortical involvement.

Osseous consolidation of a fracture should be assessed **clinically** first. The radiographic signs usually lag behind the clinical signs.

The clinical signs of an osseous consolidation (not to be equated with complete fracture healing) are:
- stability on physical examination,
- lack of pain,
- ability to bear weight.

Radiographic Signs of Osseous Consolidation

- The osseous bridging of the fracture is solid.
- The fracture callus is of homogeneous density.
- The density of the fracture callus equals the density of the cortex.
- These findings must be seen in at least two projections.

Caution: Underexposed films overestimate the degree of osseous bridging.

Basic Principles of Fracture Treatment

The **conservative** (closed) treatment follows three approaches:
1. Primary functional treatment (without cast). This requires adequate axial relationships and exercise stability; for example, a subcapital fracture of the humerus in an elderly person.
2. Repositioning and immobilization by casting, for instance, a distal radial fracture.
3. Repositioning and immobilization by means of traction; for instance, a femur fracture.

The goals of **operative** (open) therapy are to restore the normal anatomic relationship of the axial planes and articular surfaces and to stabilize fracture fragments. Several approaches are available and can be combined.
- Internal fixation by screws; for example, avulsion of juxta-articular or joint-bearing fragments,

Table 1.4 Stages of secondary osseous healing. Correlation of the pathologic and radiographic findings

Time after fracture	Healing phases	Radiographic findings
First days	Hematoma due to tearing of bone, periosteum, bone marrow and surrounding soft tissues **'Inflammation phase'** Migration of multiple cell types	**3rd – 14th day:** Demineralization of bone. The fracture line becomes clearly visible (due to bone resorption) **From the 10th day:** New periosteal callus formation begins (Fig. 1.**47**)
Up to the 3rd – 4th week	**'Granulation phase'** Fibrous conversion of the hematoma caused by proliferating tissue with collagenous fibers and capillary growth. Differentiation (migration) of osteoblasts (→ bone formation), chondroblasts (→ cartilage formation). Formation of 'soft' callus	**From the 14th day:** Increasing bone density in the fracture gap. Indistinct fragment borders. Cuff-like density around the fracture
From the 3rd – 4th week to the 3rd – 4th month	**'Conversion to hard callus'** Mineralization of the matrix Formation of woven bone	**From the 6th – 8th week:** Bridging and consolidation The bone is well demarcated and dense
From the 4th month	**'Modeling' and 'remodeling'** Conversion of woven bone into lamellar bone (modeling) Restoration of normal bone contour and of the marrow space	Complete incorporation of the bone until complete restoration (Figs. 1.**48**, 1.**49**)

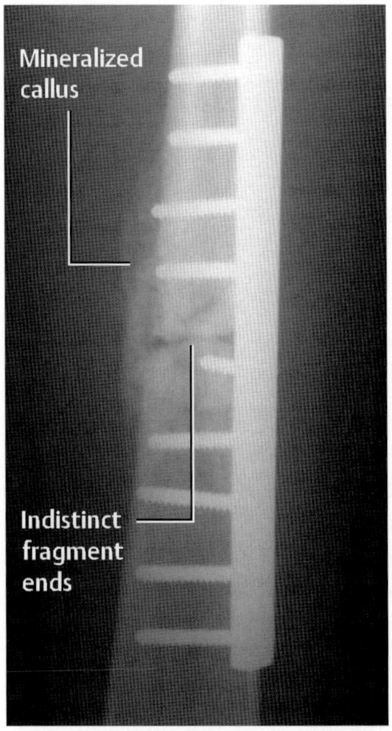

Fig. 1.**47** Callus formation following internal fixation of a femoral fracture. Indistinct fracture line.

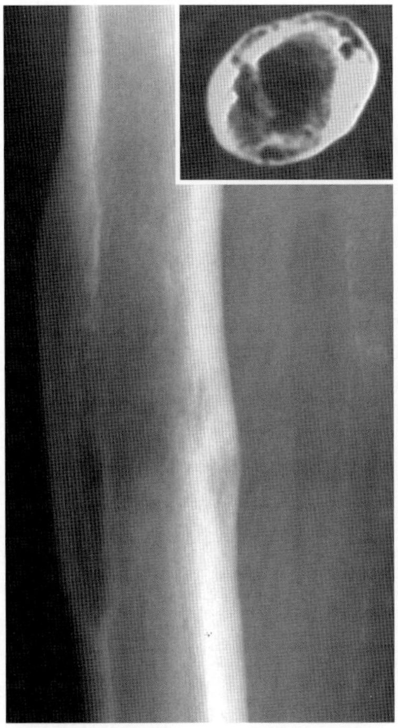

Fig. 1.**48** Status 4 years post-femoral fracture. Since the history of previous trauma was not known, the finding was initially diagnosed incorrectly as metastasis from the patient's known breast carcinoma.

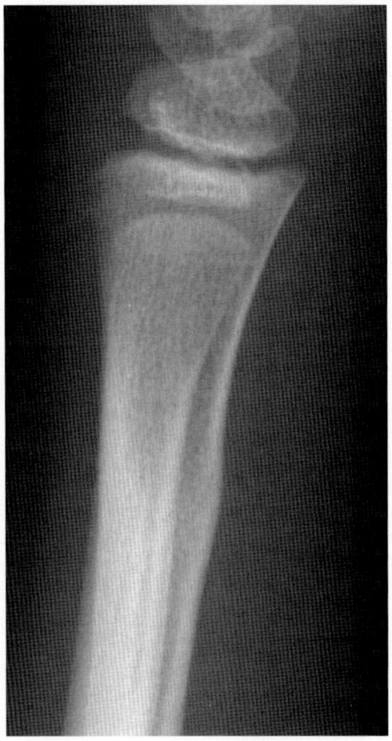

Fig. 1.**49** Status 3 years post-greenstick fracture. Subtle post-traumatic cortical thickening.

- Internal fixation by compression plates and screws,
- Internal fixation by wire fixation (cerclage); for example, the olecranon and patella,
- Intramedullary fixation; for example, by rod and pins,
- External fixation; for example, the compound fracture of the lower leg.

Delayed Fracture Healing

Delayed fracture healing takes place in the following situations:
- extension of the fracture into the joint,
- elderly patients with slow osseous metabolism,
- poor alignment of the fracture fragments,
- inadequate immobilization of the fracture fragments,
- extensive soft-tissue injury (poor condition for perfusion!).

Fracture healing is categorized as **delayed (impaired)** if the time of healing exceeds twice the expected time period (about 4 to 6 months). The primary causes are:
- inadequate immobilization,
- impaired perfusion,
- infection.

A delay in fracture healing can result in a pseudarthrosis.

Pseudarthrosis

Non-union refers to absent healing after about 6 to 8 weeks. Both primary and secondary fracture healing can develop into pseudarthroses (Figs. 1.**50**, 1.**51**).

Causes

- inadequate immobilization,
- soft tissues interposed in the fracture gap,
- extensive loss of osseous substance,
- inadequate blood supply,
- infection (with/without sequestration).

Classification

Based on appearance (descriptive):
- hypertrophic form,
- atrophic form,
- defect with pseudarthrosis.

Based on viability (biologic):
- biologically reactive pseudarthroses.
  This type is caused by bridging of the fracture gap by fibrous tissue or inadequate callus formation, resulting in mobility of the fragments.
- biologically nonreactive pseudarthroses.
  This group represents nonviable pseudarthroses with severely impaired blood supplies directly beneath the ends of the fracture fragments. They are usually caused by large defects, necroses, and infections. The therapeutic goal is to restore stability with autologous cancellous bone grafts. Ultrasound may also be used for that purpose.

X-RAY *Hypertrophic type:*
- The fracture fragments are smoothly outlined and sclerotic.
- The surrounding bone is eburnated.
- There is no evidence of osseous bridging.
- The fracture fragments are widened ('elephant foot').
- The fracture fragments can be rounded.

Atrophic type:
- There is only minimal evidence of sclerosis of the ends of the fracture fragments.

Complications after Fractures

Infection

Infection can be a primary complication of the injury or a secondary complication after operative therapy. See Post-traumatic Osteomyelitis in Chapter 2.

Avascular Necrosis (AVN)

Avascular necrosis develops if a fracture or dislocation deprives the bone of an adequate blood supply.

Predilection: femoral head, scaphoid, humeral head (Figs. 1.**52**, 1.**53**).

Avascular necrosis of the femoral head constitutes the most frequent complication of a subcapital femoral neck fracture, hip dislocation, or slipped femoral epiphysis.

The diagnostic evaluation of patients in whom AVN is suspected includes conventional radiography, MRI, and bone scintigraphy (see Avascular Necrosis, pp. 218 ff).

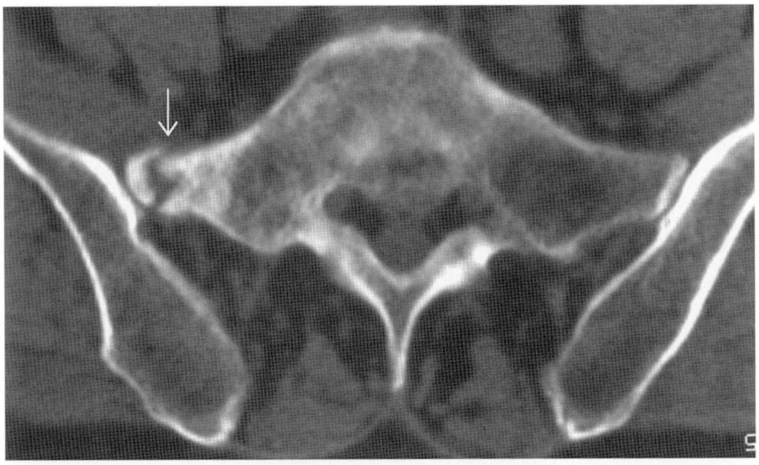

Fig. 1.**50** Pseudarthrosis following insufficiency fracture 2 years ago. Chronic back pain.

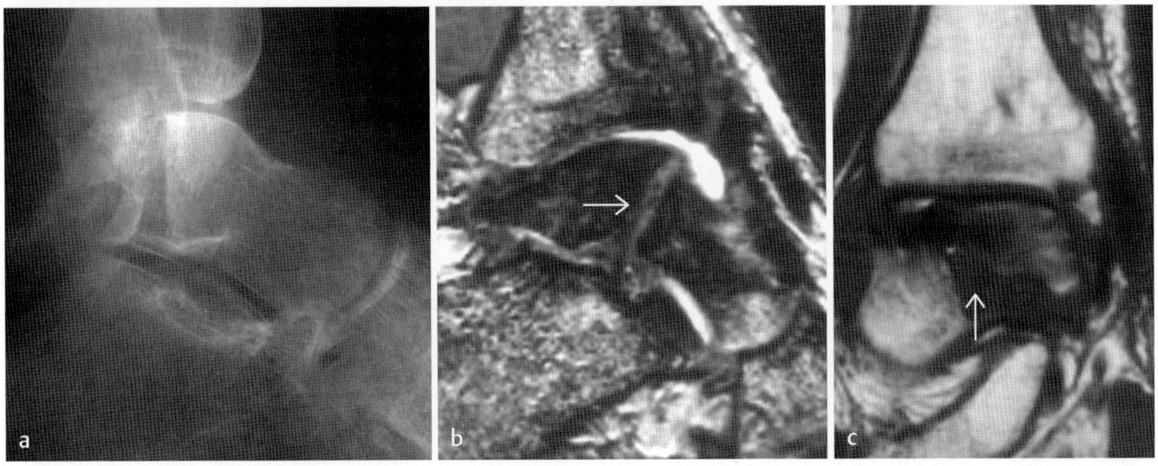

Fig. 1.**51** **a** Surgically treated talar fracture with development of a pseudarthrosis. Metallic fixation device removed. **b** T2-weighted GRE sequence. **c** T1-weighted SE sequence.

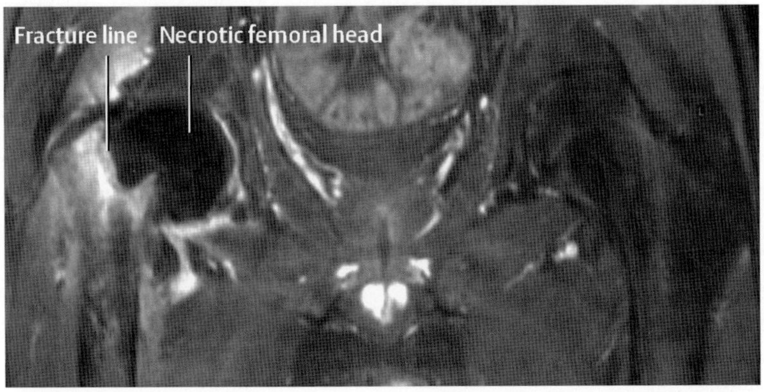

Fig. 1.**52** Avascular necrosis of the right hip following medial subcapital fracture of the femoral neck. There is no perfusion of the femoral head on the T1-weighted sequence with fat suppression following enhancement.

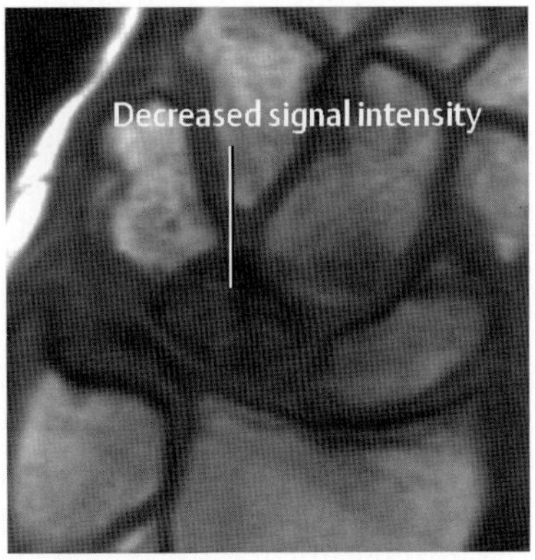

Fig. 1.**53** Avascular necrosis (osteonecrosis) of the lunate (Kienböck's disease), T1-weighted SE image.

Myositis Ossificans

Heterotopic ossification of the soft tissues adjacent to bone is referred to as myositis ossificans. It is post-traumatic, but can occur in the absence of a fracture. Typically, it appears as diffuse ossification in the soft tissues with corresponding changes on conventional radiographs, CT and MRI. (See Myositis Ossificans, pp. 286 ff).

Disuse Osteoporosis

Disuse osteoporosis is an acute form of demineralization due to immobilization.

It can have the following radiographic manifestations:
- Decreased bone density confined to the cancellous bone without cortical involvement. The small trabeculae resolve, with thickening and indistinctness of the remaining trabeculae.
- Patchy decrease in bone density seen as ovoid and round, but also irregularly outlined, radiolucencies. These changes are frequently observed in older patients and in the hands and feet.
- Radiolucent lines. They are usually juxta-articular, and are most frequently seen along the old growth plates.
- Punctate and patchy radiolucencies with the cortex (enlarged Haversian canals).

These changes generally are combined in different degrees (Fig. 1.**54**).

DD **Senile osteoporosis:** This is a diffuse loss of bone not confined to one extremity. It can be excluded only by comparing radiographs of both the normal and the immobilized extremities. **Sudeck's atrophy:** This is primarily a clinical diagnosis (see next section). The radiographic findings are almost identical to those of disuse osteoporosis.

Post-traumatic Degenerative Osteoarthritis

This complication occurs most frequently following fractures involving the articular surface or after chondral or enchondral fractures. It is caused by the incongruity of the articular surface which leads to premature abrasion and subsequent destruction of the cartilage. The resultant secondary degenerative osteoarthritis follows the stages found in primary degenerative osteoarthritis (Fig. 1.**55**).

Any altered axial orientation after a fracture changes the weight bearing of the joint. This is another mechanism that can induce degenerative osteoarthritis, particularly in the weight-bearing joints.

Post-traumatic Growth Disturbance in Children and Adolescents

Bone growth can be affected by many different situations. Any traumatic change involving a growth plate can potentially cause growth **acceleration,** generally explained by the hyperemia from trauma. This growth acceleration is transient and compensated by subsequent growth retardation.

Post-traumatic growth **retardation** has greater clinical implications. It is generally caused by an ossified growth plate. Partial involvement of the growth plate will induce asymmetric growth retardation while involvement of the entire growth plate will shorten the affected limb.

Partial fusion of the central region of the growth plate causes so-called 'cupping', which consists of cone-like widening of the epiphyses toward the metaphysis of the affected tubular bone.

Foreign Body Reaction

Foreign material retained in tissue generally becomes encapsulated and causes no irritation. However, it can represent a source of chronic irritation with subsequent bone resorption and reactive sclerosis (Fig. 1.**56**). In joints, foreign bodies generally will induce chronic synovitis.

Post-traumatic Cyst Formation around the Fracture Site

Large encapsulated hematomas that do not contribute to the healing process can form within fractures. Rarely, they can create large cystic osseous defects within a stable and load-bearing fracture. This phenomenon is encountered in greenstick fractures but can also occur in 'normal' fractures. The radiographically visualized radiolucency can be central or peripheral (Fig. 1.**57**) and any differential diagnostic problems can usually be solved by MRI. These post-traumatic cysts regress spontaneously at a slow rate over several years.

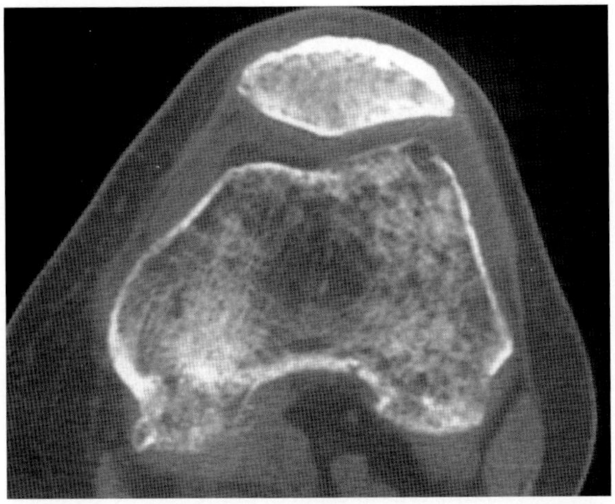

Fig. 1.**54** Severe disuse osteoporosis following femoral neck fracture with long immobilization.

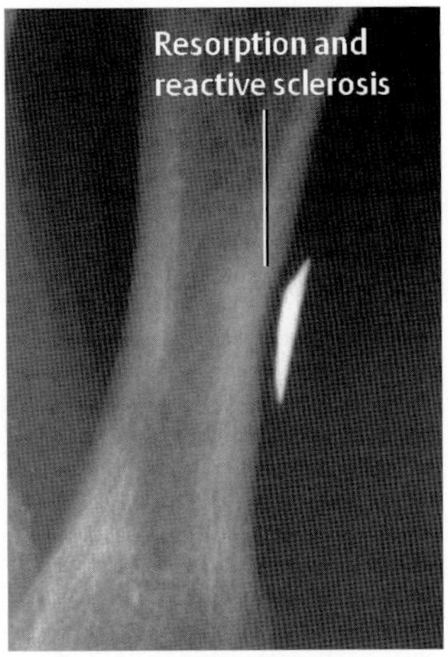

Fig. 1.**56** Osseous reaction to retained metallic foreign body.

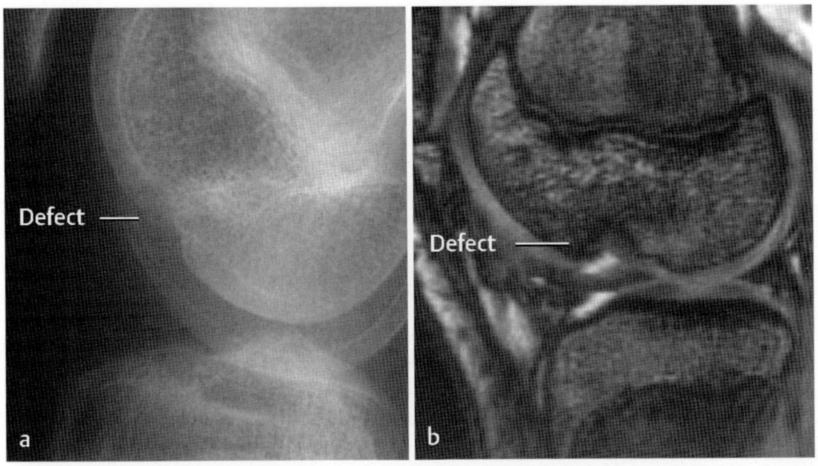

Fig. 1.**55** Residual defect following osteochondral fractures 2 years earlier. There is a predisposition to degenerative osteoarthritis in this setting.

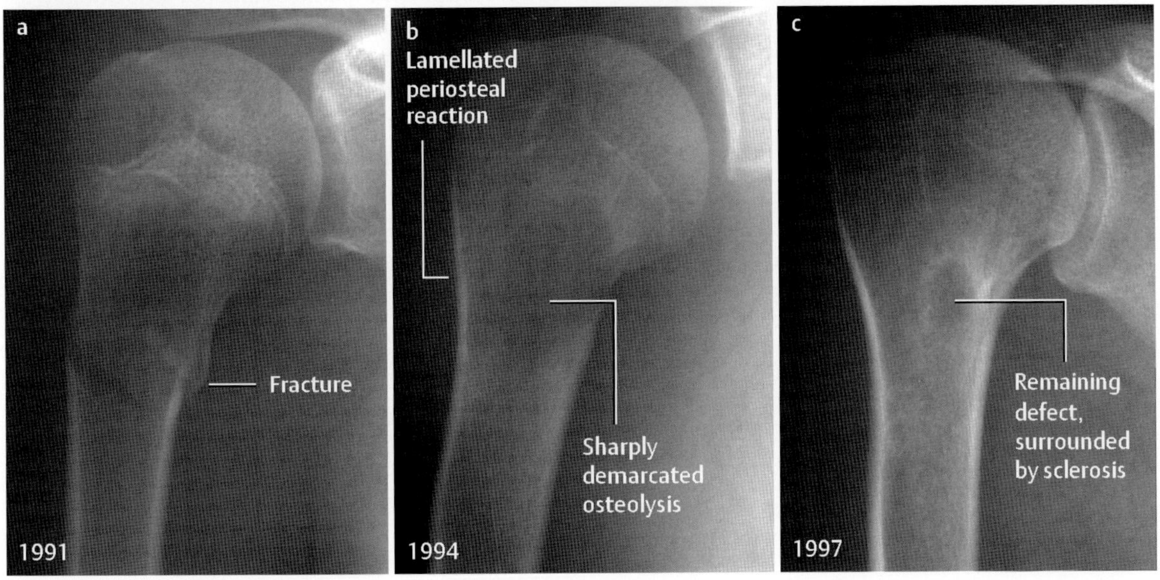

Fig. 1.**57** **a** Proximal humeral fracture in a 13-year-old girl. **b** 3 years later: large central radiolucency caused by a hematoma. Lamellated periosteal reaction as evidence of repair. **c** After a further 3 years: incomplete resolution of the osteolytic area.

Reflex Sympathetic Dystrophy (RSD)

Synonyms: Sudeck disease, Sudeck's atrophy, algodystrophy.
Causalgia: Manifestation of reflex sympathetic dystrophy with severe pain.
Shoulder-hand syndrome: Reflex sympathetic dystrophy of the hand secondary to humeroscapular periarthritis.

Because of its still unexplained pathogenesis and unspecific presentation, reflex sympathetic dystrophy is known under various names. According to the latest definition published by the American Association of Hand Surgery, reflex sympathetic dystrophy is a pain syndrome associated with functional loss and detectable autonomous dysfunction. The original description by Sudeck seems to express the relevant findings best:

> ■ Reflex sympathetic dystrophy is a painful acute osteoporosis with soft-tissue swelling or atrophy. ■

PATH Reflex sympathetic dystrophy is usually posttraumatic, typically following distal radial or tibial fractures, but it can be induced by a variety of other conditions including myocardial infarction and cerebrovascular accidents. In some cases, no predisposing condition can be found.

The pathophysiology of this condition is unclear but the most frequently postulated theory proposes that afferent pain stimulates a hyperactive sympathetic nerve system to induce a change in blood flow that increases bone resorption. Recent research supports Sudeck's original hypothesis of excessive regional inflammatory reaction.

CLINIC The diagnosis is made if four of these five clinical criteria are fulfilled:

- diffuse pain,
- change in skin color,
- diffuse soft-tissue edema,
- different skin temperature,
- limited range of active motion.

The complaints increase with weight bearing.
Clinical course: Three stages are observed:

I. Inflammatory stage: burning pain, soft tissue swelling, weakness and hyperesthesia.
II. Dystrophic stage: vasospasm or vasodilatation, skin changes (atrophy, pigmentation, hyperhidrosis, nail changes), contractures.
III. Atrophic stage: skin atrophy, resolution of other symptoms.

Therapy: Conservative therapy, initially with lymph drainage, cryotherapy, later with thermotherapy and active physical therapy.

X-RAY The radiographic changes are nonspecific and, depending on the stage, can consist of **soft-tissue swelling** or **atrophy,** as well as **regional osteoporosis.** Initially, the osteoporosis is patchy or band-like and later changes to a more uniform demineralization with indistinct texture of the cancellous bone (Figs. 1.**58,** 1.**59**). The subchondral lamella is frequently lost and the cortex can show subperiosteal, intracortical, or endosteal resorption.

In rare cases, a fracture is superimposed on reflex sympathetic dystrophy.

NUC Bone scintigraphy with Tc 99 m diphosphonate shows typical changes in the soft-tissue phase (5–15 minutes after the injection of tracer) and in the bone phase (at about 3 hours) (Fig. 1.**60**). Increased uptake around the joint, predominantly along the cortex, often extends to the entire affected extremity with accentuation distally.

In the third (atrophic) stage, the scintigraphic findings can return to normal.

MRI MRI shows soft-tissue swelling (T1-weighted images, STIR sequences) and soft-tissue enhancement. Bone marrow changes are rare (Fig. 1.**61**).

DD **Arthritis:** The regional osteoporosis is confined to the affected joints, the soft-tissue swelling is fusiform, the joint space is narrowed, and osseous erosions are found.
Disuse osteoporosis: It cannot be distinguished on the basis of the demineralization pattern. The disuse osteoporosis is painless and not associated with soft-tissue swelling. Bone scintigraphy does not show hyperperfusion.
Bone contusion: The finding is localized and seen as bone marrow edema on MRI.
Acute and chronic osteomyelitis: MRI invariably shows bone marrow changes which are absent in reflex sympathetic dystrophy.

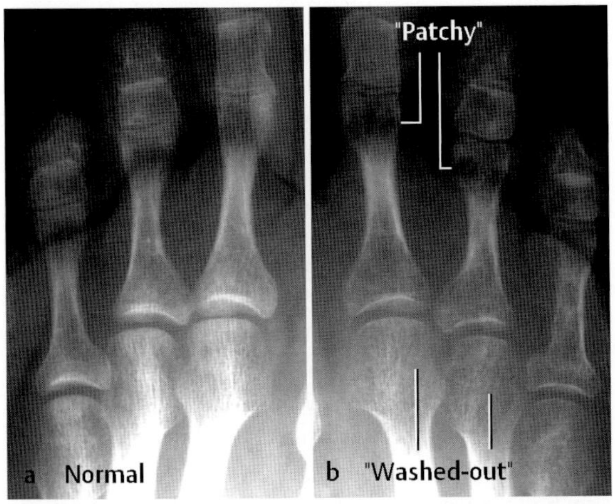

Fig. 1.58 Reflex sympathetic dystrophy with osteoporosis, right foot (**b**). Contralateral normal foot for comparison (**a**).

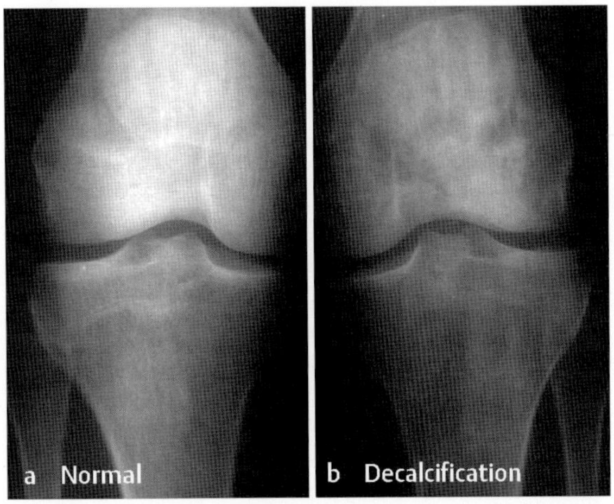

Fig. 1.59 Reflex sympathetic dystrophy of the left leg with patchy and striate radiolucencies.

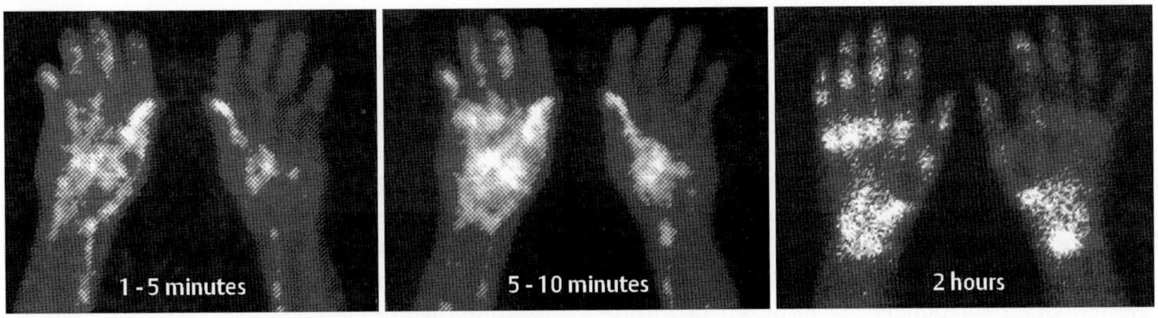

Fig. 1.60 Reflex sympathetic dystrophy following partial fasciectomy for Dupuytren contracture. The typical bone scan findings are diffuse hyperemia as well as lateralization of the early and late blood pool images, followed by increased uptake in the carpal and metacarpal bones in the bone phase.

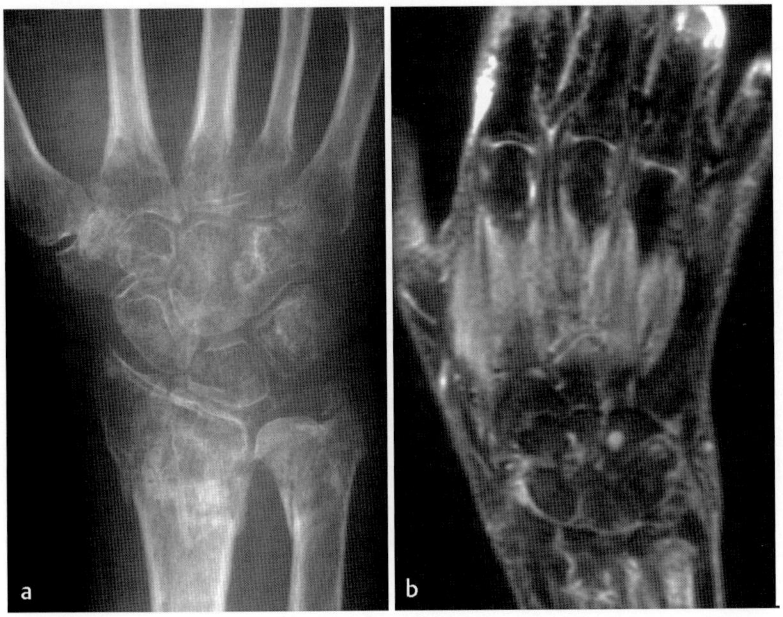

Fig. 1.61 Reflex sympathetic dystrophy of the right hand three months following a distal radial fracture. Osteoporosis with indistinct trabecular lines and patchy radiolucencies. The STIR sequence (**b**) shows increased signal intensity of the soft-tissues and an absence of bone marrow edema.

Trauma-induced Soft-Tissue Changes

Tendon Injuries

Tendons attach muscles to bone, usually bridge a joint, and have a high tensile strength. To function normally, they need an intact gliding bed, usually formed by a coarsely textured layer of connective tissues. Where the gliding range is wide, the tendons are surrounded by a sheath (e.g., fingers).

PATH Traumatic rupture of the tendon results in tendon and muscle retraction. Small gaps can be spontaneously bridged by the ingrowth of soft tissues.
Mechanism of trauma:
- separation,
- rupture,
- degeneration (age, sports-induced stress, inflammation, long-term corticosteroid therapy, hypercholesteremia, diabetes mellitus).

MRI Acute injuries to the tendons are easily detected by MRI. Since these injuries are diagnosed clinically, MRI is rarely performed.

On T2-weighted images there is increased signal intensity seen in an irregular gap of low or absent intensity in the tendon (Fig. 1.**62 b**). The gap is filled with fluid and/or enhancing granulation tissue and the tendon is surrounded by localized or diffuse edema or hemorrhage.

The so-called 'chronic tear' of ligamentous degeneration is seen as a focal area of increased intensity in a diffusely thickened tendon on T2-weighted SE MR images. Postoperatively, the sutured tendon is thickened and shows heterogeneously increased signal. The site of the suture often shows strong enhancement.

SONO A retracted tendon is easily detected ultrasonographically by comparison with the contralateral side (Figs. 1.**63**, 1.**64**). A tendon with degenerative changes is more difficult to evaluate. In general, the tendon is hypoechoic.

Ligamentous Injuries

Direct visualization of ligamentous structures requires MRI or sonography. Functional radiographic views (e.g., 'stress views') only provide indirect evidence of ligamentous lesions.

MRI Ligaments are of low signal intensity on both T1-weighted and T2-weighted images. A complete tear, best appreciated on STIR or T2-weighted SE MR images, appears as a high signal area (edema, blood) within the substance of the ligament. The tear may also be seen on the short TE images (T1-weighted or proton density). Images should be obtained in the plane that most optimally displays the ligamentous anatomy (see Special Traumatology: Knee, Ankle).

SONO Sonography is well suited to diagnose ligamentous injuries. While normal ligaments are seen as echogenic structures, injuries at the ligamentous insertion and involving the ligament itself are not only seen as continuity breaks but also as diffuse thickening and decreased echogenicity.

Muscle Injuries

Muscle fibers do not regenerate after injuries and muscular injuries result in a scar, which has less functional strength.

Types of injuries:
- Strain: Stretching of the muscle without exceeding its tensile strength. Hemorrhage occurs within the muscle.
- Crush: Blunt external force ruptures muscle fibers, possibly inducing areas of muscular necrosis.
- Rupture: This can occur after trauma to normal or degeneratively predamaged muscle. The muscle is partially or completely severed, but complete loss of function is rare.

MRI Diffuse edema and hemorrhage are the characteristic findings of acute as well as repetitive trauma and are easily identified as diffusely increased signal intensity on STIR and T2-weighted images (most conspicuous on turbo-SE sequences with fat suppression). The differentiation between sprain and (partial) tear rests on detecting a break in the ligamentous continuity. Tears result in large localized (hemorrhagic) fluid accumulations. MR findings are rarely seen in sprain or crush injury.

With immobilization of the affected extremity, the signal changes of a tear generally resolve within 14 days.

Intra- or intermuscular hematomas have a typical signal pattern which is related to the age of the hematoma. The signal intensity can be high on T1-weighted and T2-weighted images. If the T1-

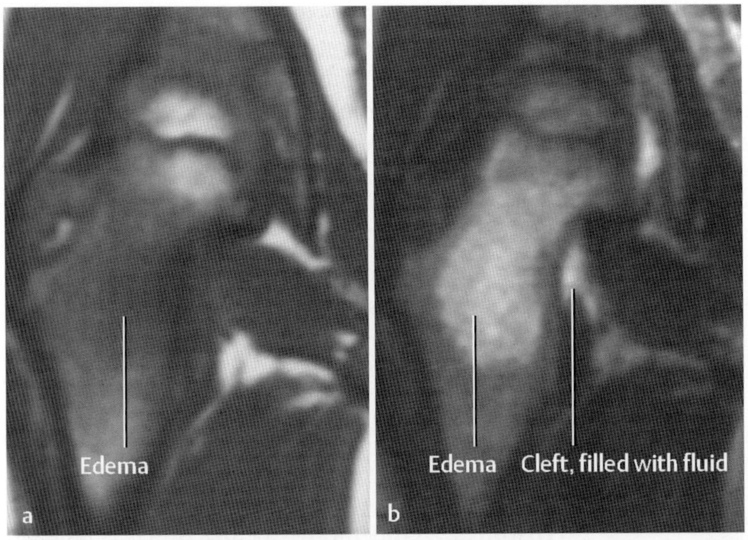

Fig. 1.**62** Avulsion trauma of the internal obturator with reactive bone marrow edema, after a fall in the bathtub 14 days previously. Patient presented with hip pain and limping. (T1-weighted [**a**] and T2-weighted [**b**] sequences.)

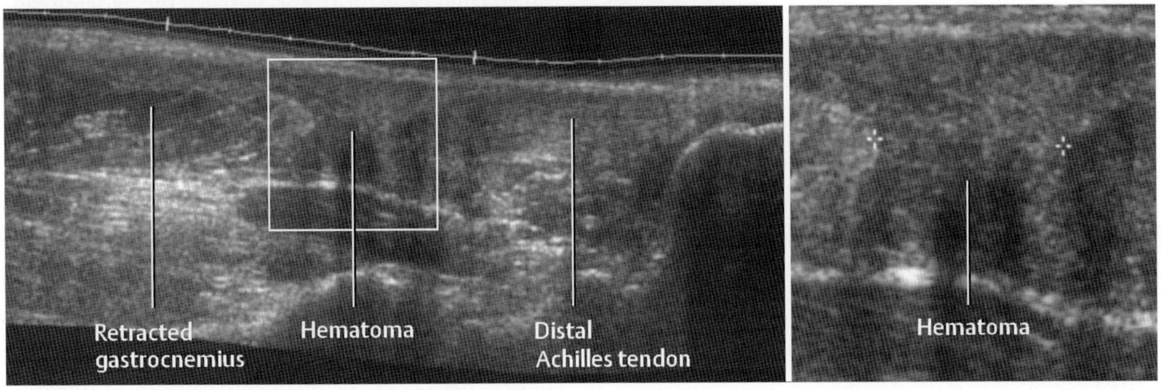

Fig. 1.**63** Sonographic visualization of an Achilles tendon tear.

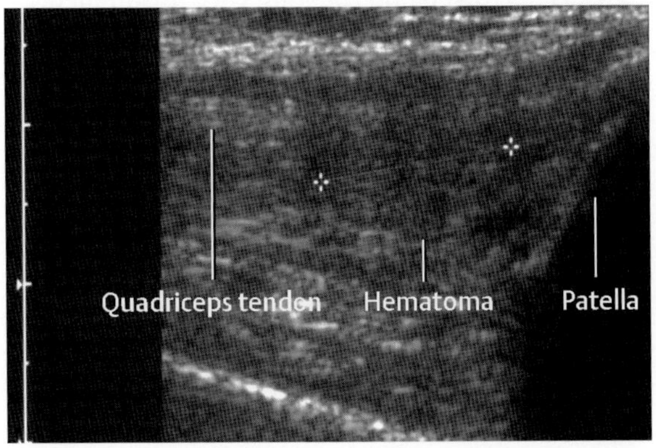

Fig. 1.**64** Small hematoma as manifestation of a partial tear of the quadriceps tendon.

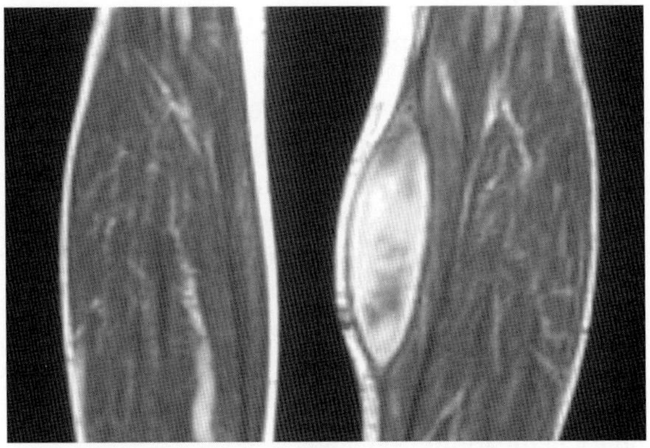

Fig. 1.**65** Subfascial hyperintense hematoma of the calf without known injury. Clinical and sonographic findings were suggestive of tumor (T1-weighted sequence).

weighted images show a signal of higher intensity than that of normal fluid (edema), the diagnosis of a hemorrhage is established (Fig. 1.**65**, 1.**66**). Older hematomas are surrounded by a rim of a signal void, which is attributed to hemosiderin deposits. This finding has to be differentiated from calcification, which appears as signal void as well. (The conventional radiograph helps to make this distinction.)

SONO A hematoma is sonographically detected as a hypoechoic or sometimes anechoic fluid accumulation. The musculature also loses its normal pennate texture. Often the hematoma cannot reliably be differentiated from synovial fluid extruded from a ruptured Baker cyst in the calf.

Rhabdomyolysis

The possible causes of loss of cellular integrity of muscle tissue are strain, trauma, burn, and exposure to toxins (drugs).

MRI may show no changes or only a slight decrease in signal intensity on the T1-weighted image. In contrast, the affected muscle exhibits a marked increase in signal intensity on the T2-weighted image (Fig. 1.**67**).

Myositis Ossificans

Soft-tissue injuries can lead to traumatic myositis ossificans (see pp. 286 ff).

Compartment Syndrome

The compartment syndrome refers to injury in an anatomically confined muscular compartment if elevated tissue pressure (caused by hematoma, edema) leads to decreased perfusion and subsequent ischemia. The end result is often hemorrhage and necrosis. MRI can display these changes and determine the extent of the soft-tissue damage (Fig. 1.**68**). Late complications of the compartment syndrome are radiographically visualized dystrophic calcifications (Fig. 1.**69**).

Glossary

Burns: Burn-induced osseous and articular changes usually depend on the size of the burned area.

The radiographic findings reflect the effect of ischemia (endothelial capillary damage) and the concurrent hyperemia of the remaining vascularized tissue:

- Focal or regional osteoporosis (immobilization or vasomotor reflex as probable cause).
- Periosteal reaction, similar to that of hypertrophic osteoarthropathy.
- Periarticular calcifications and ossifications, especially around hip, elbow, and shoulder.
- Progressive joint destruction, probably due to subchondral osteonecrosis along the articular fossa.
- Acro-osteolysis

Caution: Extensive burns frequently lead to secondary infections. They cause a multifarious picture and complicate the above-mentioned radiographic findings.

Frostbites: Temperatures below 8 – 12 °C damage soft tissues and nutrient vessels by causing decreased blood flow, erythema, and edema. The affected parts are usually the most distal ends of the extremities.

The most prominent radiographic sign of frostbitten bones is subchondral osteonecrosis, especially in the phalanges of the hands and feet, as well as in the metacarpal and metatarsal bones.

The findings can progress to osteolysis (e.g., acro-osteolysis) (Fig. 1.**70**).

Freezing-induced arthropathy is known in forest workers. The small tubular bones (fingers, toes) show evidence of (erosive) polyarthritis with cystic transformation of the articulating bones, subchondral sclerosis, and marginal osteophytes. The joint space is narrowed and the joints are misaligned.

Changes caused by freezing have been described in the ossification centers of the growing skeleton of adolescents.

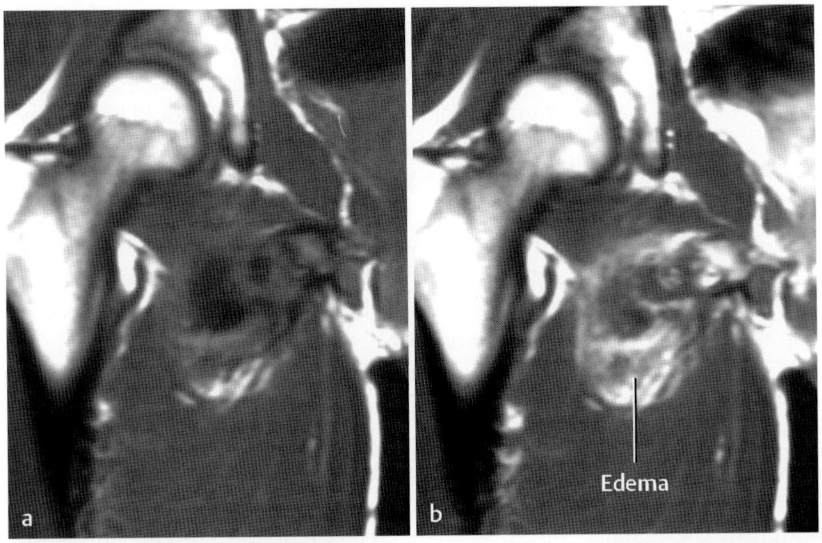

Fig. 1.**66** Muscle avulsion at the ischial tuberosity (T1-weighted sequence before [**a**] and after [**b**] administration of contrast medium).

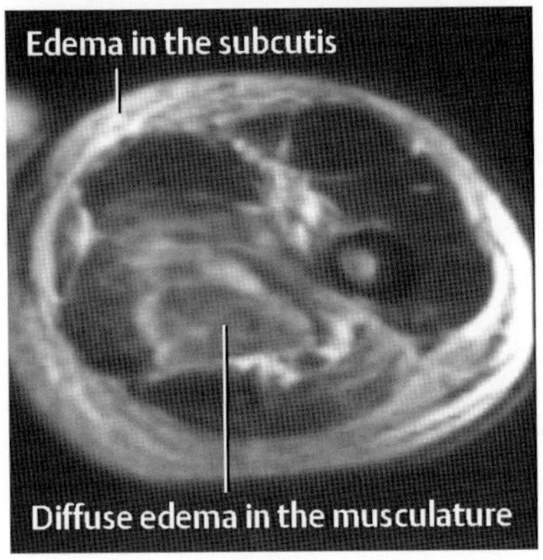

Fig. 1.**67** Rhabdomyolysis in a drug addict (T2-weighted image).

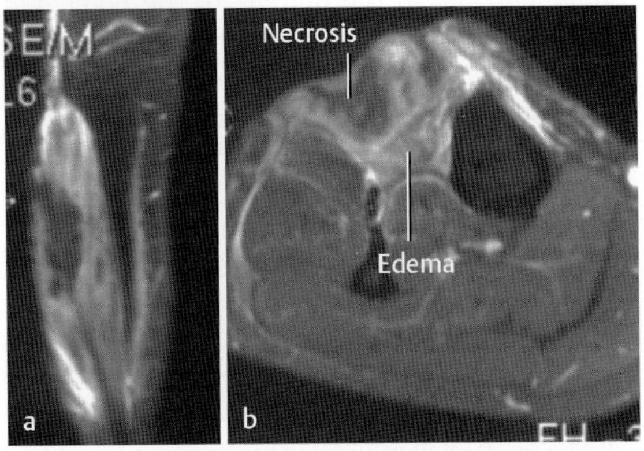

Fig. 1.**68** Muscle necrosis in compartment syndrome (T1-weighted sequence after frequency selected fat suppression and enhancement). **a** Coronal, **b** axial imaging plane.

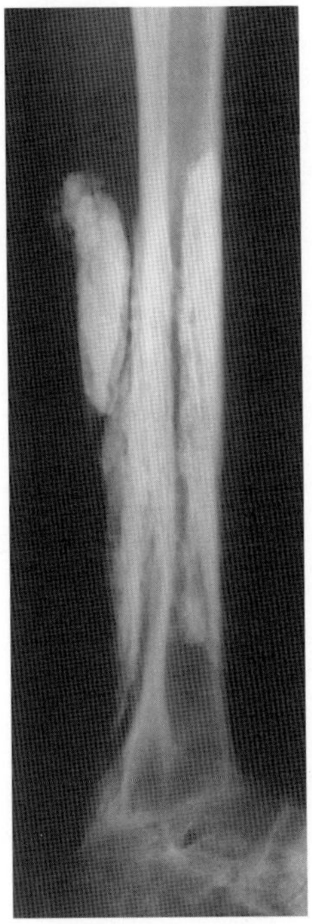

Fig. 1.**69** Soft-tissue calcifications following compartment syndrome 24 years previously.

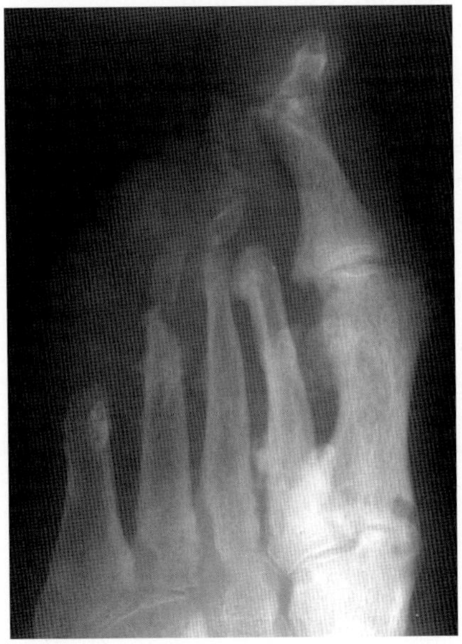

Fig. 1.**70** Severe osteolysis of the second to fifth ray after frostbite.

Radiologic Reporting of Fractures

The radiologic report should address the following items:
- Where is the fracture? To describe the level of the fracture, the long tubular bones should be divided into three equal parts (e.g., at the junction of middle and distal thirds).
- What type of fracture? The direction of the fracture line (transverse, oblique, spiral, etc.) should be stated (see Fig. 1.**20**).
- Where are the fracture fragments? The position of the **distal** fragment should be described in relation to the proximal fragment. Any angulation or tilt should be expressed in degrees. Varus position refers to medial angulation of the distal fragment toward the midline of the body, and valgus position refers to lateral angulation of the distal fragment away from the midline of the body. Additional anterior or posterior angulation in the second plane is seen on the lateral projection.
- Any translational displacement of the fracture fragments should be described (e.g., the distal fragment is displaced laterally, medially, etc., by one shaft width or one cortex width).
- Are the articular surfaces involved? Is there any associated dislocation or subluxation?
- Is the fracture complete or incomplete?

Follow-up radiographs should address:
- Position of the fragments in comparison with the initial and preceding examination.
- Amount of callus formation.
- Extent of osseous bridging and remodeling.

Search for possible complications:
- Osteomyelitis: Did radiolucent areas appear? Are indistinct radiolucent halos seen around internal fixation devices (e.g., screws, nails, pins)?
- Is there any evidence of osteonecrosis?

What Should Be Avoided?

Judgmental terms, such as 'good', 'adequate', 'acceptable', or similar expressions, should be avoided.

Likewise, statements describing the osseous bridging as 'solid,' 'delayed,' 'partial,' or 'absent' should not be used. These statements require an intimate familiarity with the clinical condition. Instead, the callus should be described by its **appearance** (how does the callus look?) and it should be stated **whether** its appearance indicates osseous bridging or not. Furthermore, it should be stated whether the fracture line is still visible.

It should be kept in mind that it is difficult to judge any possible rotation of the fragments on conventional radiographs. If a clinically relevant rotation is suspected, CT or MRI should be recommended.

Table 1.**5** Average time for fractures to heal

Fracture	Average time for healing
Skull Clavicle, scapula Sternum, ribs Humeral head Distal humerus Elbow Radial head Distal forearm Metacarpals, fingers Metatarsals, toes	3 – 6 weeks
Humeral shaft Radial and ulnar shaft Distal tibia and fibula	6 – 8 weeks
Tibial shaft Femoral shaft	8 – 10 weeks
Carpal bones Femoral neck Pelvis Distal femur Tibial plateau Tarsal bones/calcaneus	10 – 14 weeks

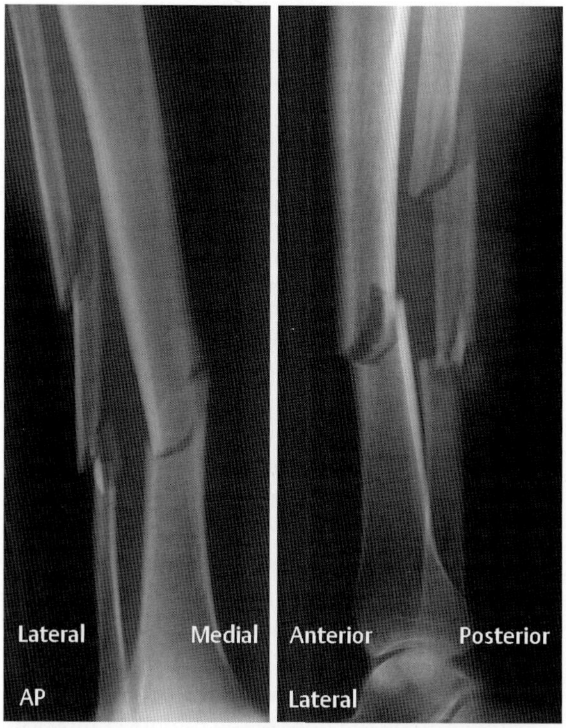

Fig. 1.**71** Typical findings: fracture of the lower leg. Segmental fracture of the middle third of the fibula with dorsal displacement of the fracture fragment by one-half shaft width, oblique fracture of the tibia at the transition of middle and distal thirds. There is about 10 degrees posterior and 15 degrees lateral angulation.

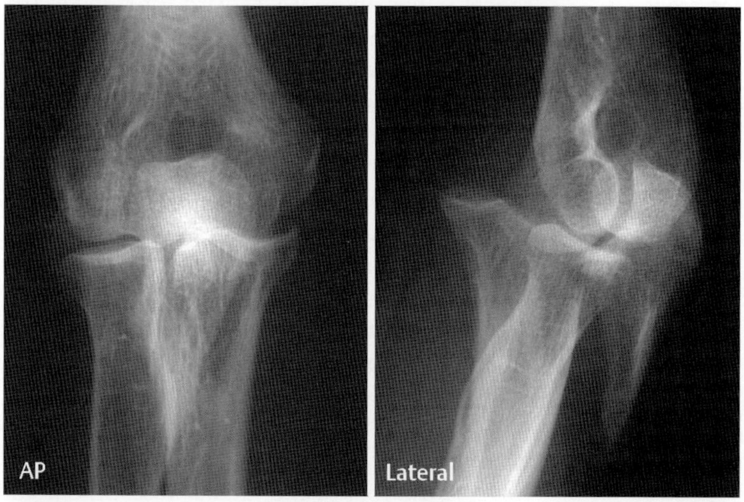

Fig. 1.**72** Typical findings: trauma films. Oblique fracture of the proximal ulna with articular involvement and anterior ulnar dislocation. There is no displacement of the olecranon fragment.

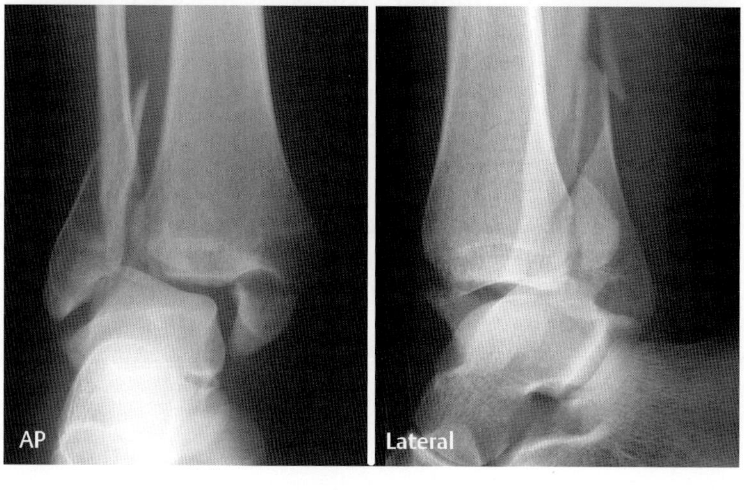

Fig. 1.**73** Typical findings: trauma films. Trimalleolar fracture-dislocation of the ankle with posterolateral displacement and medial angulation of the talus. There is a fibular fracture at the level of the ruptured interosseous membrane with medial angulation (approximately 20 degrees). The fractured medial malleolus is displaced laterally by about 8 mm and the posterior cortical fragment of the tibia (Volkmann triangle) is displaced upward by 5 mm.

Special Traumatology

Skull and Spine

Fractures of the Cranial Vault

Fractures of the cranial vault are differentiated according to location, mechanism, and configuration. Depending on the severity and type of causative force, three fracture types can be distinguished:
- linear fractures (Figs. 1.**74**, 1.**75**),
- depressed or comminuted fractures (Fig. 1.**76**),
- punched-out fractures.

Linear Fractures

These represent 80% of all fractures of the cranial vault and generally are temporoparietal, occipital, and frontal in location. Only the presence of intracranial complications (bleeding, edema, intracranial air, etc.) requires therapeutic intervention.

Caution: Linear fractures can be mistaken for sutures or vascular grooves; fracture lines cross sutures and vessels, are sharply delineated, and do not have a sclerotic rim (Fig. 1.**74**).

! Fractures that cross the groove of the middle meningeal artery can cause an epidural hematoma.

Depressed and Comminuted Fractures

These fractures generally are diagnosed by conventional radiography, but a complete diagnostic evaluation requires computed tomography to delineate the true extent of the intracranial displacement of the osseous fragments as well as any associated cerebral involvement (Fig. 1.**76**).

Punched-out Fractures

Depending on its angle and velocity, the penetrating force can result in a depressed, punched-out, or burst fracture.

Fractures of the Cranial Base

These fractures primarily involve the orbital roof, petrous pyramid, and occipital bone. The central areas of the cranial base are less often involved. Since the neurovascular structures pass through an aperture in the mechanically weak sites of the central cranial base, these fractures can be associated with considerable clinical findings (brain stem paralysis, paresthesia, vision loss, CSF fistula).

CT has become the exclusive imaging modality for the evaluation of the cranial base (Fig. 1.**77**).

Fractures of the Temporal Bone

Classification of Temporal Bone Fractures

Historically, these fractures have been categorized relative to the longitudinal axis of the temporal bone as longitudinal, transverse, and mixed fractures. This categorization is arbitrary, however, since many fractures follow a winding course through the temporal bone.

1. **Longitudinal fractures** account for 70–80% of all fractures of the temporal bone and run along the longitudinal axis of the petrous pyramid (Fig. 1.**78**). Beginning in the region of the mastoid with involvement of the tegmen tympani (roof of the middle ear cavity), external auditory canal and temporomandibular fossa, the fracture line extends along the floor of the middle cranial fossa, continues anteriorly toward the apex of the pyramidal bone, and terminates at the carotid canal, foramen lacerum, foramen spinosa, or musculotubal canal. A fracture line directed toward the internal auditory canal (risk of facial nerve palsy) or even jugular foramen is less frequently observed. Longitudinal fractures are frequently associated with dislocated or fractured ossicles and almost invariably result in conductive hearing loss.
2. **Transverse fractures** account for about 20% of all fractures of the temporal bone (Fig. 1.**79**). These fractures always follow the path of least resistance and run perpendicular to the long axis of the petrous pyramid. Thus, the fracture lines traverse the roof of the jugular fossa, the inner ear (with involvement of cochlea and vestibule), and finally the petrous ridge. The clinical findings depend on the course of the fracture line, with the spectrum ranging from hematotympanum, vertigo, and vestibular nystagmus, to complete hearing loss. The facial nerve is injured in 50% of cases.
3. **Complex or mixed fractures** exhibit longitudinal and transverse components and often occur in conjunction with severe head trauma. Cerebrospinal fluid otorrhea or herniation of cerebral tissue through the fracture line are typical complications.

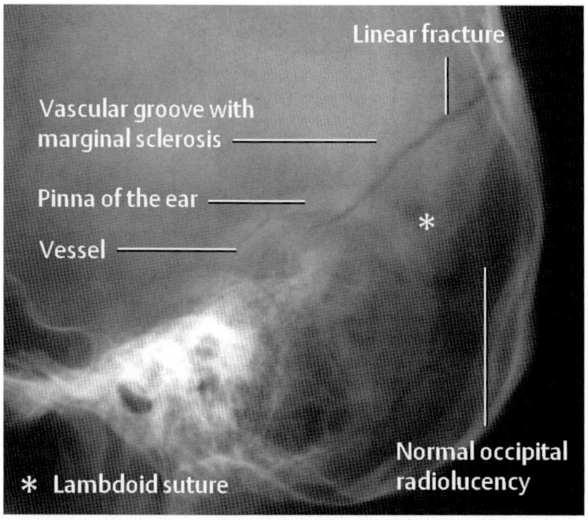

Fig. 1.**74** Typical linear fracture of the calvaria. Notice the sharp contour of the fracture line and absence of a sclerotic border, in contrast to a suture or vascular channel.

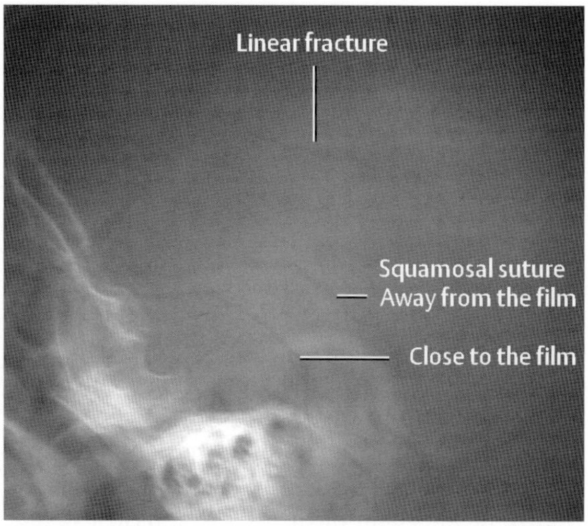

Fig. 1.**75** Linear fracture in a child.

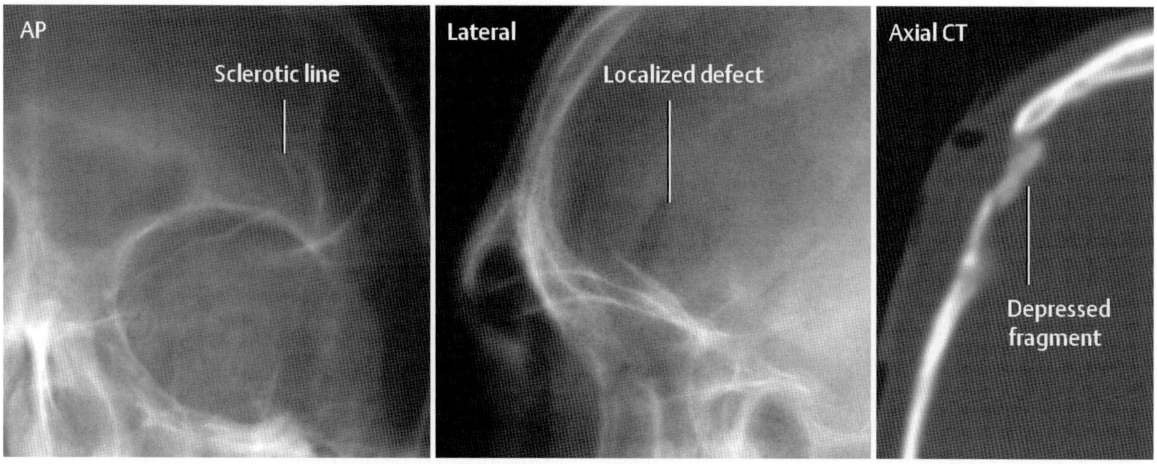

Fig. 1.**76** Depressed fracture of the calvaria. **Caution!** This case illustrates that searching for radiolucent fracture **lines** is not adequate. A CT scan is necessary to determine the extent of the impression and to exclude intracranial injuries.

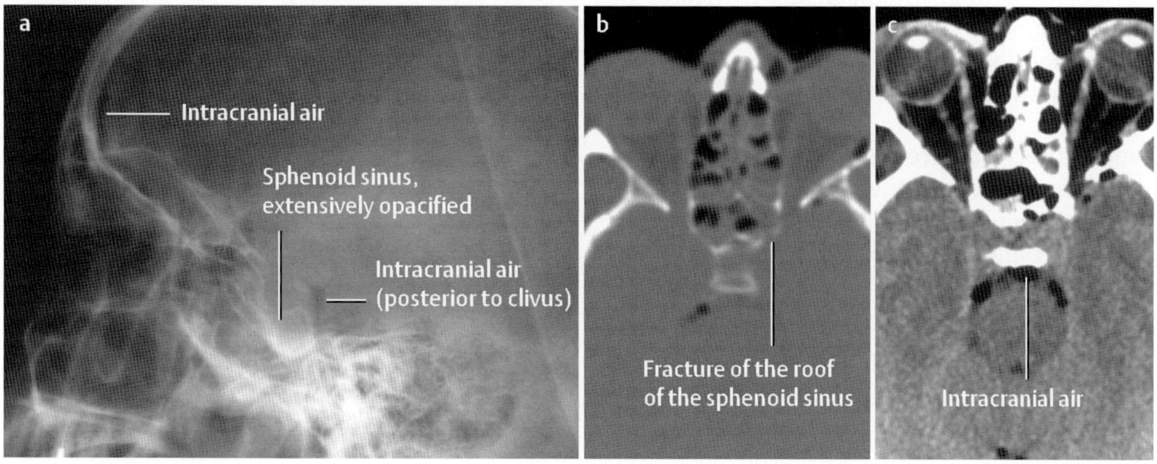

Fig. 1.**77** Fracture of the sphenoid sinus as seen on conventional radiographs (**a**) and on axial CT (**b** bone window, **c** soft-tissue window). The conventional radiograph only provides indirect evidence of a fracture of the cranial base.

X-RAY Conventional radiography is still the basic examination, comprising AP, lateral, and submentovertical projections as well as special projections, such as Law and Stenvers views and, occasionally, the Mayer view. Fractures of the temporal bone can be diagnosed on the basis of direct fracture signs (radiolucent line, contour break), indirect fracture signs (opacification of the mastoid cells, sphenoid sinus, external auditory canal, middle ear cavity), or by local pneumocephalus.

CT This is the imaging method of choice for the evaluation of the traumatized temporal bone. The fracture signs are the same as those for conventional radiography. Furthermore, a change of the chain of the auditory ossicles (subluxation, dislocation, fracture) might be detected. Traumatic lesions of the stapes, however, are rarely adequately visualized.

MRI MRI is only indicated when injuries of intracranial structures or cranial nerves dominate the clinical findings or are otherwise suspected together with fractures of the temporal bone.

Fractures of the Facial Bones

Because of their pathogenesis, fractures of the facial bone are frequently multiple and complex.

The classification is always somewhat artificial since the traumatic pattern varies from patient to patient. It is clinically appropriate to make a distinction between localized and midfacial fractures, since midfacial fractures have to be considered unstable and need stabilization by surgery (Table 1.**7**).

X-RAY Conventional radiography is used as the primary screening imaging method. The information that can be derived from it depends on the type of fracture (Table 1.**6**).

Typical **direct fracture signs** are:
- Contour break with or without step deformity,
- Radiolucent line,
- Double contour or increased density due to overlapping fragments,
- Linear density reflecting a transversely oriented fragment.

Table 1.**6** The role of conventional radiographs for the detection and localization of facial fractures

Projection	Fracture site
Skull, AP and lateral	Anterior and posterior wall of frontal and maxillary sinus, mandible
Orbits, PA	Orbits, paranasal sinuses
Paranasal sinus series	Paranasal sinuses, orbit, zygoma
Orbit, Rheese projection	Optical canal
Cranial base, submentovertical	Maxillary and sphenoid sinuses, mandible
Zygomatic arches, tangential projection	Both zygomatic arches
Panoramic tomography, pantomography, rotational tomography	Mandibular and maxillary dental arches

Typical **indirect fracture signs** are:
- Soft-tissue swelling,
- Opacification or air-fluid level in the paranasal sinuses, middle ear, mastoid air cells,
- 'Teardrop sign' as a manifestation of a blow-out fracture of the orbital floor,
- Intracranial air,
- Clinical signs: double vision, cerebrospinal fluid rhinorrhea.

The extent and severity of injury are generally underestimated without three-dimensional display. Conventional tomography for the evaluation of facial injuries is **obsolete.**

CT CT is the **most important** imaging method in this setting and permits the evaluation of bones and soft tissues. It has replaced conventional radiography for the evaluation of facial trauma in most centers. Thin sections (1–2 mm) should be obtained in the axial and coronal planes.

MRI MRI does not play a role in the diagnostic evaluation of facial fractures.

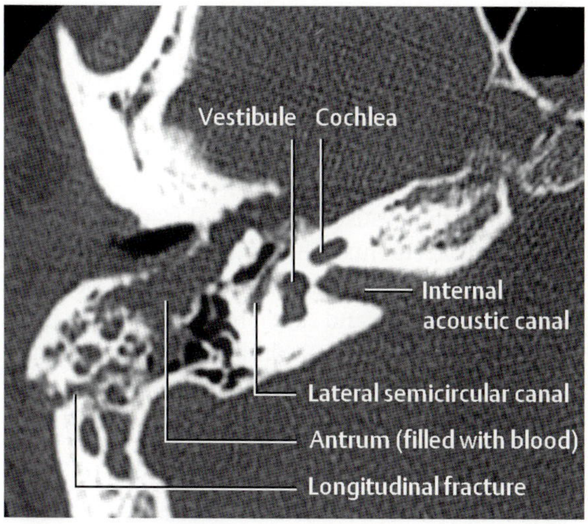

Fig. 1.**78** Longitudinal fracture of the temporal bone as seen on axial CT.

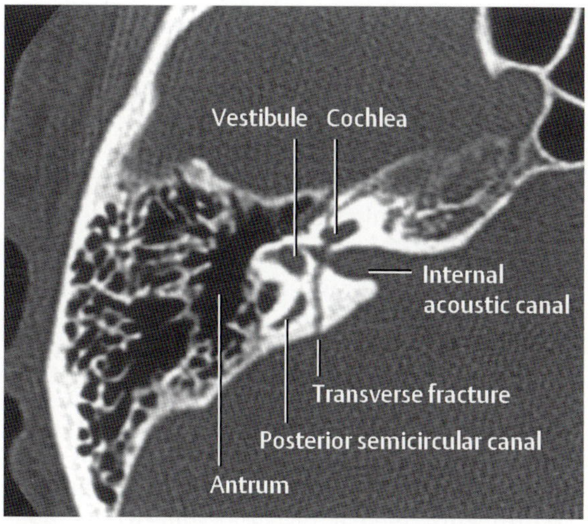

Fig. 1.**79** Transverse fracture of the temporal bone on axial CT.

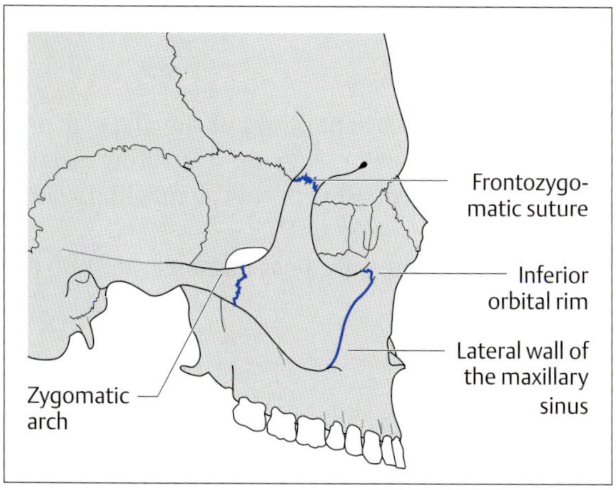

Fig. 1.**80** Schematic diagram of the zygoma and the four typical fracture sites.

Table 1.**7** Classification of facial fractures

1. Localized fracture	
Solitary fracture:	Complex fracture:
Nasal bone (> 50%)	Zygomaticomaxillary complex (ZMC)
Zygomatic arch	Naso-ethmoidal, nasofrontal
Isolated wall of the sinus cavity	Blow-in, blow-out (orbit)
Mandible	Fronto-orbital
2. Transfacial fracture	
Le Fort I	
Le Fort II	
Le Fort III	
Combinations	

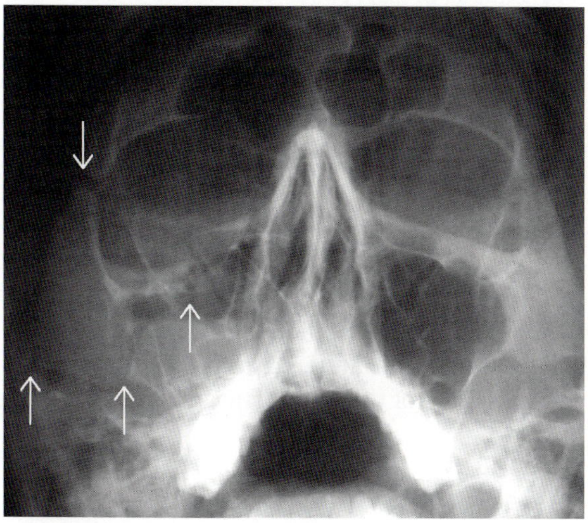

Fig. 1.**81** Fracture of the right zygoma with a fracture line at all four typical sites (compare with Fig. 1.**80**). Hemorrhage into the maxillary cavity with air fluid levels suggests osseous trauma, even without definite delineation of fractures.

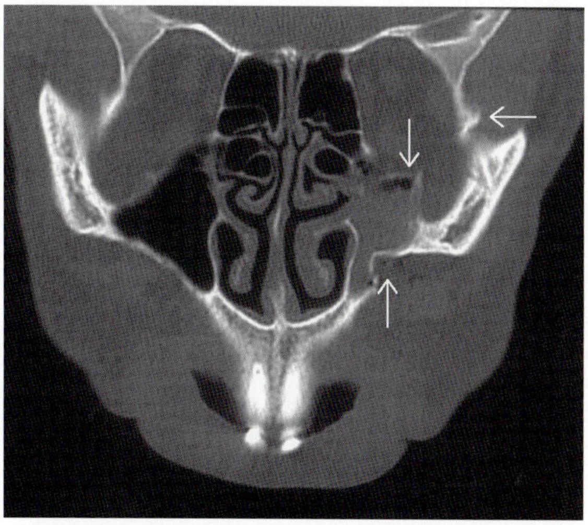

Fig. 1.**82** Fracture of the zygoma with separation of the zygoma from its maxillary, frontal, and orbital connection (arrows).

Localized Fractures of the Facial Bones

Fracture of the Nasal Bones

This is the commonest localized facial fracture and the extent of injury depends on the direction and severity of the traumatic blow. The spectrum ranges from a widened nasofrontal suture and a simple nasal fracture to a comminuted fracture with involvement of the orbit and base of the frontal bone.

Fracture of the Zygoma

This is the second commonest facial fracture. The mechanically weakest point is the zygomatic arch. The most frequent manifestation is a depressed fracture with medial displacement of the fragments.

Clinically, the lateral facial structures are asymmetric, and involvement of the temporomandibular joint causes impaired movement of the mandible.

Fracture of the Zygomaticomaxillary Complex (ZMC)

Synonym: Tripod or quadruped fracture

Four osseous sites are fractured, separating the zygoma from its temporal, frontal, and maxillary fixation (Figs. 1.**80** – 1.**82**).

Blow-out Fracture

A sudden increase in intracranial pressure (e.g., blow with a fist, ball, or stick) causes the thin osseous walls (orbital floor, medial orbital wall) to fracture and the osseous fragments to be displaced into the maxillary sinus or ethmoid air cells (Fig. 1.**83**, 1.**84**).

Frequent complications of this injury are herniated or entrapped intraorbital fat or extraocular muscles, hemorrhage into the vitreous body, and traumatic cataract (Fig. 1.**84**).

The clinical findings include double vision, hematoma, enophthalmos, paresthesias (involvement of the infraorbital nerve), and eyelid edema.

X-RAY This fracture characteristically produces a 'teardrop' along the roof of the maxillary sinus (Fig. 1.**83**), an air-fluid level in the maxillary sinus (blood) and, possibly, periorbital soft-tissue swelling. Orbital emphysema can be an indirect sign of this injury. Fracture of the thick and relatively strong infraorbital rim is rare. A definitive evaluation of the fracture can be achieved by CT, which also reveals the extent of any possible herniation of fat and muscle into the maxillary sinus (Fig. 1.**84**).

Blow-in Fracture

This causes intraorbital displacement of osseous fragments and soft tissues.

Midfacial Fractures

The commonest cause of midfacial fractures is motor vehicle accidents. The Le Fort classification is used for midfacial fractures, which can occur in any combination and are frequently associated with other fractures ('complex midfacial fractures'). One should, however, remember that midfacial fractures always include the pterygoid process (Fig. 1.**85**).

> **!** Midfacial fractures are unstable and are characterized by involvement of the pterygoid process.

Le Fort I

This injury involves separation of the alveolar process from the maxilla, causing a 'floating palate'. The basal aspects of **all** walls of the maxillary sinus are fractured.

Le Fort I fractures are best demonstrated by coronal CT (Fig. 1.**86**).

Le Fort II

This injury involves separation of a pyramidal fragment of the central portion of the face. The fracture line traverses the nasal base and the medial orbital wall bilaterally with extension to the orbital floor and infraorbital rim. The medial wall of the maxillary sinus is preserved (in contrast to the Le Fort I fracture, Fig. 1.**86**).

Complications: Damage to the infraorbital nerve in 80% of cases, entrapment of the extraocular inferior rectus muscle, damage to the nasolacrimal duct.

Le Fort III

This is complete separation of the facial bones from the skull. The fracture line traverses the nasal base, medial orbital wall and floor of the orbit bilaterally, and extends to the lateral orbital wall with an additional fracture of the zygomatic arch and pterygoid process.

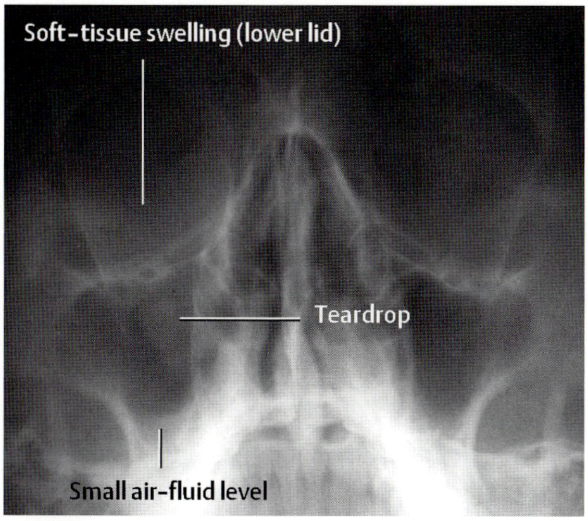

Fig. 1.**83** Blow-out fracture of the orbit with the typical 'teardrop' soft-tissue density.

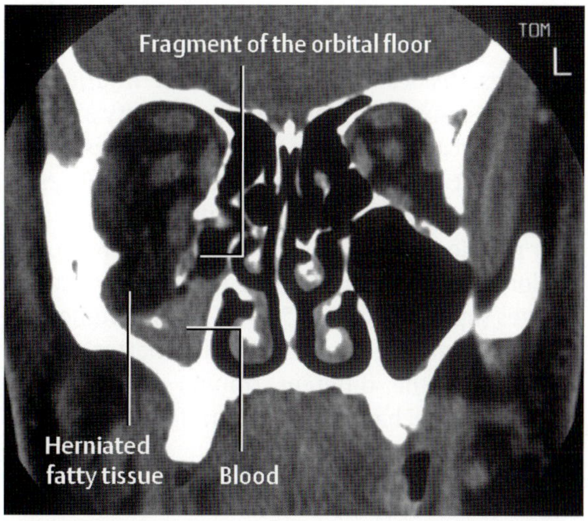

Fig. 1.**84** Blow-out fracture of the orbit as seen on coronal CT. The herniation of intraorbital fat and inferior rectus muscle is clearly displayed.

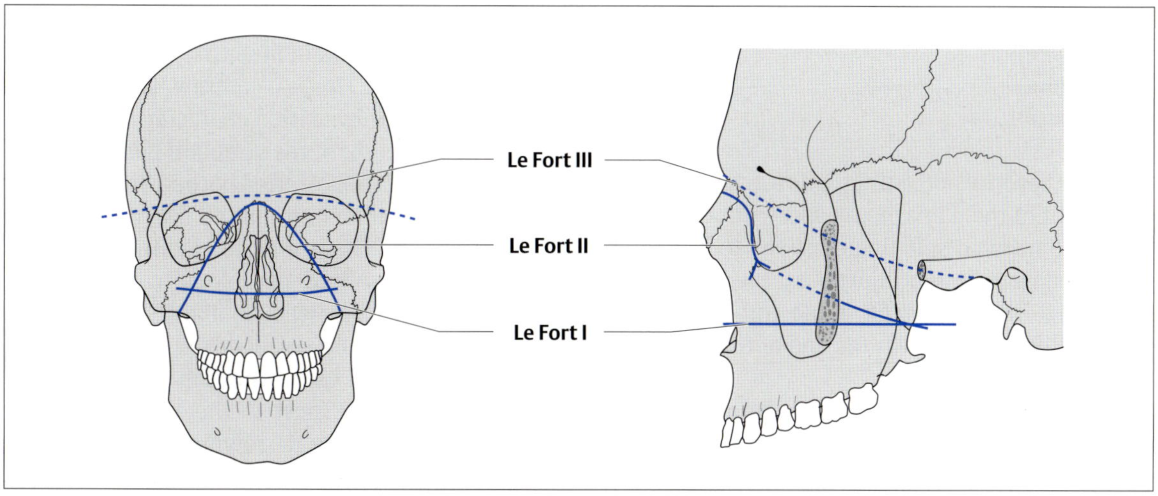

Fig. 1.**85** Schematic diagram of the fracture lines of Le Fort fractures.

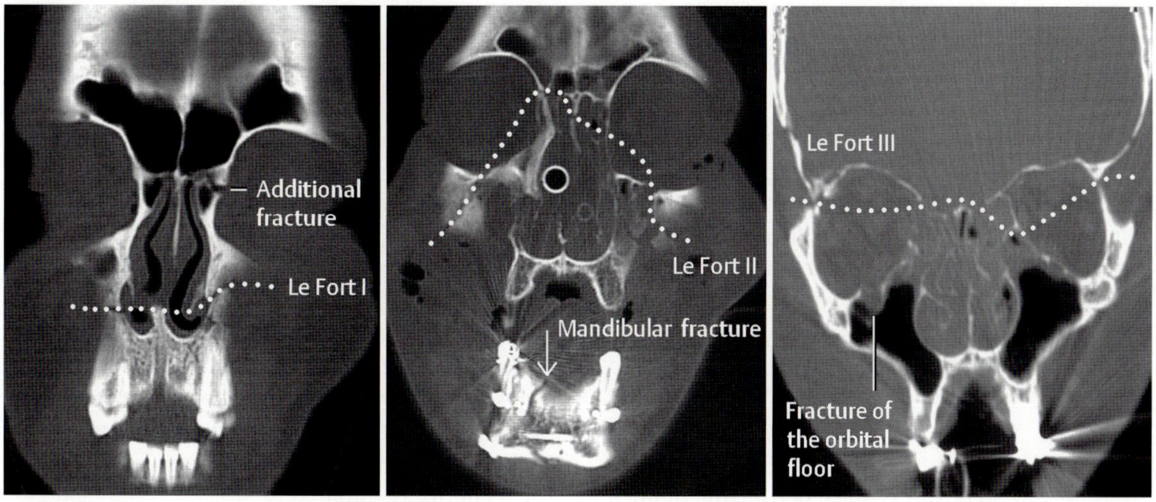

Fig. 1.**86** Le Fort fractures I–III, coronal CT. These fractures are invariably associated with other facial bone injuries. A combination of the different Le Fort fracture types is common. The involvement of the left medial orbital wall of the Le Fort III fracture is best seen on more anterior sections.

Spine

Fractures, dislocations and soft-tissue injuries can affect the spine at any level. In the majority of cases, clinical and radiologic findings can readily establish the correct diagnosis. Insufficient experience, as well as inadequate image quality (mobile units, poor positioning of immobile patients), is responsible for the relatively high rate of missed vertebral injuries (approximately 25–50%). Improvement in detection can be expected from a better understanding of the different trauma patterns and pathogenic mechanisms and from familiarity with the radiographic approach.

Classification of Spinal Fractures

Spinal injuries can be categorized according to the traumatic forces that cause them:

- Compression,
- Flexion,
- Extension,
- Rotation,
- Translation.

Since the severity of the traumatic force determines the extent of the damage, the spectrum of damage varies from trivial soft-tissue lesions to severe osseous and ligamentous injury.

Distinguishing between stable and unstable injuries will be discussed at the end of the chapter.

X-RAY Conventional radiographs remain the best screening examination for vertebral trauma. The standard projections most suitable for the various anatomic regions are listed in Table 1.**8.** The lateral view is most important and should be obtained prior to moving the patient or taking the patient off the trauma board.

CT CT has effectively replaced conventional tomography and is also superior to conventional radiography in diagnosing spinal injuries. CT provides excellent visualization of the bones and soft tissues and is capable of multiplanar image reconstruction. Its most important indication is assessing any involvement of the posterior border of fractured vertebral bodies (stability) and any cord compression by displaced fragments or hematomas.

MRI The advantage of MRI is its superb visualization of soft tissues, permitting delineation of diskoligamentous and cord injuries (edema, hematomyelia, transection).

Flexion Fractures

1. **Teardrop fracture:** A tear of the anterior longitudinal ligament causes avulsion of a teardrop-shaped fragment at the anterior inferior end plate with dislocation of the affected vertebral body into the spinal canal. On the lateral view, the osseous fragment is smaller in height than in width, which is considered an (uncertain) criterion differentiating a flexion teardrop fracture from an extension teardrop fracture (see below). This fracture is most commonly seen in the lower cervical spine (in 70% at C5, Fig. 1.**87**). It is completely unstable and leads to vertebral dislocation with paraplegia in more than 80% of cases.
2. **Compression fracture:** This a relatively common fracture of the anterior vertebral corner with wedging of the vertebral body. It is stable since the posterior aspects of the spine (including ligaments) remain intact.
3. **Burst fracture:** This is a common fracture of the thoracolumbar transition characterized by anterior loss of height of the vertebral body and fragmentation of its posterior border. The posterior fragments of this comminuted fracture are often displaced into the spinal canal with a high incidence of associated neurologic complications. The resultant narrowed AP diameter of the spinal canal generally correlates with the severity of the neurologic symptoms (Fig. 1.**88**). The diagnostic evaluation (best in the acute setting by CT) must assess any narrowing of the spinal canal and associated soft-tissue changes (cord, disk, ligaments).
4. **Chance fracture** or **seat-belt injury:** This is a flexion injury with the fulcrum in the region of the anterior abdominal wall. Severe abdominal injuries also occur in 15% of cases. It was once a common injury in motor vehicle accidents when only lap-type seat belts were used; it has become relatively rare today following the introduction of the shoulder strap. Radiographically, a horizontal fracture is seen through the vertebral body (predominantly of L1–L3), with involvement of both pedicles, the arch, and the spinous process (Fig. 1.**89**).
5. **Clay shoveler's fracture:** This fracture, originally described in clay or coal shovelers, represents an avulsion fracture of the spinous process at the insertion of the supraspinous ligament (C6–T3). This injury is stable.
6. **Anterior subluxation and dislocation:** The **segmental** rupture of the posterior ligament causes

Table 1.**8** Anatomic structures that can be evaluated on conventional radiographs

Projection	Anatomic structure
AP	Vertebral body, pedicle, spinous process, intervertebral disk space, paravertebral space
Dens AP (open mouth odontoid view)	Atlas, axis (including dens), atlantoaxial articulation
Lateral	Vertebral body (height, posterior border), intervertebral space, prevertebral soft tissues
Swimmer's view	C5 – T2
Oblique views	Facet joints, spondylolysis
Functional views	Instability (only with cooperative patients and normal initial views)
Tomography	Dens, cervicothoracic and thoracolumbar transition

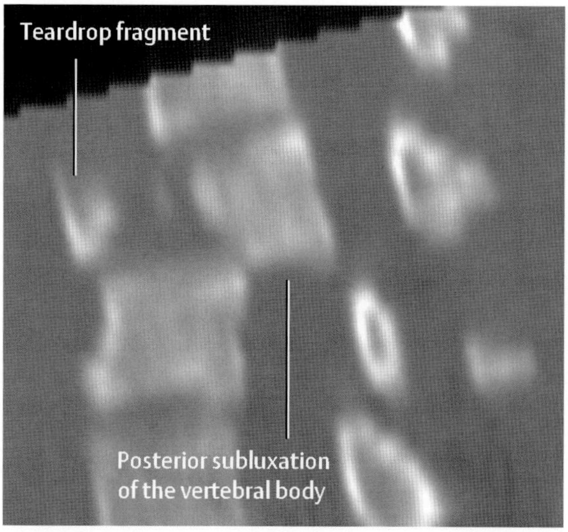

Fig. 1.**87** Flexion distraction injury (teardrop fracture). Reformatted sagittal CT image shows marked narrowing of the spinal canal by the retropulsed vertebral body fragment.

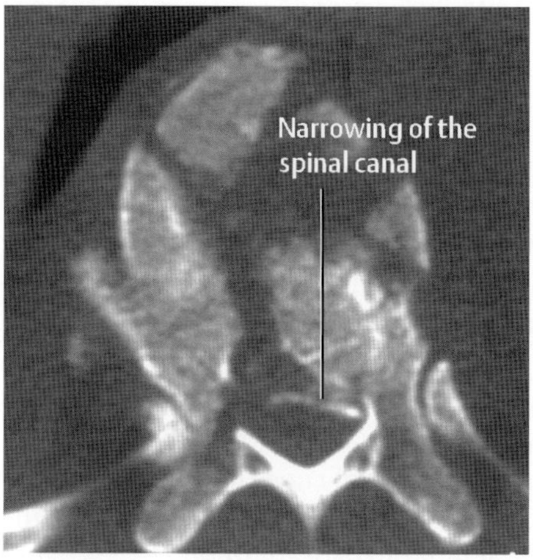

Fig. 1.**88** Burst fracture (T11) with the posterior fragment displaced into the spinal canal.

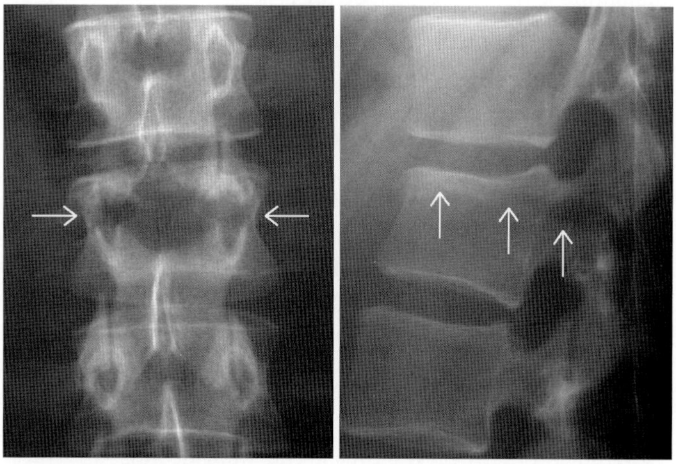

Fig. 1.**89** Chance fracture. The L2 vertebral body is divided by a horizontal fracture through the vertebral body and both arches.

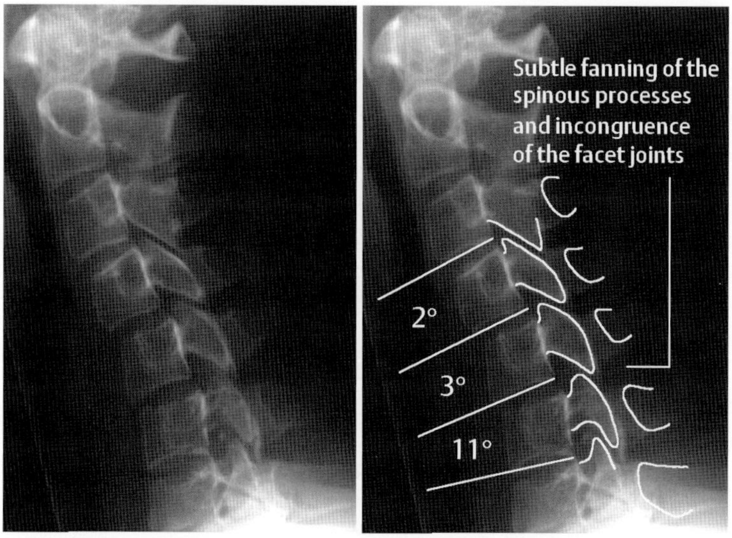

Fig. 1.**90** Segmental hypermobility of C5 – 6. The 11-degree angulation by itself is not pathologic, but the associated severe segmental kyphosis is. Such a finding:

- **can** represent a normal variant,
- **can** be caused by muscle spasm following whiplash injury,
- but is **strongly suspicious** for an anterior subluxation.

A reliable differentiation is **not** possible with conventional radiography.

an anterior angulation of a vertebral body relative to the subjacent vertebral body with fanning of the spinous processes, incomplete articulation of the facet joints, and possible anterior displacement of the subluxated vertebra (Fig. 1.**90**). The stability is determined by the extent of angulation and translation. The most important diagnostic criterion is the hypermobility of **one** segment observed in an otherwise hypomobile spine. A subtle anterior subluxation cannot be diagnosed by conventional radiography and, if clinically suspected, requires an MRI.

7. **Bilateral facet joint dislocation (blockade):** This injury complex is predominantly seen in the lower cervical spine. Caused by severe distraction of the dorsal ligaments with resultant anterior dislocation of the more cephalad vertebra, it leads to spinal canal stenosis and is often associated with neurologic symptoms (Fig. 1.**91**).

Radiographic Hints: Flexion Fractures

- Interrupted posterior cervical line: displacement, rotation, angulation, absence, and doubling are abnormal,
- Increased interpedicular width on the AP view (secondary to fracture of the lamina),
- Forward displacement,
- Segmental hypermobility,
- Subluxation or dislocation of the facet joints,
- Narrowed intervertebral disk space – usually above the fractured vertebra.

Extension Fractures

1. **Anterior avulsion fracture** (also referred to as 'extension teardrop fracture'): The anterior longitudinal ligament avulses a fragment from the anteroinferior or superoanterior edge of the vertebral end plate (Fig. 1.**92**). On the lateral view, the height of the avulsed fragment is usually equal to or larger than its width. In contrast to the flexion fracture, this extension fracture generally affects the upper cervical spine (most frequently at C2) and is stable on flexion. Neurologic deficits are rare.
2. **Hangman's ('Hangee's') fracture:** Frequently seen after motor vehicle accidents, this injury represents a distraction fracture of both posterior arches of C2 (Figs. 1.**92, 1.93**).
   Type I (65%): Nondisplaced fragment through the pedicle – the C2/3 disk is intact.
   Type II (30%): Additional anterior displacement of C2 (> 3 mm) or angulation (> 15°) with rupture of the C2/3 disk. This is an unstable injury.
   Type III (5%): Like type II plus a unilateral or bilateral dislocation of the facet joints. This is a highly unstable fracture.
3. **Posterior subluxation or dislocation:** This injury is caused by tears of the anterior and posterior longitudinal ligaments and the disk. Subluxation or dislocation of the facet joints or fractures through the pedicles causes the loss of an articulating connection. The most affected levels are C4 through C6 and the thoracolumbar junction. It is unstable and associated with severe neurologic deficits.

Radiographic Hints: Extension Fractures

- Avulsion fracture of the anterior end plate (Fig. 1.**92**),
- Widened subjacent disk space,
- Posterior displacement representing rupture of the anterior and posterior longitudinal ligament and disk,
- Fracture with dislocation of the facet joints.

Rotation Fractures

Torsion forces result in an unstable vertebral injury with a high incidence of spinal cord injury. Dislocation or fracture of the facet joints indicates a rotational component, and rotatory and/or translatory misalignment is frequent.

1. **Unilateral facet joint blocking:** This is the result of hyperflexion superimposed on torsion flexion and frequently occurs in the lower cervical spine. It is associated with a fracture of the articular process in only one third of cases. Neurologic complications secondary to narrowed intervertebral foramina are common.

Radiographic Hints: Rotation Fractures

- Dislocated and rotated fracture fragments (Fig. 1.**94**),
- Fracture of the transverse process and ribs,
- Fracture and dislocation of the facet joints,
- Interrupted posterior cervical line,
- Possible anterior displacement.

Shear Fractures

These fractures are caused by a horizontal or oblique impact (Fig. 1.**95**). They usually occur with the body's lower half fixed and the spine exposed to and moved by the impact. These injuries are frequently associated with severe neurologic findings.

Location: The thoracolumbar and craniovertebral junctions as a manifestation of the atlanto-occipital dislocation (rare).

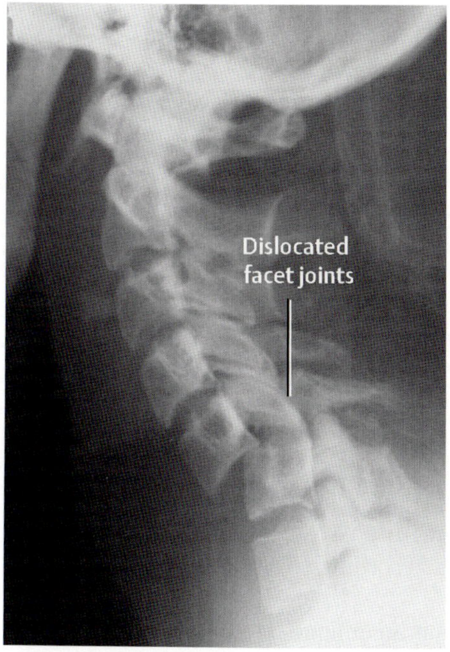

Fig. 1.**91** From a 16-year-old female patient in a motor vehicle accident. There is distraction of the posterior ligamentous complex with anterior dislocation of C5 and bilateral facet joint 'locking'. Note the marked spinal canal stenosis.

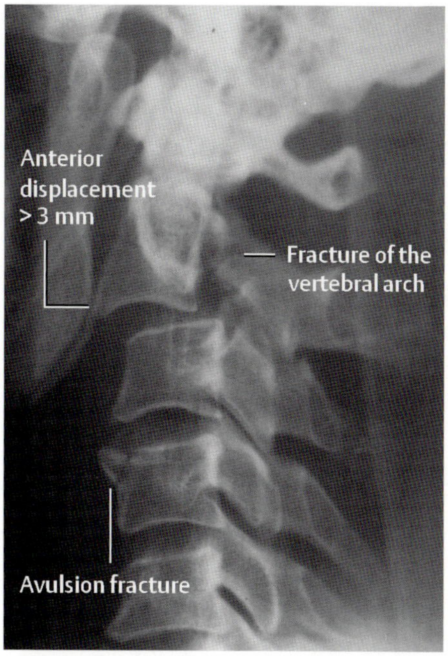

Fig. 1.**92** 'Hangman's fracture' Type II. Hyperextension together with distraction leads to bilateral fracture of the vertebral arches with anterior displacement of the axis. In addition, an avulsion fracture of C4 can be seen.

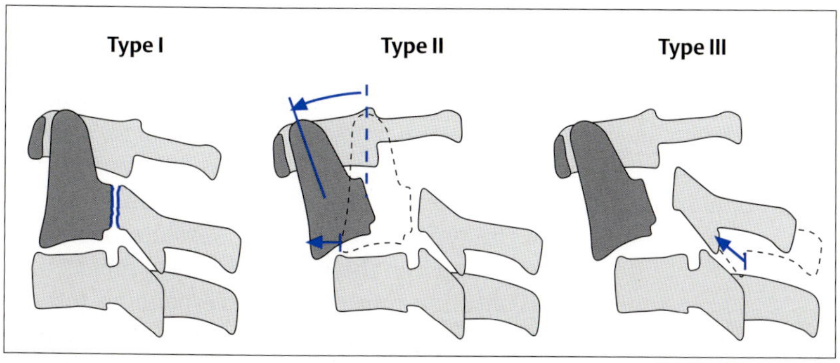

Fig. 1.**93** Schematic representation of the different types of 'hangman's (hangee's) fracture'.

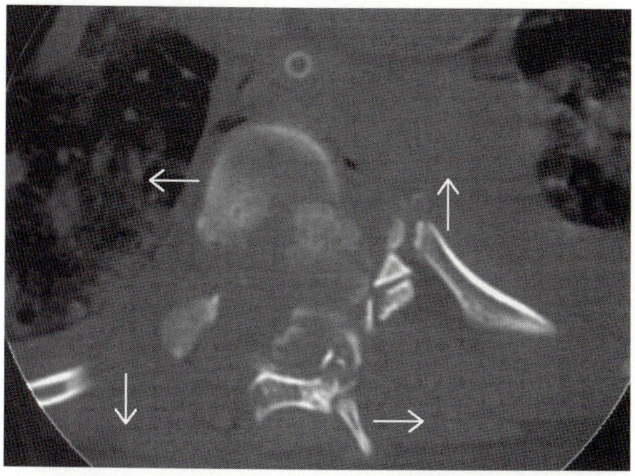

Fig. 1.**94** This 40-year-old patient suffered a motor vehicle accident. The fracture fragments are displaced into the spinal canal, and the transverse processes are fractured. The rotational component of the injury is clearly displayed.

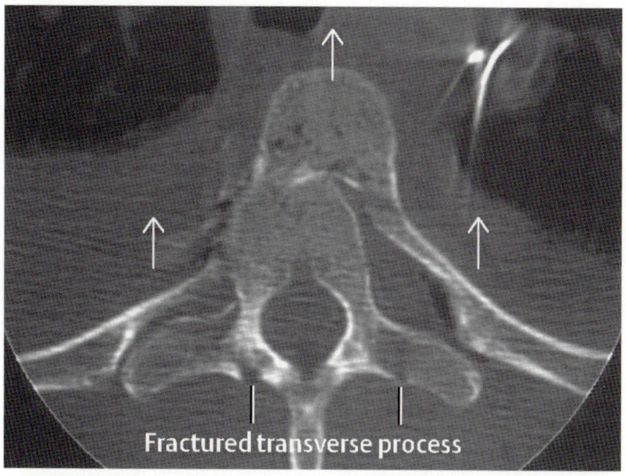

Fig. 1.**95** This 27-year-old patient suffered a motor vehicle accident. When the lower half of the body is fixed, a horizontal impact leads to anterior displacement of the vertebral body.

Radiographic Hints: Shear Fractures

- Horizontal fracture (especially at the thoracolumbar junction) with lateral dislocation and displacement,
- Fracture of the vertebral body, articular processes, transverse processes, and ribs,
- Interrupted posterior spinal canal.

Special Traumatology of the Cervical Spine and Craniocervical Transition

Since 65% of spinal injuries affect the cervical spine, correct interpretation of cervical spine radiographs is of great importance. Special attention should be given to the following:

1. The auxiliary lines on the lateral view should be smooth and uninterrupted (Fig. 1.**96**). The interspinal line (distance between adjacent spinous processes) should not vary more than 2 mm.
2. Prevertebral soft-tissue swelling is recognized by a widened retropharyngeal space (in the adult, this is pathologic if it measures > 2 mm at the level of C2, > 5 mm at the level of C3/4, and > 22 mm at the level of C6) and by displacement of the paravertebral fat stripe or trachea (Fig. 1.**96**).
3. All segments should be checked for the correct position of the facet joints.

Fracture of the Occipital Condyles

This occurs frequently in combination with fatal injuries of the brain stem, usually is bilateral and is associated with other fractures of the occipital and temporal regions (Fig. 1.**97**).

Fracture of the Atlas

Neurologic deficits are rare with fractures of the atlas since both the sagittal and transverse diameters of the spinal canal are increased.

Type I: anterior arch – often occurs together with a dens fracture.

Type II: posterior arch – most frequent manifestation, with the posterior arch fractured by being squeezed between the occiput and C2.

Type III: anterior and posterior arch ('Jefferson fracture') – caused by a significant axial blow to the extended head. It is frequently associated with a tear of the transverse ligament of the atlas and is unstable (Fig. 1.**98**). The lateral masses are displaced because of the loss of the atlas ring and these findings can frequently be seen on the AP view of the dens (malposition relative to articular surface of the axis).

Type IV: lateral masses

Type V: transverse process

Atlantoaxial Dislocation, Subluxation, and Rotation

Dislocation: Anterior, posterior, and lateral dislocations are distinguished. The diagnosis is made on the lateral radiograph. The normal distance between anterior arch and dens measures 2.5 – 3 mm in adults and 3 – 4 mm in children (Fig. 1.**96 b**):

Causes: trauma (most common), inflammation, or congenital.

Subluxation: Causes: inflammation (rheumatoid arthritis), trauma (often concurring with dens fracture since the transverse ligament provides stability).

Fracture of the Axis: Dens Fracture

The dens fracture is conventionally classified into three types according to **Anderson and D'Alonzo** (Fig. 1.**99**):

Type I: This is an oblique fracture through the **apex of the dens** caused by avulsion of the alar ligaments and is extremely rare.

Type II: Transverse fracture through the **base of the dens** (Fig. 1.**100**), **unstable.** This is the most frequent type of fracture and, with dislocation, pseudarthrosis develops in up to 70% of patients (Fig. 1.**101**).

Type III: Fracture through the **body of the axis,** with frequent involvement of the atlantoaxial articular surface and anterior dislocation in 90% of patients. This fracture is mechanically unstable but generally does not form a pseudarthrosis.

Since the type I fracture is an absolute rarity, the classification into three types has been replaced by a classification into upper (corresponding to type II) and lower (corresponding to type III) fractures of the dens.

Caution!

1. The os terminale might not fuse with the apex, mimicking a type I fracture.
2. The fusion between the dens and the body of the axis along the subdental synchondrosis can be delayed and mimic a type II fracture. Helpful distinguishing criteria: The 'os odontoideum', a manifestation of absent fusion, has a smooth outline and is generally rounded. The anterior arch of the atlas also shows a compensatory prominence.

Fracture of the Axis: 'Hangman's ('Hangee's') Fracture'

Since this is a classical extension fracture, it is discussed with the other extension fractures.

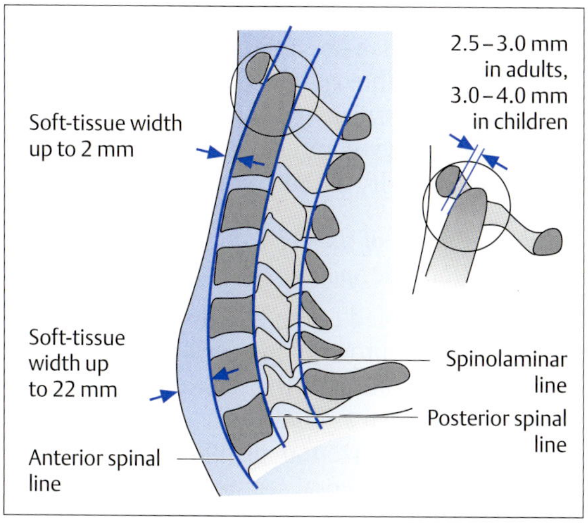

Fig. 1.**96** **a** Schematic representation of the cervical spine with auxiliary lines for the evaluation of alignment. **b** Normal position of the dens within the atlas ring.

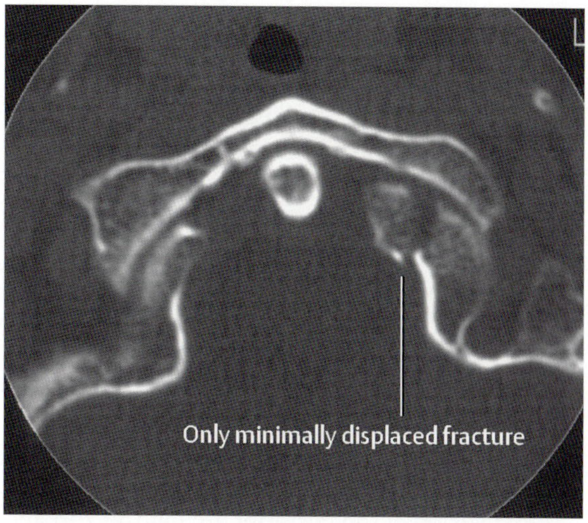

Fig. 1.**97** Fracture through the left occipital condyle. The ligaments are intact, and there is no narrowing of the spinal canal.

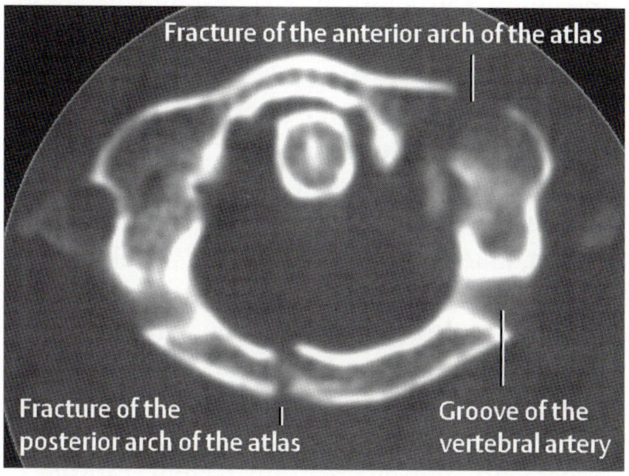

Fig. 1.**98** Jefferson fracture. The fracture involves the anterior and posterior arch of the atlas, and there is no narrowing of the spinal canal.

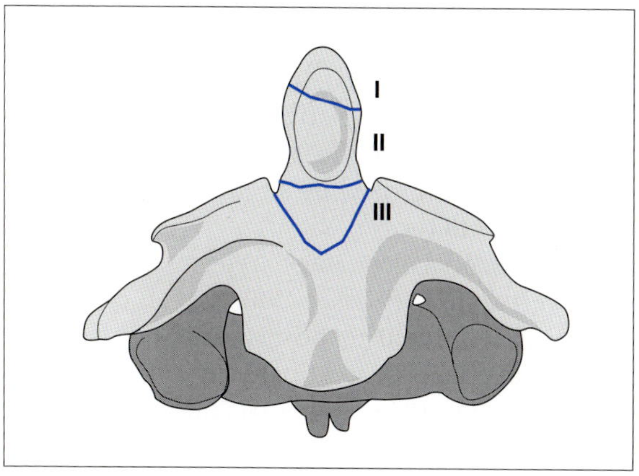

Fig. 1.**99** Schematic representation of the types of dens fractures. Type II is most frequent and unstable.

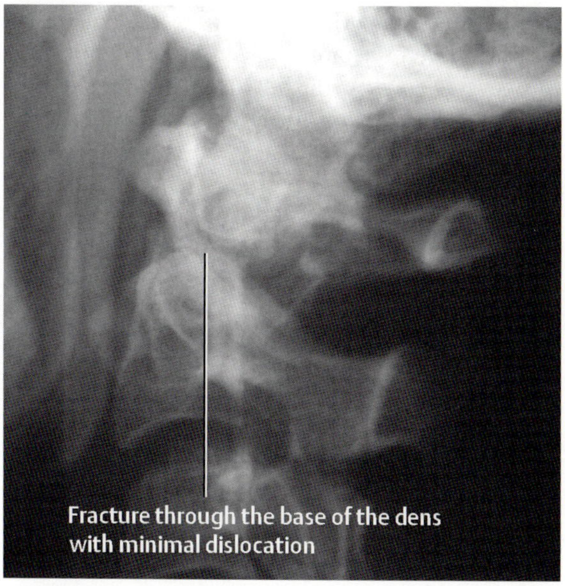

Fig. 1.**100** Type II dens fracture.

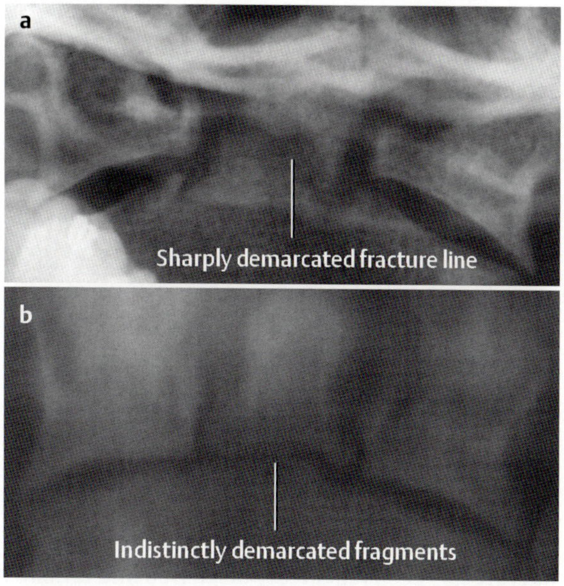

Fig. 1.**101** **a** Acute Type II dens fracture. **b** Old fracture with pseudarthrosis (conventional tomography).

Pediatric Considerations

In children, the osseous and ligamentous structures are still highly elastic, and osseous injuries are uncommon even in the presence of neurologic deficits caused by trauma. Interpretation of images must consider several features unique to the pediatric spine:

1. A still incomplete ossification or fusion of the ossification centers should not be mistaken for a fracture. Significant ossification benchmarks are:
   Atlas: Ossification of the posterior arch at the end of the 4th year, complete fusion between the 7th and 10th years.
   Axis: Fusion of the posterior arch in the 2nd and 3rd year, and its fusion with the body of the axis in the 7th year. The os terminale of the dens fuses about the 11th to 12th year. The subdental synchondrosis can persist until adolescence (mimicking a type II dens fracture).
2. In about 20% of children, a physiologic anterior displacement of C2 relative to C3 or of C3 relative to C4, or both, can be seen. This 'pseudodislocation' is characterized by an intact spinolaminar line (Fig. 1.**103**).
3. Based on an inadequate pharyngeal distension, a prevertebral soft-tissue fullness is often observed and should not be mistaken for a hematoma. If in doubt, an additional view in inspiration should reveal the normal variability.

Fractures of the Sacrum and Coccyx

These fractures, generally resulting from direct trauma (e.g., falls) and rarely presenting as an isolated finding, characteristically occur in conjunction with pelvic fractures.

Isolated sacral fractures normally have a transverse course, while sacral fractures as part of pelvic fractures frequently are vertically oriented. Fractures through the neural foramina frequently cause neurologic findings.

Insufficiency fractures frequently involve the sacrum.

X-RAY Most fractures are diagnosed on AP and lateral radiographs, although overlying bowel gas can pose considerable problems. If a fracture of the sacrum is suspected, CT should be considered early in the diagnostic evaluation.

Stable or Unstable Fracture?

Differentiating between a stable and an unstable fracture has been repeatedly discussed and remains a controversial topic. Stability is defined as the ability of the spine to maintain integrity under physiologic stress. A **stable** spine requires integrity of the osseous elements, disks, facet joints, and ligaments. An **unstable** spine requires surgical intervention to restore the integrity of these structures.

Instability Criteria of the Cervical and Upper Thoracic Spine

Universally accepted criteria do not exist for determining the stability of the **cervical and upper thoracic spine** injuries although the following two criteria can be used as guidelines:

- > 3.5 mm of horizontal displacement between two adjacent vertebral segments.
- > 11° angulation between two adjacent vertebrae.

An anterior marginal avulsion has to be critically assessed as to whether it is part of a flexion teardrop injury. This injury implies absolute instability.

The model of three structural columns proposed by Denis is used to determine the stability of the **lower thoracic and lumbar spine** (Fig. 1.**102**). This model divides the spine into

- **anterior column:** anterior longitudinal ligament, anterior two-thirds of the vertebral body and disk,
- **central column:** posterior longitudinal ligament, posterior one-third of the vertebral body and disk,
- **posterior column:** vertebral arch, interspinous ligaments and ligamentum flavum, capsule of the intervertebral joints.

Injuries with loss of one column are considered stable, and injuries with loss of two or three columns are considered unstable. Since injuries confined to the central column do not exist, involvement of the central column invariably implies instability.

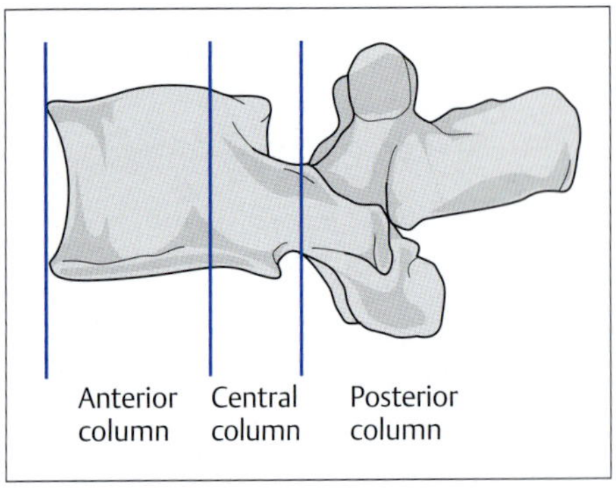

Fig. 1.**102** Three-column model according to Denis.

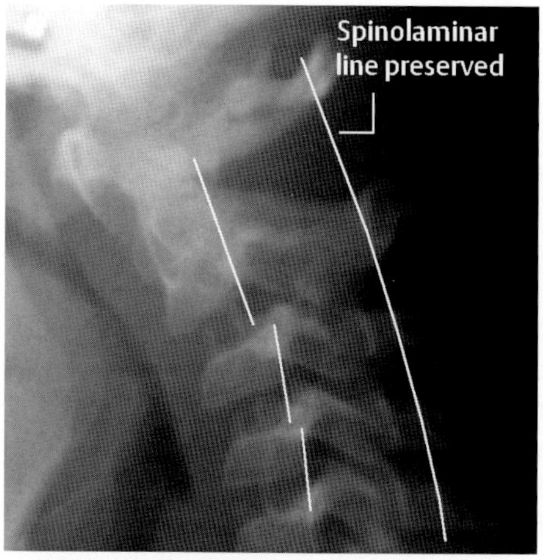

Fig. 1.**103** Pseudosubluxation of C2/3 and, less severe, of C3/4 in a 4-year-old child representing a normal variant.

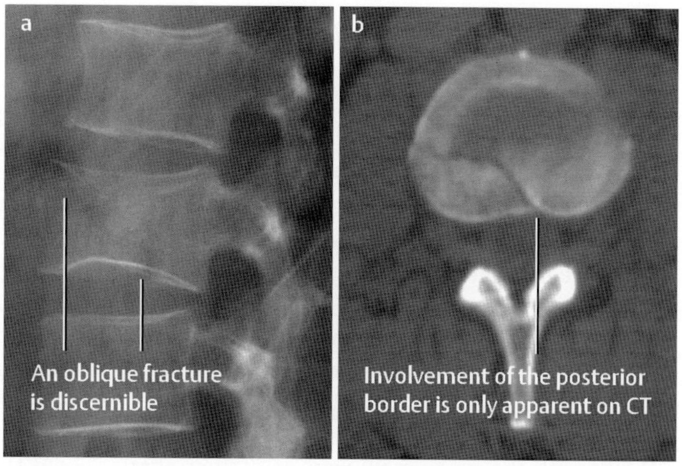

Fig. 1.**104** Fracture of a lumbar vertebral body with involvement of the posterior border. **a** Conventional radiograph shows only an anterior fracture, whereas CT (**b**) delineates involvement of the posterior border, indicating relative instability.

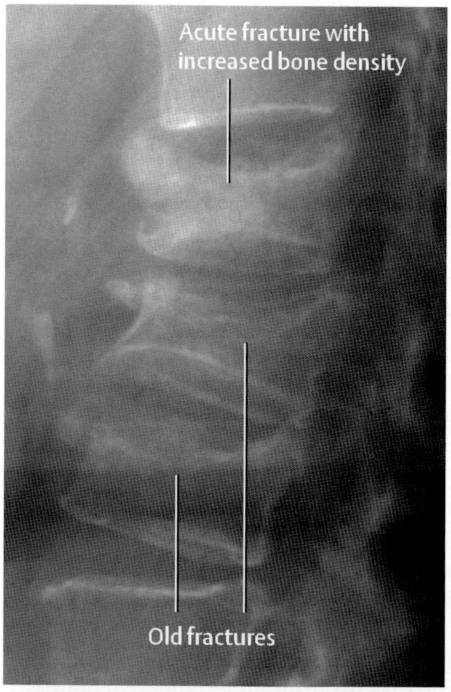

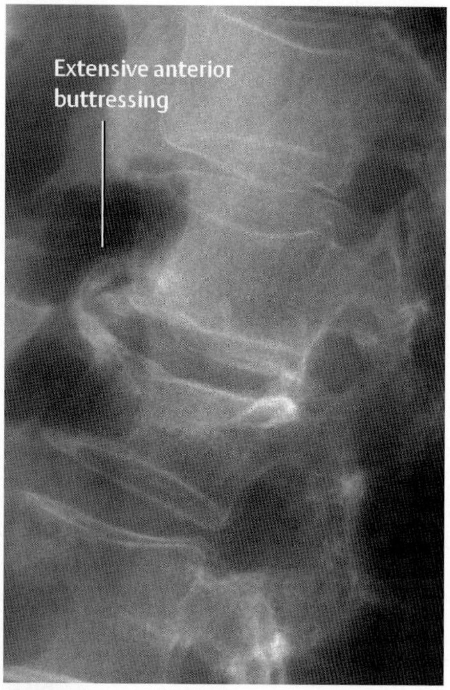

Far left:
Fig. 1.**105** Comparison of an acute and old vertebral fracture.

Left:
Fig. 1.**106** Osteophyte formation with partial osseous bridging as supporting reaction following a remote osteoporotic compression fracture.

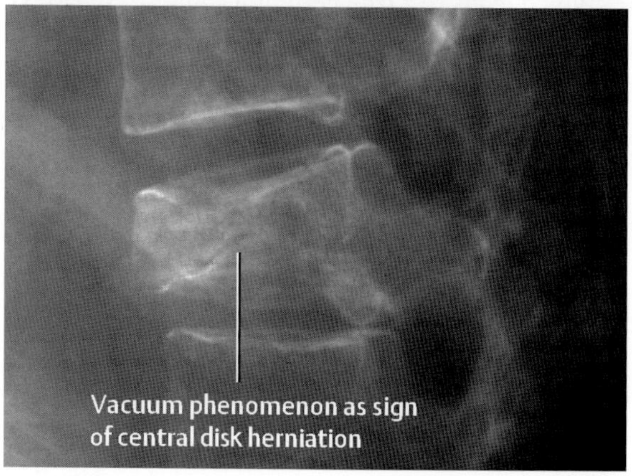

Fig. 1.**107** Old osteoporotic compression fracture of the T12 vertebral body with central disk herniation and vacuum phenomenon in the indented end plate.

Instability Criteria of the Lower Thoracic and Lumbar Spine

- Involvement of the posterior border of the vertebral body,
- Post-traumatic kyphosis exceeding 30°,
- Rib fractures, costovertebral dislocations,
- Sternal fractures,
- Fracture dislocations.

Hints for the evaluation of the posterior border:

1. Anterior and posterior heights should not differ more than 2 mm.
2. Compare the posterior height of the vertebral body with the posterior height of the vertebral body above and below.

Caution: Involvement of the posterior border of the vertebral bodies is often not recognized on conventional radiographs, and an apparent 'anterior compression fracture' might actually represent an unstable fracture. Therefore, the indication for CT should be rather generous (Fig. 1.**104**).

New or Old Fracture?

This common dilemma cannot be definitively answered in all cases, but the following criteria are helpful (Figs 1.**105** – 1.**107**).

Signs of an Old Vertebral Fracture

- Clinical history,
- Degenerative osseous apposition (supportive buttressing reaction),
- Narrowed intervertebral disk,
- Absence of paravertebral soft-tissue swelling,
- MRI: Fat signal and lack of edema within the vertebral body indicate an old fracture as cause of the vertebral deformity (Figs. 1.**109,** 1.**110**).

Traumatic, Osteoporotic, and Metastatic Fracture?

This is a question frequently raised in elderly patients with an uncertain history of trauma or with a history of inadequate trauma. A reliable differentiation can often be achieved because a vertebral body weakened by osteoporosis or metastasis collapses differently than a normal vertebral body. However, a differentiation between a fractured osteoporotic or metastatic vertebral body is not always possible since all proposed criteria have been found unreliable. Biopsy may be required in many cases depending on the clinical situation (Figs. 1.**108,** 1.**109**).

Signs of an Osteoporotic Fracture

- Typical location: midthoracic spine, upper lumbar spine,
- Characteristic 'fish mouth' or 'convex' configuration,
- Additional and possibly older compression fractures are seen in the remaining spine,
- Osteoporotic fractures exhibit a 'harmonic' configuration (indentation of superior **and** inferior end plates),
- Vacuum disk (Fig. 1.**107**),
- Band-like thickening along the end plates (= callus formation),
- At the most, only a thin (< 10 mm) diffuse paravertebral soft-tissue swelling (only observed in acute osteoporotic fractures),
- MRI: Acute fracture: diffuse bone marrow edema, minimal rim-like paravertebral soft-tissue edema (not obligatory). Old fracture (see Fig. 1.**110**).

Signs of a Metastatic Fracture

- Increased uptake on bone scan,
- Heterogeneous density of the vertebral body as evidence of metastatic deposits,
- Involvement of the pedicles,
- Location at atypical level: e.g., solitary fractures above T7 are suspicious for metastases,
- Often unilateral loss of height on the AP view,
- CT: Focal or epidural soft-tissue masses,
- MRI: Detection of an enhancing soft-tissue structure (space-occupying process), which projects beyond the borders of the vertebral bodies (frequently asymmetric) and/or involves the pedicles.

! Since the tumor cannot simply 'disappear into the air,' any vertebral collapse 'squeezes' the tumor into the paravertebral soft tissues. This is the most important criterion that distinguishes underlying metastatic disease from underlying osteoporosis, which leads to a true vertebral collapse (see MRI).

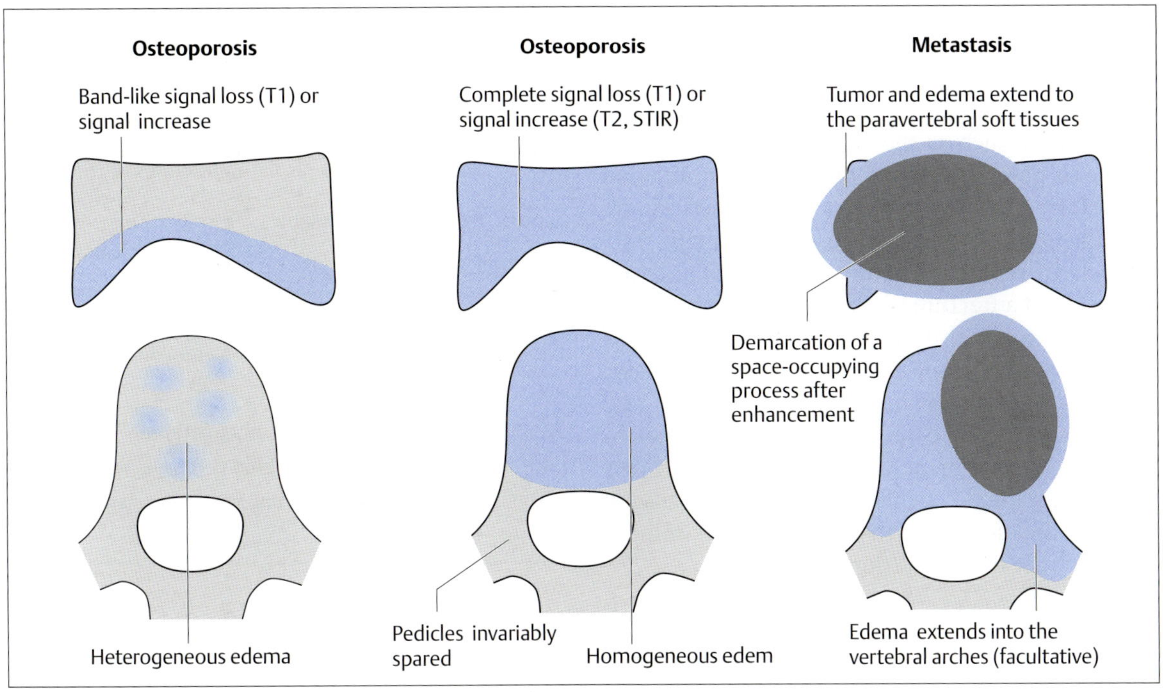

Fig. 1.**108** Differentiation between osteoporotic and metastatic vertebral fractures by MRI.

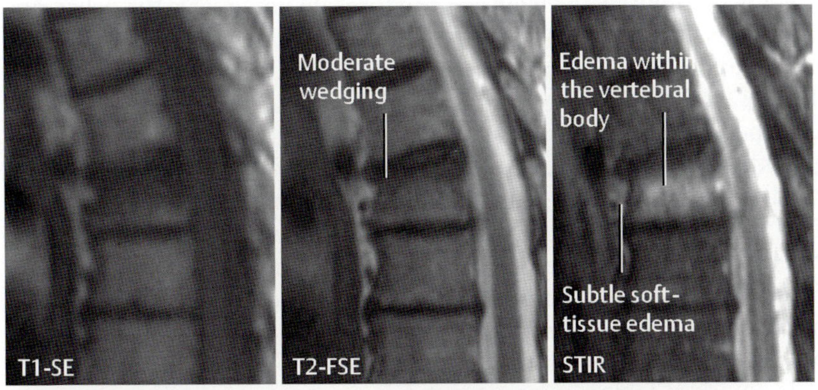

Fig. 1.**109** Acute osteoporotic fracture on MRI (T1, T2, STIR).

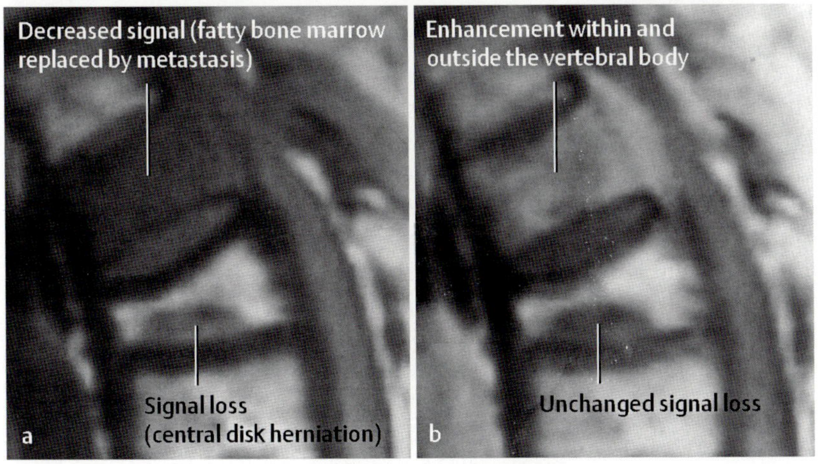

Fig. 1.**110** Concomitant finding of an old osteoporotic vertebral fracture and a vertebral metastasis. T1-weighted SE image before (**a**) and after administration of contrast medium (**b**).

Pelvis

X-RAY The radiographic diagnosis generally begins with an AP view of the pelvis. Additional views, such as the butterfly view of the sacrum, an oblique view of the obturator foramen (Fig. 1.**111**), and a lateral view of the sacrum, are often needed to detect iliac crest or pelvic ring fractures with **certainty** or to exclude any fracture extension of a fracture into the acetabulum. Useful information can also be obtained from the inlet/outlet views proposed by Pennal. The inlet views (40° craniocaudad angulation of the center ray) show anterior and posterior dislocations of the anterior and posterior pelvic ring. The outlet views (40° caudocraniad angulation) can assess sacral fractures and determine the extent of displacement in the craniocaudal direction (Fig. 1.**116**).

Table 1.**9** Classification of pelvic disruption according to Tile

Type A:	**Stable**
A1:	Fracture of the pelvis not involving the ring
A2:	Stable, minimally displaced fractures of the ring
Type B:	**Rotationally unstable**, vertically stable
B1:	Anteroposterior compression: open book injury
B2:	Lateral compression: ipsilateral injury of the anterior and posterior pelvic ring
B3:	Lateral compression: contralateral injury of the anterior and posterior pelvic ring
Type C:	Rotationally and **vertically unstable**
C1:	Unilateral, rotationally and vertically unstable
C2:	Bilateral, rotationally and vertically unstable
C3:	Associated with an acetabular fracture

Pelvic Injuries

Severe injuries of the pelvic ring remain a challenge for all involved specialties. Because of frequently associated extensive injuries, severe pelvic injuries have a relatively high mortality. Ruptures of the diaphragm and intra-abdominal and retroperitoneal organs, and hemorrhage from the presacral venous plexus, pierced spongiosal vascular spaces, and pelvic arteries are life-threatening. Furthermore, concomitant injuries of the bladder and urethra are frequently associated with pelvic fractures.

The most frequent causes of pelvic fracture are falls from a height, motor vehicle crashes, and motor vehicle accidents involving pedestrians. The direction of the impact determines the trauma pattern. (See classification of pelvic injuries, Table 1.**9**.) Clinical examination must search for the different types of potential instability (external rotation, internal rotation, vertical instability) by pulling and pressing on both anterior superior iliac spines and by applying manual traction to the legs.

Classification of Pelvic Injuries

Of the many classifications of pelvic ring fractures, the classification proposed by Tile has become generally accepted since it considers the mechanism of trauma (direction of impact), the clinical stability, and the morphology (radiologic diagnosis) (Table 1.**9**). The severity of injury increases from Type A to C:

Type A: This type includes all **stable** pelvic fractures (fractures of the pelvic rim; stable, minimally displaced fractures of the anterior pelvic ring, Figs. 1.**112**, 1.**113**).

Pelvic rim fractures do not involve the pelvic ring (Fig. 1.**112**), and the pelvic ring remains stable. Isolated fractures of the iliac wing and crest, as well as fractures of the coccyx and transverse fractures of the lower sacrum, are the result of direct blows. Avulsion fractures, caused by extreme muscular contraction, are most commonly seen in sports injuries during the adolescence years. Nondisplaced fractures of the superior or inferior pubic bone are also included. Some authorities question whether fractures of the obturator foramen can be isolated, implying an additional, radiographically occult fracture in these cases.

Type B: This type includes all pelvic fractures that are **rotationally unstable,** but vertically stable. These are caused by anteroposterior or lateral compression.

Anteroposterior compression causes external rotation of one hemipelvis or both hemipelvises ('open book' mechanism) and the symphysis pubis is frequently disrupted (Fig. 1.**114**). Lateral compression causes an inward rotation of one hemipelvis (Fig. 1.**115**). Both mechanisms cause a disruption of the anterior and posterior pelvic rings.

It is important to note that neither traumatic mechanism completely disrupts the posterior pelvic ring since, depending on the actual mechanism, either the posterior ('open book' mechanism) or anterior (lateral compression) sacroiliac ligament re-

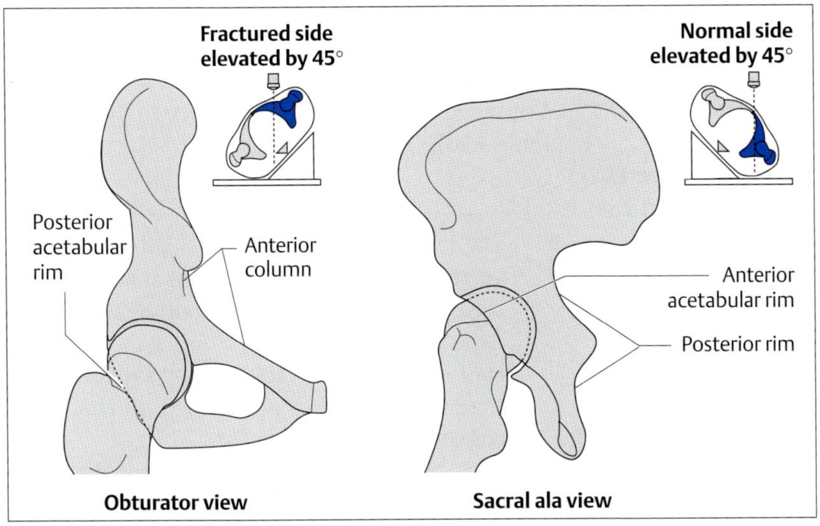

Fig. 1.**111** Oblique views according to Judet.

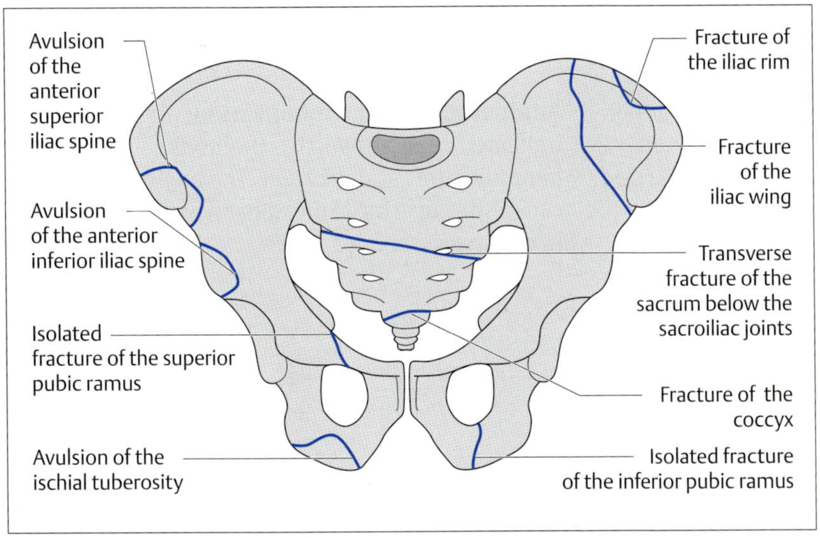

Fig. 1.**112** Pelvic fractures (Type A1 trauma according to Tile).

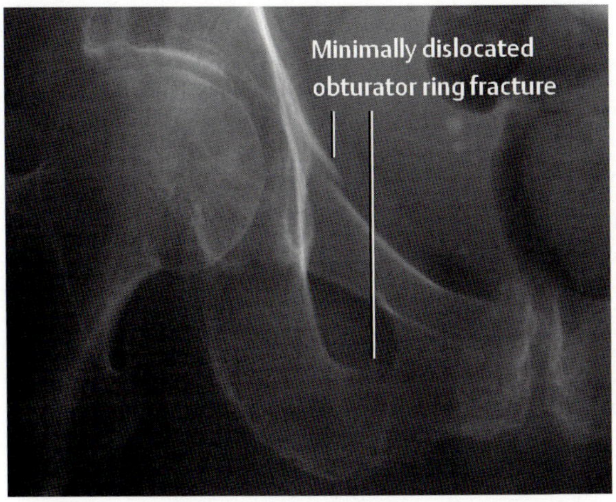

Fig. 1.**113** Type A2 trauma according to Tile. **Stable** fracture without involvement of the posterior pelvic ring.

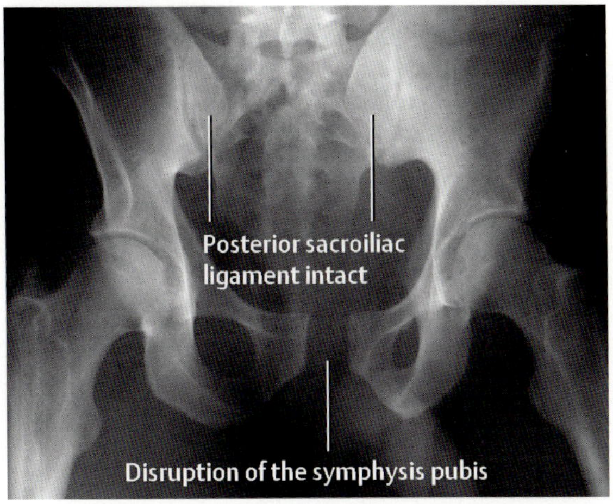

Fig. 1.**114** Type B1 trauma according to Tile caused by anteroposterior compression. **Rotational instability.**

mains intact and stabilizes the posterior pelvic ring. This trauma type causes a partial instability, i.e., rotational instability with preserved vertical stability (Figs. 1.**114**, 1.**115**).

Type C: This type of injury is rotationally and **vertically unstable** (translation instability). The vertical shear force elevates one hemipelvis, which is only conceivable with a **complete** posterior and anterior osseous or ligamentous disruption of the pelvic ring (including sacrospinal and sacrotuberous ligaments, Fig. 1.**116**). The SI joints and sacral foramina are anatomic regions prone to fracture in this type of pelvic injury (Fig. 1.**117**). Even **severe** external forces acting as anteroposterior compression ('open book' mechanism) can cause complete posterior and anterior osseous or ligamentous disruption and lead to a Type C injury. Transacetabular fractures of the pelvic ring are classified as Type C even in the absence of vertical instability since acetabular involvement worsens the prognosis of pelvic ring fractures.

Pelvic ring fractures can be further characterized by stating the site of the injury (Fig. 1.**117**).

CT

If the diagnosis is inconclusive by conventional radiography, CT is mandatory.

CT can also provide a more definitive assessment of the severity of ligamentous injury to the SI joints (Table 1.**10**).

!

- The transverse processes of the lower lumbar vertebrae must be checked for fracture. Fractures here are a frequent indication of a Type C injury (Fig. 1.**116**).
- Half of the sacral fractures and two-thirds of the SI joint injuries are missed on the initial conventional radiographs.
- CT is clearly superior to conventional radiography in the detection and accurate assessment of sacral fractures (Figs. 1.**115**, 1.**116**) and injuries of the SI joints.

Angiography and Embolization: Angiography is indicated if all supportive methods fail to achieve hemodynamic stabilization. The angiogram can localize sites of arterial bleeding, which can be embolized if necessary.

Table 1.**10** Classification of the severity of ligamentous injuries of the SI joints by CT

First-degree injury

Distortion of the sacroiliac ligaments with preserved joint space, vacuum phenomenon due to negative pressure

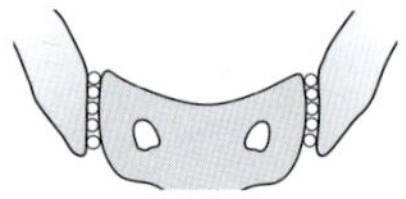

Second-degree injury

Rupture of the anterior sacroiliac ligament with widened joint space anteriorly

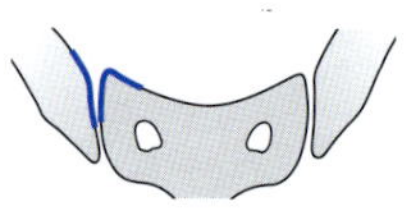

Third-degree injury

Unilateral dislocation of the SI joint with rupture of all sacroiliac ligaments and complete disruption between sacrum and ilium

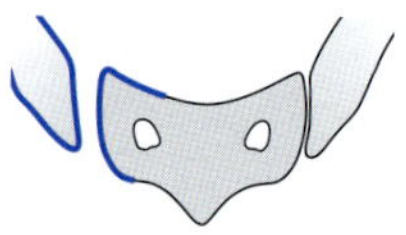

Fourth-degree injury

Bilateral third-degree injury

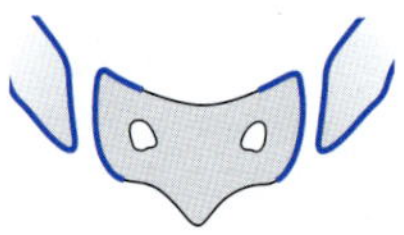

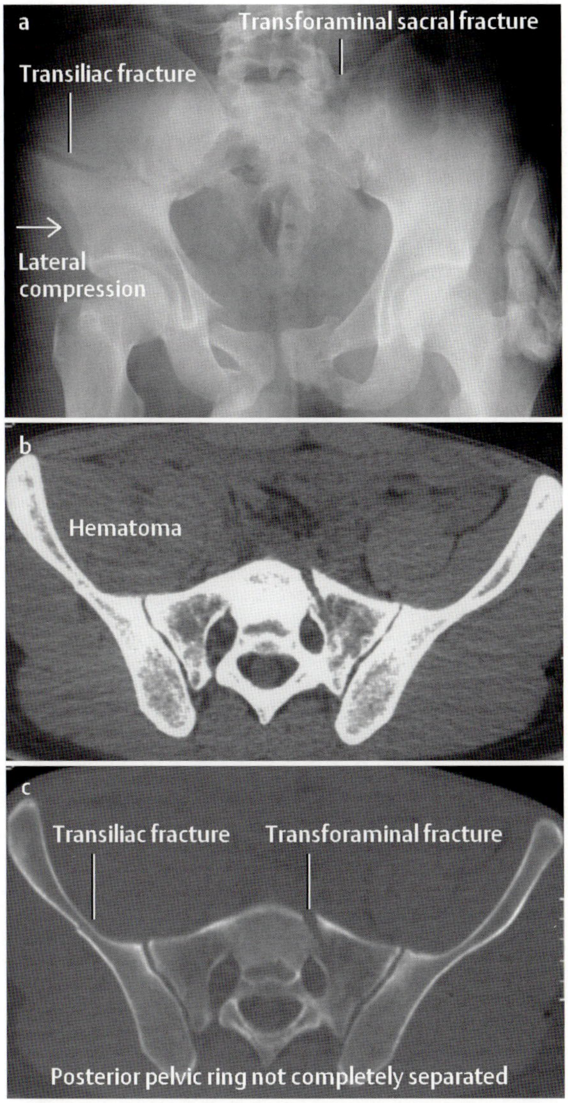

Fig. 1.**115** Type B3 trauma (transforaminal fracture of the left sacral ala, right iliac fracture, and bilateral transpubic fracture). **Rotational instability.** The horizontal transiliac fracture on the right does **not** cause vertical instability.

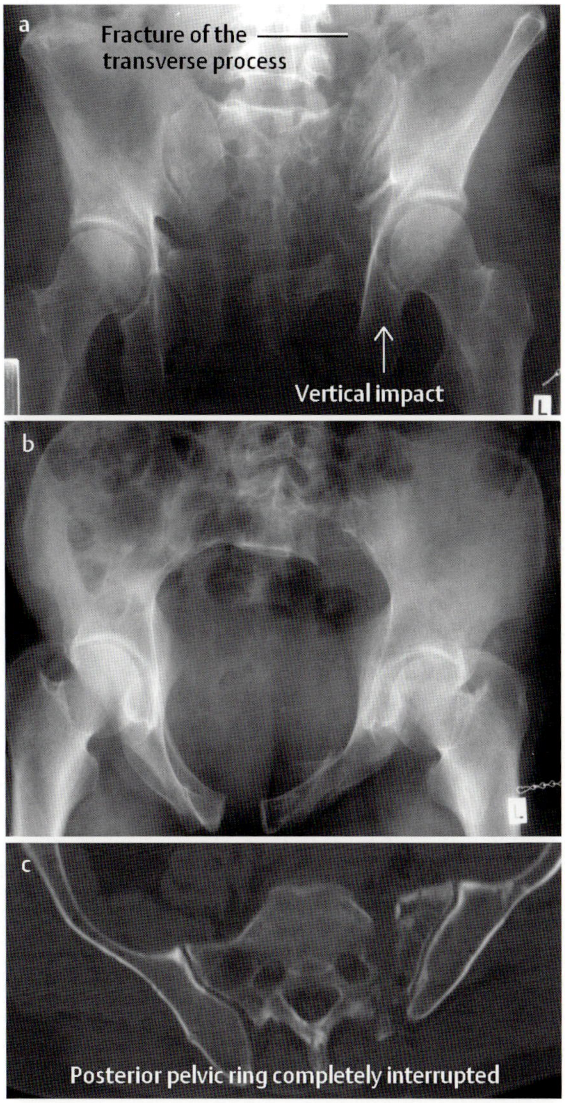

Fig. 1.**116** Type C1 trauma according to Tile. **Rotational and vertical** instability. (Fracture through the left sacral ala, left transpubic fracture and separation of the pubic symphysis). **a** Outlet view, **b** inlet view, **c** CT.

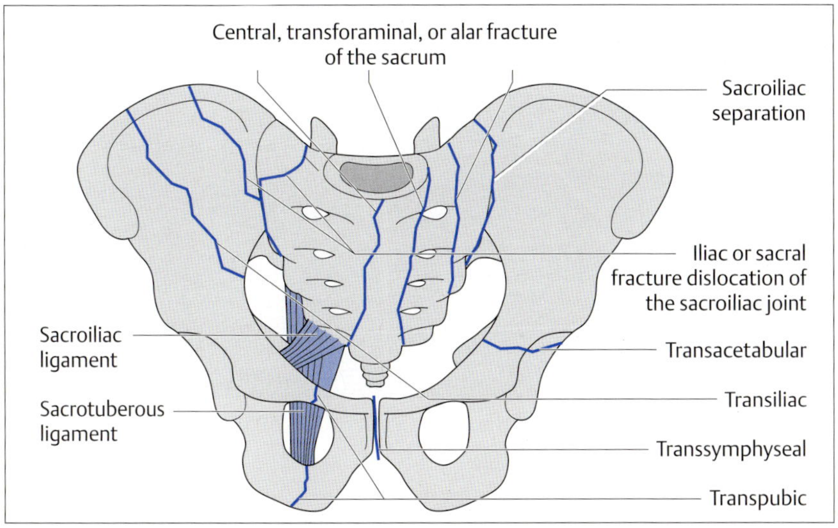

Fig. 1.**117** Fracture lines of pelvic ring fractures.

Acetabular Fractures

X-RAY The AP view of the pelvis must be supplemented by an angled view of the sacrum and oblique views of the obturator foramen for the best overall assessment of osseous pelvic integrity (Fig. 1.**111**). For the analysis of the AP view it is helpful to use six auxiliary lines, which should not be interrupted (Fig. 1.**118**). The assessment of the weight-bearing dome in the presence of an acetabular fracture has far-reaching therapeutic implications (Fig. 1.**121**).

Characteristically seen in the setting of motor vehicle accidents, acetabular fractures are caused by severe trauma in which the impact on the foot, knee, or greater trochanter is transmitted to the acetabulum. Through the transmission of this traumatic impact, other fractures (midfoot, calcaneus, femoral neck, and femoral head) and ligamentous injuries frequently occur. Secondary changes often associated with this injury are post-traumatic degenerative osteoarthritis, periarticular heterotopic ossifications, and, rarely, avascular necrosis of the femoral head, leading to pain and impaired mobility.

Classification of Acetabular Fractures

The classification of acetabular fractures proposed by Judet and Letournel in 1964 is the one most widely used today. It was developed before the CT era and is based on conventional radiographs (AP and bilateral oblique views). According to this classification, acetabular fractures are divided into two large groups: basic types and combination types. These groups are further divided into five subtypes (Fig. 1.**120**), with the understanding of the classification dependent upon the concept of anterior and posterior columns (Fig. 1.**119**). Each fracture type can occur together with a dislocation of the femoral head, which usually is posterior but can be central with the combination types.

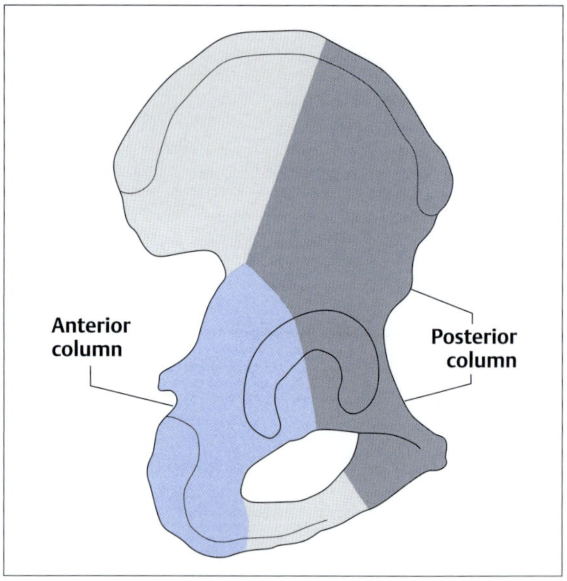

Fig. 1.**119** Right hemipelvis seen from the side. Columns according to Judet and Letournel.

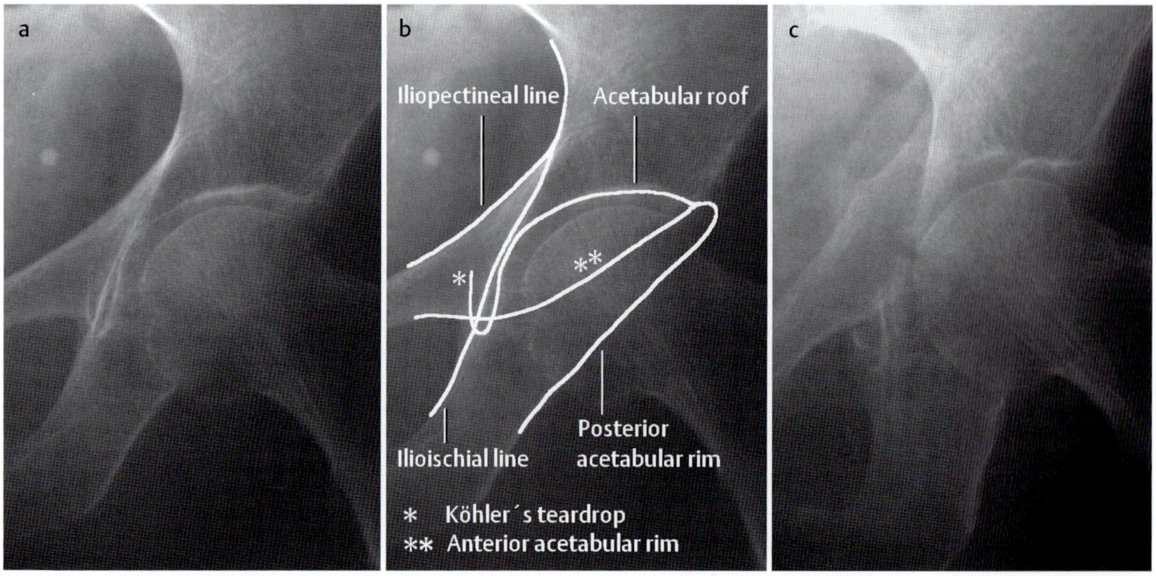

Fig. 1.**118** The six auxiliary lines used to assist in the evaluation of the acetabulum on the AP view (**a, b**). An acetabular fracture showing discontinuity in multiple areas (**c**).

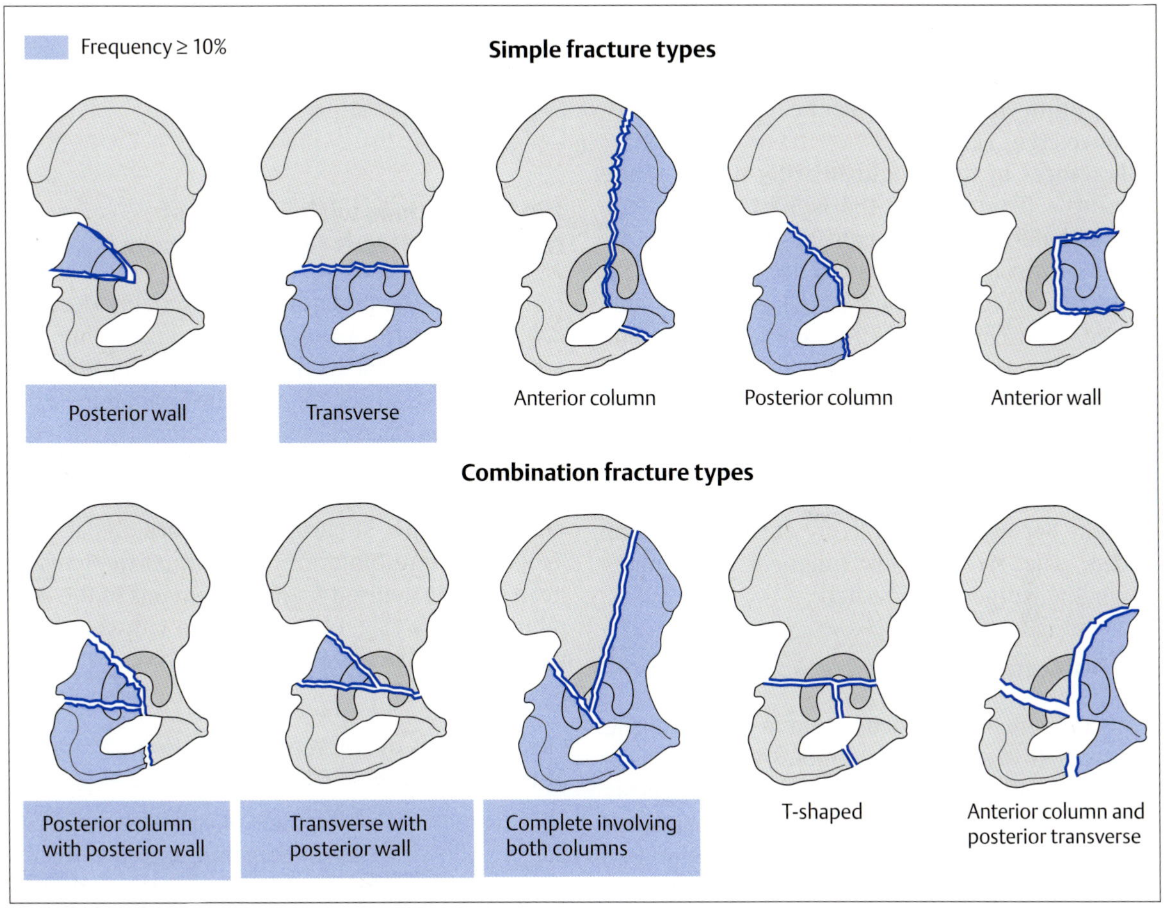

Fig. 1.**120** Acetabular fractures according to Judet and Letournel.

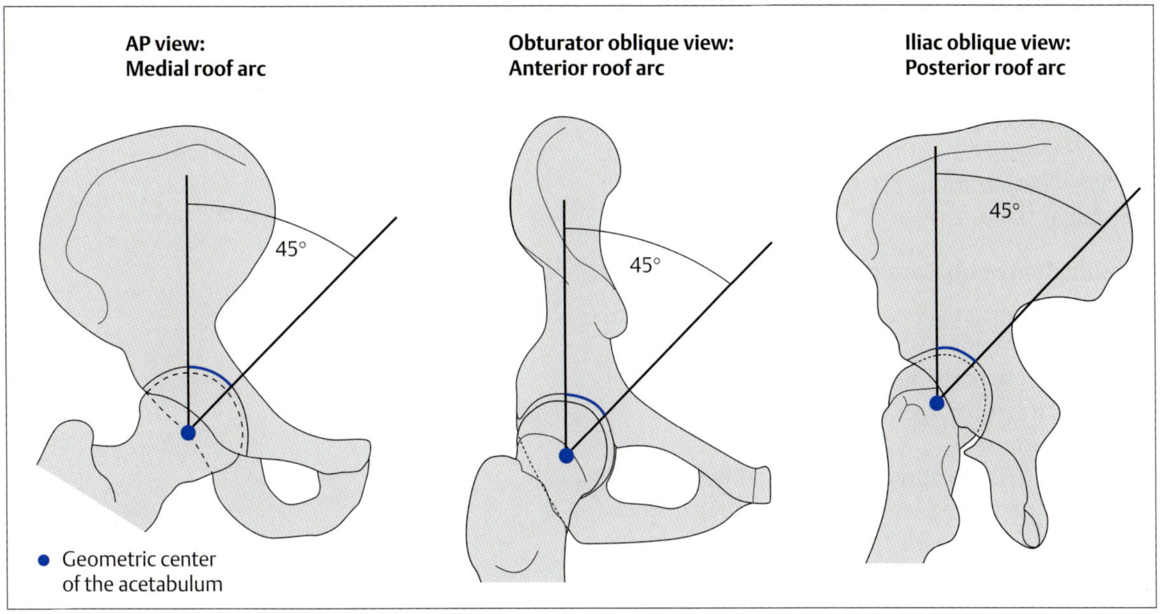

Fig. 1.**121** Evaluation of the force per unit area or pressure on the acetabulum (acetabular roof arcs as proposed by Matta) as integral part of the treatment decision. Nonoperative therapy should be considered if:

- the fracture lines fall outside the roof arc measurements,
- the femoral head remains congruent to the acetabular roof in all three projections.

CT CT provides important information:

1. Detection of **small free osseous fragments in the joint,** which must either be reattached or removed (Fig. 1.**122**).
2. **Fractures of the weight-bearing dome of the joint** – 10 mm below the highest point of the acetabulum – which might be undetectable by conventional radiography. If the CT shows no fracture in this segment of the acetabular surface, then conservative therapy is appropriate. CT of the acetabulum should be obtained with contiguous thin sections (e.g., 2 mm) through this region of the acetabular roof.
3. Detection of **femoral head** fractures.
4. Assessment of the size and degree of dislocation of the dorsal avulsion fracture of the **acetabular rim.** The size of this fragment determines whether surgery is indicated.

Hip Dislocation Without Acetabular Fracture

It takes severe trauma such as that in motor vehicle accidents to dislocate the femoral head from its deep position in the acetabulum. This diagnosis can be suspected clinically when the patient presents with a leg in an abnormally fixed position. Associated fractures of the lower extremity (femoral neck, pilon fracture) are also often associated with this injury. The dislocated femoral head must be immediately reduced to minimize cartilage damage and to improve its compromised vascular supply in order to decrease the incidence of avascular necrosis. If there are interposed capsular or labral components or osseous fragments in the joint, an open instead of closed reduction may be required. The late complications are the same as found with acetabular fractures.

Classification of Hip Dislocations Without Fracture

Hip dislocations are divided into **posterior** and **anterior** types. A special type is the central dislocation of the femoral head into the lesser pelvis through a fractured acetabulum.

X-RAY Hip dislocation can invariably be diagnosed on the AP radiograph. Iliac dislocation, the most frequent type, can mimic a normal articulation on the AP view if the femoral head is dislocated directly posterior to the acetabulum. The oblique view, however, definitively shows the dislocated femoral head. It is imperative to look for osseous injuries that are typically associated with hip dislocations, such as acetabular fractures and, in particular, avulsions of the posterior acetabular rim and femoral head fractures.

CT See acetabular fractures.

Hip Dislocations with Fracture of the Femoral Heads (Pipkin Fractures)

Fractures of the femoral head invariably occur in conjunction with a posterior hip dislocation and are rare compared to the number of hip dislocations. Fracture-dislocations of the femoral head occur when the knee is impacted anteriorly with the hip in flexion, as with a dashboard injury in motor vehicle accidents. When the femoral head displaces posteriorly the superoposterior acetabular rim avulses an anteroinferior fragment off the femoral head and the avulsed fragment remains in the acetabular cavity (Fig. 1.**123**). Possible late complications are the same as observed with acetabular fractures.

Classifications of Fracture-Dislocations of the Femoral Head (Fig. 1.**124**)

This diagnosis is easily made on the AP view of the pelvis. Following closed reduction, angled and oblique views (Fig. 1.**111**) and CT are necessary to provide additional information as to the position and size of the femoral head fragment and any possible acetabular rim fragment.

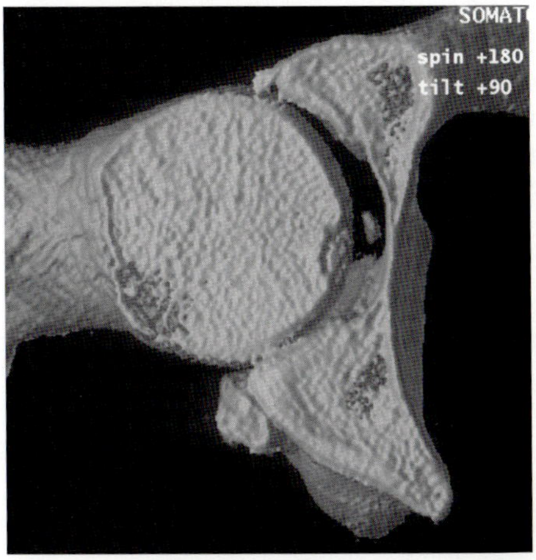

Left:
Fig. 1.**122** 3-D CT of the acetabulum revealing a small osseous fragment in the acetabular fossa (S/P posterior acetabular roof fracture).

Below:
Fig. 1.**123** Fracture dislocation of the left femoral head (Pipkin IV).

Bottom:
Fig. 1.**124** Classification of the fracture dislocations of the femoral head according to Pipkin.

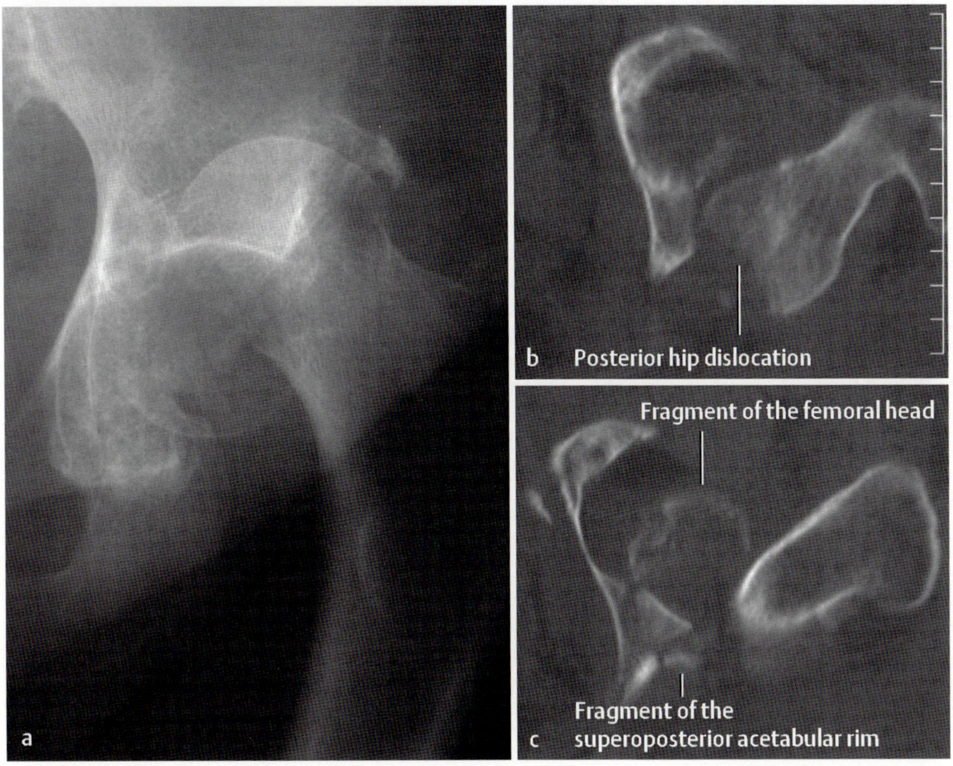

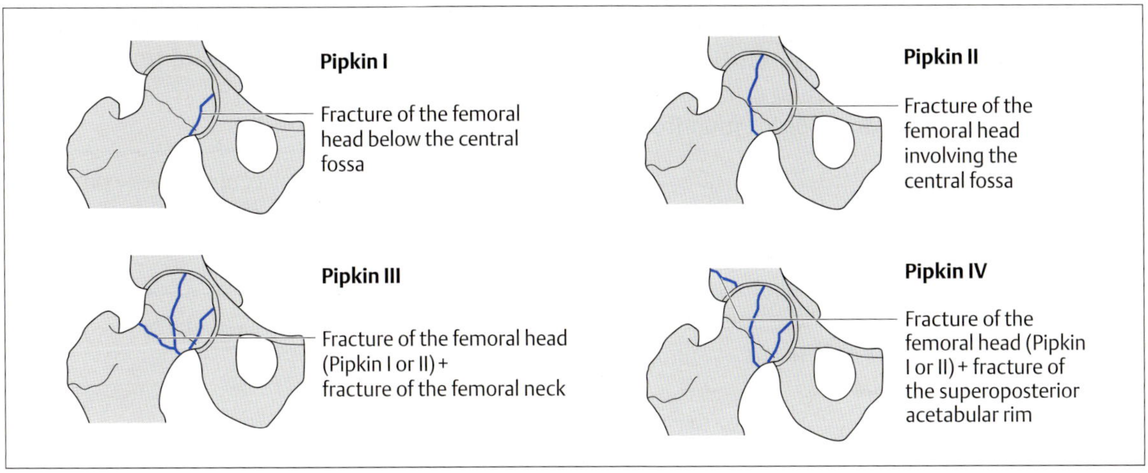

Shoulder Girdle

Sternoclavicular Dislocation

■ In sternoclavicular dislocation the medial clavicular end is most often displaced anteriorly and, less frequently, posteriorly or superiorly. ■

PATH The actual articulation between the medial end of the clavicle and the sternal manubrium is small but the joint is stabilized by strong ligaments. The dorsal ligaments are considerably thicker than the anterior ones (Fig. 1.**125**). This is the major reason that the clavicle most often dislocates anteriorly. Sternoclavicular dislocations are usually caused by a blow to the shoulder girdle, and are seen most often after motor vehicle accidents and sports injuries. Direct trauma is less frequently a cause of this injury. The rare posterior dislocations can potentially cause severe injuries to the major vessels, nerves, lung, trachea, or the esophagus.

X-RAY Technique: AP projection with 40° craniocaudad or caudocranial angulation. The straight AP view is generally unrevealing because of superimposed structures.

! The medial clavicular epiphysis ossifies between the ages of 18 to 28 and fuses at about 25 years of age. Until then, epiphyseal injuries and sternoclavicular dislocations are difficult to diagnose by conventional radiography.

CT CT offers excellent visualization of sternoclavicular dislocations, and coronal reformatting may be helpful in some instances.

SONO Sonography can distinguish between soft-tissue swelling and clavicular dislocation.

MRI MRI should be reserved for chronic injuries. Its major advantage is direct coronal display and the visualization of soft-tissue structures, including the intra-articular disk. It may also be helpful in differentiating a dislocation from infection or tumor.

DD In the acute stage, a fracture of the medial aspect of the clavicle should be considered clinically in the differential diagnosis. A chronic subluxation or dislocation of the medial clavicle can also be mistaken for soft-tissue swelling due to inflammation or neoplasm.

! The acute sternoclavicular dislocation is rare, and its radiographic visualization difficult. The rare posterior dislocation can be associated with serious injuries to adjacent structures. A chronic subluxation can be clinically mistaken for a soft-tissue tumor or inflammation.

Clavicular Fracture

■ Based on its geometry and rigidity to flexion and torsion, 80% of clavicular fractures involve the middle third of this bone. ■

PATH Most clavicular fractures are caused by indirect trauma (axial impact with bending and torsion of the clavicle, as occurring with a fall on the outstretched arm or a direct lateral blow on the shoulder). Only about one-fifth of clavicular fractures are caused by direct trauma. Characteristically, the lateral clavicular fragment is pulled down by the weight of the arm and by the pectoralis major and latissimus dorsi muscles, and the medial clavicular fragment is pulled upward by the sternocleidomastoideus muscle. The displacement of the fragments of the medial and lateral fractures is determined by the integrity of the adjacent ligaments (especially of the costoclavicular ligament and coracoclavicular ligament).

Complications are rare and consist primarily of injuries to the brachial plexus, subclavian artery and veins in the costoclavicular space, or pleuropulmonary injuries. The incidence of associated rib fractures is probably underestimated.

X-RAY The clavicle appears more-or-less straight on the AP or PA views, but is S-shaped when viewed from above. The clavicle and any possible fracture can be adequately visualized on conventional radiographs, especially with the central ray of the AP view angled caudocranial about 15° (Fig. 1.**127**). Additional views are necessary only to address specific clinical questions.

CT CT is especially useful in differentiating a medial clavicular fracture from a sternoclavicular dislocation.

! The medial ossification center fuses completely between the ages of 22–25. Up to this age, epiphyseal fractures can be mistaken for sternoclavicular dislocation.

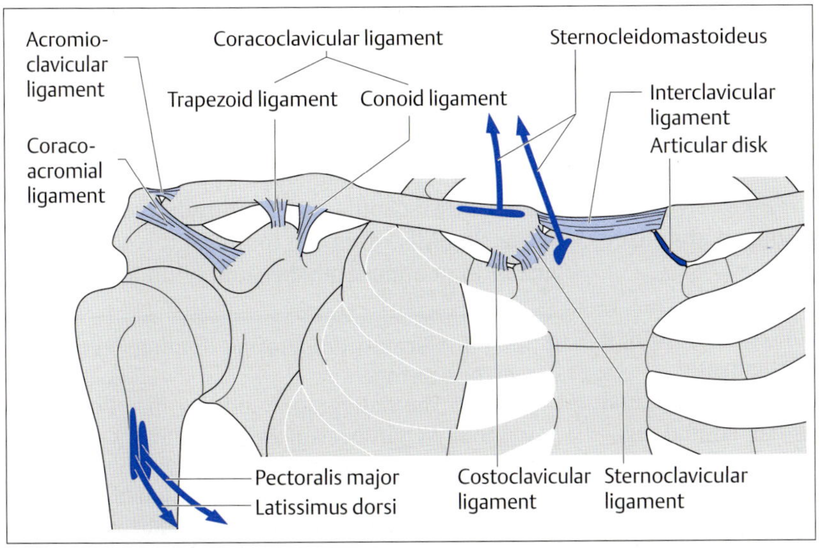

Fig. 1.**125** Normal anatomy of the sternoclavicular and costoclavicular joints.

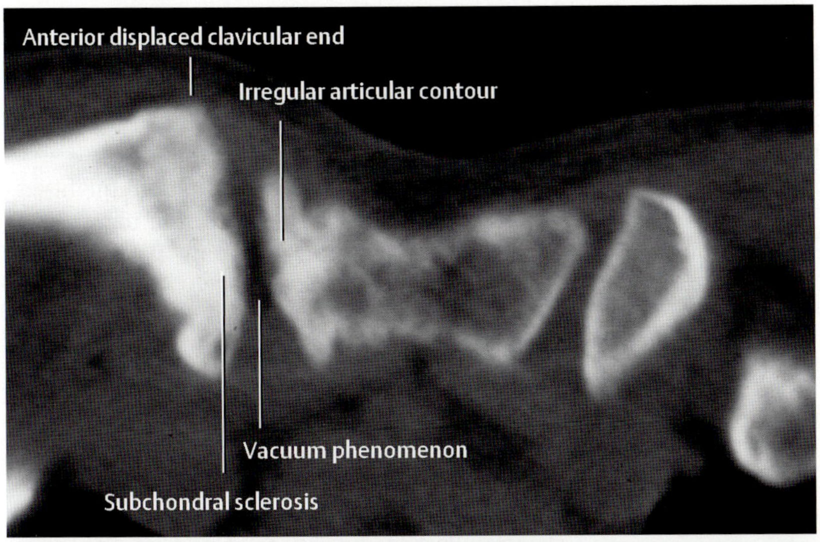

Fig. 1.**126** Post-traumatic anterior subluxation with secondary degenerative osteoarthritis.

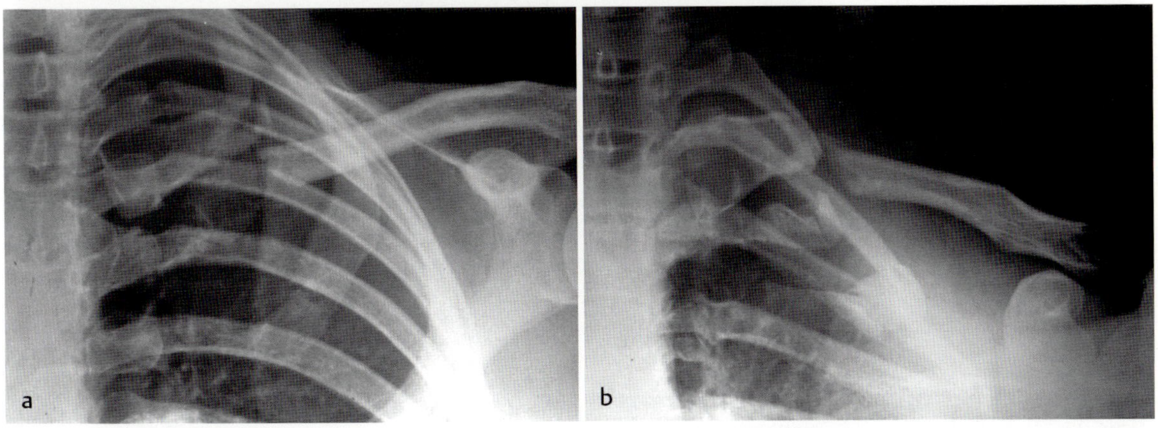

Fig. 1.**127** Fractures of the medial third of the clavicle and the first rib. **a** AP and **b** apical lordotic projections.

Acromioclavicular Separation

■ Acromioclavicular joint separation can be caused by direct or indirect trauma, with the lateral clavicular end displaced superiorly or, rarely, inferiorly. ■

Anatomy: The acromioclavicular joint is stabilized by (Fig. 1.**125**)
- the joint capsule,
- the acromioclavicular ligaments, constituting a superior enforcement of the joint capsule,
- coracoclavicular ligaments, comprising a lateral trapezoid ligament and a medial conoid ligament.

Classification according to Tossy et al.
Type I: Tear of the capsular ligaments, with the extracapsular ligaments remaining intact.
Type II: Tear of the capsular ligaments and the acromioclavicular ligament. The coracoclavicular ligament has been stretched, but remains intact.
Type III: Both the acromioclavicular and the coracoclavicular ligaments are torn.

Rockwood et al. (1996) expanded this classification by adding rarely occurring types: *Type IV,* with displacement of the clavicle into or through the trapezius muscle; *Type V,* with gross superior displacement of the clavicle (extreme version of the *Type III* injury); and *Type VI,* with subacromial or subcoracoid positioning of the inferiorly displaced clavicle.

Patients with acromioclavicular injuries frequently develop coracoclavicular ossifications which occur after conservative or operative treatment (Rockwood et al., 1996). Post-traumatic osteolysis of the distal clavicle is a rare late complication that can develop after a single or repetitive trauma (Fig. 1.**128**). The osteolysis affects only the clavicle and not the acromion.

X-RAY Technique: AP views of both shoulders for comparison, with 5 – 10 kg (10 – 20 lb) weight in each hand and the arms in slight external rotation. For optimal results, the weights should hang from the wrist. The central ray should be angled 10 – 15° caudocranially to prevent superimposition of the scapula. Standard radiographic views of the shoulder often fail to image the acromioclavicular joint adequately because of underexposure.

! *Tossy I:* Normal radiographic findings even with weight bearing.
Tossy II: The radiographic finding may be normal without weight bearing but is definitely abnormal with weight bearing. There is widening of the acromioclavicular joint and elevation of the clavicle by up to one-half clavicular shaft width. The distance to the coracoid is widened at most by 50% compared to the normal.
Tossy III: Elevated scapula. With weight bearing, the acromioclavicular separation exceeds that of Type II and the distance to the coracoid is widened by more than 50%.

DD Acromioclavicular separation might escape radiographic detection on standard views if the ligaments are only partially torn.

Establishing the correct diagnosis is more difficult because of the widely variable appearance of the acromioclavicular joint. The width of the joint usually measures 1 – 3 mm, but has been shown to vary in normal individuals from 0.5 mm (especially in elderly patients) to as wide as 6 – 7 mm.

Clinically, acromioclavicular separation can be mistaken for a fracture of the lateral aspect of the clavicle. Post-traumatic osteolysis of the distal clavicle can be confused with the osseous resorption (usually bilateral) seen in rheumatoid arthritis, scleroderma or hyperparathyroidism.

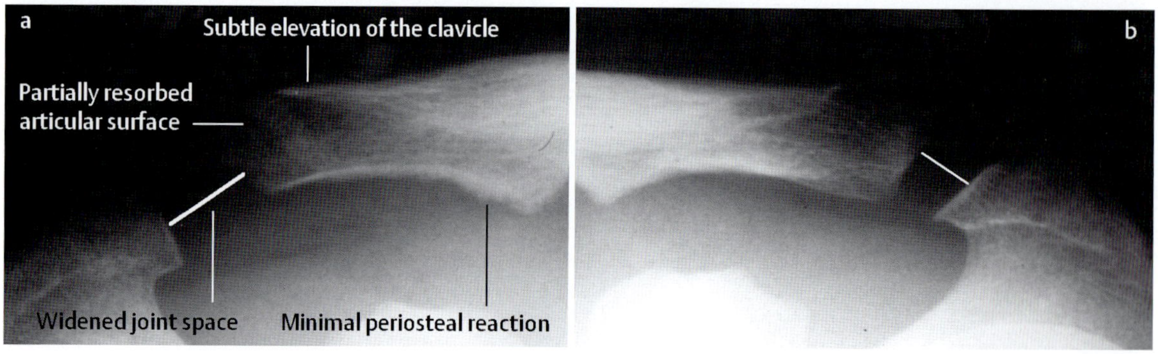

Fig. 1.**128** **a** AP projection of the right shoulder with weight bearing 5 months after acromioclavicular separation. **b** Normal contralateral acromioclavicular joint.

Impingement and Rotator Cuff Rupture

■ Shoulder impingement syndrome is caused by compression of the rotator cuff (especially the supraspinatus muscle) against the anterior aspect of the acromion or coracoacromial ligament or, at times, against the acromioclavicular joint, when the arm is in abduction. This compression of the cuff results in degeneration and, later, rupture. Rotator cuff ruptures, however, can also occur without impingement as the direct result of acute trauma. ■

PATH Four muscles, which arise on the anterior and posterior scapular surface and insert at the humeral head, make up the rotator cuff (Fig. 1.**129**):

- the subscapularis inserts at the lesser tuberosity (internal rotation, adduction),
- the supraspinatus inserts at the proximal aspect of the greater tuberosity (supports the deltoid muscle with abduction and external rotation),
- the infraspinatus and teres minor insert at the middle and inferior portion of the greater tuberosity (external rotation).

According to Neer, the impingement syndrome is divided into three stages:

- **Stage I** is primarily seen in patients younger than 25 years of age and is characterized by **edema** and **hemorrhage** in the supraspinatus tendon.
- **Stage II** is characteristically observed in patients between the ages of 25 and 40 years and is characterized by **tendinitis** and **fibrosis** of the rotator cuff and fibrotic thickening of the subacromial bursa. The term 'tendinitis' is commonly used but is controversial since histologically, the tendon shows no inflammation, but does exhibit changes of degeneration.
- **Stage III** almost exclusively occurs in patients older than 40 years of age and represents a **tear** of the rotator cuff.

Special Types of Impingement

Subcoracoid shoulder impingement is caused by a decreased distance between the humeral head and the coracoid process and can be idiopathic, iatrogenic (coracoid repositioning), or post-traumatic.

Posterosuperior impingement occurs with overhead throwing. In the throwing position (the humerus in external rotation and in 90° abduction), the supra- and infraspinatus insertions at the posterior upper glenoid rim are squeezed. Morphologically, this leads to a partial tear of the rotator cuff at the greater tuberosity (a nonspecific sign of degeneration) and degenerative changes of the posterior glenoid rim and labrum.

Rotator Cuff Lesion

A rotator cuff lesion occurs together with a traumatic dislocation almost exclusively in patients older than 40 years. Recognizing this association is relevant since the inability of abduction after traumatic dislocation due to the associated rotator cuff lesion is otherwise incorrectly attributed to axillary nerve palsy.

Glenohumeral instability can also lead to secondary impingement since anterior subluxation or dislocation causes the humeral head to impinge on the acromioclavicular arch. Likewise, a rotator cuff tear can lead to secondary glenohumeral instability.

CLINIC The clinical examination in a patient with impingement characteristically reveals tenderness, crepitus, and weakness, with the severity of these findings depending on the size of the ligamentous tear. Small tears (up to 1 cm) are mainly characterized by pain. A pseudopalsy with flexion and abduction is present in

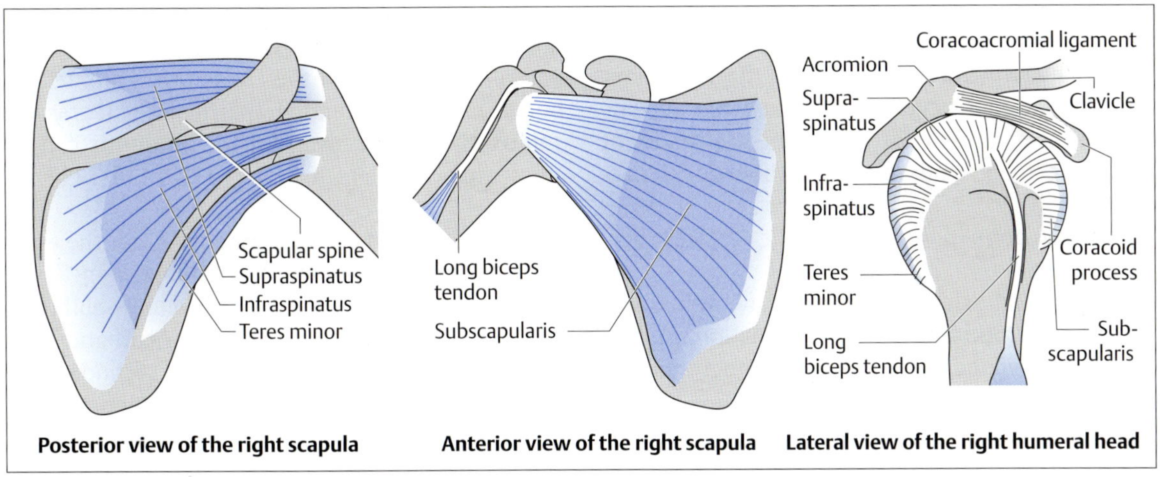

Fig. 1.**129** Schematic diagram of the rotator cuff.

about one-sixth of these patients. Half of the patients with tears up to 2 cm report of pain only. The other half complain of pain and additional pseudopalsy. As the size of the tear increases, pain as the isolated clinical finding decreases, and the incidence of pseudopalsy increases. Advanced stages with radiographically recognizable degenerative changes of the glenohumeral articulation invariably cause a pseudopalsy.

Rotator cuff pathology can be tested with the 'impingement test'. A positive test is elicited when a local anesthetic injected beneath the acromion eliminates or markedly reduces the pain elicited by forced forward elevation of the humerus against the acromion. Pain caused by this maneuver in other conditions is usually not relieved. Diagnosing impingement syndrome on the basis of clinical presentation alone can be difficult. Furthermore, the extent of the morphologic changes does not strictly correlate with the clinical findings. This is why imaging plays an important role in the objective assessment and quantification of the pathologic findings as well as in the differential diagnosis.

X-RAY **Technical considerations:** In general, conventional radiography is performed first if impingement syndrome or a rotator cuff lesion is suspected. The AP view of the glenohumeral articulation is obtained with the patient in the 45° posterior oblique position and the central ray craniocaudally angled by 12–15° to visualize the subacromial space without superimposition. Because of the high variability of the acromial morphology, some authors have suggested fluoroscopic guidance for correct positioning. The second projection should be the view proposed by Neer (or any modification of this view). This view visualizes the glenohumeral joint *en face* by rotating the patient so that the central ray is parallel to the scapular ala (Fig. 1.**130**). Craniocaudal angulation of the tube, usually about 10°, is again necessary for visualization of the subacromial space without superimposed structures. These views reveal the shape of the acromion, which correlates with the extent of the impingement: about one-fourth of acromia are flat, about two-thirds curved, and the remainder hooked. The more curved or hooked the appearance of the acromion, the higher the probability of an impingement syndrome. The radiologic findings are:

- cyst formation in the region of the greater tuberosity,
- subchondral sclerosis of the greater tuberosity and subacromial osteophyte formation, in particular if related to the origin of the acromioclavicular ligament.

Shoulder impingement syndrome can partially or completely obliterate the peribursal fat stripe. The distance between the humeral head and acromion, which normally measures 9–10 mm, decreases with a rotator cuff tear. In middle-aged patients, a distance of less than 6 mm is considered pathologic. (Caution! The subacromial space should be assessed only on technically adequate projections.)

Arthrography: Shoulder arthrography is generally performed as a double contrast examination with injection of a few milliliters of contrast medium and about 10 ml of air. The contrast coating can visualize additional cartilage defects and capsular lesions. Arthrography should be used only if metal implants preclude CT or MRI arthrography. Extension of the contrast medium into the subacromial bursa is a sign of a complete rotator cuff tear (Fig. 1.**131**).

SONO Examining both shoulders makes it easier to evaluate the rotator cuff. The following signs have been found to be reliable evidence of a rotator cuff tear:

- focal interruption of the rotator cuff,
- loss of the rotator cuff,
- focal thinning of the rotator cuff,
- small hypoechoic band replacing the normal structure.

Echogenic foci are by far less informative and have a positive predictive value of 50% or lower. Such foci can be caused by zones of degeneration and calcifications, as well as the intra-articular segment of the long biceps tendon. A rotator cuff defect can remain undetected sonographically if it is partially or completely filled with granulation tissue, debris-containing fluid and tendon remnants. Likewise, superimposed osseous structures (in particular, the acromion and acromioclavicular joint) can interfere with sonographic visualization of all components of the rotator cuff.

If correctly performed and judiciously interpreted, sonography can provide clinically relevant information, especially in differentiating an intact rotator cuff from a complete tear and diagnosing pathologic changes of the subacromial/subdeltoid bursa and biceps tendon (particularly tears and subluxations). Moreover, calcific tendinitis can be sonographically detected (Fig. 1.**132**, 1.**133**, 1.**134**).

CT Standard CT is less important for the evaluation of shoulder impingement syndrome and rotator cuff lesions despite its ability to visualize large defects of the rotator cuff and fatty degeneration of the musculature secondary to chronic tears. CT arthrography is more appropriate, especially for subscapular lesions, which are difficult to diagnose with conventional arthrography. The supraspinatus muscle can also be imaged and evaluated directly or on coronal reconstructions.

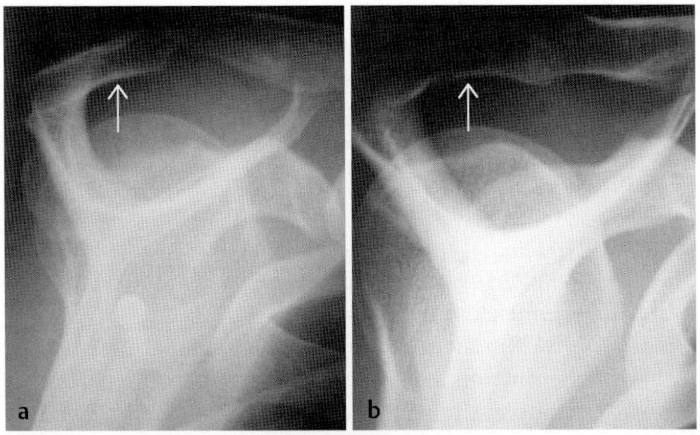

Fig. 1.**130** Neer projection with straight (**a**) and curved (**b**) acromion.

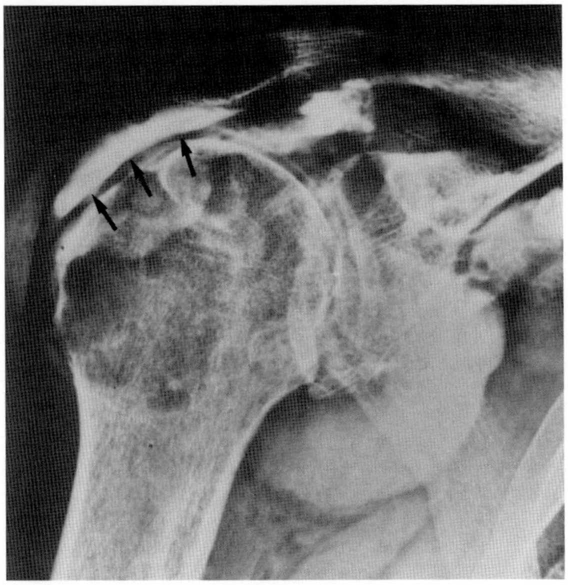

Fig. 1.**131** Arthrography of full-thickness rotator cuff tear. The narrowed space between the acromion and humeral head is filled with contrast medium (arrows).

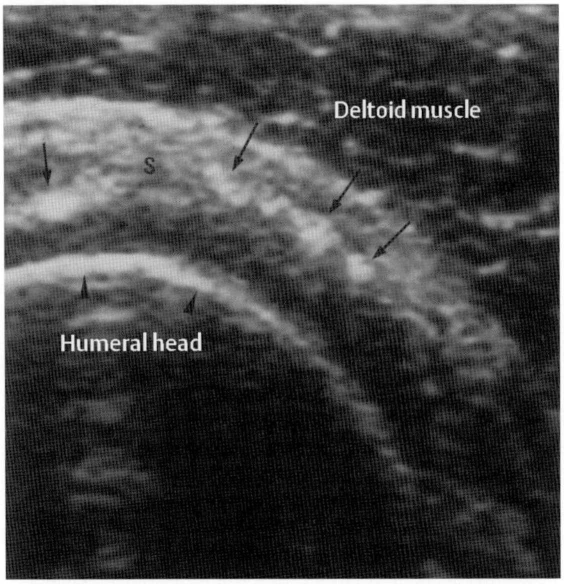

Fig. 1.**132** Sonography (perpendicular to the directions of the fibers of the supraspinatus) in calcific tendonitis with intact supraspinatus. Arrows: echogenic calcifications, **s:** supraspinatus tendon.

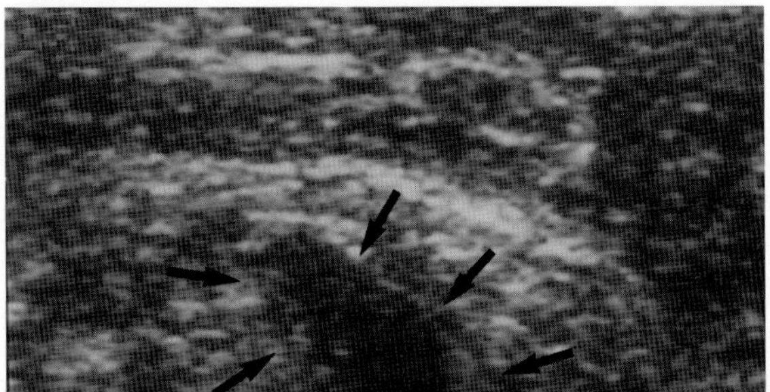

Fig. 1.**133** Sonography of small full-thickness tear of the supraspinatus. The muscle is thickened and indistinctly demarcated from the deltoid, and there is a large hypoechoic defect (arrows).

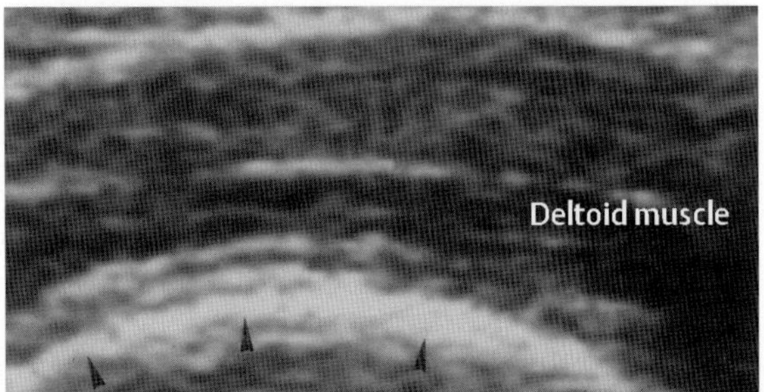

Fig. 1.**134** Sonography of full-thickness tear of the supraspinatus, with the transducer in a position comparable to that in Fig. 1.**132**. The supraspinatus tendon is completely absent.

MRI MRI and MRA (MR arthrography) provide the most informative visualization of the rotator cuff and surrounding structures.

Technical considerations: The oblique orientation of the glenohumeral articulation should be considered when selecting the image plane. In addition to the axial plane, the oblique coronal plane (perpendicular to the glenoid fossa or parallel to the supraspinatus muscle, Figs. 1.**135** – 1.**137**) and the oblique sagittal plane (parallel to the glenoid fossa) have become standard. In view of the small size of many structures (biceps tendon, labrum), a small field of view should be selected, and the section thickness should not exceed 4 mm. In general, oblique coronal T1-weighted or proton density and T2-weighted spin echo sequences are used. T2*-weighted gradient echo sequences seem to overestimate pathologic changes of the rotator cuff. Oblique sagittal images are used to determine size and location of the tear and to visualize the acromial shape. Axial images are needed for the subscapular muscle, the intertuberculous portion of the biceps tendon and the intra-articular structures (labrum, capsule) (Fig. 1.**138**).

Direct MRA is generally performed with highly diluted (1 : 250) gadolinium-based contrast medium. Gradient echo and fat-suppressed T1-weighted SE sequences are employed (Figs. 1.**136,** 1.**138,** 1.**139**).

Indirect MR arthrography is based on the diffusion of intravenously injected contrast medium into the joint capsule, producing an 'arthrographic' effect. This diffusion is best accomplished by post-injection mobilization of the joint for 10 minutes prior to imaging.

The accuracy of MRI for rotator cuff lesions depends on the examiner, examination technique and patient selection, and the results have improved markedly over the last few years because of technological advances. Compared to sonography MRI has a higher sensitivity and specificity (for complete tears, 90 – 100% as compared to 90%).

Conceivable sources of diagnostic difficulties are the zones of increased signal within the rotator cuff, as often seen on T1-weighted and proton density sequences. These lesions have been attributed to a variety of causes, especially to the orientation of the tendon relative to the magnetic field ('magic angle') and to partial volume effect of the different components of the tendon. They can, however, reflect degeneration, which causes hyperintensity on T1-weighted and isointensity on T2-weighted images, without altering the contour of the rotator cuff or the peribursal fat stripe. True substance defects (acute partial or complete rotator cuff tears) can generally be distinguished from these conditions by a sharper demarcation and hyperintensity on T2-weighted images (mainly caused by the joint effusion). Remote and chronic tears are not hyperintense on T2-weighted images because there is no edema, but they are associated with an increase in the signal intensity of muscle on the T1-weighted sequences because of fatty atrophy induced by loss of muscle function.

MRA offers advantages over standard MRI in the distinction between degeneration and partial or complete tear. The complete tear is diagnosed by extension of contrast medium into the tendon region, therefore increasing the specificity of MRI (Figs. 1.**136,** 1.**138**). In comparison with direct MR arthrography, indirect MR arthrography cannot distend the joint capsule (which is particularly useful for evaluating the labrum and ligaments). Another disadvantage of indirect MR arthrography is extra-articular enhancement that should not be mistaken for a pathologic extension of contrast medium.

DD The clinical differential diagnosis of Stage I shoulder impingement syndrome includes subluxation of the glenohumeral joint and acromioclavicular joint changes with calcific tendinitis or adhesive capsulitis appearing in Stage II. Stage III shoulder impingement syndrome, which corresponds to a rotator cuff tear, must be differentiated from pathologic changes of the cervical spine and neoplasms in the shoulder region.

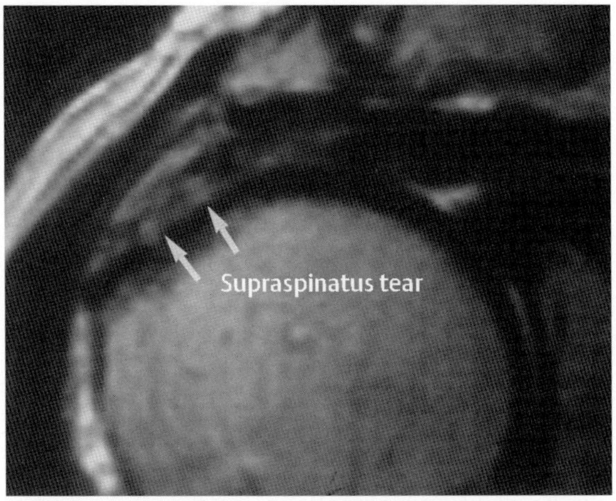

Fig. 1.**135** Oblique coronal T2-weighted MR image shows a full-thickness tear of the supraspinatus tendon close to its osseous insertion. The zone of increased signal intensity represents a tear.

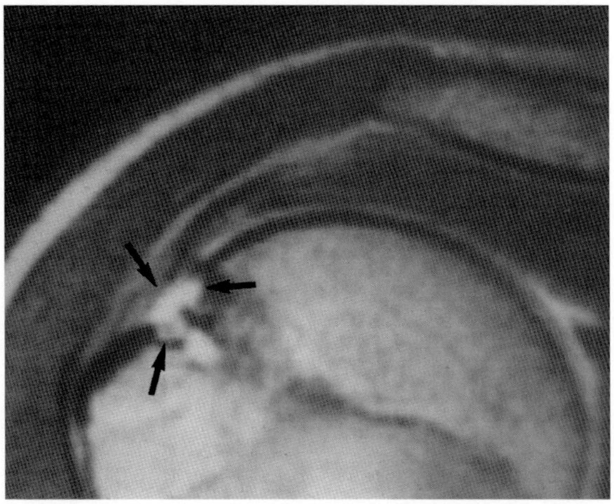

Fig. 1.**136** MR arthrography of a **partial** tear of the supraspinatus tendon. The arthrogram shows the exact extent of the tear (arrows). Contrast medium does not enter the subacromial bursa (compared to Fig. 1.**137**).

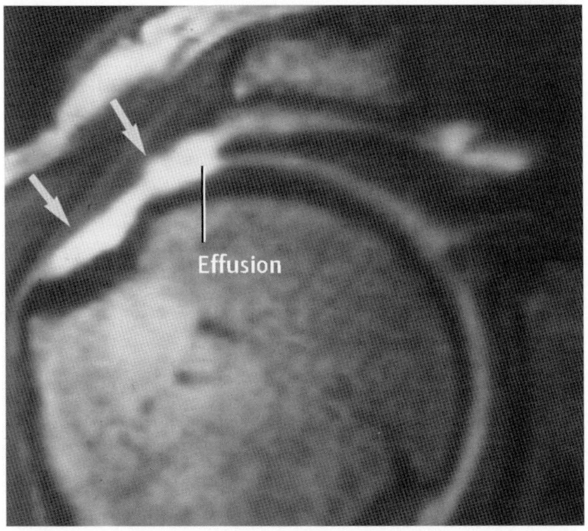

Fig. 1.**137** MRI (T2-weighted image) of a full-thickness tear of the supraspinatus (arrows). The effusion serves as a natural contrast medium.

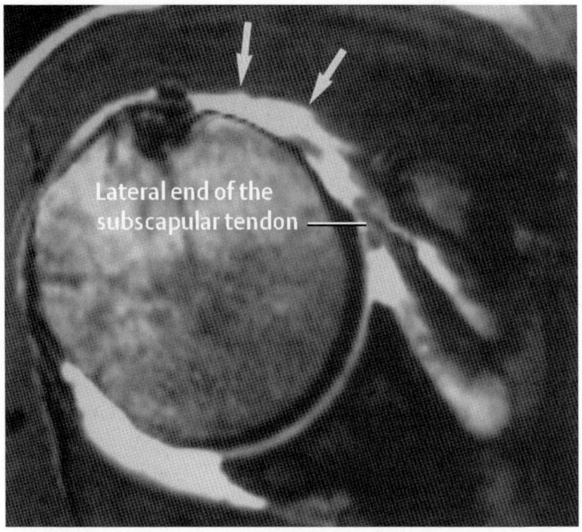

Fig. 1.**138** MR arthrography (axial GRE image) visualizing a tear of the subscapularis tendon.

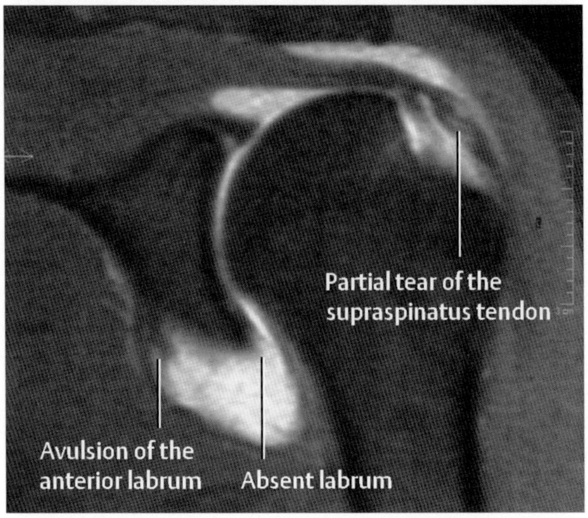

Fig. 1.**139** MR arthrography. Avulsion of the inferior glenoid ligament and anterior labrum ('ALPSA lesion'). These structures are displaced anteromedially. Partial tear of the supraspinatus tendon.

Shoulder Dislocation, Shoulder Instability

■ The shoulder is the most unstable joint of the body, dislocates most commonly and accounts for almost one half of all dislocations. ■

Shoulder dislocations can be classified by direction (anterior, posterior, multidirectional, and rarely superior), extent (dislocation vs. subluxation), chronology (acute, chronic, recurrent), and mechanism (traumatic vs. nontraumatic), as well as by the patient's role (deliberate vs. accidental). Classification by the direction of displacement is most frequently used. Posterior dislocations are rather rare and seen mainly in the setting of seizures (e.g., epilepsy and alcoholism). Subluxations are often transient, and intentional dislocations occur in the context of multidirectional instabilities (general laxity). Chronic dislocations are more frequent than generally expected (Fig. 1.**140**, 1.**141**).

Bankart lesion: This is a lesion of the anterior capsulolabral complex and often also refers to fractures of the antero-inferior glenoid rim.

Hill-Sachs lesion: This is a depression of the posterolateral aspect of the humeral head caused by anterior shoulder dislocation.

PATH The glenohumeral joint is inherently unstable. Its osseous enclosure is limited, and additional stabilization is provided by the joint capsule, glenohumeral ligaments, labrum, and rotator cuff. Various conditions can lead to instability. The most common cause is probably traumatic damage to the joint capsule, labrum, and osseous glenoid rim, but constitutional factors have been implicated, such as capsular laxity, torsion of the humeral head, and the anatomic position of the glenoid.

CLINIC The patient might experience a subluxation only by the vague feeling of abnormal function. In unclear cases, it might be useful to apply several clinical stress tests to elicit symptoms and physical findings.

In a traumatic anterior dislocation, the patient can usually recall the time and event. The mobility of the shoulder is restricted by pain, and the arm is in a fixed position with the position determined by the location of the displaced humeral head. Inspection reveals deformity of the soft tissues. A posterior dislocation can be overlooked clinically.

Chronic dislocations are most common in patients over 50 years old. These patients complain of an impaired range of motion and shoulder pain. This type of dislocation might not be apparent clinically. Trauma is not always remembered (but should be considered a trigger mechanism in many cases).

X-RAY The AP view (with the involved shoulder in the posterior oblique position) and Neer view constitute the basic radiographic evaluation. The transthoracic view can be used to supplement the Neer view, but its image quality is often suboptimal. Obtaining an axial view of a dislocated shoulder is not always feasible, although if obtained it is almost diagnostic. The view proposed by Bernageau (fluoroscopically guided view, obtained axial to the anterior inferior glenoid rim) can visualize an osseous Bankart lesion. Tangential views of the posterosuperior humeral head are suitable to search for a Hill-Sachs lesion (Fig. 1.**142**). The conventional view is important for visualizing additional osseous injuries, such as a fracture of the greater tuberosity or the rare fractures of the coracoid and acromion.

SONO Sonography does not play a major role in evaluating shoulder instability, though it can confirm any clinical instability if the humeral head is moved with one hand and the probe is held in the other hand. Sonography can also show the Hill-Sachs lesion.

CT Standard CT (without arthrography) can show osseous **Bankart** and **Hill-Sachs** lesions, as well as other osseous lesions (Figs. 1.**143**, 1.**144**). Morphometry of the proximal humerus and scapula, which should be reserved for specific questions, measures the rotation of the humeral head relative to the epicondyles and the position of the articular surface of the glenoid process relative to the axis of the scapular ala.

CT arthrography plays a major role by visualizing the relevant soft-tissue structures, such as the labrum, joint capsule and glenohumeral ligaments. It can be performed as single contrast (air or iodinated contrast medium alone) or as a double-contrast examination. Iodinated contrast medium should be diluted (with physiologic sodium chloride solution or with a local anesthetic) to avoid beam-hardening artifacts on the CT images. The needle can be inserted under CT guidance, but usually is placed under fluoroscopic guidance. The total amount of contrast medium is about 15 ml. Increasing this amount often causes extravasation of contrast medium under the subscapular muscle medially.

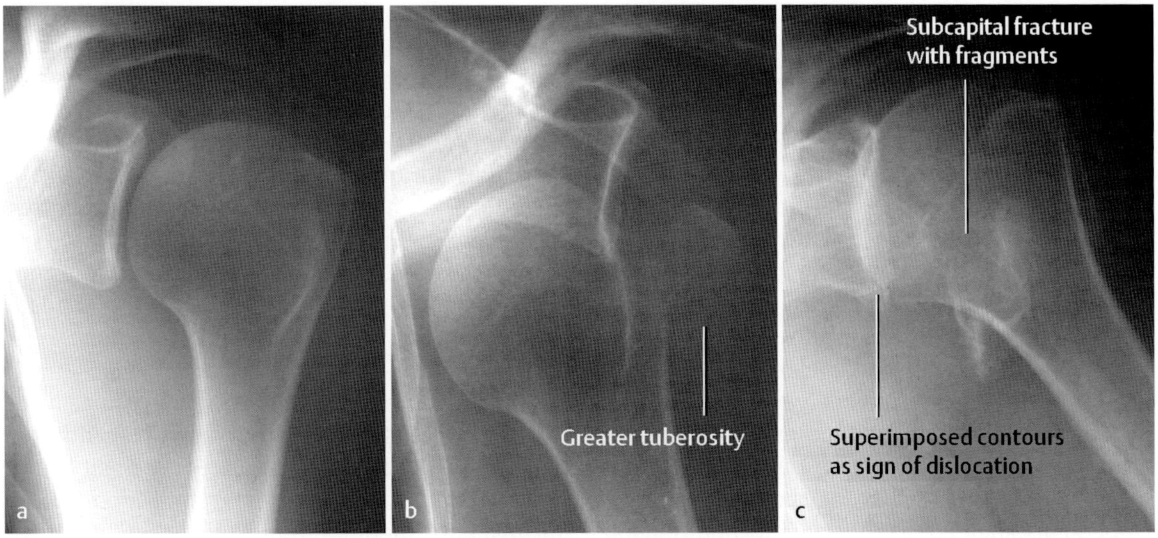

Fig. 1.**140** Rotated and craniocaudally angled anteroposterior view of the shoulder. **a** Normal finding, humeral head and glenoid process are not superimposed. **b** Anterior dislocation, avulsed greater tuberosity (a common concomitant injury). **c** Posterior dislocation with subcapital humeral fracture: superimposed glenoid process and humeral head.

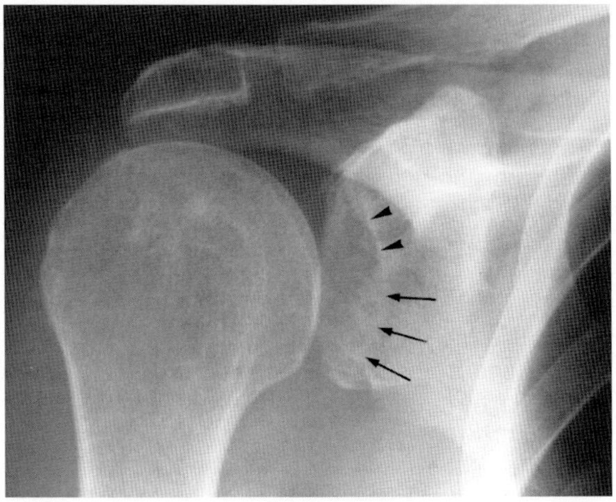

Fig. 1.**141** S/P anterior shoulder dislocation with blunted anterior inferior glenoid rim (arrows), in contrast to the normal superior glenoid rim (arrowheads).

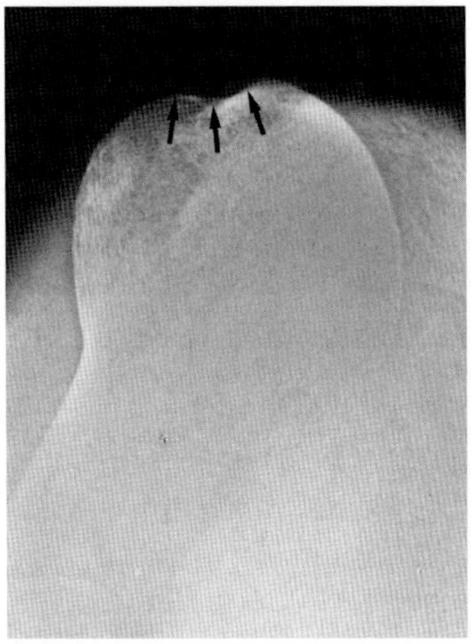

Fig. 1.**142** Tangential radiographic projection of the humeral head with Hill-Sachs defect (arrows).

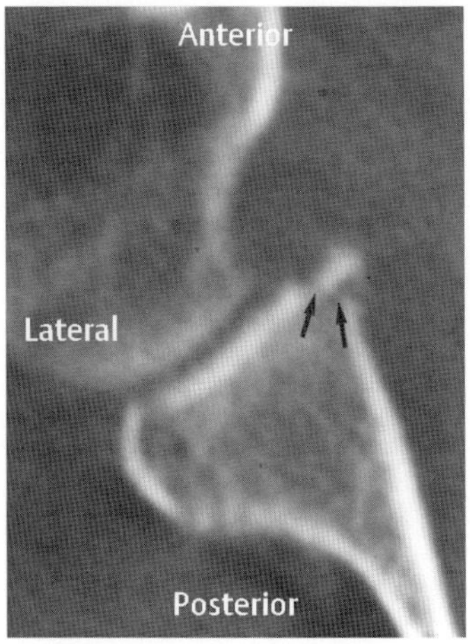

Fig. 1.**143** Axial CT showing a fracture of the anterior glenoid rim following dislocation (arrows).

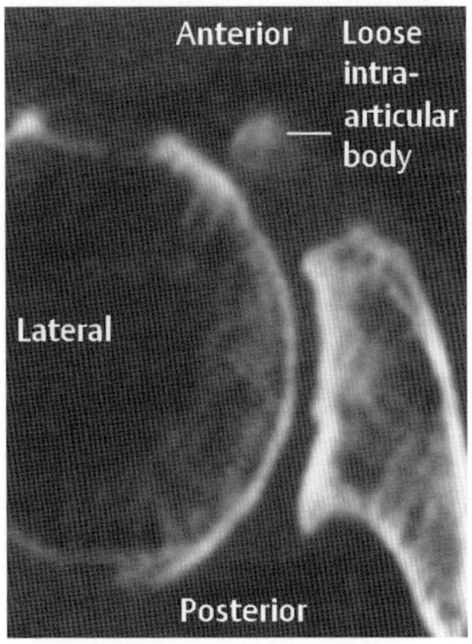

Fig. 1.**144** Axial CT showing a glenoid dysplasia with retroversion of the glenoid process and a loose intra-articular body.

When evaluating the labrum, its variable size and shape must be kept in mind. Although classically thought to be triangular in shape, the anterior labrum has been shown to have rounded, cleaved, or notched configurations. A nondisplaced tear along its base can be mimicked by a crescent variant of the supero-anterior labrum, not to be mistaken for a flap lesion. A tear in the other labral segments with or without degeneration can be diagnosed with greater confidence.

The anterior capsule usually inserts immediately medial to the labrum and blends with its base (Type I) or slightly more medially but no more than 1 cm from it (Type II). A capsular insertion along the scapular neck (Type III) has been described as a congenital condition with predisposition to glenohumeral instability or as an acquired condition following shoulder dislocation. The posterior capsule normally inserts at the tip of the labrum or immediately medial to it.

MRI Standard MRI (without intra-articular contrast medium) can visualize the morphologic changes found in instability. Most important are the axial views for the evaluation of the anterior and posterior labrum. For lesions of the upper and lower labrum, coronal sections perpendicular to the glenohumeral joint space are indicated. There is no uniform agreement about the appropriate MR sequences. Gradient echo sequences are well suited because of their high contrast between labrum, articular cartilage, and joint fluid. T2-weighted sequences are generally used for acute injuries, since the joint effusion often found after trauma serves as natural contrast medium (Figs. 1.**145**, 1.**146**, 1.**147**). A labral tear is visualized as increased signal intensity along its base, with or without displacement (Fig. 1.**148**).

Without a joint effusion, evaluation of the joint capsule and labrum is limited by standard MRI alone. Another limitation is the fact that small fractures of the glenoid rim that occur together with cartilage lesion (representing an **osseous** Bankart lesion) can be overlooked.

MR arthrography has the advantage of showing the capsule, glenohumeral ligaments, and labrum and can detect nondisplaced labral avulsions and ligamentous and/or capsular tears. The criteria are the same as those for CT arthrography. The advantages of MRI are the better contrast visualization of the labrum and capsuloligamentous structures, as well as the multidirectional image display. The risk of overlooking small osseous Bankart lesions is the same for MR arthrography as for standard MRI (Fig. 1.**148**).

DD Dislocations can be mistaken clinically for various conditions, such as contusion, fracture (especially of the greater tuberosity), and rotator cuff tear. A recurrent subluxation can be mistaken for shoulder impingement syndrome, rotator cuff tear, free intra-articular fragment, and degenerative osteoarthritis of the glenohumeral articulation, as well as for a 'clicking' scapula. Imaging plays a major role in evaluating these diagnostic possibilities and in surgical planning.

Differentiating normal variation from pathologic conditions is crucial for correct interpretation.

! The morphology of the glenohumeral joint found in shoulder dislocation or instability primarily depends on the direction of the dislocation, and much less on the number and severity of dislocations.
Because of the frequency of normal variation in the glenoid labrum and joint capsule, the findings of CT arthrography and MRI must be interpreted diligently (and always in context with the clinical findings).

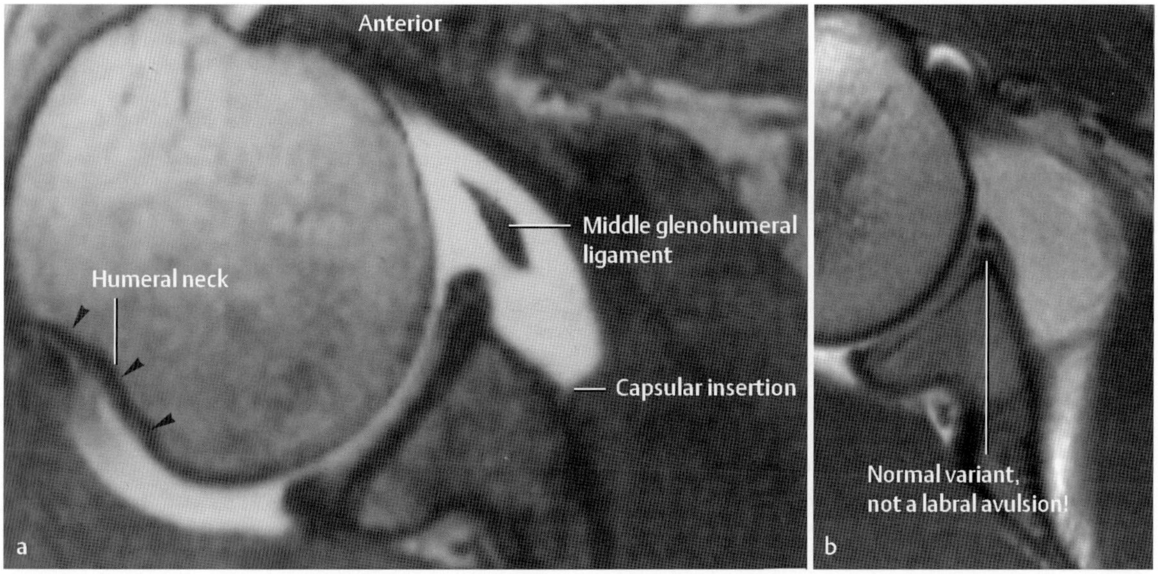

Fig. 1.**145** MR arthrography, normal findings. **a** The anterior capsule may insert far medial to the labrum as a normal variant and the anterior and posterior glenoid labra are rounded. The middle glenohumeral ligament anterior to the anterior labrum can mimic a labral tear. The posterior indentation of the humerus corresponds to the normal humeral neck and does not represent a Hill-Sachs defect! Rule of thumb: an indentation should be called a Hill-Sachs defect only if it is seen at the level of or higher than the coracoid process. **b** Normal variant of the anterior labrum.

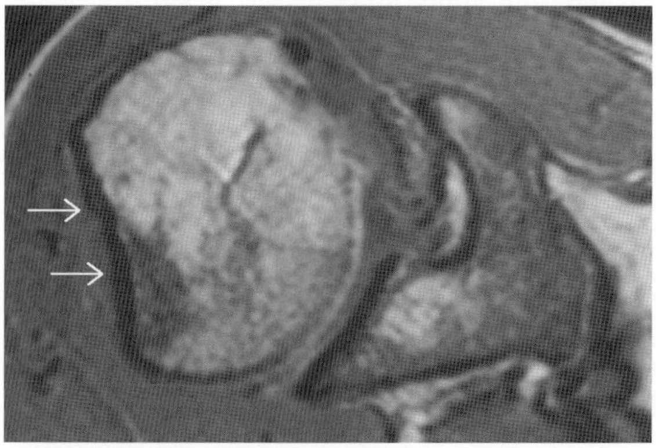

Fig. 1.**146** Standard MRI examination (GRE technique) with large Hill-Sachs defect (arrows).

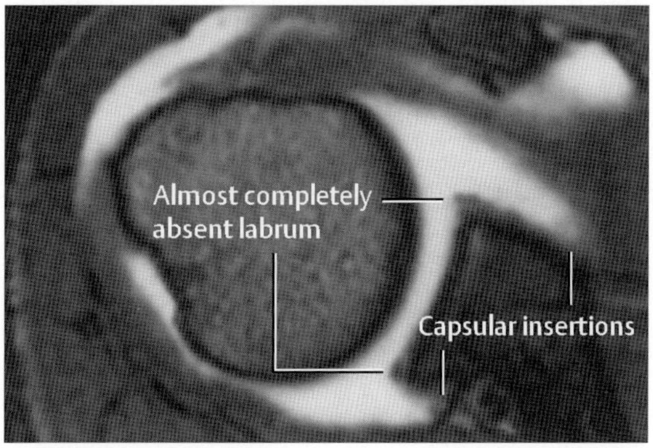

Fig. 1.**147** MR arthrography of multidirectional instability with complete absence of the anterior and posterior glenoid labrum. Anterior and posterior capsule show a definite medial insertion.

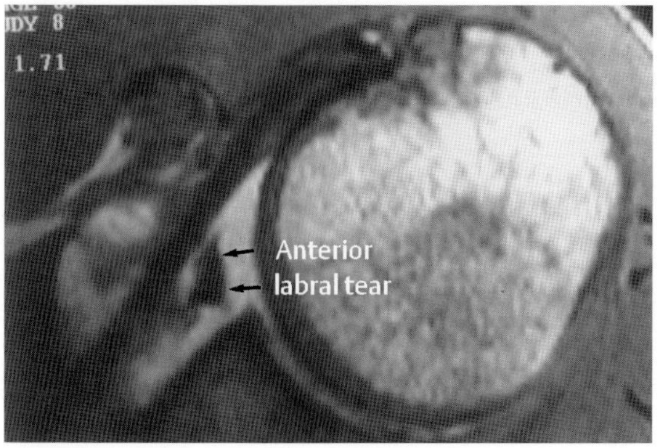

Fig. 1.**148** MR arthrography of an avulsed anterior glenoid labrum.

Upper Extremity

Humeral Fractures

Proximal Humeral Fractures

Proximal humeral fractures include intra- and extra-articular fractures of the humeral head and fractures of the metadiaphyseal region.

A universal classification of these fractures is not available, but the classification proposed by Neer is most often used. It differentiates among six fracture types with different therapeutic implications. The humeral head, including the proximal humeral metaphysis, is divided into four segments (Fig. 1.**149**). The classification considers the displaced fracture fragments only, regardless of the actual number of fractures. A segment is considered 'displaced' if it is either displaced by more than 1 cm or angulated by more than 45°.

When no displaced segment is identified, the fracture is classified as **Type I.**

If **one** fracture is displaced, the fracture is classified according to the displaced fragment as **Type II–V** (Fig. 1.**150**). In addition, one should note that two fragments are present to indicate that the humeral head is broken into two relevant 'pieces' only. Additional fractures without displacement or involving the fragments are not included.

If **several** fragments are displaced, one should note whether the fracture consists of three or four fragments since the higher fracture type determines the classification. For example, a fracture with a displaced greater tuberosity and displaced shaft fragment would be 'a three-fragment fracture, Type IV' (Fig. 1.**151**).

A fracture dislocation is always classified as Type VI.

X-RAY Technical considerations: It is necessary to visualize all fragments in two projections perpendicular to each other.

AP and axillary views are mandatory. An additional transscapular or transthoracic view might be necessary.

SONO Sonography might delineate concomitant injuries, such as tears of the rotator cuff or long head of the biceps tendon, or a joint effusion.

CT CT might complement the fracture evaluation, especially if intra-articular fragments are suspected. However, CT is not necessary in most cases.

! Fractures of the proximal humerus are rare in children. If they occur, they consist of epiphyseal separation with a metaphyseal fragment. Inconclusive findings can be further evaluated by comparison with the contralateral side.

Humeral Shaft Fractures

Humeral shaft fractures include diaphyseal fractures with and without dislocation. The displacement of the major fragments depends on the level of the fractures and the muscular pull on them. The classification of the AO group is based on the orientation of the fracture line and displacement pattern (Fig. 1.**152**).

! In about 25% of cases concomitant injuries can be found in the shoulder and forearm.

X-RAY Radiographic views in two projections (AP and transthoracic) are sufficient. The neighboring joints must be visualized to exclude concomitant injuries.

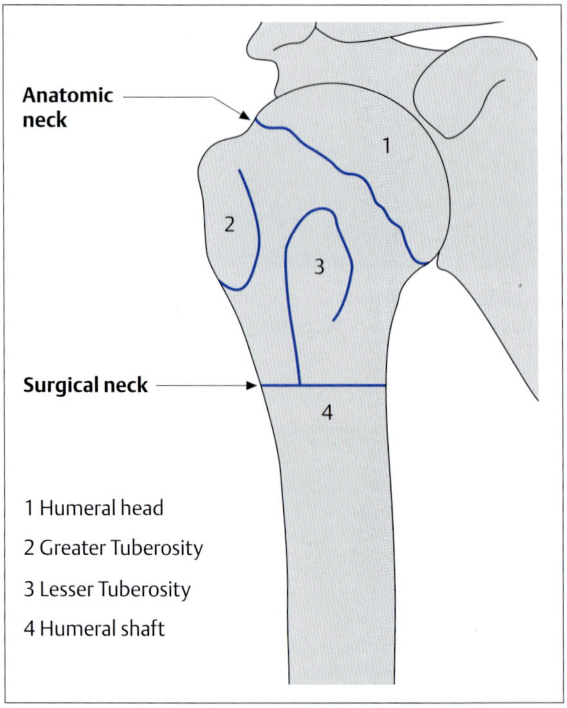

Fig. 1.**149** Segmental division of the humeral head.

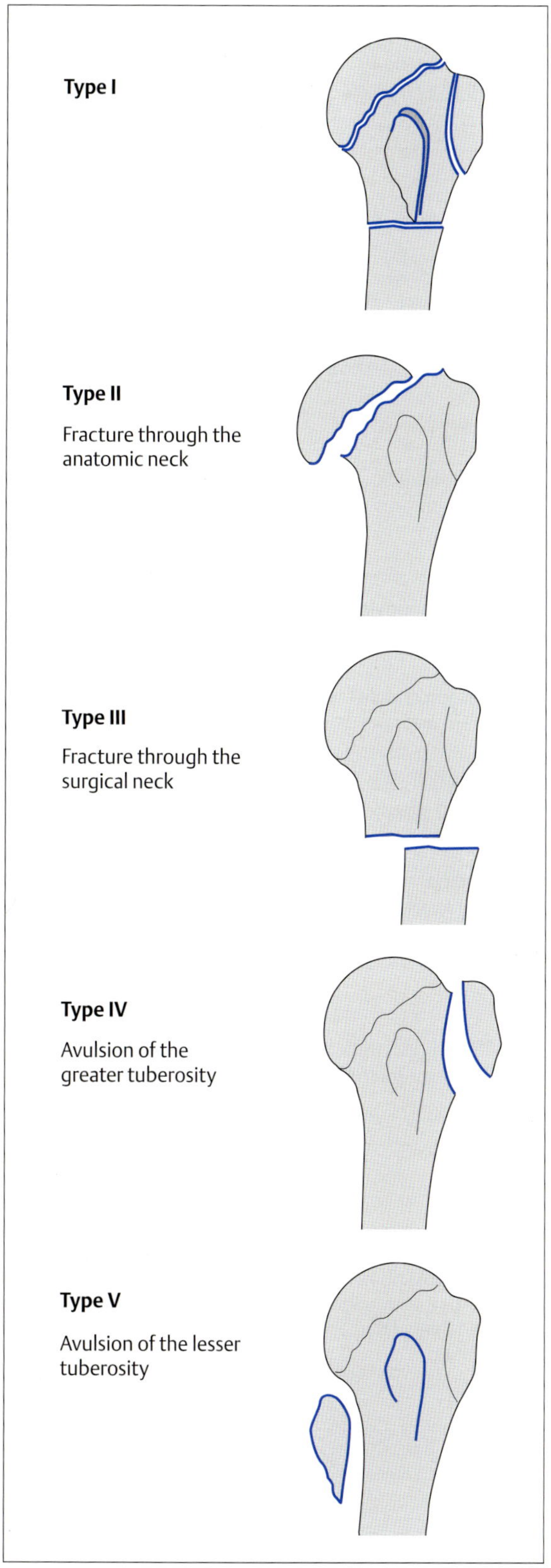

Fig. 1.**150** Modified Neer classification of the proximal humeral fractures according to the AO system.

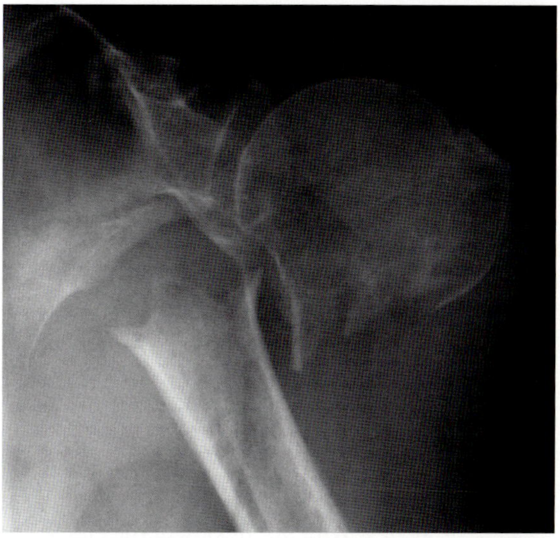

Fig. 1.**151** Example of a three-segment fracture, Type IV.

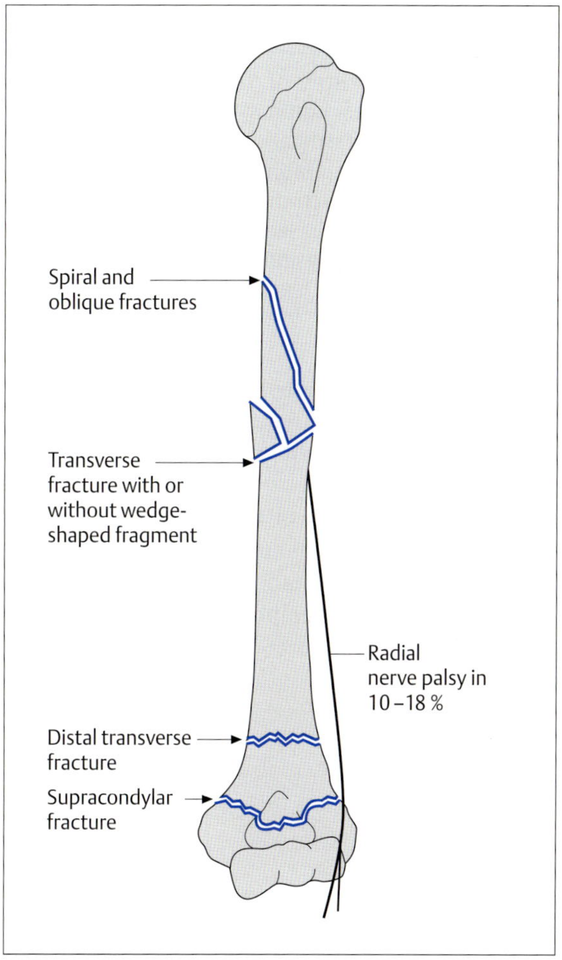

Fig. 1.**152** Typical fractures of the humeral shaft.

Distal Humeral Fractures

Fractures of the distal humerus are divided into metaphyseal and intra-articular fractures.

> **!** In adults, 90% of distal humeral fractures show articular involvement. In contrast, supracondylar fractures are the most frequent fractures found in children (3 – 10 years).

The classification of these fractures follows the recommendations of the AO group and determines the surgical procedure and approach (Fig. 1.**156**).

X-RAY Technical considerations: AP view and lateral view with 90° flexion of the elbow are mandatory. A nondisplaced fracture can be occult on AP views, so indirect signs of fracture must be considered (Fig. 1.**153**).

> **!** Diagnosing fractures of the distal humerus in children requires familiarity with the development of the ossification centers (Fig. 1.**154**). Though avulsed metaphyseal fragments are frequently present, such injuries might only be differentiated on the basis of displaced ossification centers. If the findings remain unclear, MRI should be the next imaging text performed.

Rotational malposition should be looked for in children. The lateral view frequently suggests rotation by showing an apparent widening of the rotated fragment.

The correct position of the humeral capitellum can be determined with auxiliary lines (Fig. 1.**155**). This is especially important in the child with a suspected distal humeral epiphyseal separation.

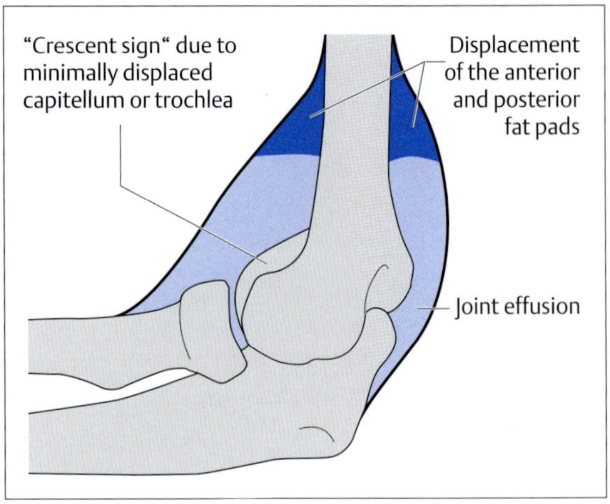

Fig. 1.**153** Radiologic evidence of hard-to-see fractures of the distal humerus and elbow joint.

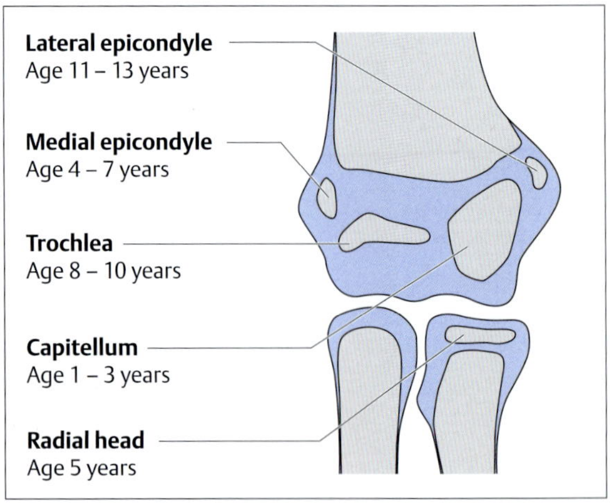

Fig. 1.**154** Presentation of the ossification centers in the distal humerus related to the child's age.

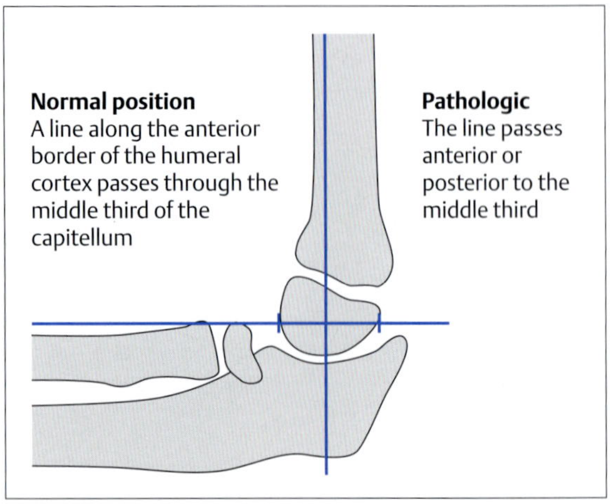

Fig. 1.**155** The anterior humeral line aids in determining the normal position of the capitellum.

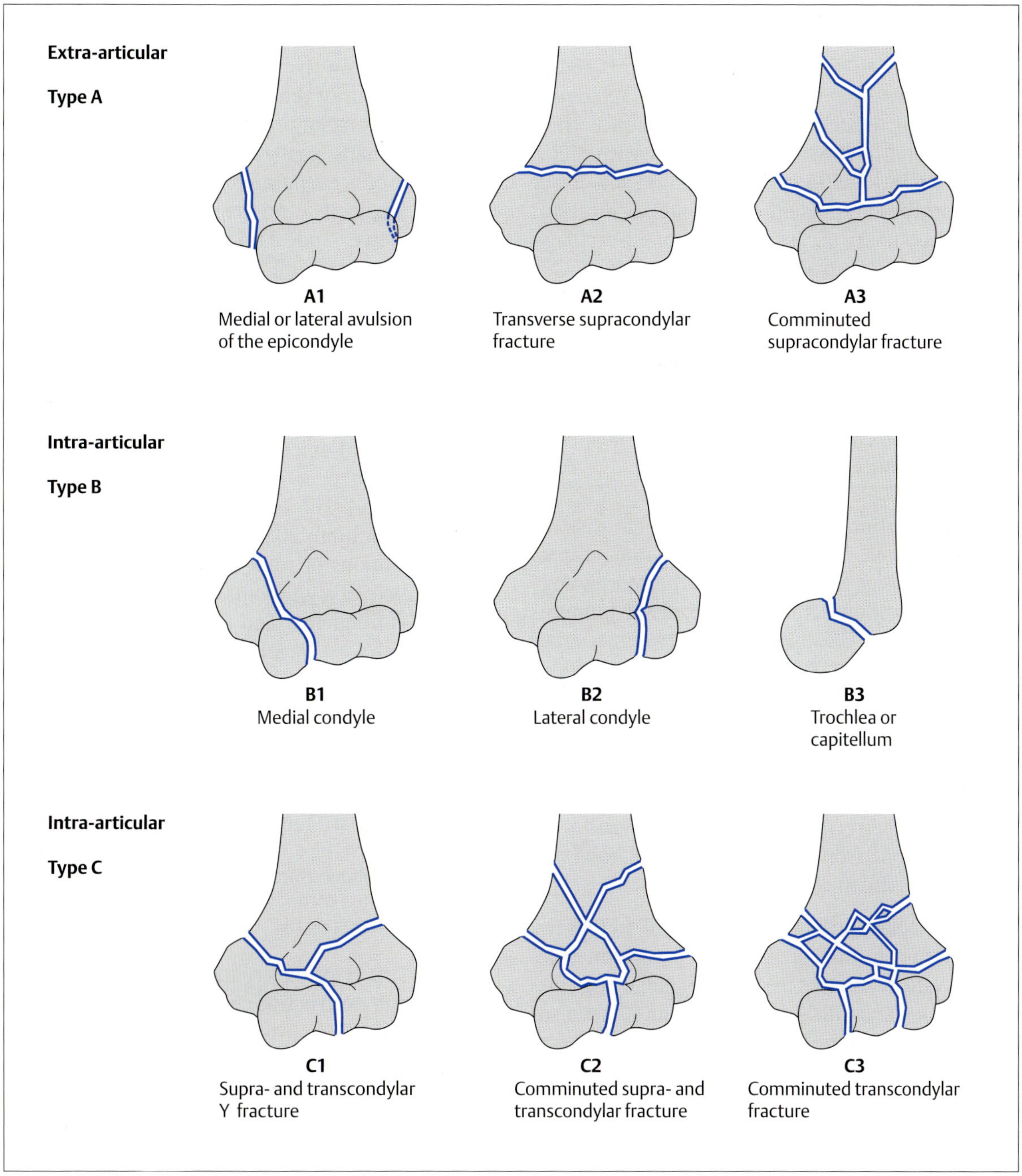

Fig. 1.**156** Classification of the distal humeral fractures according to the AO group.

Dislocation of the Elbow

The classification of elbow dislocations is based on the displacement of the radius and ulna relative to the humerus. Posterior radial dislocation is most frequent, and fractures are associated with elbow dislocation in 30–50% of cases. Because soft-tissue injury is invariably present, soft-tissue calcifications occur in about 90% of cases. Damage of the cartilage, nerves, and vessels is also frequently observed.

> ! A special type of elbow dislocation is displacement of the radial head accompanied by a fracture of the ulnar shaft, the so-called Monteggia fracture. If radial head dislocation or forearm fracture is suspected clinically, the elbow must be included in the entire forearm.

Elbow dislocations are the most frequent dislocations in children. Interpretation of the radiographic findings requires familiarity with the morphology of the ossification centers of the distal humerus (see Fig. 1.**154**).

X-RAY Technical considerations: Necessary views are the AP view in supination, if the clinical condition permits, and the lateral view in 90° flexion with the thumb pointing upward. Conventional tomography might visualize displaced fragments to better advantage, particularly after reduction. Comparison views of the contralateral side might be helpful in children.

SONO Sonography might be helpful to identify free intra-articular bodies (flexion side) and to evaluate injuries in children (radial head dislocation?). The ossification centers can be seen sonographically before they are detected by radiographs. For suspected vascular injuries, color-coded Doppler sonography is indicated.

MRI MRI plays a role only in the evaluation of chronic post-traumatic conditions (cartilage, free loose bodies) and in the pediatric age group.

CT CT with 2-D and 3-D reconstructions can achieve a more accurate visualization of associated complex fractures and soft-tissue injuries.

DD It can be difficult to differentiate between elbow dislocation and complete separation of the distal humeral epiphysis. If the humeral capitellum is ossified, the preserved extension line between the radius and capitellum indicates an epiphyseal lysis (Fig. 1.**157**). For inconclusive findings, MRI should be used.

Subluxation of the Radial Head (Chassaignac)

A sudden pull on the forearm can cause the radial head to slip out of the annular ligament, with subsequent blockage of pronation (Fig. 1.**158**). This minor and usually easily reduced injury generally does not produce a pathologic or radiologic finding (clinical diagnosis!) and the radiographic examination serves to exclude a fracture.

> ! Subluxation of the radial head is a frequent injury of the pediatric elbow up to age 5 years.

Tennis Elbow

Lateral humeral epicondylitis is caused by stress-induced damage at the fibro-osseous transition (enthesopathy). The extensor carpi radialis brevis is involved in up to 90% of cases and microtrauma to the tendinous or teno-osseous segments is the major cause of symptoms. Medial epicondylitis occurs less frequently and is often associated with sports such as javelin throwing or golfing (Fig. 1.**159**).

X-RAY Technical considerations: AP or oblique views using soft-tissue technique. The radiograph is frequently normal or only shows subtle changes (compare Table 1.**11**).

NUC About one-third of the cases of radiographically occult epicondylitis have increased radionuclide accumulation on the three-phase bone scan.

SONO This is primarily used to exclude erosive and destructive changes.

MRI MRI can detect thickened, thinned, or partially torn ligamentous structures, as well as reactive osseous changes such as edema or microfracture (Fig. 1.**160**).

> ! Intraoperatively, the tenomuscular transition of the extensor carpi radialis shows fibrous or edematous changes in 97% of cases. Macroscopically, a rupture or partial rupture is found in 35% of cases.

Partial ruptures (thinning of the tendinous insertion and surrounding edema) and complete ruptures are clearly shown with MRI. Since both conditions occur following failed conservative therapy, the MRI findings are crucial and often prompt a change in the therapeutic approach.

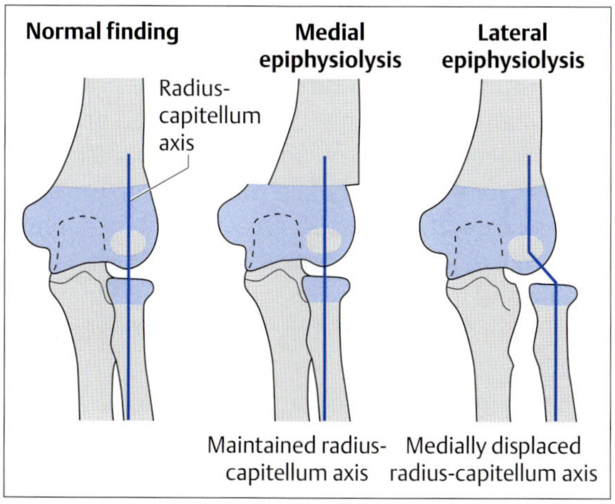

Fig. 1.**157** Abnormal relationship of the radius to the humeral capitellum and epiphysiolysis of the distal humerus in contrast to dislocation of the pediatric elbow.

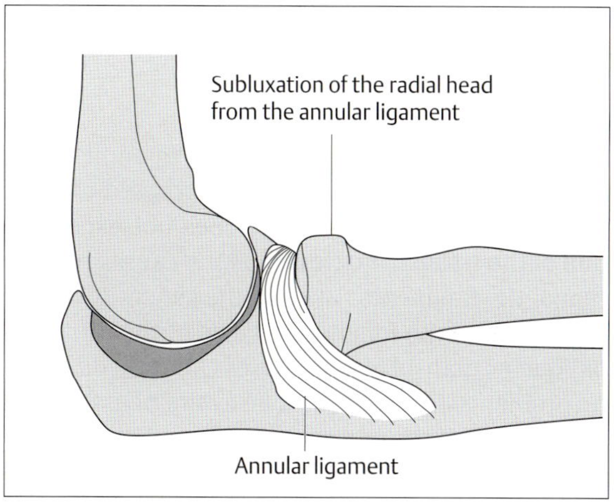

Fig. 1.**158** Example of Chassaignac injury.

Table 1.**11** Spectrum of the radiographic findings of epicondylitis

Radiologic findings
Enlarged soft-tissue structures
Round, coarse or intraligamentous, longitudinally oriented calcific deposits adjacent to the epicondyles. Possible epicondylar demineralization
Osseous overgrowth along the epicondyle
Indistinct, frayed outline of the osseous overgrowth, especially along its course

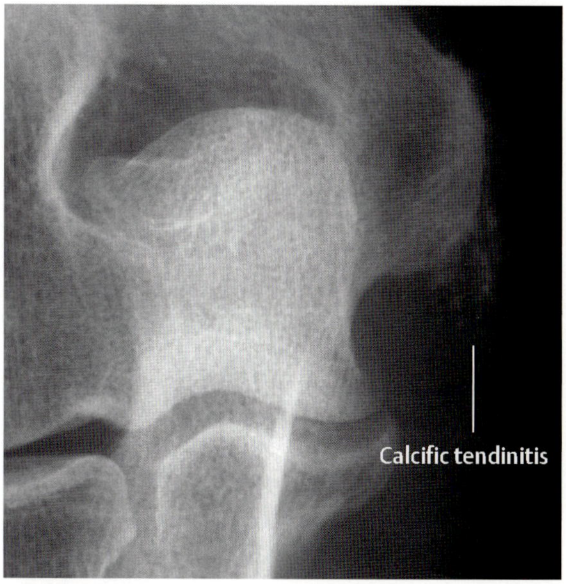

Fig. 1.**159** Golfer's elbow with calcification and osseous reaction (proliferation) at the insertion of the extensor carpi ulnaris at the lateral epicondyle.

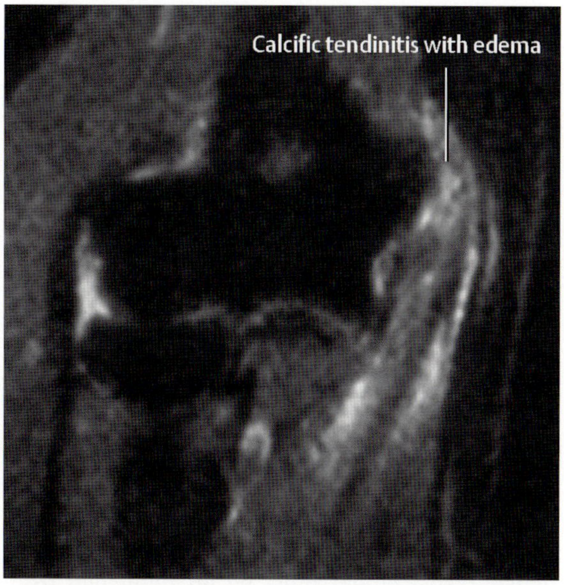

Fig. 1.**160** MRI STIR sequence of patient shown in Fig. 1.**159** exhibiting soft-tissue edema in the region adjacent to the lateral epicondyle.

Fractures of the Proximal Forearm

Olecranon Fractures

Fractures of the olecranon are frequent adult elbow injuries (up to 20%). A uniformly accepted classification of these fracture types does not exist. The pull of the triceps muscle frequently causes separation of the fragments. The fracture generally occurs transverse to the longitudinal axis of the ulna, but oblique or undisplaced fractures can pose diagnostic problems. One must also be aware of associated dislocations of the elbow, which can involve the radius, or ulna, or both. A well-recognized combination is the fracture of the ulnar shaft with dislocation of the radial head **(Monteggia fracture)** (see page 82).

Fractures of the **coronoid process** are generally secondary to posterior elbow dislocations. Isolated avulsion fractures at the insertion of the pectoralis muscle are less frequent.

Since the coronoid process maintains the posterior stability of the elbow joint, these injuries must be searched for after closed or spontaneous reduction since the risk of recurrent dislocation with this injury is high.

X-RAY Radiographs in two views (AP and lateral with the forearm flexed) are generally adequate to diagnose osseous injuries. For nondisplaced fractures, oblique views might be needed.

! An olecranon fracture has to be distinguished from the patella cubiti, a sesamoid bone in the triceps tendon.

Fractures of the Radial Head and Neck

Fractures of the radial head and neck are the most frequent injuries of the elbow in adults, accounting for about 50% of all elbow injuries. They are generally caused by indirect trauma such as a fall on the outstretched hand with compression of the radial head against the capitellum. The appearance of these fractures is quite variable, and several classification schemes have been proposed.

About 50% of the fractures are nondisplaced and might not be visible radiographically.

The compression fracture with minimal intra-articular displacement must be distinguished from the sagittal fracture of the radial head and neck (chisel fracture) (Fig. 1.**161**).

Extra-articular fractures of the radial neck and comminuted fractures also can occur.

In comminuted fractures of the radial head with radial shortening, or in severely displaced proximal radial fractures, the so-called Essex-Lopresti fracture has to be considered. In this rare fracture type, the radial shortening causes a concomitant subluxation to a dislocation of the distal radioulnar articulation and interosseous membrane tear. Mnemonic aid: **a**cute **l**ongitudinal **r**adio-**u**lnar **d**issociation = 'ALRUD.'

With any radial head fracture, avulsion fractures of the capitellum must be excluded.

X-RAY Technique: Radiographs in two projections, AP view and lateral view, if possible, with 90° flexion of the elbow.

! If the soft tissues are abnormal (effusion, hematoma) and a fracture is not discernible on these standard two views, a 45° oblique view should be obtained to search for a nondisplaced fracture of the radial head.
Comminuted fractures of the radial head always require further radiographic evaluation of the distal forearm, including wrist, to exclude an Essex-Lopresti injury.

Compression fractures might present only as a subchondral radiodense band and joint effusion (Fig. 1.**162**).

CT In selected cases, 2-D or 3-D reconstructions can better demonstrate complex fractures and detect intra-articular fragments with a high degree of accuracy (Fig. 1.**163**).

MRI If radiographs of the elbow and proximal forearm are negative, MRI may be helpful since its visualization of soft-tissue injuries without osseous involvement (e.g., medial and lateral collateral ligaments or muscles) is unsurpassed. However, performing an MRI in the acute setting is not always feasible. MRI is also the best imaging method to detect occult fractures and bone bruises, as well as chondral or osteochondral injuries, and osteochondritis dissecans. Finally, it is the best technique available to differentiate fracture fragments from accessory ossicles.

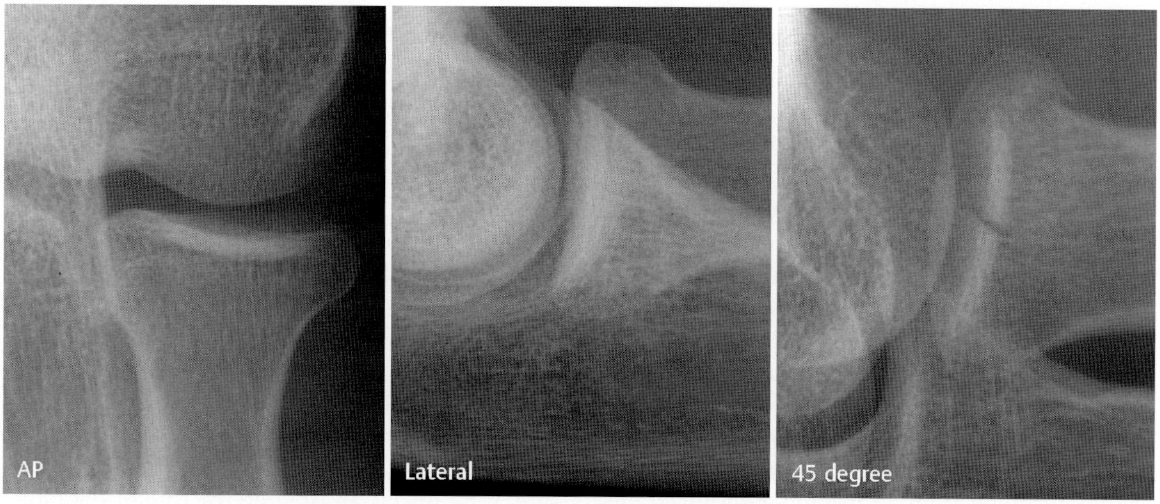

Fig. 1.**161** Chisel fracture of the radial head with articular involvement. Seen only in the 45° projection.

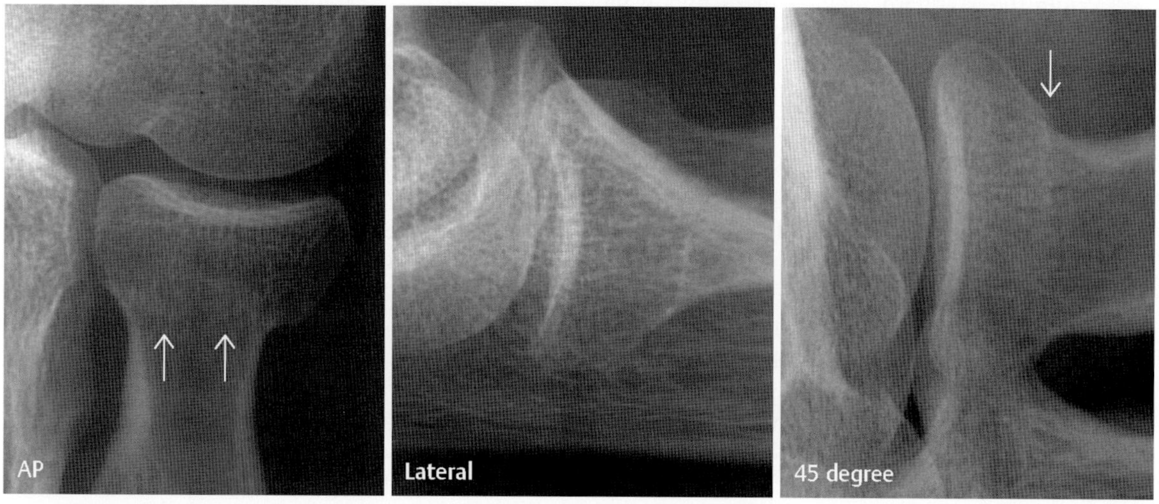

Fig. 1.**162** Nondisplaced extra-articular fracture through the neck of the radial head. The AP view shows the fracture solely as a line of increased density. The oblique view reveals a subtle cortical step-off.

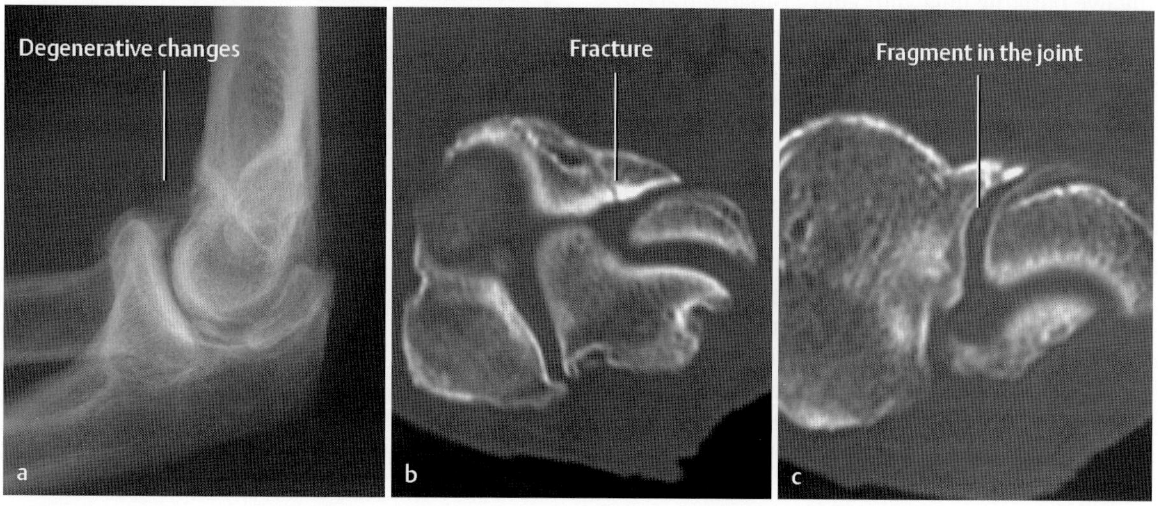

Fig. 1.**163** Olecranon fracture with free intra-articular bodies that are only seen by CT (**b, c**).

Special Considerations in the Pediatric Age Group

Proximal fractures of the ulna (about 6%) and fractures of the radial head (15%) are less frequent in children and adolescents than in adults.

In the pediatric age group, fractures of the olecranon are frequently associated with fractures of the radial head or neck, and vice versa.

An incomplete olecranon fracture in children can lead to a Monteggia fracture, and the position of the radial head should always be noted.

Fractures rarely involve the articular surface of the radial head and present more frequently as Salter-Harris type II epiphyseal injuries (Fig. 1.**164**).

It is important to differentiate an epiphysiolysis of the olecranon from an incompletely fused epiphysis.

X-RAY If the standard views are inconclusive, comparison views of the contralateral side should be obtained.

SONO Greenstick fractures that are not apparent radiographically can be visualized sonographically. Bilateral sonography can further evaluate epiphyseal injuries, and especially if epiphysiolysis is suspected.

MRI MRI can differentiate Salter-Harris type I and II epiphyseal injuries of the radial head from Salter-Harris type III epiphyseal injuries, which are associated with a higher incidence of growth disturbances.

Forearm Fractures

Fractures of the forearm are frequent and generally involve both the ulna and radius. Isolated fractures of either the radius or ulna are rare. Occasionally, if one bone is not fractured there is an associated subluxation or dislocation involving the proximal or distal radio-ulnar articulation.

A generally accepted classification of these fracture types does not exist. The AO classification differentiates between transverse fractures (Type A), fractures with a triangular fragment (Type B) and comminuted fractures (Type C). The presence or absence of displacement as well as any abnormal rotation and angulation should be recorded, and the location of the fracture can be described as involving the proximal, mid, or distal shaft.

Fractures Specific to the Forearm

The **Monteggia** fracture is a fracture of the ulnar shaft or olecranon associated with dislocation of the radial head, and there are four distinct variations according to Brado (Table 1.**12**).

DD The Monteggia fracture must be differentiated from anterior dislocation of the elbow associated with a proximal ulna fracture. The trauma pattern of the Monteggia fracture is more extensive since it entails a tear of the proximal radio-ulnar ligaments (Fig. 1.**165**).

The **Galeazzi** fracture (or reverse Monteggia fracture, Fig. 1.**166**) is an isolated fracture of the radial shaft combined with a posterior ulnar subluxation or dislocation at the distal radioulnar articulation.

X-RAY Radiographic views must include the elbow and the wrist. Exact positioning of the lateral view is extremely important whenever a fracture of the radial head or distal radio-ulnar dislocation is suspected (also see Distal Forearm section).

CT Subluxation and rotatory misalignment, especially of the distal radio-ulnar articulation, are most clearly identified on axial sections.

Special Considerations in the Pediatric Age Group

Fractures of the forearm are frequent in children and most often involve the distal third of the forearm. The so-called **greenstick fractures** are also very common.

! Greenstick fractures are shear fractures and present as a unilateral cortical break with a maintained periosteal cover. Because of therapeutic ramifications, they must be distinguished from torus (compression) fractures.

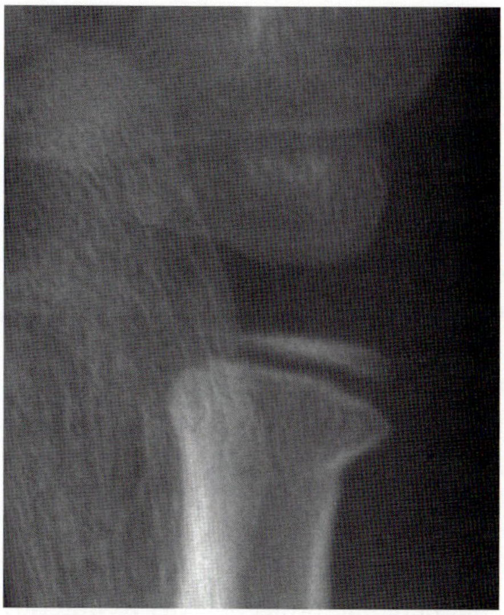

Fig. 1.**164** Salter-Harris Type II fracture of the proximal radial metaphysis.

Table 1.**12** Four distinct variations of Monteggia fractures (according to Brado)

Type 1	Fracture of the ulnar diaphysis with anterior dislocation of the radial head (about 65%)
Type 2	Fracture of the ulnar diaphysis with posterior dislocation of the radial head (about 18%)
Type 3	Fracture of the ulnar metaphysis with lateral dislocation of the radial head (about 16%)
Type 4	Fracture of the proximal one-third of the radius and ulna with anterior dislocation of the radial head

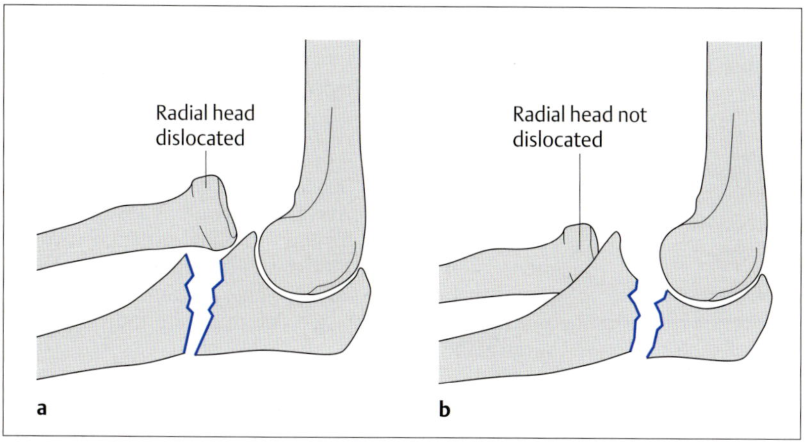

Fig. 1.**165** Comparison of Monteggia fracture Type I (**a**) and anterior fracture-dislocation of the elbow (**b**).

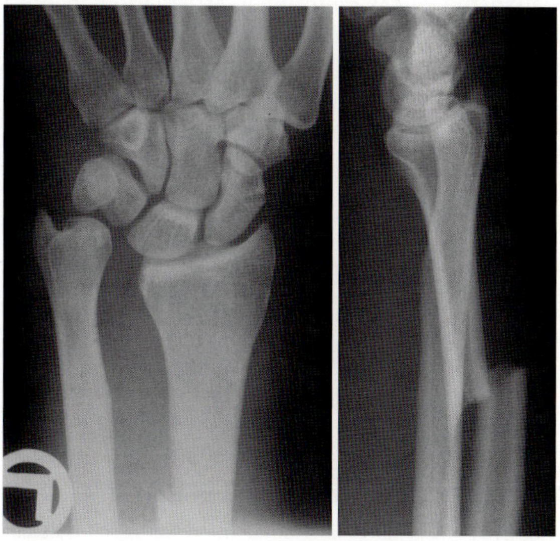

Fig. 1.**166** Galeazzi fracture: radial fracture and distal ulnar dislocation.

Distal Forearm Fractures

Distal forearm fractures are the most common type fractures in adults. Since these fractures are almost never confined to the epiphyseal region of the ulna, they can be viewed as injuries of the distal radius, with or without involvement of the ulna. Hyperextension fractures predominate (85% of cases) and age, gender (osteoporosis) and type of trauma all contribute to the degree of fracture.

Orientation of the fracture line and associated injuries determine the degree of stability or instability of the fracture and the resulting therapeutic approach (Table 1.**13**).

Table 1.**13** Radiologic criteria of instability of distal radial fractures

Definite signs of instability
– Fracture of the ulnar styloid process (= avulsion)
– Radioulnar subluxation or dislocation, intra-articular fracture of the distal radioulnar articulation (= radioulnar separation)
– Comminution of the metaphysis
– Displaced intra-articular fracture or fracture dislocation
Signs suggestive of instability
– Radial shortening > 3 mm
– Posterior angulation of the distal radial fragment > 20°

Fractures of the distal forearm are generally divided into extra- and intra-articular types.

Extra-articular fractures characteristically occur 3–4 cm proximal to the radiocarpal articulation, without involvement of the radiocarpal or distal radio-ulnar articulation. With severe displacement of these fractures, however, the radio-ulnar ligaments are torn.

Intra-articular fractures involve the radiocarpal or radio-ulnar joint, or both.

Classification: Numerous systems have been proposed for classifying these fractures on the basis of conventional radiographic findings.

The AO classification divides the fractures into three major groups, A to C (extra-articular, partial articular, completely articular), each with three subgroups and additional discriminating criteria. These extremely detailed subdivisions according to morphologic pattern and prognostic implication, however, have proved too complicated in the clinical setting.

Since the classification of intra-articular fractures proposed by **Melone** (Type I–IV) is determined by the extent and direction of the displacement of the fragments, it is the categorization most commonly used in the surgical literature.

The old and eponymous classifications of distal radial fractures (Smith, Colles, Barton, etc.), which primarily consider the mechanism of trauma and the direction of displacement (Fig. 1.**168**), are commonly used in clinical practice. However, they neither distinguish between extra- or intra-articular fractures nor include other prognostically relevant criteria (e.g., avulsion of the ulnar styloid process). In particular, the Colles and Smith fractures are better categorized by the system proposed by Frykman (Fig. 1.**169**). Though this classification disregards the lateral radiographic projection (as to anterior or posterior angulation) and the number or displacement of the fragments, it has proven to be a useful treatment guide since it provides an accurate assessment of articular involvement and fracture stability.

The Type VIII **Frykman** fracture has the worst prognosis.

CLINIC **Therapy:** Displaced fractures should be reduced. Conservative therapy is justified if the fracture is stable and shows minimal articular involvement (step deformity of the radiocarpal articulation of less than 1 mm). Instability, signs of ligamentous injuries and marked articular step deformity are indications for surgical intervention.

X-RAY **Technical considerations:** The initial diagnosis is made on radiographs obtained in two views (PA and lateral). It is imperative to visualize the distal radio-ulnar articulation in both projections as this is the only way to exclude radio-ulnar misalignment and to appreciate the orientation of the fracture line through the radio-ulnar articulation (Fig. 1.**167**).

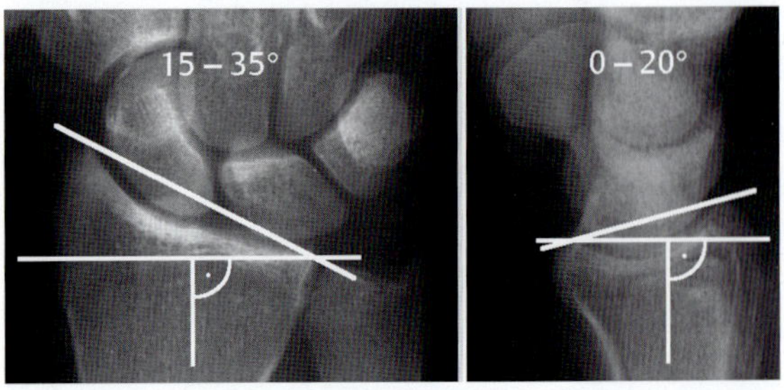

Fig. 1.**167** Normal inclination of the distal radial articular surface.

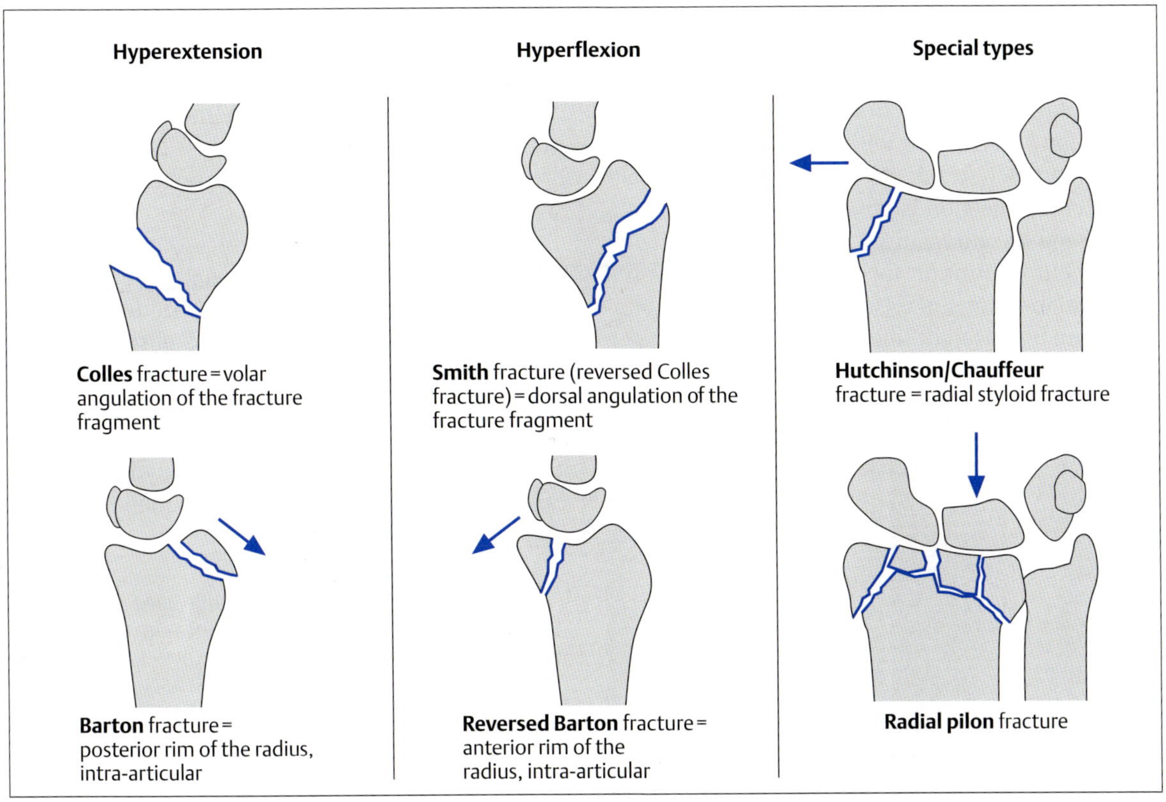

Fig. 1.**168** Classification of distal forearm fractures from a clinical perspective. The arrow indicates the direction of the radiocarpal dislocation associated with the various fractures.

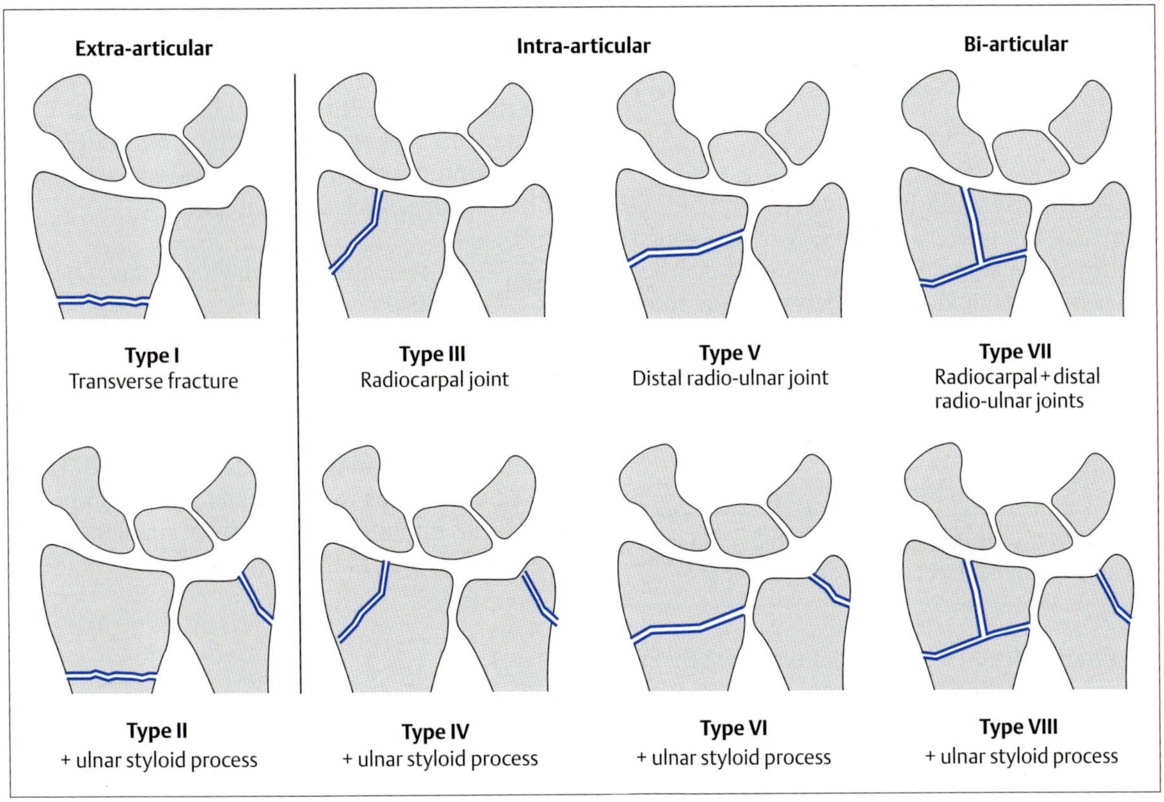

Fig. 1.**169** Classification of distal radial fractures according to Frykman.

To achieve a correct, standardized view of the distal forearm, the forearm must be in **neutral position** for both projections. For the standard PA projection, this implies a 90° abduction of the shoulder and a 90° flexion of the elbow, with the wrist and forearm placed completely flat on the examination table. The lateral projection is obtained with the arm abducted and the elbow in 90° flexion. The forearm is in the neutral position for the lateral projection if the distal forearm, lunate, capitate, and third metacarpal are in a straight line (Fig. 1.**170**).

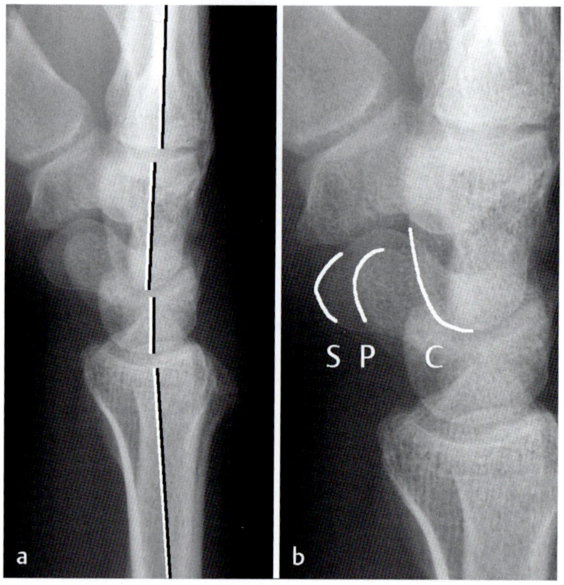

Fig. 1.**170** Criteria for exact positioning of the lateral view of the wrist.

Viewing the relationship between scaphoid, pisiform, and capitate is another way of assessing the quality of the lateral view. The anterior contour of the pisiform should project between the anterior contour of the upper scaphoid pole and the anterior contour of the capitate (SPT = scaphopisocapitate alignment). The ulnar styloid process projects over the posterior one third of the distal radius (Fig. 1.**170**).

! Incorrect positioning for these radiographic views can lead to incorrect diagnosis.

The prognostically relevant relationship of the relative lengths of the radius and ulna can be measured in the neutral position of the wrist only since their relative lengths vary with the position of the forearm. The ulna is relatively longer in supination (ulna plus variance) and shorter in pronation (ulna minus variance) (Fig. 1.**171**).

Radiographically occult fractures of the distal radius can become apparent as hematoma in the palmar muscle compartment with loss of the fat stripe of the pronator quadratus (pronator quadratus sign) (Figs. 1.**172**, 1.**173**).

DD Post-traumatic ulnar elongation must be differentiated from intrinsic ulna plus or minus variance. Comparison views of the contralateral side might resolve any ambiguity.

SONO This is especially useful in the pediatric age group. Step deformities of the cortex can be diagnosed with high-frequency probes (Fig. 1.**174**).

NUC The three-phase radionuclide bone scan can detect occult fractures with focal increased accumulation of tracer being present as early as two days after trauma. Differentiation between soft-tissue injury and bone injury can be difficult, thus limiting the usefulness this technique.

CT CT has replaced conventional tomography since it images the articular region and the surrounding bones and soft tissues without superimposition of other structures. With multiplanar reconstruction, complex fracture lines can also be visualized to better advantage.

Furthermore, CT can show radiographically occult fractures, as well as small intra-articular fragments, and makes an additional contribution by demonstrating rotational malpositions associated with fractures of the distal forearm.

MRI T1-weighted SE sequences and fat-suppression sequences (e.g., STIR) can delineate occult fractures, osteochondral injuries, involvement of the articular surface, and stress fractures (Fig. 1.**175**). Depending on the level and thickness of the slices, associated injuries of ligaments and the triangular fibrocartilage complex (TFCC) can be detected as well. MRI and CT are competing modalities for the definitive evaluation of inconclusive conventional radiographic findings.

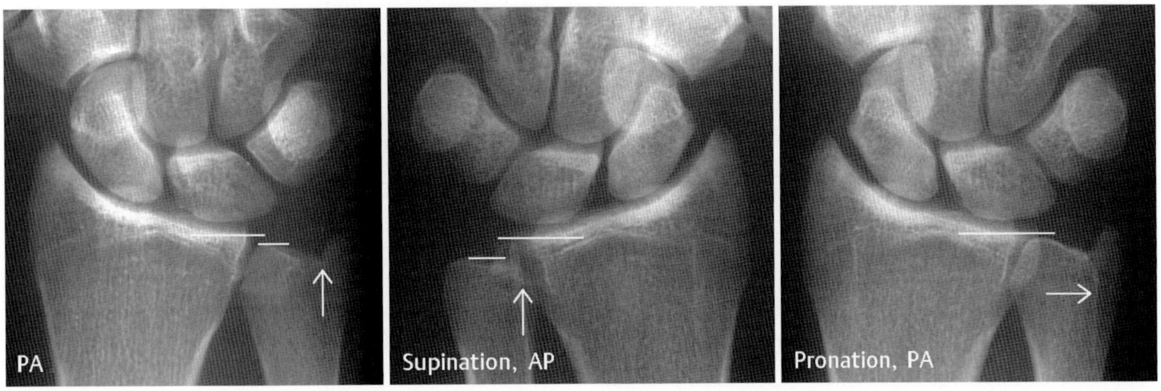

Fig. 1.**171** Ulnar variance related to radiographic positioning, normal findings. **a** Correct PA projection: the groove of the extensor carpi ulnaris is between the ulnar styloid process and ulnar articular surface. **b** Projection in supination shows relative shortening of the ulna. The groove of the extensor carpi ulnaris moves toward the radius. **c** Projection in pronation with relative lengthening of the ulna. The groove of the extensor carpi ulnaris is seen as a linear structure and is displaced toward the ulna.

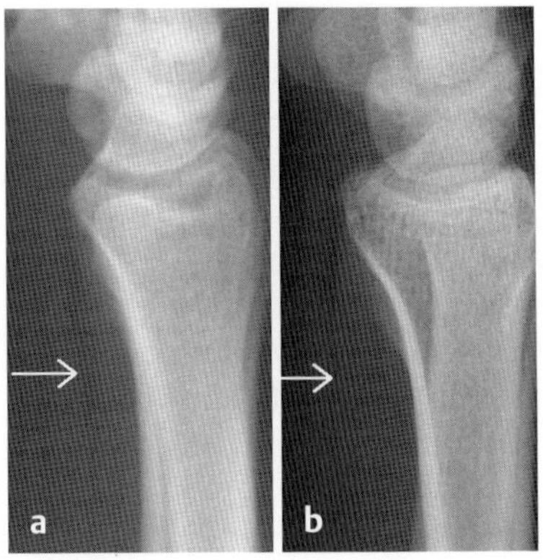

Fig. 1.**172** Normal (**a**) and pathologic (**b**) pronator quadratus fat plane on the lateral radiograph. In **b** the fat stripe is obliterated and displaced anteriorly.

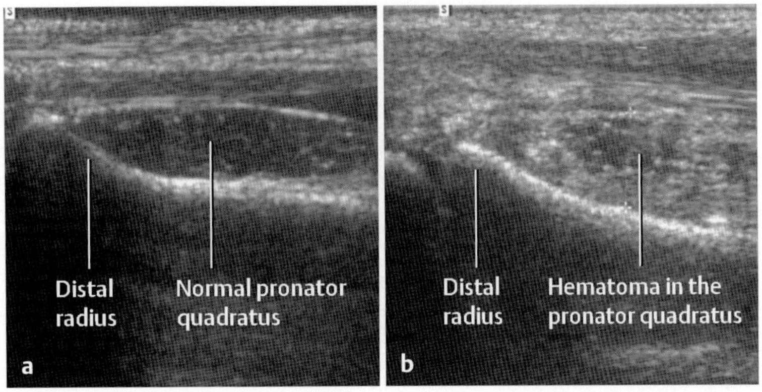

Fig. 1.**173** Normal (**a**) and pathologic (**b**) pronator quadratus by sonography (same patient as in Fig. 1.**172**). Thickening and increased echogenicity of the pronator quadratus indicate hemorrhage.

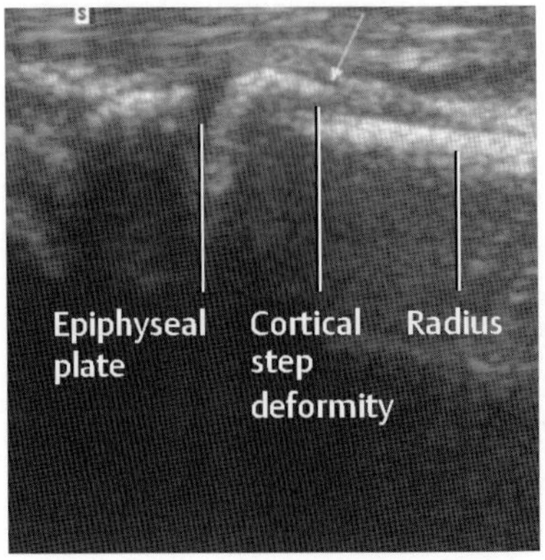

Fig. 1.**174** Sonography of a distal radial fracture in a child (Salter-Harris Type II).

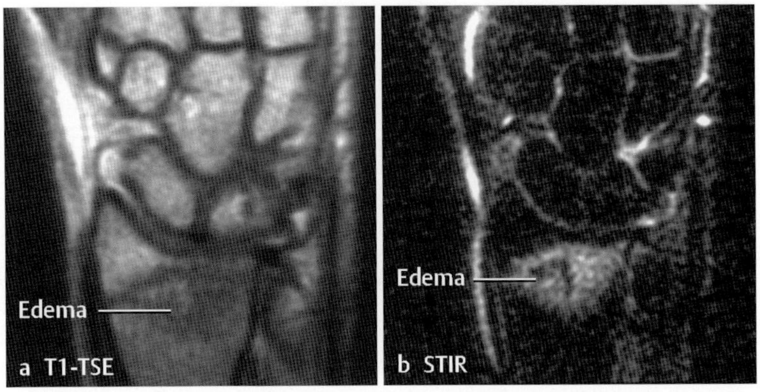

Fig. 1.**175** MRI: (**a**) T1-weighted image and (**b**) STIR image show trabecular fractures with definite bone marrow edema. The patient's radiograph was entirely normal.

Dislocation of the Distal Forearm

■ By definition, distal radio-ulnar derangement with a remaining articular contact of more than 50% is a subluxation whereas articular contact of less than 50% is a dislocation. ■

Distal radio-ulnar and radiocarpal subluxations or dislocations are mainly associated with fractures, including the dislocation of the ulna as part of the Galeazzi fracture-dislocation and the radiocarpal dislocation in all directions as part of the Barton, reversed Barton, or Hutchinson (chauffeur) fractures.

Radiocarpal dislocations imply severe and complex ligamentous ruptures.

These injuries must be distinguished from the isolated distal radial subluxation or dislocation **without** fracture. They are caused by forced pronation or supination with tears of the radio-ulnar ligament and triangular fibrocartilage complex (TFCC). Since the ulna is the fulcrum around which the distal radius rotates in pronation and supination, it is the **radius** that dislocates anteriorly or posteriorly.

X-RAY Radiocarpal and radio-ulnar misalignment can usually be diagnosed with technically adequate views (Table 1.**14**).

CT Sagittal sections demonstrate the axial displacement of any radiocarpal subluxation and dislocation without superimposition of other structures. In comparison to conventional radiography, intra-articular fragments and concomitant injuries are better seen. To grade any distal radial dislocation, axial CT should be compared to the contralateral side, with each side imaged in pronation and supination, particularly in cases with inconclusive radiographic findings. This approach might demonstrate strictly functional instabilities. At the level of the radial tuberosity, the tangents to the dorsal and volar radial contour normally enclose the entire ulna (Fig. 1.**176**).

Injuries of the Triangular Fibrocartilage Complex (TFCC)

Synonyms: ulnar fibrocartilage complex or ulnocarpal meniscus homologue.

■ The TFCC constitutes a complex of various ligaments and an articular disk that serves to connect the distal ulna, distal radio-ulnar joint, and proximal carpal row (Fig. 1.**178**). Lesions of the TFCC primarily cause pain on the ulnar aspect of the wrist. ■

Degenerative lesions (due to overuse or positive ulnar variance) can occur after the age of 30 years and frequently involve the disk centrally. Traumatic lesions, especially if they are part of distal radial fractures with involvement of the ulnar styloid process, involve the sites of the radial and ulnar attachment and usually are vertically oriented. TFCC lesions are generally described using the classification proposed by **Palmer**.

X-RAY Radiographic views serve to exclude osseous lesions and to detect anomalies (ulna plus variance).

Arthrography (injection of contrast medium usually into the radiocarpal **and** radio-ulnar joint compartment) generally shows TFCC defects as extension of the contrast medium into the disk. However, a definitive differentiation between a traumatic or degenerative injury is not possible and any concomitant soft-tissue injuries are not demonstrable. One advantage of arthrography is being able to follow the dynamics of the distribution of the instilled contrast medium during fluoroscopy and stress views. An additional benefit is the high resolution of even small marginal defects (Fig. 1.**177**).

! To evaluate the TFCC for post-traumatic lesions, especially when medicolegal questions have to be answered, comparison arthrography of **both** wrists is often necessary.

MRI With suitable echo sequences (3-D gradient echo sequences, coronal plane, 0.6–1.0 mm slice thickness), lesions of the triangular fibrocartilage are often shown as areas of hyperintense defects. But even MRI cannot offer a reliable morphologic differentiation between degenerative and traumatic changes.

Direct (Fig. 1.**179**) or indirect MR arthrography is increasingly applied for clarification because of its presumed superior sensitivity to conventional MRI. Compared to conventional arthrography, MR arthrography has the advantage of demonstrating the surrounding soft tissues, cartilage, trabecular bone (occult fracture?), and ligaments, but it has not yet achieved the accuracy of conventional arthrography and arthroscopy. At the present time, no generally accepted clinical recommendation for utilization of these imaging techniques in the wrist can be offered.

Table 1.**14** Radiologic findings of distal radio-ulnar dislocation

Fracture through the base of the ulnar styloid process
Widening of the radioulnar joint space (> 3 mm) in the PA projection
Deviation of the ulna in the AP projection
Shortening of the radius of more than 5 mm relative to the ulna after radial fracture

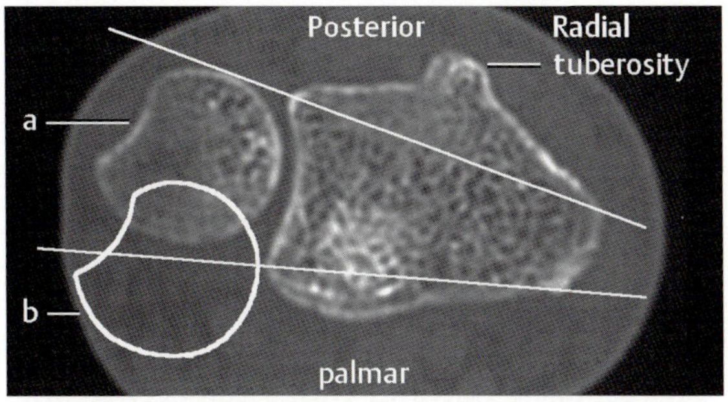

Fig. 1.**176** Normal articulation of the distal radio-ulnar joint on axial CT at the level of the radial tuberosity. **a** Normal finding, the ulna lies within the radial tangents. **b** Posterior dislocation of the radius.

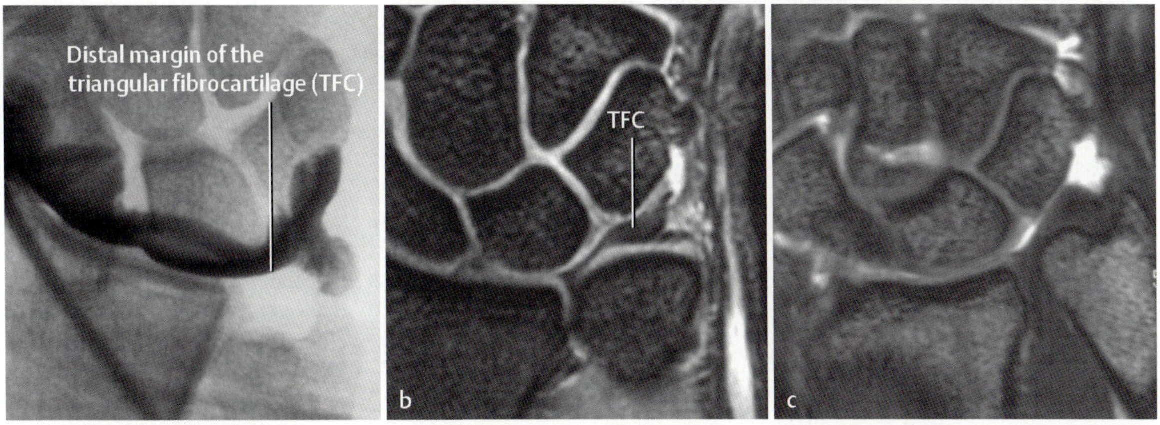

Fig. 1.**177** Normal proximal arthrographic delineation of the triangular fibrocartilage (**a** radiocarpal injection). Normal triangular fibrocartilage on MRI (**b** GRE sequence) and MR arthrography (**c** GRE sequence).

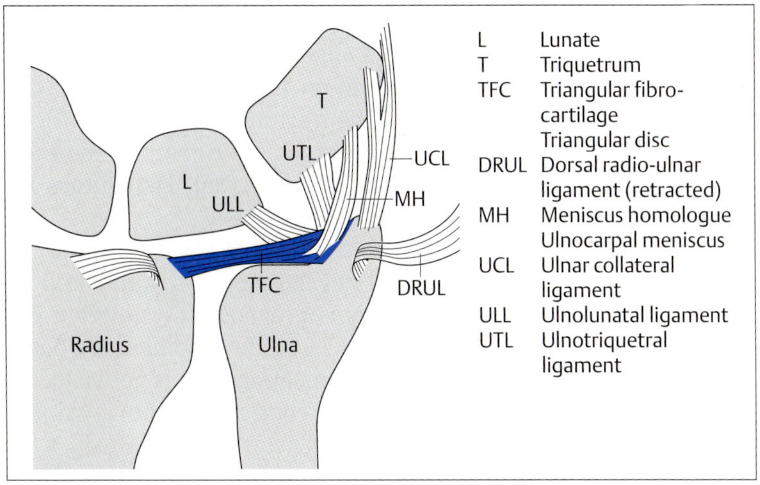

L	Lunate
T	Triquetrum
TFC	Triangular fibrocartilage Triangular disc
DRUL	Dorsal radio-ulnar ligament (retracted)
MH	Meniscus homologue Ulnocarpal meniscus
UCL	Ulnar collateral ligament
ULL	Ulnolunatal ligament
UTL	Ulnotriquetral ligament

Fig. 1.**178** Anatomic diagram of the ulnocarpal triangular fibrocartilage complex (TFCC), seen from the dorsum of the wrist.

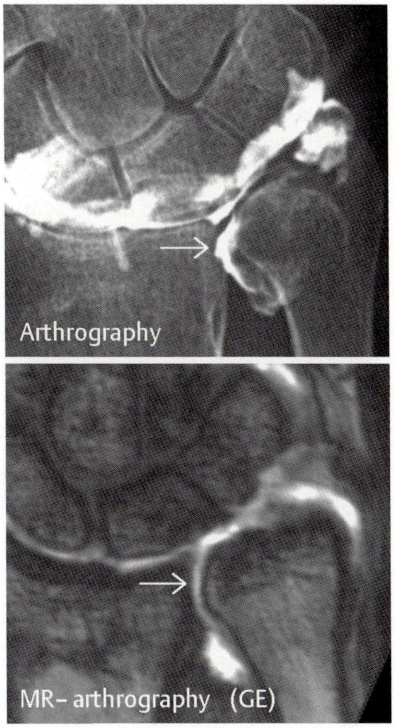

Right:
Fig. 1.**179** Lesion of the triangular fibrocartilage. After radiocarpal injection, extension of contrast medium into the distal radio-ulnar joint (arrow).

Fractures of the Carpal Bones

About 70% of fractures of the carpal bones affect the scaphoid, with two-thirds of the fracture lines traversing the middle segment. Transverse fractures are most frequent. Because of the decreasing arterial supply from distal to proximal, proximal fractures have a high propensity to become osteonecrotic and form a pseudarthrosis.

All complete fractures with a gap between the fragments of more than 1 mm are considered unstable, and up to 50% result in a pseudarthrosis after conservative therapy. Associated injuries of the radial styloid process, lunate, and capitate are not infrequent, as well as ligamentous lesions with scapholunate disassociation or perilunate dislocation. A special type is the transscaphoid perilunate fracture dislocation of de Quervain (Fig. 1.**180**).

Isolated fractures of the remaining carpal bones are less frequent (< 1 – 15%); of these the ligamentous avulsion fracture of the triquetrum is the most common. Complex carpal fractures are increasingly diagnosed because of the improvement in diagnostic techniques, especially CT.

X-RAY **Technical considerations:** The standard views of the wrist in two projections must often be supplemented by additional views determined by the clinical findings. Special navicular views may show an initially undetected fracture.

! As an alternative to the navicular views, a coned-down view as proposed by **Stecher** can be helpful. This radiograph is obtained in ulnar deviation with the fist clenched and displays an optimal longitudinal profile of the scaphoid (Fig. 1.**181**).

The so-called 'scaphoid fat pad sign' can also be helpful as a fracture-induced hematoma will obliterate this fat stripe along the radiocarpal collateral ligament.

In addition to documenting the fracture site, the displacement and number of fragments should be recorded, as well as any signs of ligamentous instability.

! Since fractures of the carpal bones are frequently not detected, even with the help of special views, further evaluation is indicated if the radiographs are normal and the clinical suspicion of a fracture remains strong.

NUC The three-phase bone scan has been proposed as a sensitive method to detect radiographically occult fractures of the carpal bones, and a negative study 72 hours after injury virtually excludes fracture. The role of nuclear medicine has declined with the increasing utilization of CT and MRI.

CT High-resolution CT (1 mm slice thickness) can detect subtle fractures not seen on conventional radiography. The advantage of CT is the exact assignment of the dislocated fragment to its site of origin, the delineation of even the smallest intra-articular fragments, and the assessment of associated subluxation and dislocation (Figs. 1.**182**, 1.**183**).

CT reformation can show the articulations in various planes and allow analysis of even complex injury patterns.

! CT is the method of choice to evaluate the often complex injuries of the carpal **bones.** For occult scaphoid fractures, CT is often preferred to MRI since it allows an exquisite assessment of the healing process (especially of scaphoid fractures). Not infrequently, this can shorten the period of wrist immobilization.

MRI Even in the acute phase immediately after trauma, MRI can establish a definitive diagnosis. However, the presence of edema alone cannot be equated with a fracture, since it may merely represent trabecular microfractures (Fig. 1.**184**). The edema appears of high signal intensity on STIR images and on T2-weighted images with fat suppression. The fracture line may be difficult to see within edematous bone marrow. Furthermore, MRI can reveal associated ligamentous injury.

A considerable advantage of MRI is its ability to assess the viability of the proximal scaphoid fracture fragment. This is prognostically relevant because of the high risk of the development of a pseudarthrosis if the proximal fragment is not viable. In this setting injection of contrast medium is mandatory.

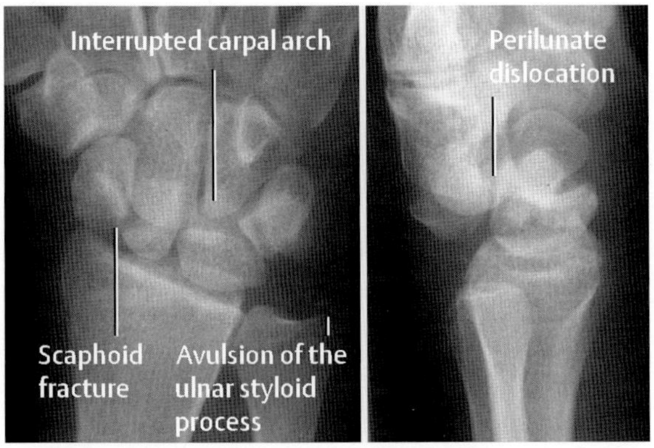

Fig. 1.**180** De Quervain fracture-dislocation.

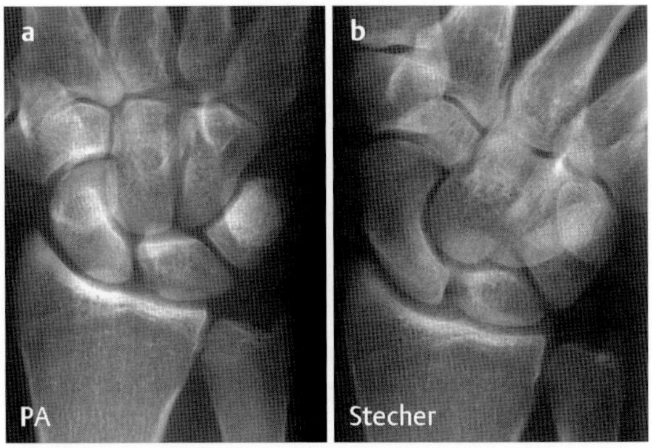

Fig. 1.**181** Comparison of the PA view (**a**) with the special navicular (Stecher) view (**b**). Normal finding.

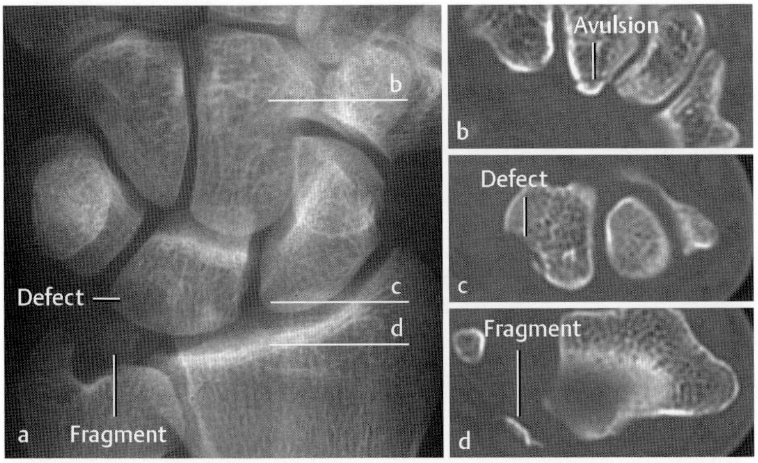

Fig. 1.**182** Osseous avulsion of the lunate. **a** The radiograph shows the displaced fragment as well as the defect in the lunate. CT (**b–d**) reveals an additional dorsal avulsion of the capitate.

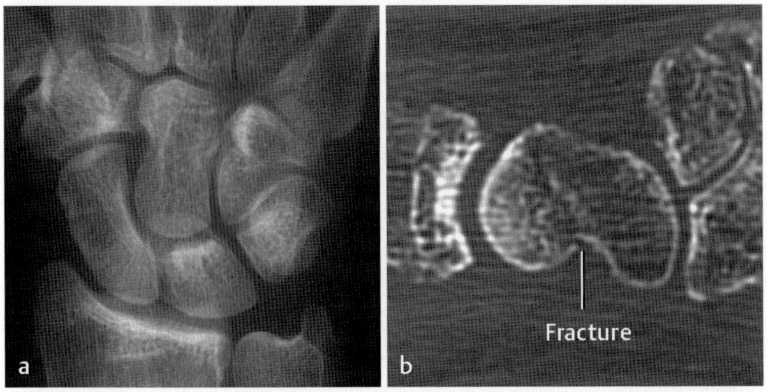

Fig. 1.**183** CT (**b** examination performed with a cast in place) of an acute navicular fracture. The fracture is not visualized on the conventional radiograph (**a**).

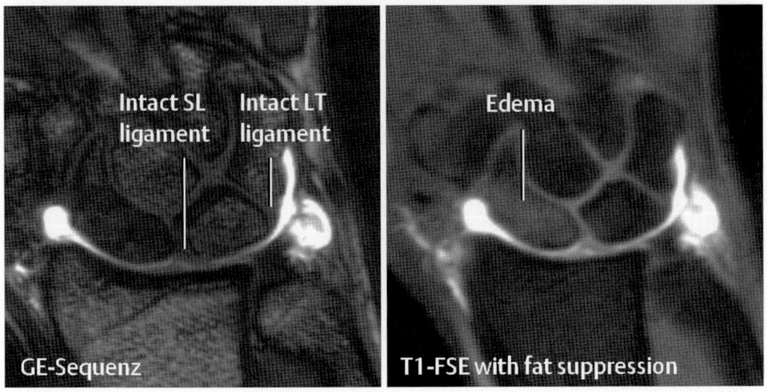

Fig. 1.**184** Because of a clinically suspected injury of the scapholunate (SL) ligament and a normal radiographic examination, direct MR arthrography was performed. It showed intact ligaments, but there is a trabecular fracture within the scaphoid.

Carpal Derangements

Carpal derangements refer to misalignment of the carpal bones relative to each other. They are usually post-traumatic (predominately hyperextension trauma) but can be degenerative, developmental, or inflammatory in origin.

Anatomic considerations (Fig. 1.**186**): Misalignment is invariably caused by ligamentous lesions. The functionally separate proximal carpal row (scaphoid, lunate, and triquetrum) and distal carpal row (trapezium, trapezoid, capitate, and hamate) are connected to each other through 'intrinsic' intercarpal ligaments. They are connected to the distal forearm and the metacarpals by 'extrinsic' ligaments. The most important stabilizers are the scapholunate (SL) ligament and lunatotriquetral (LT) ligament, both of which are intrinsic and interosseous.

Clinical severity separates the static misalignment (at rest) from dynamic misalignments (elicited only with motion). Using the **proximal** carpal row as a reference, the most complex trauma pattern can be classified as follows (Table 1.**15**):

- carpal instability dissociation **(CID)** of the proximal row with lesions of the SL and/or LT ligaments,
- carpal instability nondissociation **(CIND)**,
- carpal instability complex **(CIC)**.

! Increasingly sophisticated ligamentous reconstruction surgery mandates early detection of ligamentous injuries and instabilities.

X-RAY Alignment of the carpal bones, axial orientation, and relative congruence are determined with the help of auxiliary lines (Fig. 1.**187**).
Important: Since the proximal and distal carpal rows slide in opposite directions with radial and ulnar deviation and, in addition, the proximal carpal row is dorsiflexed in ulnar deviation and palmar flexed in radial deviation, PA and lateral views must be obtained with the wrist exactly in neutral position. Faulty positioning may mimic a functional tilt of the lunate.

In the lateral view, the lunate is in an intercalated segment that serves as the axis of rotation. The radiolunate angle is used to describe the instability pattern of the proximal row (Fig. 1.**185**):

- dorsiflexion exceeding 15° corresponds to a dorsal intercalated segmental instability **(DISI)**,
- palmar flexion exceeding 15° corresponds to a volar intercalated segmental instability **(VISI)**.

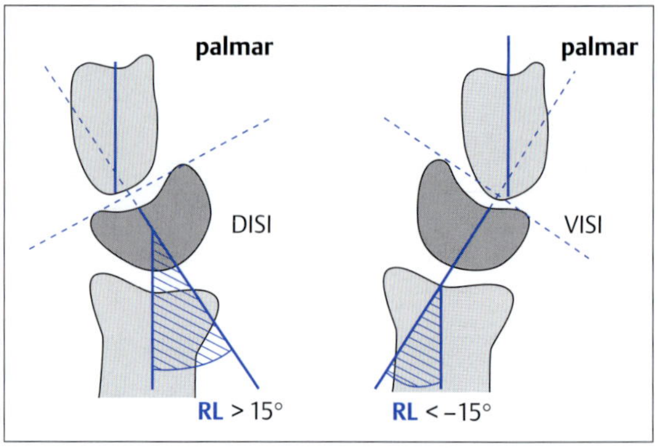

Fig. 1.**185** Determination of the direction and angulation of instability on the lateral radiograph.

Additional radiographic views include PA projections in maximal radial and ulnar deviation, as well as lateral views in full palmar flexion and dorsiflexion.

Cinematography is indicated if the clinical findings suggest a dynamic instability. Manipulation of the wrist during fluoroscopy (with video recording) can reveal instabilities that are not evident on other conventional radiographic views.

Arthrography: With the injection of contrast medium, disruptions of the intercarpal ligaments can be demonstrated by the unidirectional or bidirectional flow between the compartments of the wrist joint. The clinical importance of these findings remains controversial since abnormal flow of contrast medium can also be seen in asymptomatic patients older than 30 years as a manifestation of premature ligamentous degeneration. Nevertheless, three-compartment arthrography (midcarpal, radiocarpal, and distal radioulnar carpal compartments) is still considered the gold standard for the evaluation of ligamentous disruptions. Ideally, the asymptomatic contralateral side should be examined for comparison, but this is not always practical.

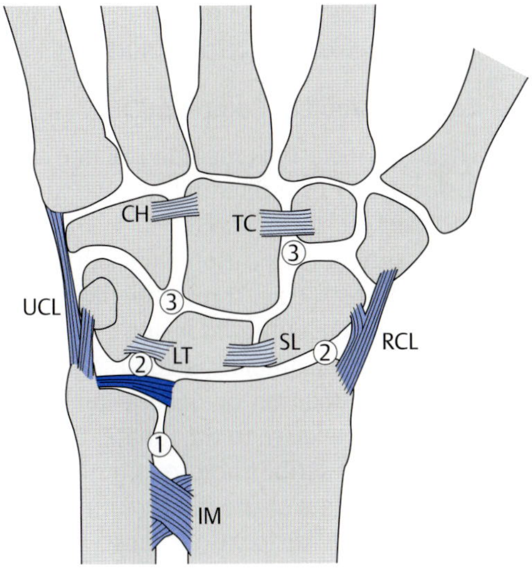

Fig. 1.**186** The most important interosseous (intrinsic) ligaments and compartments of the midcarpal and radiocarpal articulations.

Table 1.**15** Classification of carpal instability

Category	Subcategory	Primarily affected ligaments/trauma pattern
CID	SL dissociation	Rupture of the SL ligament
	LT dissociation	Rupture of the LT ligament
CIND	Radiocarpal instability, posterior	Radiocarpal ligaments (often in a misaligned healed radial fracture)
	Midcarpal instability	Rupture of the triquetrocapitate ligament
	Ulnar translocation	Lesion of the radiocarpal ligaments (also seen in rheumatoid arthritis)
CIC	Perilunate dislocation	Scapholunate/radioscapholunate ligament
	Transscaphoid, perilunate fracture-dislocation	Radioscaphocapitate ligament

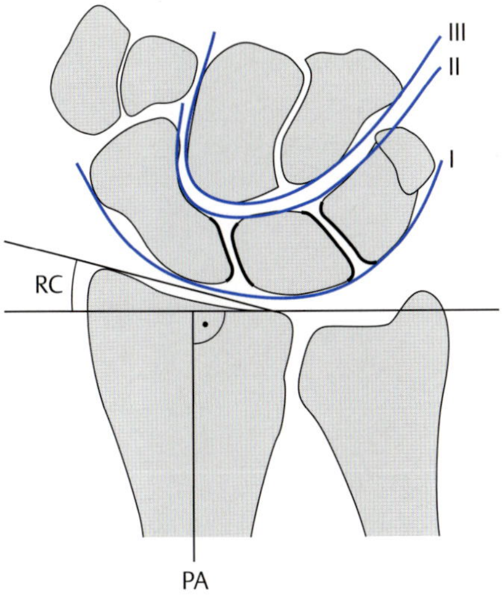

Fig. 1.**187** The most important auxiliary lines for the evaluation of the PA radiograph of the wrist.

MRI MRI has become more important in the diagnostic evaluation of ligamentous injuries of the wrist because of its ability to directly delineate the majority of the ligamentous structures. However not all of the ligaments are invariably visualized (e.g., radioscaphoid lunate ligament and radiolunate ligament). Thin coronal sections achieve the best delineation of the lunotriquetral (LT) and scapholunate (SL) ligaments, but only 50% to 70% of ruptures of these ligaments are detected by this technique. Failure to visualize individual ligaments should not be assumed to be evidence of rupture in all patients.

MR arthrography with direct (intra-articular) or indirect (intravenous) administration of gadolinium-based contrast medium can increase the detection rate of ligamentous injuries (Fig. 1.**188**). Indirect MR arthrography has been found to display ligamentous ruptures as sites of contrast enhancement, but the experience so far is inadequate to justify routine clinical use.

Carpal Instability Disassociation (CID)

The most frequent CID is the scapholunate disassociation, referring to an increased separation between the scaphoid and lunate due to a rupture of the SL ligament. On the PA view, it is only recognized if the scapholunate joint space is widened by more than 3 mm ('Terry-Thomas sign' or, more currently, 'David Letterman sign', Fig. 1.**189**) and suggests a DISI misalignment. Stress views or cinematography can detect this lesion at an earlier stage.

Lunatotriquetral disassociation following rupture of the LT ligament is less frequent and is primarily characterized by a static VISI misalignment with conventional radiography.

Carpal Instability Nondissociation (CIND)

Essentially, a distinction is made between radiocarpal CIND (between radius and proximal carpal row) and midcarpal CIND (between proximal and distal carpal rows).

Functional testing usually elicits a snapping or clicking sensation on wrist motion. The underlying causes are congenital ligamentous weakness (e.g., Madelung deformity) and post-traumatic or post-arthritic changes (e.g., rheumatoid arthritis).

Radiocarpal dissociations (in DISI or VISI misalignment) are most frequent after distal radial fractures. In most cases, the radiographic findings are often suggestive, and the most revealing information is provided by cinematography, which also best differentiates the osseous movement patterns.

Misalignment at rest is best evaluated by CT and MRI because of the superior delineation of any incongruence of the articular surfaces.

Carpal Instability Complex (CIC)

These dissociations include isolated and combined dislocations of individual or several carpal bones, and fracture-dislocations.

Perilunate dislocations and perilunate fracture-dislocations (e.g., transscaphoid) are the most frequently encountered lesions. Perilunate dislocations often accompany distal radial fractures, usually as subluxation or dislocation of the scaphoid or capitate relative to the lunate. Despite staging, it is best to describe the direction of the dislocation and orientation of the fracture line.

Perilunate dislocation must be distinguished from true lunate dislocation (Fig. 1.**190**).

Dislocations and fracture-dislocations of the distal carpal row and carpometacarpal articulations are best grouped under the heading of axial trauma patterns. The description is based on the displacement and axial deviation of the affected bone.

X-RAY Standard radiographic views in two 90° projections can establish the diagnosis in the majority of cases if radiocarpal auxiliary lines are applied. Care should be taken to distinguish radiocarpal misalignment from perilunate and lunate dislocations (Fig. 1.**191**).

CT If the dislocation pattern or the presence of associated fractures is inconclusive on the radiographs, CT can be helpful especially with the use of direct sagittal sections. In addition, sagittal planes can be reformatted from coronal or axial sections and in selected cases, 3-D reconstructions may influence therapeutic planning.

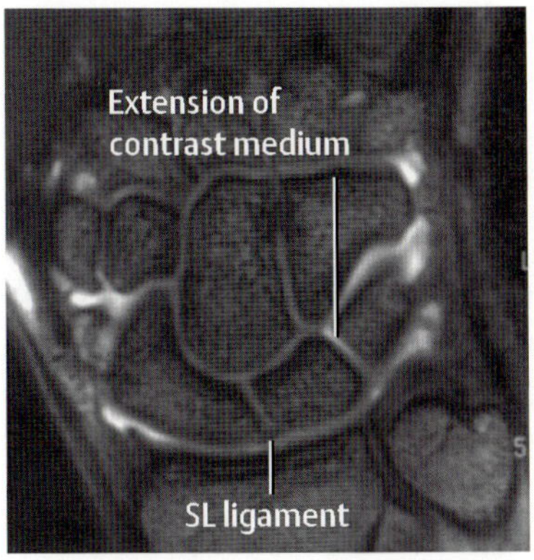

Fig. 1.**188** MR arthrography (radiocarpal injection, T1-weighted images, fat suppression) showing extension of contrast through a torn lunotriquetral (LT) ligament.

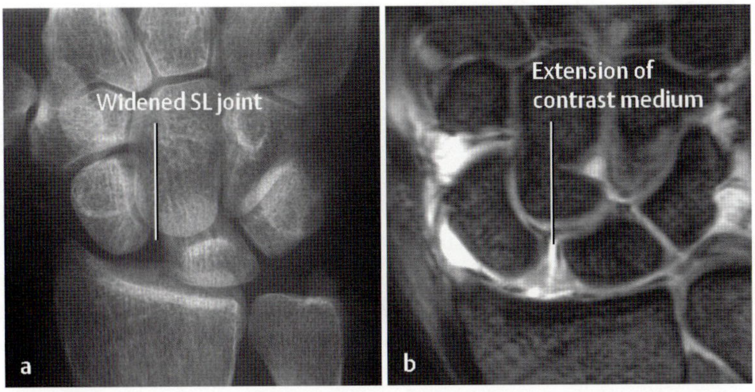

Fig. 1.**189** Scapholunate dissociation. The radiograph shows the **'Terry-Thomas sign'** or **'David Letterman sign'**, representing a widened scapholunate space of more than 3 mm. The MR arthrogram (**b** GRE sequence) shows extension of contrast into the scapholunate joint following radiocarpal injection, indicating a tear of the SL ligament.

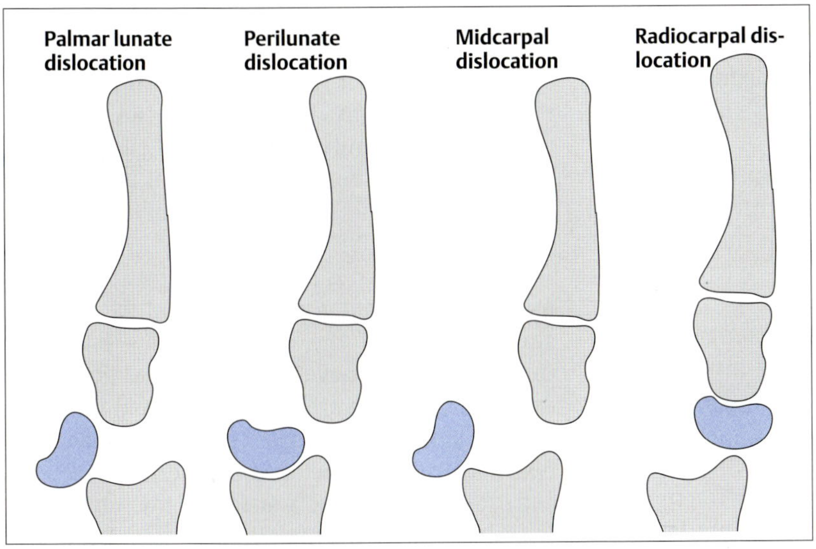

Fig. 1.**190** Manifestations of various dislocations as seen on the lateral radiograph.

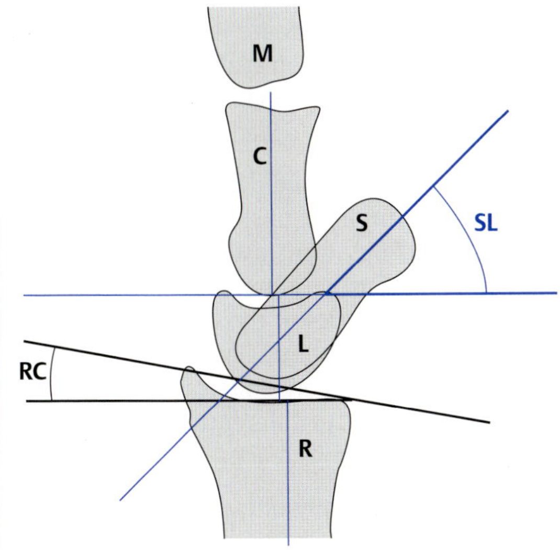

Pathologic findings of the lateral radiograph

- Deviation of the co-linearity of the axes of the third metacarpal (**M**), capitate (**C**), lunate (**L**), and radius (**R**) by more than 15°
- **SL** angle < 30°, > 60°
- **RL**, **CL** angle < −15°, > +15°
- **RS** angle < − 30°, > 60°
- **RC** angle = 0 – 20°

Fig. 1.**191** The most important auxiliary lines used for the evaluation of the lateral radiograph of the wrist.

Carpometacarpal Injuries

These injuries consist primarily of carpometacarpal intra-articular fracture-dislocations or dislocations, mainly involving the fifth ray. They are often associated with other injuries, most commonly with posterior dislocations.

A special situation is encountered with fractures involving the saddle (sellar) joint between the first metacarpal and trapezium (Fig. 1.**193**):

1. An intra-articular fracture dislocation with an oblique avulsion fracture of the metacarpal base is referred to as the **Bennett** fracture. A Y-shaped or comminuted fracture of the metacarpal base including metacarpal shortening is referred to as the **Rolando** fracture.
2. An extra-articular fracture of the first metacarpal is referred to as the **Winterstein** fracture.

X-RAY Radiography may not adequately show the trauma pattern because of the superimposition of other carpometacarpal structures. A crucial criterion confirming a normal articulation is the preserved M-shaped line formed by the carpometacarpal articular surfaces on the PA view of the hand (Fig. 1.**195**).

CT CT may adequately characterize complex trauma patterns including intra-articular extension of fractures and fracture-dislocations.

Injuries of the Metacarpals

A distinction should be made between fractures involving the base (often with concomitant fracture-dislocations) from fractures of the midcarpal shaft and subcapital region, and intra-articular fractures of the metacarpal head.

The fracture of the metacarpal head is characterized by intra-articular step deformity.

A special type of injury is the 'skier's thumb' representing a rupture of the ulnar collateral ligament, often with an osseous avulsion fracture of the proximal phalanx of the thumb (Fig. 1.**194**). Inappropriate treatment of this fracture leads to a distinct functional impairment of the thumb from an unstable metacarpophalangeal articulation.

X-RAY Conventional radiography is generally adequate, requiring two projections to determine the extent of angulation, shortening or rotation. Stress views of the first metacarpal base can be used to diagnose an injured ulnar collateral ligament by comparison with the contralateral side.

CT CT has replaced conventional tomography in evaluating fractures not adequately shown by radiograph, particularly with suspected intra-articular extension.

SONO Sonography and MRI can diagnose injuries of the ulnar collateral ligament of the thumb and distinguish between undisplaced and displaced ruptures, but neither technique has been advocated for routine clinical use at this time.

Fractures and Dislocations of the Fingers

Extra-articular fractures of the phalangeal shaft and intra-articular fractures of the phalangeal base and head must be distinguished from avulsion fractures involving the sites of tendon insertion.

Unnatural positions without detectable fractures suggest tendon ruptures.

A distal rupture of the extensor tendon or an avulsion fracture of the insertion of the tendon at the distal phalanx can produce the so-called 'swan-neck deformity'. This finding is characterized by simultaneous flexion of the distal interphalangeal (DIP) joint and hyperextension of the proximal interphalangeal (PIP) joint.

Another pattern is the so-called 'buttonhole deformity' with simultaneous flexion of the PIP joint and extension of the DIP joint. This finding is caused by a tear or avulsion of the insertion of the extensor tendon overlying the proximal interphalangeal joint. A distinction should be made between avulsions of the osseous insertion of tendon and osteochondral (intra-articular) fractures.

Dislocations of the fingers occur more frequently at the PIP joint than at the DIP joint.

X-RAY Two projections are mandatory, with the lateral projection exactly positioned since subluxations and other small juxta-articular fractures can be easily overlooked otherwise.

SONO The accuracy and dependability of sonography in distinguishing avulsions of ligamentous insertions from osteochondral fractures are improving. Furthermore, sonography can directly visualize injuries of the collateral ligaments and effusions of the interphalangeal joint in selected cases. Performing sonography as a dynamic examination also helps to differentiate complete from incomplete ligamentous tears.

MRI MRI essentially offers the same performance as sonography, with the notable exception that, unlike sonography, it cannot be executed dynamically.

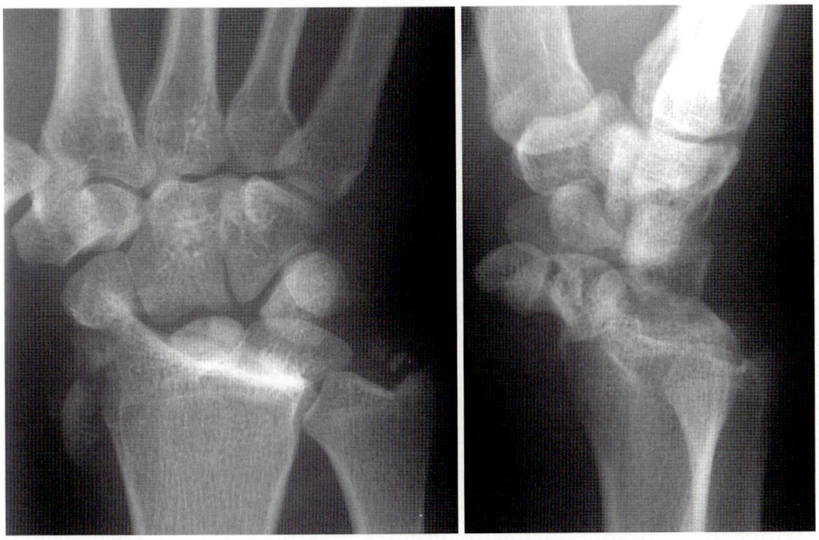

Fig. 1.**192** Complex carpal trauma. The trauma can be described as 'transcapital, transscaphoid, radiocarpal dislocation with avulsion of the ulnar styloid process and radial styloid process.'

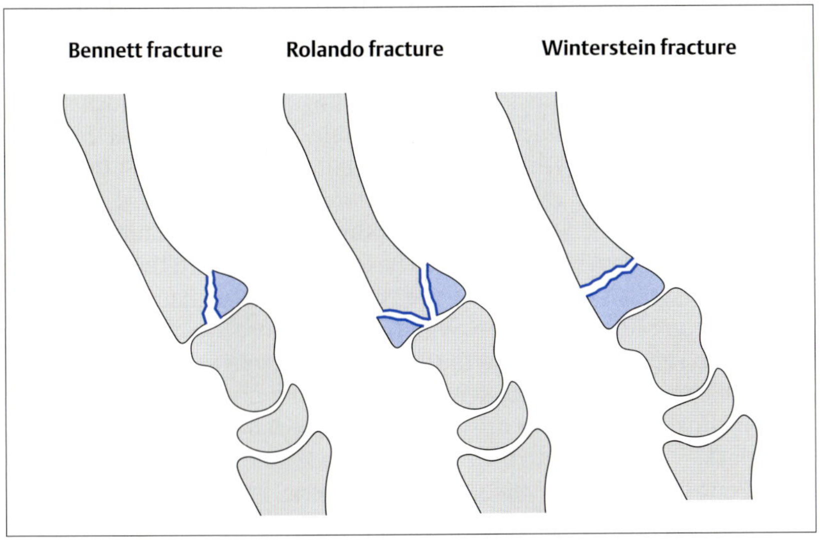

Fig. 1.**193** Typical fracture patterns encountered at the first metacarpal base.

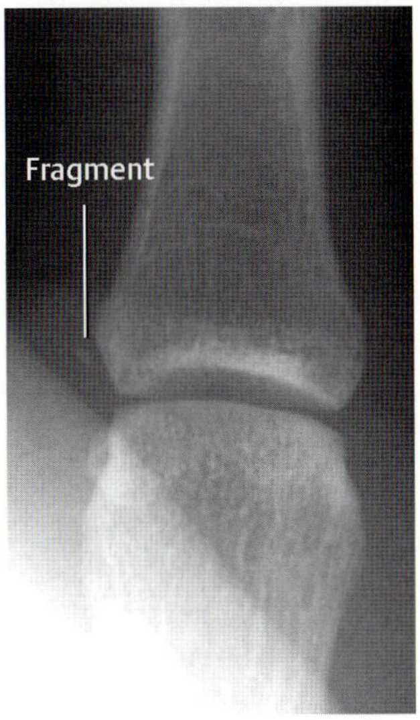

Fig. 1.**194** Skier's thumb with a small avulsed osseous fragment.

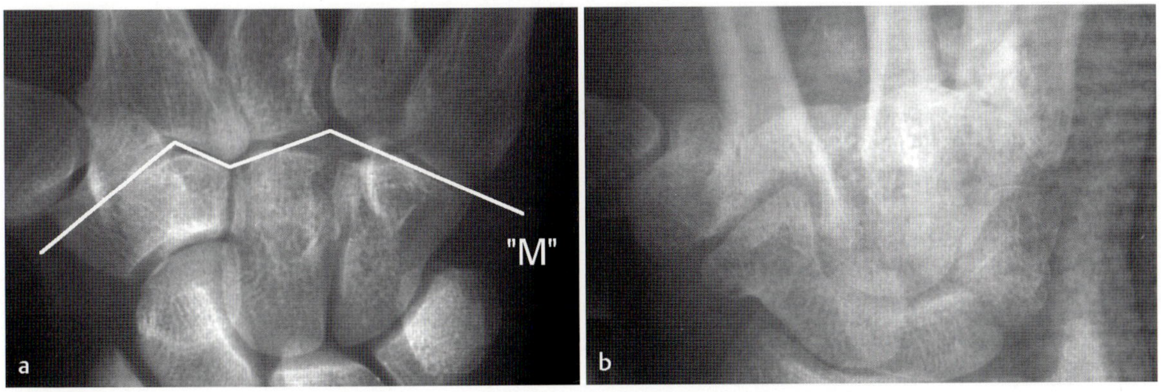

Fig. 1.**195** The 'M' line can be used to evaluate the position of the metacarpophalangeal joints.
a Normal finding.
b Dislocation of the second through fifth metacarpophalangeal joints.

Lower Extremity

Femur and Patella

Fractures of the Proximal Femur

Fractures of the proximal femur typically occur in older people. Because of diminished bone mineral density from senile osteoporosis, fractures can occur even after minor trauma, such as a fall on the hip. Stress fractures in athletes and pathologic fractures through focal osseous lesions are not as common. The classification of the proximal femoral fractures is illustrated in Fig. 1.**196**.

Subcapital Fractures of the Femoral Neck

The subcapital fracture of the femoral neck is the commonest fracture in this anatomic site and, in contrast to the basicervical fracture, it is intracapsular. Potential complications include:
- avascular necrosis of the femoral head (10–20%),
- delayed fracture healing or pseudarthrosis (5–25%)
- secondary degenerative osteoarthritis.

Classification according to Pauwels: Three types of subcapital femoral neck fractures are described and are based on the angulation of the fracture line relative to the horizontal plane (Fig. 1.**199**). The risk of femoral head slippage, pseudarthrosis, or avascular necrosis increases with greater inclination of the fracture line through the femoral neck.
Classification according to Garden: Four types of subcapital femoral neck fractures are described in this classification and are based on the displacement of the fracture fragments (Fig. 1.**200**). The risk of injury to the lateral epiphyseal vessels and the risk of avascular necrosis of the femoral head are greater with increasing fragment displacement.
Therapy: In patients older than 65 years who have a fracture type associated with a high risk of avascular necrosis of the femoral head, the fracture is primarily treated with a total hip arthroplasty. The remaining cases are treated conservatively, usually with internal fixation.

X-RAY The diagnosis and classification of fractures with displaced fragments are easily accomplished with radiography. However, nondisplaced femoral neck fractures and insufficiency fractures may show only trabecular disruption or a faint delicate radiopaque line (Figs. 1.**197**, 1.**198**). If the radiographic findings are inconclusive, CT and MRI are indicated to exclude the presence of a fracture.

MRI In cases where radiographs are inconclusive, MRI can diagnose a fracture and also uncover early signs of avascular necrosis. However, it cannot predict the **risk** of avascular necrosis at the time of acute fracture.

Intertrochanteric Fractures

These fractures occur in the region of the lesser trochanter and extend upward and laterally to the greater trochanter. In rare cases, the fracture line extends inferiorly (reverse intertrochanteric fracture). In this setting, the fragments may be displaced and result in a comminuted fracture with three, four, or more fragments. In general, these fractures require more severe trauma that causes subcapital fractures. The more severe trauma, coupled with the larger fracture surfaces, is responsible for the more extensive soft-tissue injuries and hemorrhage that accompany this type of fracture.

The classification of these fractures as ‘stable’ or ‘unstable’ is misleading since all intertrochanteric fractures are unstable without internal fixation. This description implies instead whether the surgical fixation is easy or difficult.

For the sake of simplification, a fracture with two fragments can be called stable, with the notable exception of the reversed intertrochanteric fracture. Fractures with three and more fragments are unstable, and the instability worsens with the disruption of the femoral calcar (the critical weight-bearing spur arising from the medial cortex and extending into the trabecular space) and the lesser trochanter. Reverse intertrochanteric fractures are extremely unstable.

Fractures of the Femoral Shaft

The femoral shaft is the most resilient bone in the human body. Thus, any fracture of the femoral shaft indicates considerable trauma and is usually associated with other injuries such as blood loss and shock.

Motor vehicle accidents are the commonest cause of femoral shaft fractures and are usually associated with injuries to other sites. The adductor muscles, which insert on the medial side of the femur, pull the distal fragment upward and place it in a typical varus position. Segmental fractures are common.

Fractures of the Distal Femur

Axial forces with valgus stress and rotation are responsible for fractures of the distal femur. Three types are distinguished (Fig. 1.**201**):

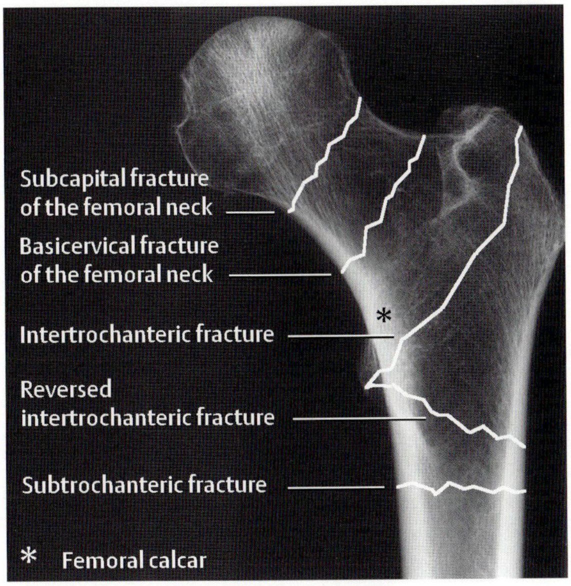

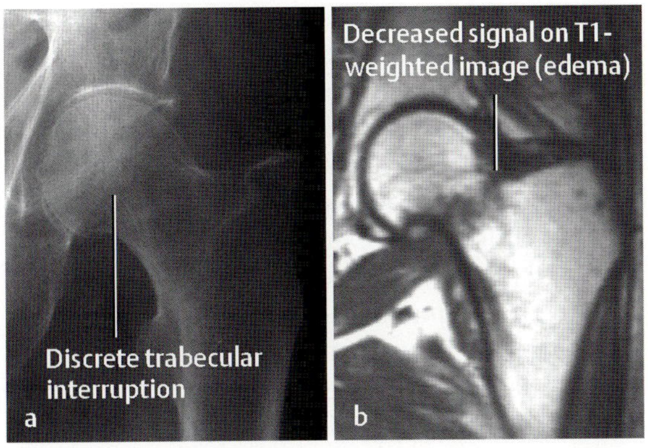

Fig. 1.**197** Radiographically barely recognizable fracture of the base of the femoral neck. MRI (T1-weighted image) reveals the linear edema of the fracture.

Left:
Fig. 1.**196** Classification of proximal femoral fractures. Specimen radiograph.

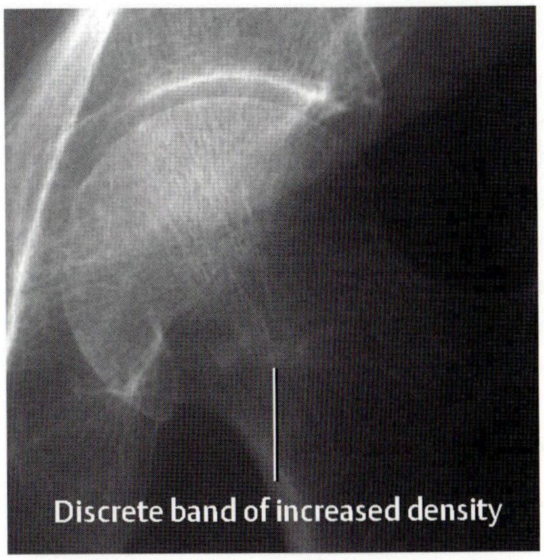

Fig. 1.**198** Femoral neck fracture. Caution! A fracture 'cleft' is not always identified.

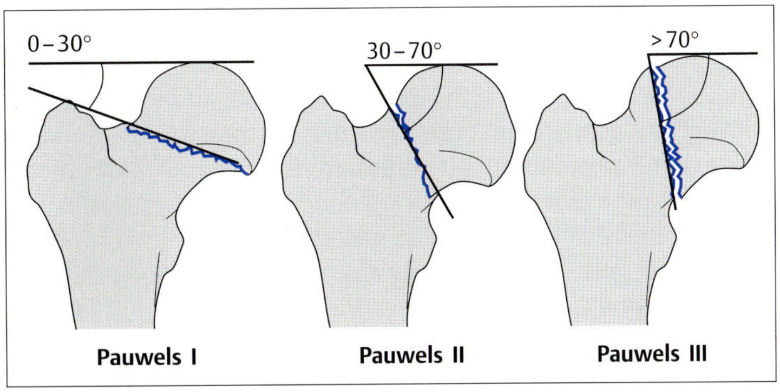

Fig. 1.**199** Classification of femoral neck fractures according to Pauwels.

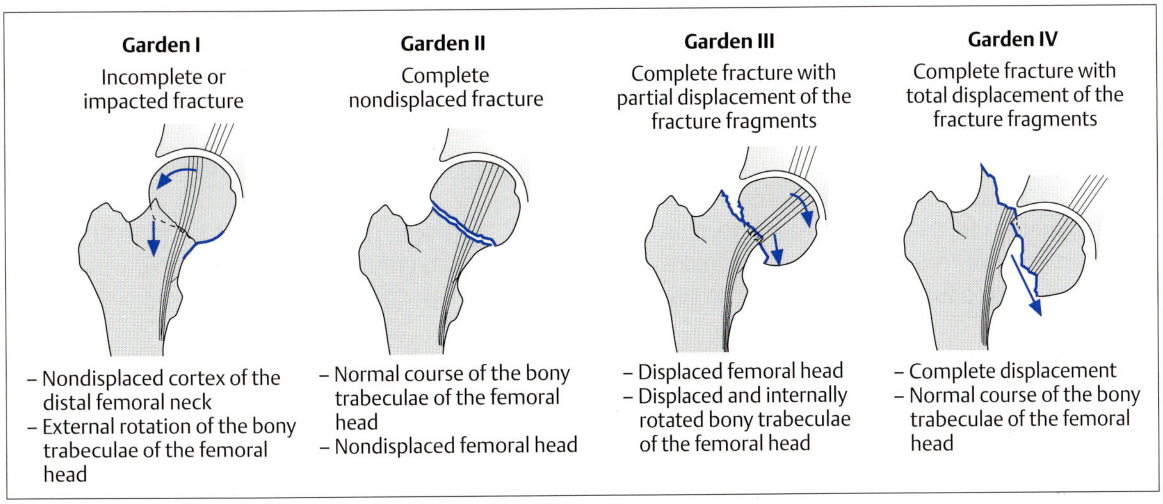

Fig. 1.**200** Classification of the femoral neck fractures according to Garden.

1. **Supracondylar fractures** are extra-articular and oriented transversely or somewhat obliquely. Displacement and comminution of the fragments are quite variable, and damage to the popliteal artery is of major concern in this setting.
2. **Intercondylar fractures** are supracondylar fractures with vertical extension of the fracture line into the knee joint (T or Y configuration or isolated). Displacement of the fragments affects incongruent femorotibial or femoropatellar articular surfaces, and oblique views may be helpful in the diagnostic evaluation.
3. **Condylar fractures** are sagittal or coronal fractures through a condyle. Detecting these fractures is rarely difficult, but assessing their extent can be challenging. In such instances, CT or MRI may be helpful.

Special Consideration in the Pediatric Age Group: Epiphysiolysis of the Femoral Head

Epiphysiolysis of the femoral head, usually idiopathic, generally follows minor trauma. Adipose children between the 10th and 15th year of life who are in a growth burst are particularly prone to this lesion. The predominant clinical finding is pain with limitation of motion.

The epiphysis generally splits posteriorly, medially and inferiorly, which is easily recognized on the 'frog leg' lateral view of Lauenstein (Fig. 1.**202 a**), but displacement of the slipped epiphysis in other directions is possible. The diagnosis can be established by sonography (Fig. 1.**202 b**), though conventional radiography is still needed for surgical planning. Only unclear cases require evaluation by MRI.

Patellar Fractures

Fractures of the patella are usually caused by a direct blow, and only rarely by a massive muscle pull. The fracture lines can traverse the patella in any or all directions. The commonest types are transverse and longitudinal fractures. Severe trauma often produces a comminuted or crush fracture.

Possible complications following a fracture of the patella include avascular necrosis of the proximal fragment and osteoarthritis of the patellofemoral articulation due to involvement and incongruence of the articular surface of the patella.

DD The **partite patella** follows two or several separate ossification centers and generally can be distinguished from fracture fragments by the following criteria (Fig. 1.**203**):
- the bipartite patella usually is superolateral in location,
- the contours are smooth and exhibit a sclerotic margin,
- the bipartite patella is mostly bilateral (compared to the contralateral side),
- fracture fragments fit together like parts of a puzzle, unlike the osseous fragments of the partite patella.

Tendon Ruptures

Ruptures of the quadriceps tendon occur predominately in elderly patients with underlying degenerative changes of the tendon. The tear usually is directly above the upper pole of the patella. Partial ruptures tend to involve the medial aspect of the tendon.

Ruptures of the patellar tendon occur in young patients as a result of sports injury, usually secondary to an underlying chronic tendonitis. The rupture usually occurs at or just below the patellar insertion. Avulsion fractures of the tibial apophysis are rare. Complete ruptures are clinically diagnosed by the striking elevation of the patella and the failure of knee extension.

Sonographically, both ruptures produce hematomas that can be seen sonographically and are associated with a retracted tendon if the rupture is complete. Inconclusive radiographic and sonographic findings require further evaluation by MRI (Fig. 1.**204**).

Traumatic Dislocation of the Patella

This relatively rare but characteristic sports injury is caused by a sudden change in direction while running or falling. The displacement is invariably to the lateral side.

This injury is associated with a partial or complete rupture of the medial retinaculum, usually near the femoral ligamentous insertion (see internal derangement of the knee). In about 5% of cases, the forced sliding of the patella over the femoral condyle causes a compression fracture of the lateral femoral condyle and a chondral or osteochondral fracture of the medial articular surface of the patella.

MRI This is the most reliable method for the detection of small chondral or osteochondral fragments, which are generally not seen radiographically.

Chronic (Recurrent) Dislocation

Chronic (recurrent) patellar dislocation refers to recurrent dislocations following minimal trauma. As with traumatic dislocations, the patella almost exclusively dislocates laterally. Predisposing factors

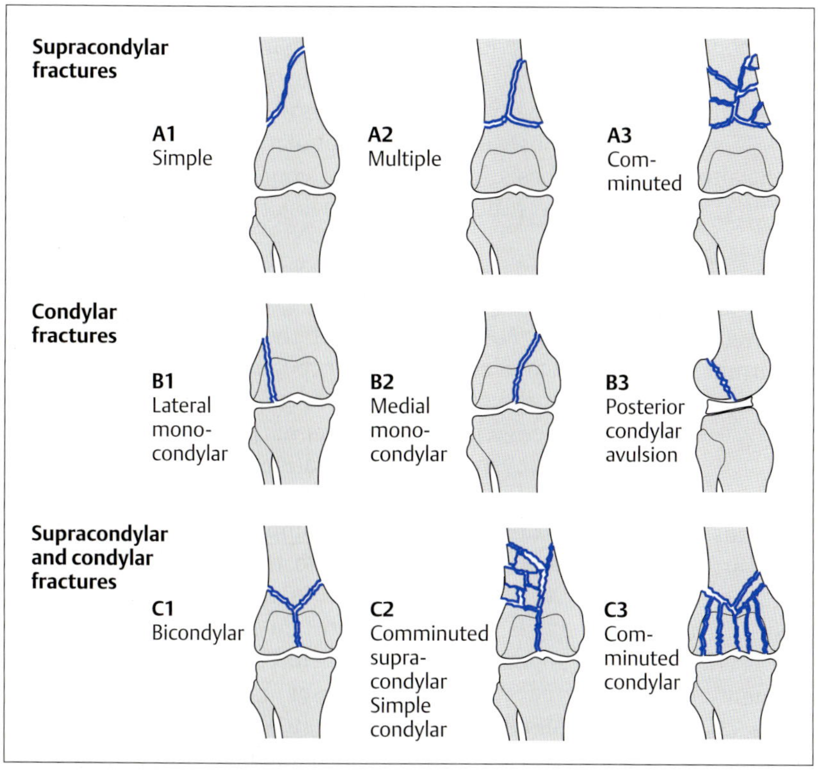

Fig. 1.**201** AO classification of the distal femoral fractures.

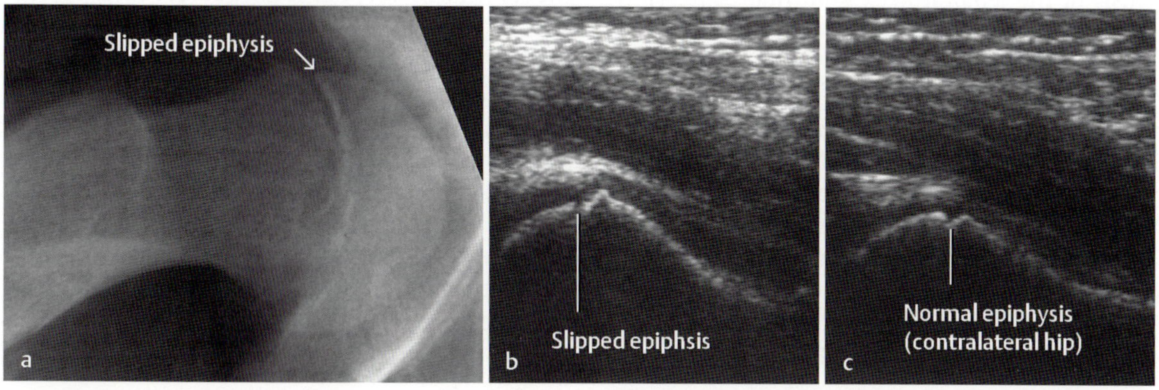

Fig. 1.**202** Typical image of epiphysiolysis of the femoral head in an 11-year-old boy. The cross-table lateral view according to Lauenstein (**a**) clearly demonstrates the posteromedial slippage of the epiphysis. The slipped epiphysis is also sonographically detectable (**b**). Sonographic image of the contralateral normal hip (**c**) for comparison.

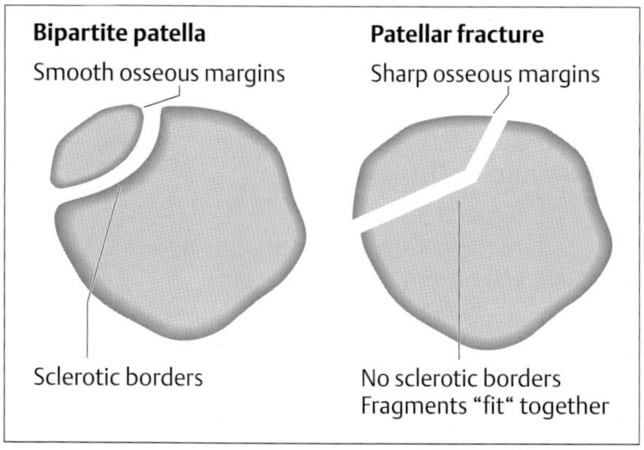

Fig. 1.**203** The partite patella has sclerotic borders and rounded contours with both components not entirely congruent.

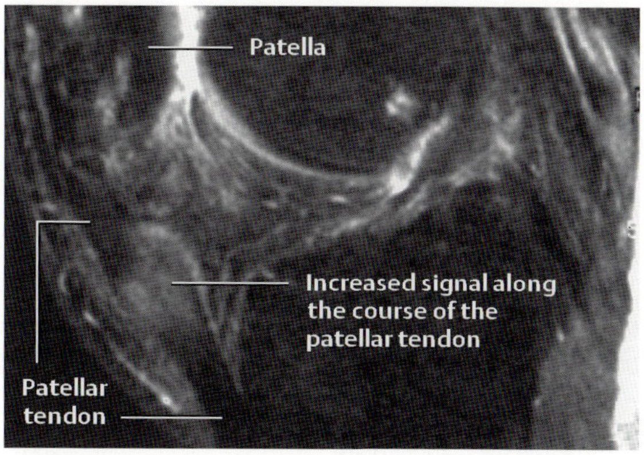

Fig. 1.**204** MRI (fat suppressed) of a partial tear of the patellar tendon in a 49-year-old patient.

for chronic (recurrent) dislocation are preceding traumatic dislocation and constitutional factors such as:
- dysplasia of the medial patellar articular surface,
- flattening of the patellar groove,
- high position of the patella (patella alta),
- genu valgum.

This clinical scenario is a nuisance for patients and can also cause osteochondral or chondral fractures, with an inherent risk of secondary osteoarthritis. It is for this reason that chronic (recurrent) dislocations are frequently surgically corrected.

The Post-Surgical Hip

The most frequent surgical interventions of the hip are insertion of a total hip prosthesis (arthroplasty) and internal fixation of fractures. The most frequent surgical procedures and their different indications are listed in Table 1.**16**.

Indication of total hip replacement following subcapital fractures of the femoral neck in elderly patients is justified by the high rate of avascular necrosis of the femoral neck following conservative therapy or internal fixation by compression screws and plate.

X-RAY It is the role of radiography to document post-surgical changes and fracture healing and to recognize early and delayed complications. Following the immediate post-surgical radiographic examination, follow-up examinations are performed with the interval determined by the surgical procedure and clinical course. In general, an AP view of the pelvis and an AP view of the hip are obtained with the film positioned low to include the entire stem of the femoral component of the hip prosthesis. Excluding the iliac wings is acceptable since there is no loss of pertinent information. If loosening of the acetabular component of the prosthesis is suspected, a coned-down view centered over the acetabular region may be helpful.

Total Hip Prosthesis

Permanent fixation of the hip prosthesis can be achieved by screws or cement. In addition, the shaft of the prosthesis can be anchored by a porous surface (with the diameter of the pores measuring 0.2 to 0.5 mm), causing fixation by ingrowth of osseous tissue. Not infrequently, the femoral component becomes partially or completely surrounded by fibrous tissue, leading to the clinical complaint of weight-bearing pain. In addition, the prosthetic shaft must have almost an exact fit to achieve permanent stability. Therefore, the prosthetic stem (or the cement, in case of a cemented prosthesis) should circumferentially abut the cortex. Cement is used primarily in pathologic fractures and patients who are very old or have severe osteoporosis.

X-RAY The radiographic criteria used in the follow-up of the postoperative total hip replacement are shown in Table 1.**17**. The extended radiographic follow-up serves to recognize dislocations, fractures, prosthetic fractures, decentralization of the acetabulum (due to wear and tear), osteomyelitis, or myositis ossificans. The most important complication, however, is loosening of the prosthesis.

Table 1.**16** The frequent surgical procedures of the hip and their indications

Surgical procedure	Indication
Prostheses	
Total hip prosthesis	Severe osteoarthritis, basicervical fracture of the femoral neck in elderly patients with osteoarthritis (Fig. 1.**205**)
Bipolar prosthesis	Basicervical fracture of the femoral neck in elderly patients without osteoarthritis (Fig. 1.**207**)
Internal fixation	
Screw-plate device	Subcapital fracture of the femoral neck without severe osteoarthritis, intertrochanteric femoral fracture
Regazzoni plate (screw-plate device with proximal plate extension for trochanteric support)	Intertrochanteric femoral fracture with avulsion of the greater trochanter (Fig. 1.**206**)
Screws	Basicervical fracture of the femoral neck in young patients
130-degree fixed angle plate	Intertrochanteric femoral fracture; rarely applied today since the compression screw is more easily inserted

Table 1.**17** Criteria of post-surgical radiographic follow-up after total hip replacement

Iatrogenic fracture	Insertion of the femoral stem can produce a longitudinal fracture (fissure), usually recognized intraoperatively and treated with cerclage wires
Dislocation	The femoral head component rarely dislocates. The acetabular component or the outer acetabular shell of a bipolar prosthesis dislocates even less frequently.
Position of the prosthesis	No relevant difference in the leg length should result. Reference line: line parallel to the tangents to both ischial tuberosities through lower border of the lesser trochanter of the healthy and operated leg (Fig. 1.**207**)
Femoral component	- The stem of a self-locking prosthesis should fit tightly in direct contact with the cortex; cemented prosthesis should be completely engulfed by cement, which should fill the entire medullary space between stem and cortex - Depending on the type of prosthesis inserted, anteversion (= angle between femoral neck and shaft, normally 15–30°) can be abnormal or absent on the axial view
Acetabular component	The acetabular entrance plane should be angulated by about 45° on the AP view and by 30–35° on the axial view (Fig. 1.**205**)

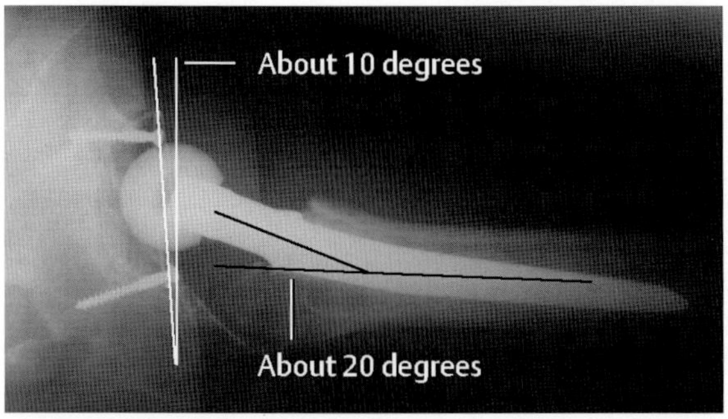

Fig. 1.**205** Axial projection of the left hip with a total hip prosthesis in place. The angle between femoral neck and prosthesis measures 20°. With a 10° angulation relative to the horizontal plane, the entrance plane of the acetabulum is tilted inadequately.

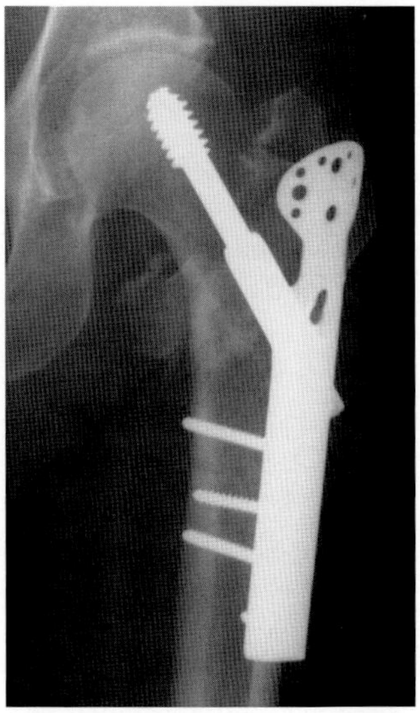

Fig. 1.**206** Status post insertion of a Regazzoni plate following intertrochanteric femoral fracture with avulsion of the greater trochanter.

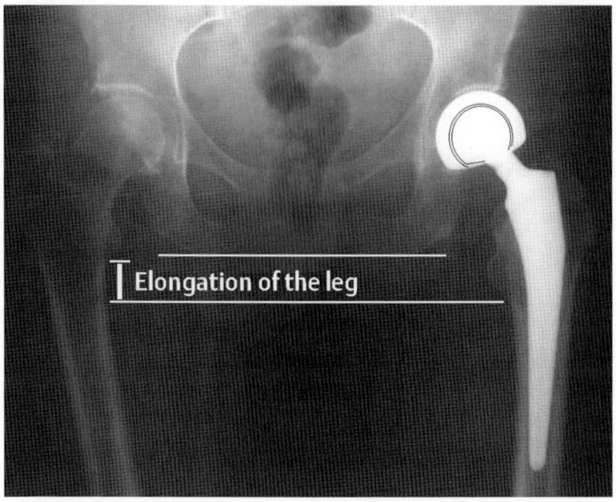

Fig. 1.**207** AP radiograph of the pelvis. After femoral neck fracture (81-year-old patient without noticeable degenerative osteoarthritis), a bipolar endoprosthesis was inserted. There is elongation of the leg by about 2 cm.

The radiographic signs of prosthetic loosening are generally ambiguous and only rarely conclusive (see Table 1.**18**). Non-cemented prostheses can have a 3 mm radiolucent halo if the fixation is exclusively fibrous. In addition, distal migration of the prosthesis up to 10 mm within the first year should not be considered pathologic.

Hip arthrography: This is best performed with the DSA technique and is highly specific if contrast medium extends along the prosthesis or cement.

NUC Prosthetic loosening can be detected scintigraphically, but the findings are not specific.

SONO Postsurgical seromas, hematomas, and abscesses can be identified sonographically and aspirated under sonographic guidance.

! Since the radiographic criteria are soft and must be viewed as 'uncertain signs of loosening,' prosthetic loosening should only be diagnosed in context with clinical findings. Findings suggesting loosening are progressive pain with weight bearing, radiating into the thigh or hip and clearly relieved without weight bearing. The pain worsens with hip rotation (loosening of the femoral stem) or flexion (loosening of the acetabular component). The clinical findings are crucial since surgical revision in the absence of clinical complaint is only indicated with massive osteolysis around the prosthesis or a fracture of the prosthesis.

In almost all cases of osteomyelitis, the prosthesis must be removed and the prosthetic bed filled with antibiotic pellets. The outcome is that of a Girdlestone procedure (Fig. 1.**213**).

Table 1.**18** Radiologic findings of prosthetic loosening

Definitive signs of prosthetic loosening	
All types of prostheses	Fracture of the prosthesis in the region of osseous contact Mobility of the prosthesis (fluoroscopy or comparison views with the patient standing and lying or, respectively, at rest and the leg pulled)
Cemented prostheses	Cement fracture (Fig. 1.**208**) Radiolucent halo between metal and cement Migration of the prosthesis (applies to the femoral component only)
Self-locking prostheses	Osseous fracture around the prosthetic stem (seen as interrupted or angulated periprosthetic sclerotic line) (Fig. 1.**209**)
Signs suspicious for prosthetic loosening	
All types of prostheses	Osseous resorption along prosthesis or cement, induced by friction of the inserted material (Fig. 1.**209**) Resolution of previously seen sclerotic changes around the acetabular component Migration of the acetabular component
Cemented prostheses	Radiolucent rim exceeding 2 mm between cement and bone. The wider the radiolucent rim relative to the entire cement-bone contact interface and the more progressive, the more likely is loosening. The more cranial the radiolucent rim around the acetabular component, the more specific (Figs. 1.**210**, 1.**211**)
Self-locking prostheses	Widened radiolucent rim (> 3 mm) and any progression with time. A more superior radiolucent rim around the acetabular component is more specific. Sclerosed spongiosa at the tip of the stem (socket sign, Fig. 1.**212**) Periosteal reaction around the tip of the stem (Fig. 1.**212**)

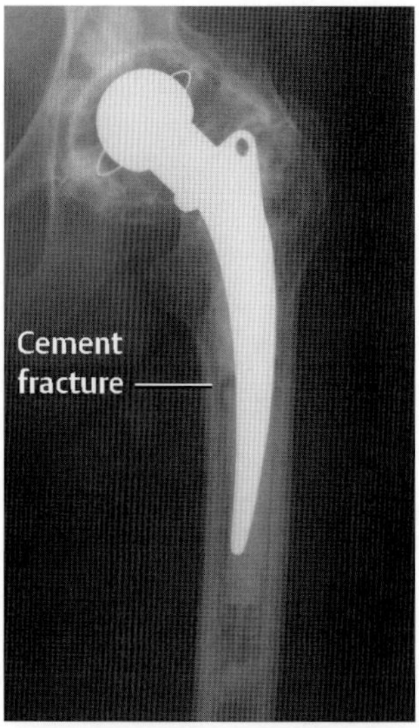

Fig. 1.**208** The cement around the femoral stem of the prosthesis is fractured, indicative of prosthetic loosening. The acetabular component remains firmly embedded.

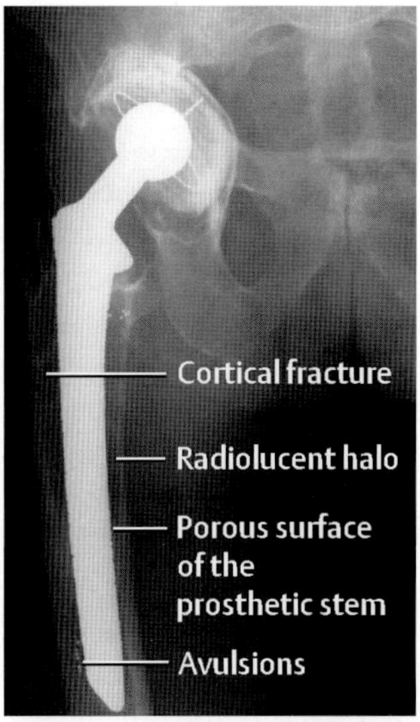

Fig. 1.**209** Cemented acetabular component and self-locking femoral component of a total hip prosthesis. Pronounced radiolucent halo around the prosthetic stem. The concomitant pathologic fracture of the lateral femoral cortex confirms the prosthetic loosening. Central protrusion of the acetabular prosthesis.

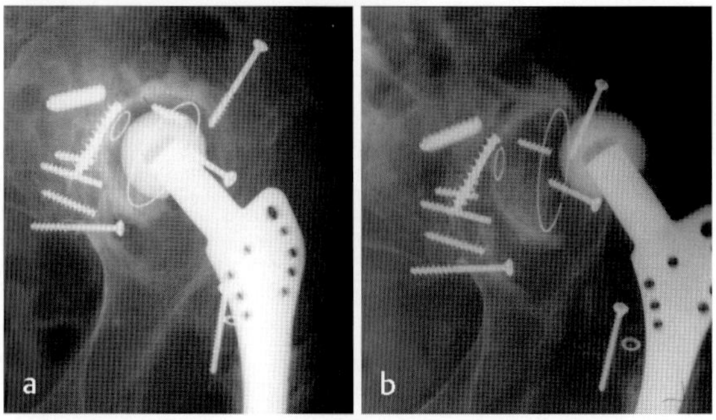

Fig. 1.**210** **a** Cemented acetabular component replacing a screwed acetabular component. Because of underlying hip dysplasia, there is dystopic location of the acetabular component with a relatively steep entrance plane of about 60°.
b About one year later, there is almost vertical orientation of the entrance plane of the acetabular component due to prosthetic migration. Increased width of the radiolucent halo is also seen along the cement at the middle and inferior aspects of the acetabular components.

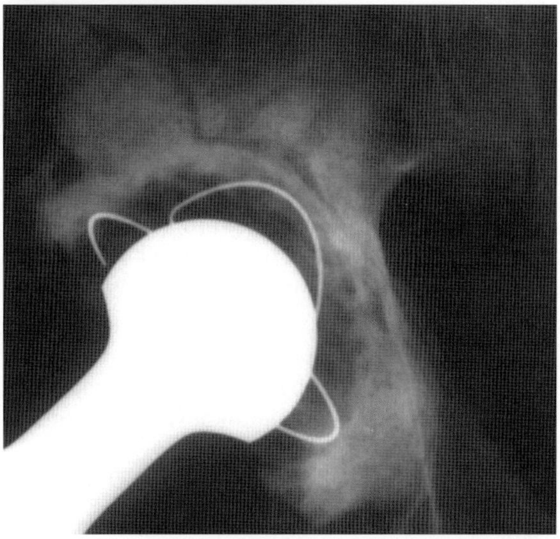

Fig. 1.**211** Radiolucent halo around the upper aspect of the cement of a loose acetabular component.

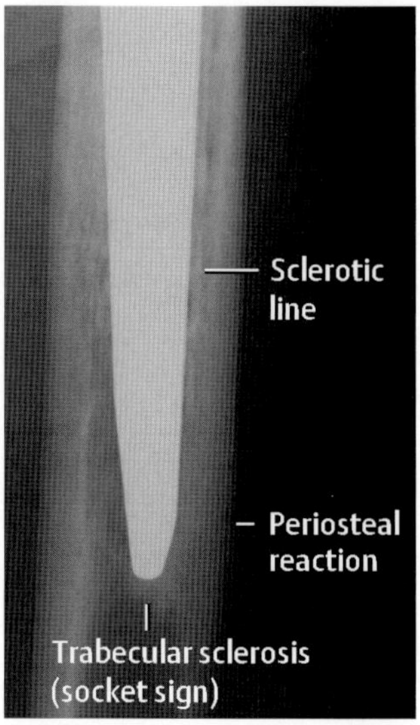

Fig. 1.**212** Inconclusive radiographic signs of loosening of a self-locking prosthesis without surgical evidence of loosening. Solid periosteal reaction and trabecular sclerosis at the tip of the prosthetic stem (socket sign) are often seen with the prosthesis in stable position. A **localized** periosteal reaction **adjacent** to the tip of the stem, however, is a sign of loosening (local weight loading).

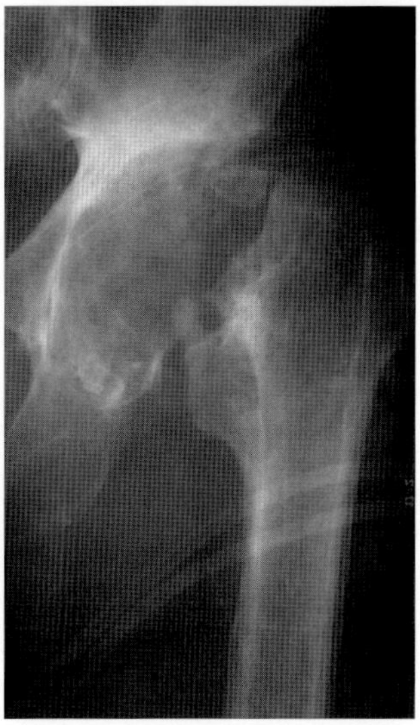

Fig. 1.**213** Status post removal of a total hip prosthesis because of periprosthetic infection (Girdlestone procedure). Drains are in place.

Internal Fixation

X-RAY The immediate post-operative radiographic examination is obtained to document the position of the fracture fragments. Normal anteversion of the femoral neck should be seen on the axial view (Fig. 1.**214**). The optimal position of the screw is inferior and somewhat posterior to the center of the femoral head. The tip of the screw should not extend beyond the subchondral bone into the joint space. The plate should lie flat along the femoral shaft with the screws completely inserted and anchored in the opposite cortex. There should be no defect along the medial cortex (in the region of the greater trochanter). The Regazonni plate should completely cover the greater trochanter. Of course, a dislocation or a refracture must be recognized.

Follow-up radiographic examinations should monitor the fracture healing and recognize any late complications (Table 1.**19**).

A decreasing distance between the fragments due to migration is not a complication and is even desirable: fracture healing is promoted by pressure on the fracture zone, which is achieved by partial or complete weight bearing of the operated hip and resultant compression of the fracture ends against each other. Internal fixation is a dynamic process, which is most evident by the lateral movement of the screws relative to the femoral shaft or trochanteric region.

NUC This can be used in diagnosing avascular necrosis of the femoral head.

MRI Though this is the method of choice for diagnosing avascular necrosis of the femoral head, it does not play a role after internal fixation because of the metal-induced artifacts.

CT This can provide information relevant for planning osteotomies to correct or reduce deformities.

Table 1.**19** Radiologically detectable late complications following internal fixation of the hip

- Avascular necrosis of the femoral head (Fig. 1.**215**)
- Pseudarthrosis
- Loosened screw (Fig. 1.**216**)
- Osteomyelitis
- Disuse osteoporosis
- Fracture or dislodgement of the fixation device
- Dislocation
- Settling of the screws into the joint
- New fracture
- Periarticular and periosseous calcifications

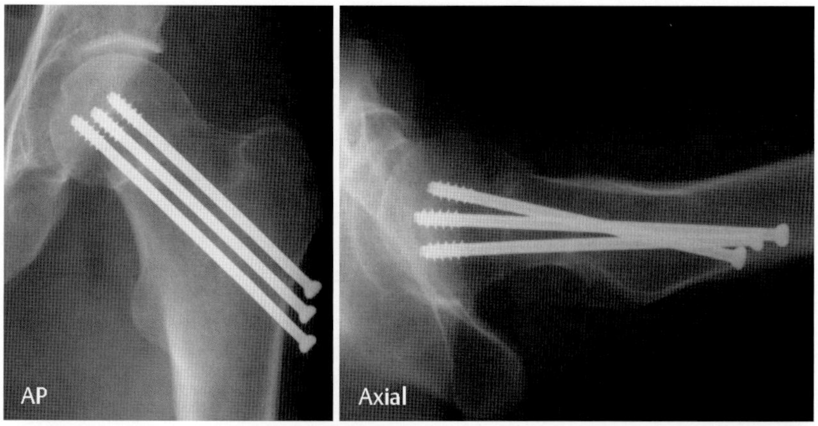

Fig. 1.**214** Internal fixation of the medial femoral neck fracture by means of three screws (46-year-old patient). Anatomic position of the fracture fragments, normal position of the screws.

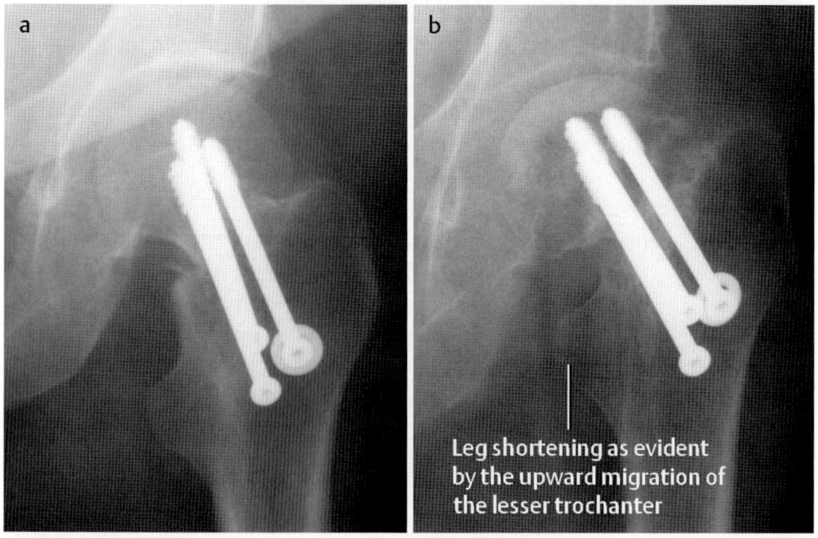

Fig. 1.**215**
a Post-surgical follow-up of a basicervical fracture of the femoral neck with internal fixation by means of three screws.
b One year later, collapse and medial slippage of the femoral head as manifestation of an avascular necrosis.

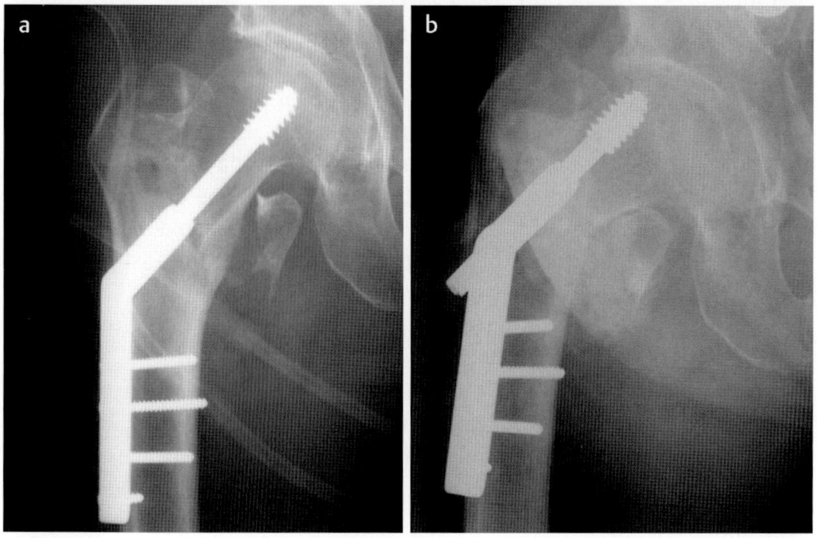

Fig. 1.**216**
a Post-surgical follow-up of an intertrochanteric fracture with internal fixation by means of screw-plate device.
b About 10 weeks later, migration of the screw within the head as well as disimpaction and medial slippage of the femoral head.

Internal Lesions of the Knee

Menisci

Anatomy: Menisci are fibrocartilaginous structures that rest on the tibial plateau. Each meniscus covers about two-thirds of its corresponding tibial articular surface and has a triangular cross section with a thick outer and a thin inner border. Each meniscus can be divided into an outer third (zone I, the only vascularized zone), middle third (zone II), and inner third (zone III).

The axial plane of the meniscus is structurally trisected into posterior horn, anterior horn and body (pars intermedia, Fig. 1.**217**).

Another division follows the '25 : 50 : 25 rule' with the inner 25 % comprising the genuine posterior and anterior horns, the middle 50 % the anterior and posterior meniscal bodies, and the outer 25 % the genuine peripheral meniscal bodies (Fig. 1.**217**).

The lateral meniscus is more C-shaped than the medial meniscus, has a shorter radius and accordingly has an increased curvature.

Trauma mechanisms: Rotation of the body with the knee flexed and the foot fixed subjects the meniscus to pressure and shearing forces. The menisci can be injured alone or as part of complex injury patterns. The menisci can also be damaged by tibial plateau fractures.

A healthy meniscus can only be harmed by sudden and considerable traumatic forces. A degeneratively altered meniscus frequently tears after even minor trauma. Longitudinal tears are more frequent than transverse tears and the medial meniscus is more commonly affected than the lateral meniscus.

CLINIC Meniscal tears cause pain (with knee extension), swelling (usually a hemorrhagic effusion), and functional impairment (restriction of extension). Forcible rotation causes pain in the joint line (Steinmann sign I), with the pain migrating posteriorly on flexion (Steinmann sign II).

! Arthroscopy and MRI are the methods of choice to evaluate any meniscal abnormalities. Conventional arthrography no longer plays an important role in the knee.

MRI Criteria for evaluating meniscal damage:
- size of meniscus,
- configuration of the meniscus and signal pattern (reference: hyaline cartilage with T1-weighting),
- depth and width of the altered signal,
- location within the meniscus.

Gradation of the Signal Alteration of the Meniscus on MRI (Fig. 1.**218**):

Grade 0: meniscus seen as homogeneous low signal intensity.
Grade I: round signal not extending to the superior or inferior articular surface.
Grade II: linear intrameniscal signal not extending to the articular surface (Fig. 1.**221 a**).
Grade III: linear intrameniscal signal extending to the articular surface (IIIa: one surface, IIIb: both surfaces, Figs. 1.**221 b – d**).

! Only Grade III lesions have clinical relevance since only these lesions represent meniscal tears.

Morphology of Meniscal Tears (Fig. 1.**219**):
Vertical tears are generally traumatic or degenerative.
Horizontal tears are predominately degenerative in nature, but can also be traumatic. They usually affect the posterior horn but can extend into the body or anterior horn.
The **bucket-handle tear** is an extensive, longitudinally oriented vertical tear with displacement of one or two meniscal fragments. The medial meniscus is more often involved than the lateral meniscus. The resultant abnormal meniscal configurations are determined by the orientation of the tear. Characteristically, the inner segment dislodges into the intercondylar fossa, or – with associated posterior meniscal capsular separation – the posterior horn folds over the anterior horn ('flipped meniscus sign', Fig. 1.**220**).
Peripheral tears: a tear within 5 mm of the meniscal periphery.
Amputating tear: truncation of the free border or the tip of the meniscus.
Meniscocapsular separation: a subtype of the meniscal tear, with separation of the posterior meniscal horn from the capsule and displacement of the posterior meniscal signal from the posterior tibial border by more than 8 – 10 mm.
Radial tears can be degenerative or traumatic and usually involve the medial meniscus.

Traumatic tears are typically observed in adolescents and young adults. They usually are caused by axial compression applied to the meniscus and run parallel to the collagenous fibers. They heal spontaneously if the patients are young and the tear is incomplete, less than 5 – 6 mm thick, and located in the peripheral vascular zone.

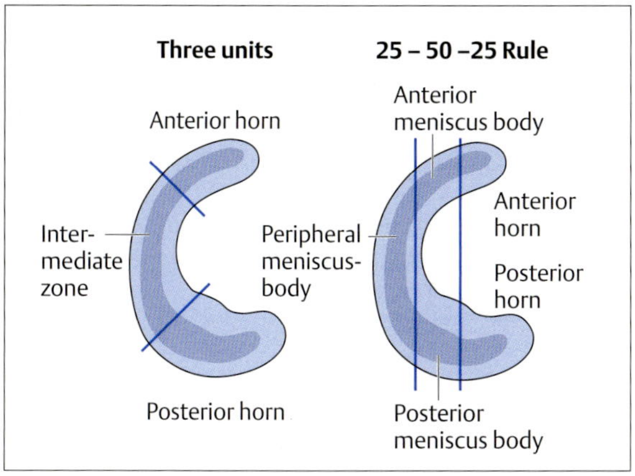

Fig. 1.**217** Meniscal anatomy.

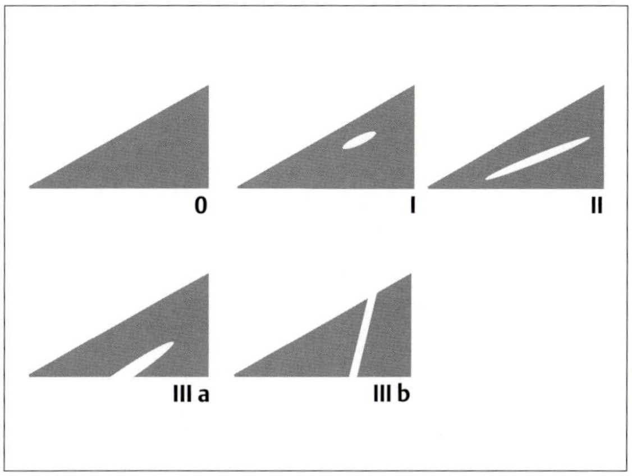

Fig. 1.**218** Grading of abnormal MRI signal in the menisci (after Stoller).

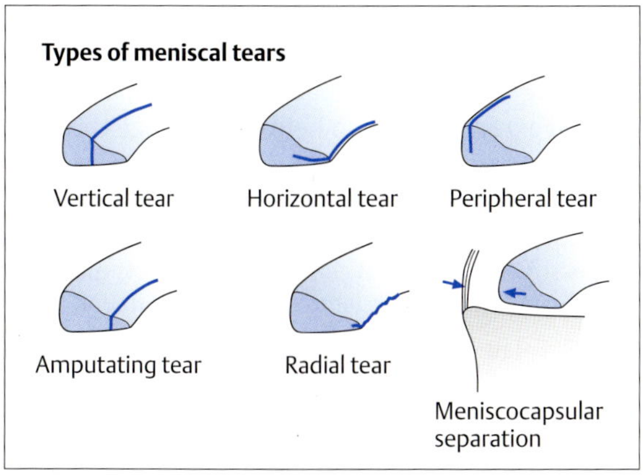

Fig. 1.**219** Types of meniscus tears.

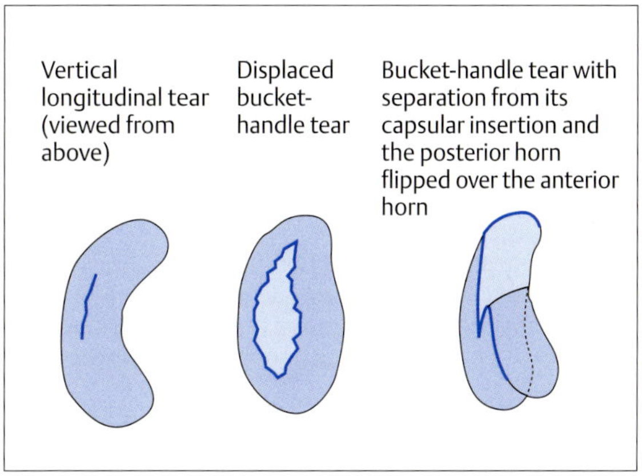

Fig. 1.**220** Schematic drawing of a bucket-handle tear.

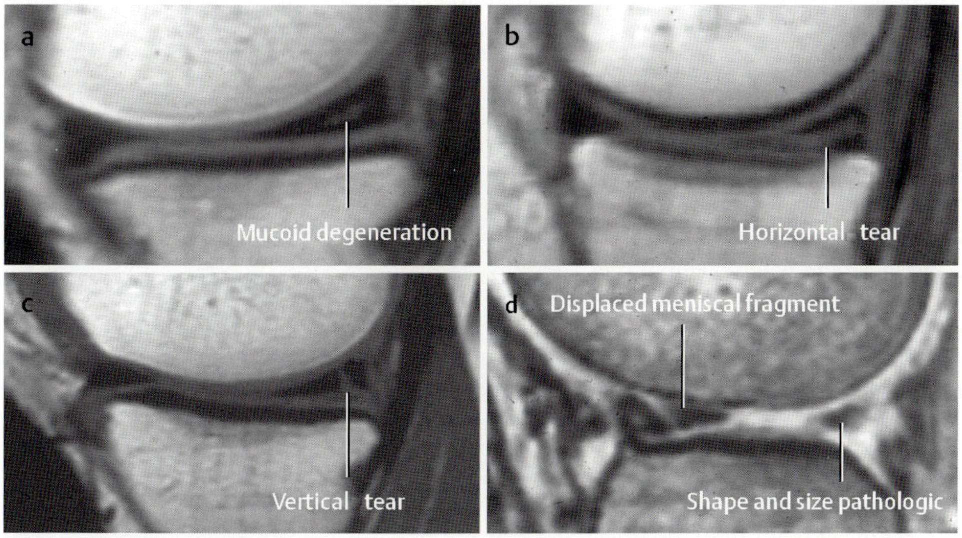

Fig. 1.**221** Several types of meniscal lesions as seen on MRI. **a** Grade II lesion. **b** Horizontal tear in the posterior horn of the medial meniscus (= degenerative tear), **c** Traumatic vertical tear, **d** Bucket-handle tear of the medial meniscus.

Ligaments of the Knee

Anterior Cruciate Ligament

The anterior cruciate ligament is an intra-articular, extra-synovial structure that extends from the anterior intercondylar region of the tibia to the inner aspect of the lateral femoral condyle. It limits anterior translation of the tibia in relation to the femur (anterior drawer) and stabilizes against hyperextension and internal rotation.

Mechanism of injury: The anterior cruciate ligament is the most frequently injured ligamentous structure of the knee. Typical causes are abrupt deceleration with internal rotation of the knee (jumping injury) as well as hyperextension in internal rotation. Combined injuries of the cruciate ligaments occur with the knee flexed and subjected to rotation and valgus stress (ski injury). In most instances there is a transient subluxation of the femur posteriorly in relation to the tibia. Injuries of the anterior cruciate ligament frequently occur in conjunction with injuries of the meniscus, injuries of the collateral ligaments, osteochondral fractures, or compression fractures.

MRI Criteria of a **complete** rupture of the anterior cruciate ligament:

Direct signs:
- complete disruption of all fibers,
- abnormal course of the cruciate ligament,
- intracapsular pseudomass as a manifestation of a hematoma in the expected position of the anterior cruciate ligament.

Indirect signs:
- acute angulation of the posterior cruciate ligament,
- drawer phenomenon,
- 'kissing contusions' of the posterolateral aspect of the tibial plateau and the anterolateral aspect of the lateral femoral condyle (Fig. 1.**222**)

Criteria of an **incomplete** tear of the anterior cruciate ligament:
- thinning of the anterior cruciate ligament (< 10 mm),
- periligamentous pseudomass related to a hematoma in the presence of intact fibers,
- increased intraligamentous signal with remnants of intact fibers.

! The anterior cruciate ligament is best seen in the oblique coronal plane (Fig. 1.**223 c**).

Posterior Cruciate Ligament

The posterior cruciate ligament extends from the posterior intercondylar area of the tibia to the inner aspect of the medial femoral condyle. It limits anterior translation of the femur in relation to the tibia (posterior drawer) and stabilizes the knee in extension.

Mechanism of injury: The posterior cruciate ligament is much less frequently injured than the anterior cruciate ligament. An isolated tear of the posterior cruciate ligament is often caused by a fall on a flexed knee and is frequently associated with an osseous avulsion fracture at the tibial ligamentous insertion.

! Clinical examination of the posterior cruciate ligament is less reliable than that of the anterior cruciate ligament, especially in combined injuries. Furthermore, the posterior cruciate ligament is less accessible by arthroscopy.

MRI Criteria of a rupture of the posterior cruciate ligament (Fig. 1.**224**):
- confined areas of increased signal intensity along the course of the ligament (= partial rupture),
- continuity disruption (complete rupture).

Caution: Several sagittal sections must be analyzed since partial volume effect can mimic tears.

Medial Collateral Ligament

The medial collateral ligament prevents medial widening of the joint space and is taut with the knee in extension. It also helps to stabilize the knee against external rotational forces.

Mechanisms of injury are valgus stress without rotational component (e.g., ice hockey) and direct trauma with valgus stress. The medial collateral ligament is more frequently injured than the lateral collateral ligament.

MRI The MRI criteria for medial collateral ligamentous injury are summarized in Table 1.**20** (Fig. 1.**225**).

! Frequent concomitant injuries include complete rupture of the anterior cruciate ligament, osteochondral injuries, bone marrow bruises, and meniscal tears (Fig. 1.**222**).

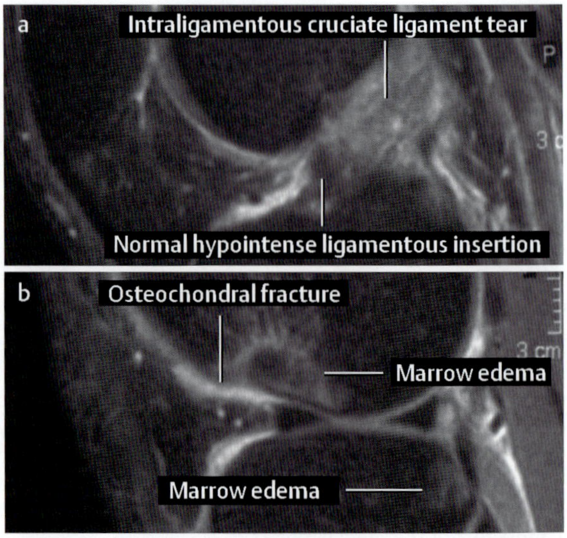

Fig. 1.**222** MRI (fat suppression) of a tear of the anterior cruciate ligament (**a**) with osteochondral and trabecular fracture in typical location ('kissing contusion') (**b**).

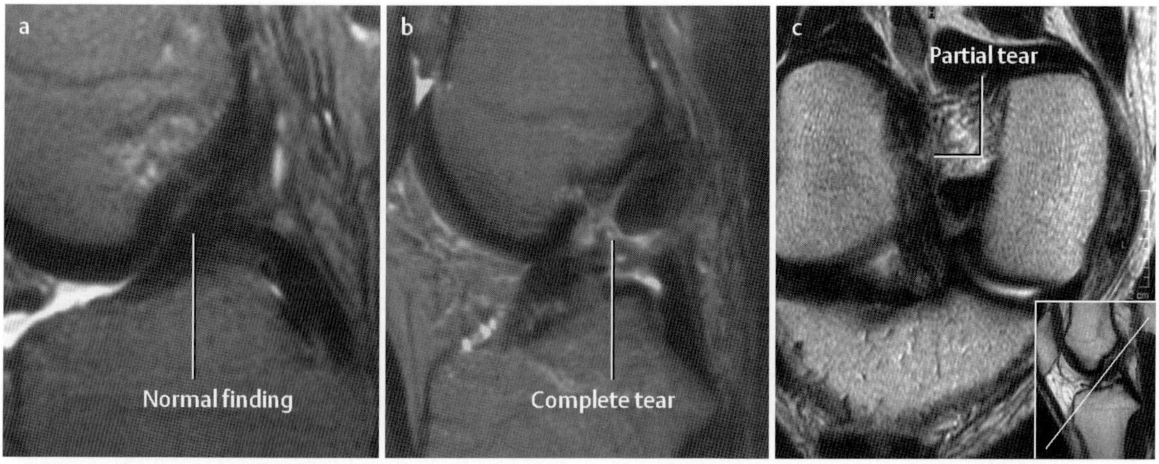

Fig. 1.**223** Anterior cruciate ligament, T2-weighted TSE sequence. **a** Normal. **b** Tear of the middle third. **c** Partial tear of the upper third (oblique coronal plane).

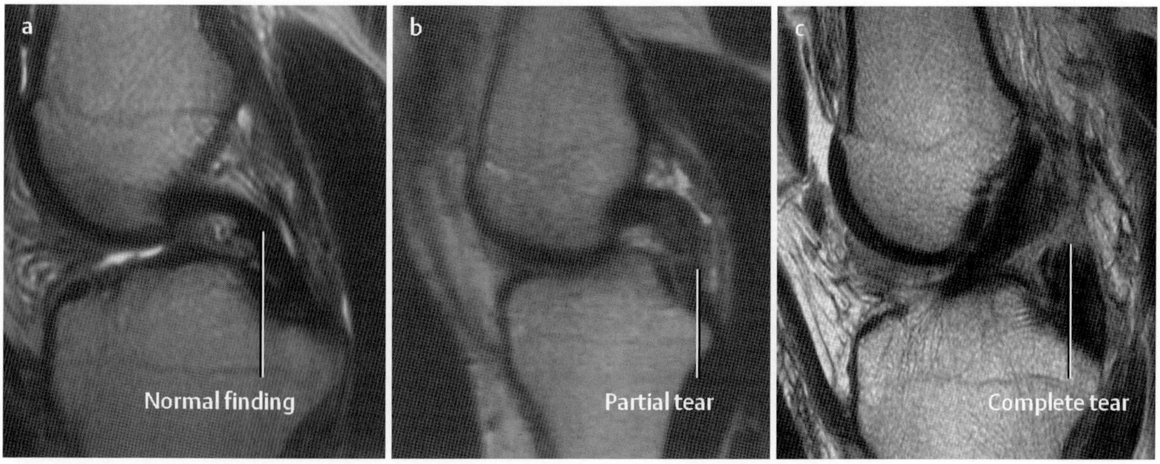

Fig. 1.**224** Posterior cruciate ligament, T2-weighted sequence. **a** Normal finding. **b** Partial tear. **c** Complete tear.

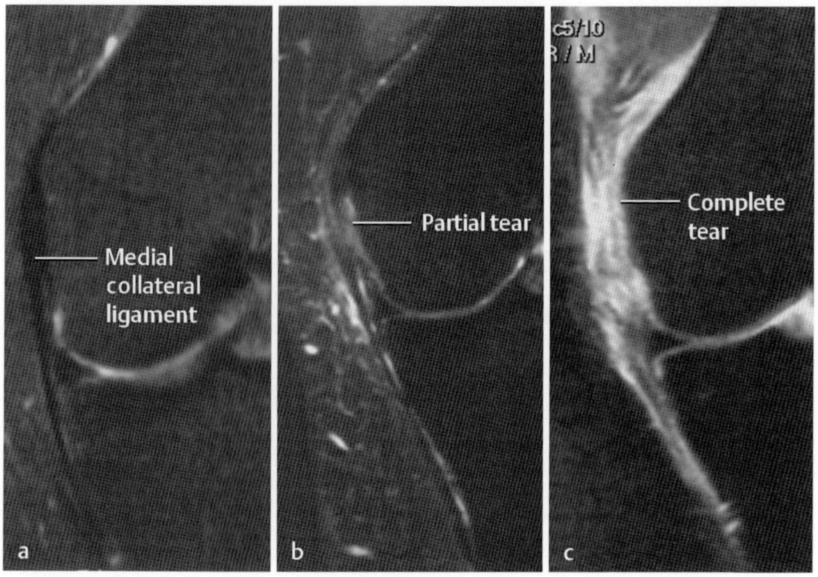

Fig. 1.**225** Fat-suppressed MRI of the medial collateral ligament.
a Normal.
b Localized thickening and increased signal intensity in the proximal portion: partial tear (grade II).
c Complete tear and extensive edema or hematoma in the proximal third (grade III).

Lateral Collateral Ligament

The lateral collateral ligament is a complex structure composed of a strong cord, the fibrous joint capsule (also referred to as lateral capsular ligament), the arcuate ligament, the iliotibial band, the popliteal tendon, the tendon of the biceps femoris muscle, the fibular collateral ligament and the conjoined tendon. It stabilizes against valgus stress and internal rotation.

Mechanism of injury: Varus stress with or without rotational component.

MRI The MRI criteria for lateral collateral ligament damage are identical to those for medial collateral ligament injury (Table 1.**20**, Fig. 1.**226**).

Meniscal Cysts

Meniscal cysts are divided into intrameniscal, parameniscal, and synovial cysts. The more frequent parameniscal cysts constitute simple or septated accumulations of fluid in the periphery of the meniscus. Parameniscal cysts are more frequent laterally than medially and in 90% of cases associated with a horizontal meniscal tear (Fig. 1.**227**). Intrameniscal and synovial cysts are rare.

Synovial Plicae

Synovial plicae are remnants of synovial tissue that divided the joint into three compartments during the early development. The plicae are most frequently suprapatellar, medial patellar, and infrapatellar. The most important pathologic changes caused by the plicae are the symptomatic thickening of the medial patella plicae and a chronic impingement with erosive changes of the patellofemoral cartilage.

A normal synovial plica is identified on T2-weighted MRI images as a thin band of low signal intensity clearly outlined by the surrounding joint fluid of high signal intensity (Fig. 1.**228**). A pathologic plicae is thickened and enhances ('plica syndrome').

Retinacula

The medial and lateral patellar retinacula are superficial fibers extending from the medial and lateral vastus muscles (Fig. 1.**229**). They flank the patella and control the gliding of the patella in the patellofemoral articulation.

The most important pathologic change is the rupture of the medial retinaculum, usually caused by a dislocated patella and only rarely as part of a torn proximal patella or distal quadriceps tendon.

On MRI the torn retinaculum does not insert into the patella and demonstrates a 'pseudotumor' representing an aggregation of torn retinacular fibers. This is associated with an edema or hematoma of high signal intensity on T2-weighted or fat-suppressed sequences (Fig. 1.**230**).

Table 1.**20** Grading of the injuries of the collateral ligaments

Grade	I	II	III	IV
MRI criteria	Thickened capsule	Thin or lamellated ligament	Rupture, edema, and retraction of the ligament	Rupture, edema, and retraction, plus meniscal tear and bone bruise
Schema	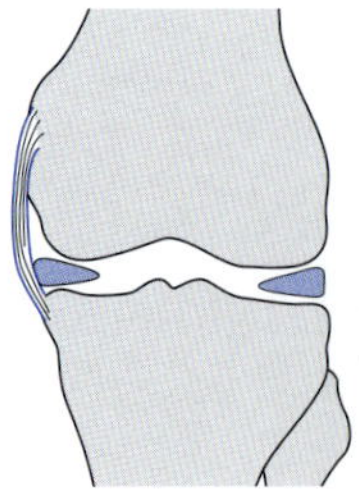	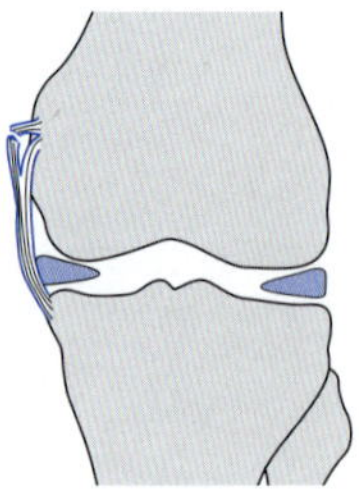	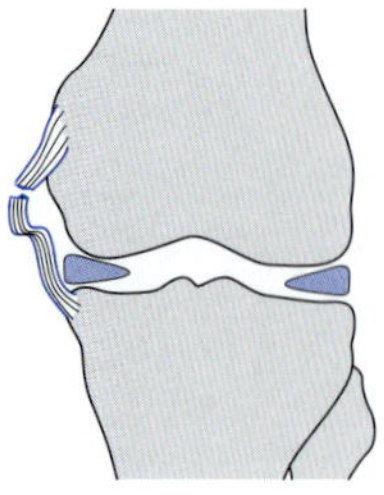	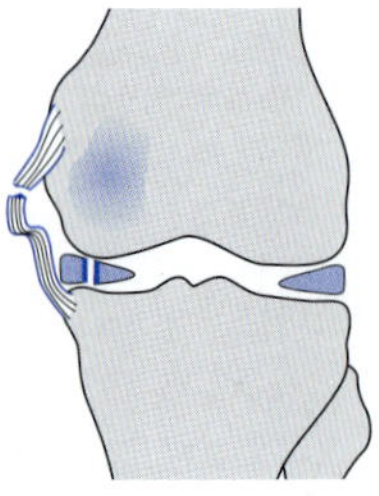

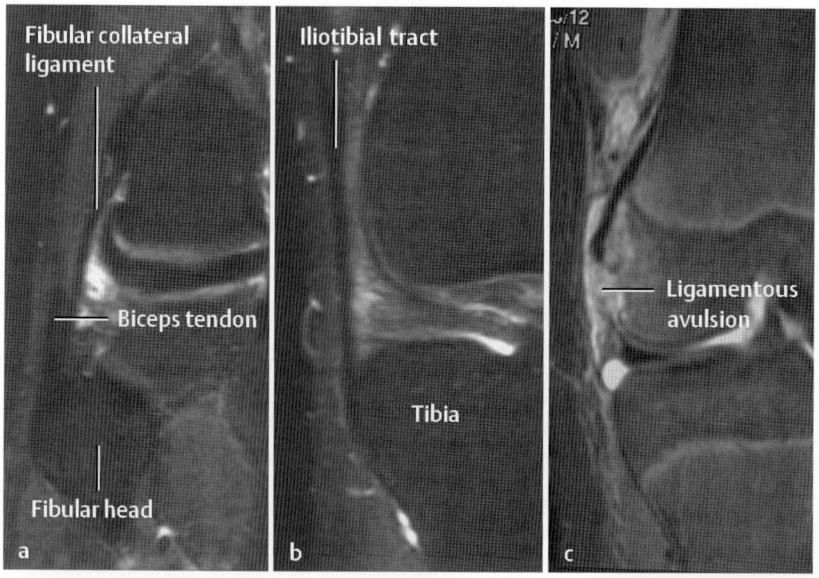

Fig. 1.**226** Fat-suppressed MR images of the lateral collateral ligament complex.

a Normal posterior portion with insertion of the fibular collateral ligament and the biceps tendon.

b Normal anterior portion with iliotibial band.

c Osseous avulsion of the lateral collateral ligament.

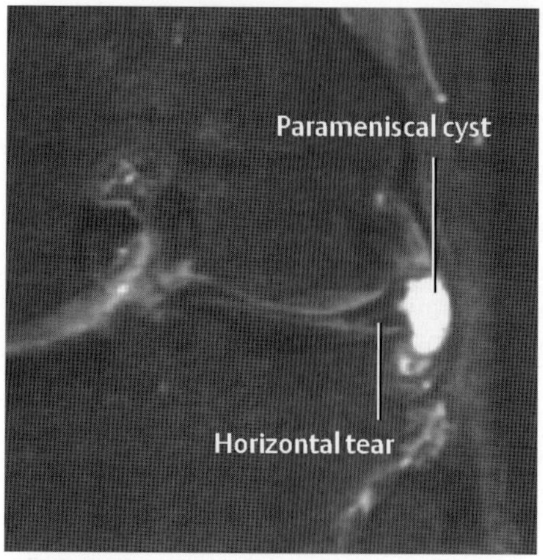

Fig. 1.**227** Lateral parameniscal cyst associated with a horizontal tear of the lateral meniscus (fat-suppressed MR image).

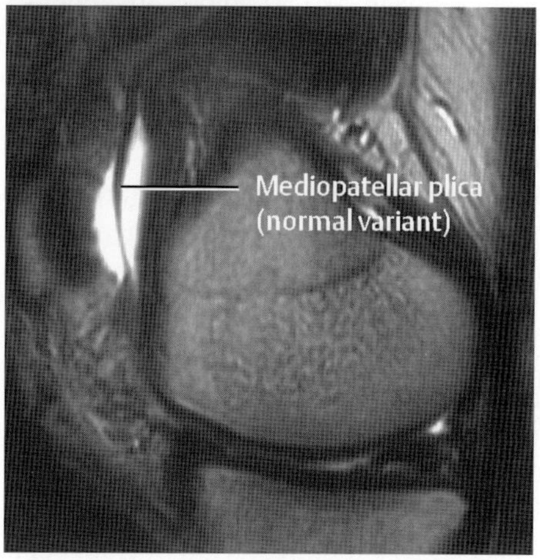

Fig. 1.**228** The mediopatellar plica is seen as a thin hypointense band in the medial patellar recess, well demarcated by the surrounding joint effusion (sagittal T2-weighted image).

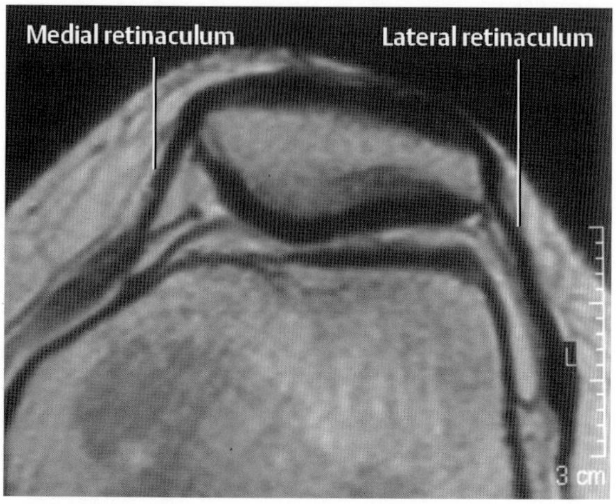

Fig. 1.**229** Axial T1-weighted image at the level of the patella with visualization of the normal lateral and medial retinacula.

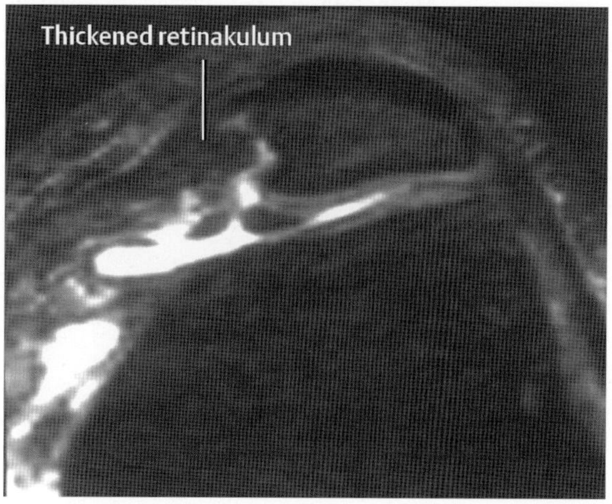

Fig. 1.**230** Axial fat-suppressed MR image. Partial rupture of the medial retinaculum seen as thickening and almost complete break in the continuity.

Tibia/Fibula

Tibial Plateau Fractures

PATH Tibial plateau fractures can be caused by axial compression of the femoral condyles on the tibial plateau combined with valgus or varus stress and also by direct blows (bumper injury).

Classification of tibial plateau fractures: Tibial plateau fractures are divided into fractures without dislocation of the knee joint (the majority of fractures, Fig. 1.**231**), and fractures with dislocations (Fig. 1.**232**). Since most dislocations have spontaneously reduced by the time of the radiographic examination, they can only be deduced if the fracture lines follow a pattern typically seen with dislocations. The fracture-dislocations follow the classification system proposed by Moore. This classification has clinical implication since the fracture type is indicative of possible concomitant ligamentous injuries (Fig. 1.**232**).

X-RAY Radiographs in two 90° views are generally adequate as the initial evaluation.

! Tibial plateau fractures are occasionally difficult to discern on conventional radiographs and CT, or MRI should be obtained in patients with negative conventional radiographs and a strong clinical suspicion of this injury. Furthermore, CT and MRI display the position of the fragments and depression of the articular surface needed for pre-operative planning (Fig. 1.**233**).

MRI In addition to delineating radiographically occult tibial plateau fractures, MRI can show bone bruises as a manifestation of trabecular fractures and associated soft-tissue injuries (Fig. 1.**234**). Isolated osseous injuries seen only on MRI do not require special therapy.

Special manifestations of fracture-dislocations are:

- Distal avulsion of the lateral capsular ligament (lateral anterior femorotibial ligament). This injury is referred to as the Segond fracture and there is a high association with anterior cruciate ligament tears. The fragment and the site of the avulsion are well seen on the AP view (Fig. 1.**237a**).
- Distal avulsion of the iliotibial tract at Gerdy's tubercle. This can be seen on the AP view only if the fragment is dislocated, and is easily mistaken for an osseous avulsion of the insertion of the lateral capsular ligament. Characteristically, the site of origin of the osseous avulsion is not detectable.

Both of these types are grouped under Type 3 (rim avulsion) of tibial fracture-dislocations (Fig. 1.**232**).

! Even if the fragments are small, the possibility of an associated ligamentous injury, especially the ACL, must be considered.

Avulsion of the Intercondylar Eminence

Avulsion of the intercondylar eminence, almost exclusively an injury of the growing skeleton, represents an osseous avulsion of the anterior cruciate ligament. Depending on the severity of dislocation, the fractures are classified as proposed by Meyers and McKeever. From a therapeutic standpoint, classifying these fractures as **incompletely** and **completely** displaced fractures is adequate (Fig. 1.**235**).

! A fracture with barely dislocated fragments may be seen easier on the lateral view.

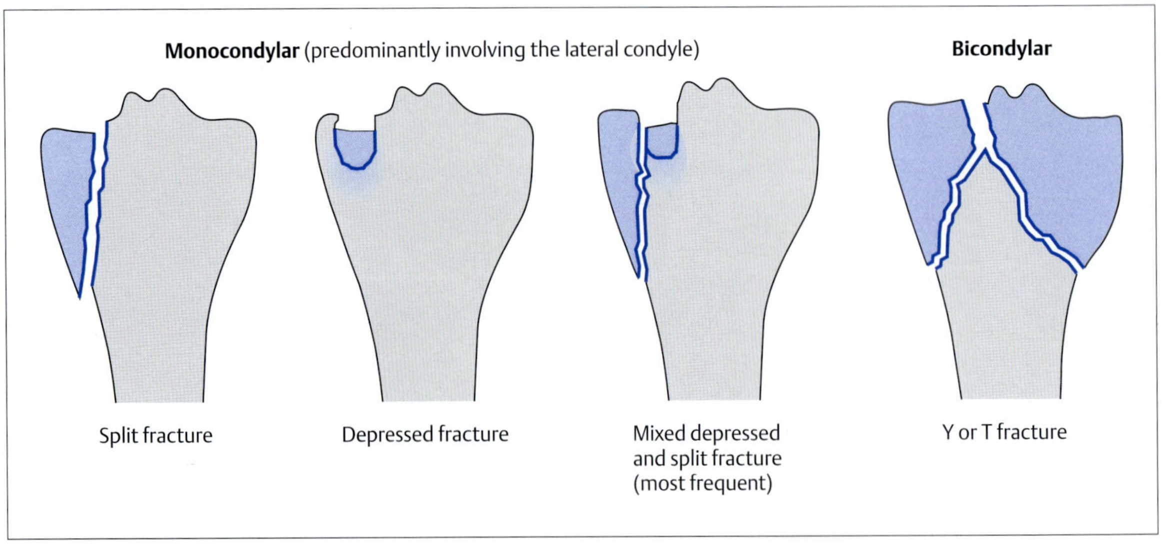

Fig. 1.**231** Fracture of the tibial plateau without dislocation of the knee.

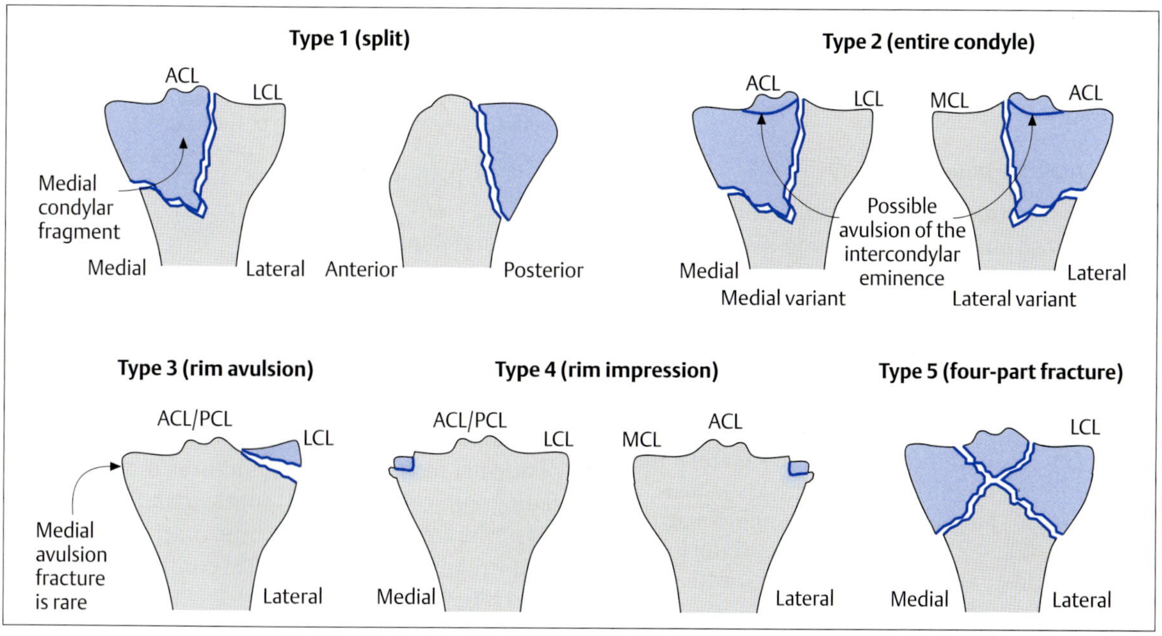

Fig. 1.**232** Fracture-dislocations of the tibial plateau, according to Moore. Possible associated ligamentous injuries and distal osseous avulsions are annotated. MCL = medial collateral ligament; LCL = lateral collateral ligament; ACL = anterior cruciate ligament; PCL = posterior cruciate ligament.

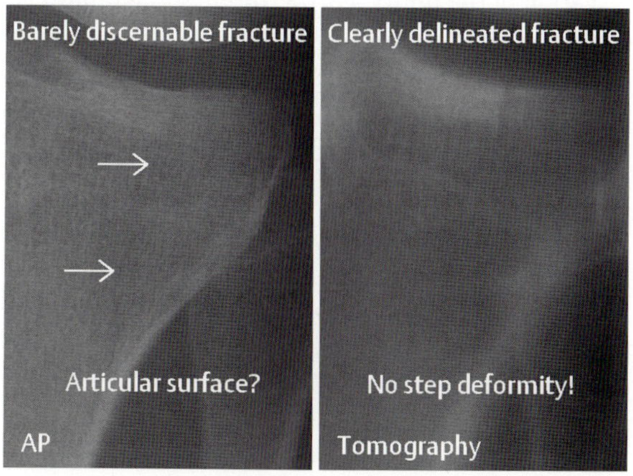

Fig. 1.**233** Exact visualization of a fracture line in the lateral tibial condyle by conventional tomography.

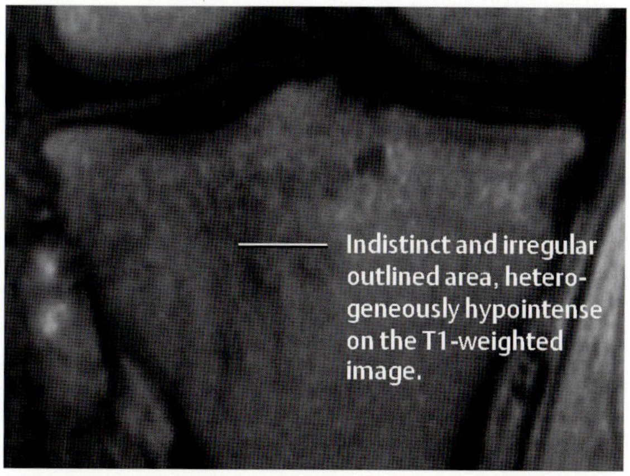

Fig. 1.**234** Bone bruise (trabecular fracture) of the lateral tibial plateau. T1-weighted MRI.

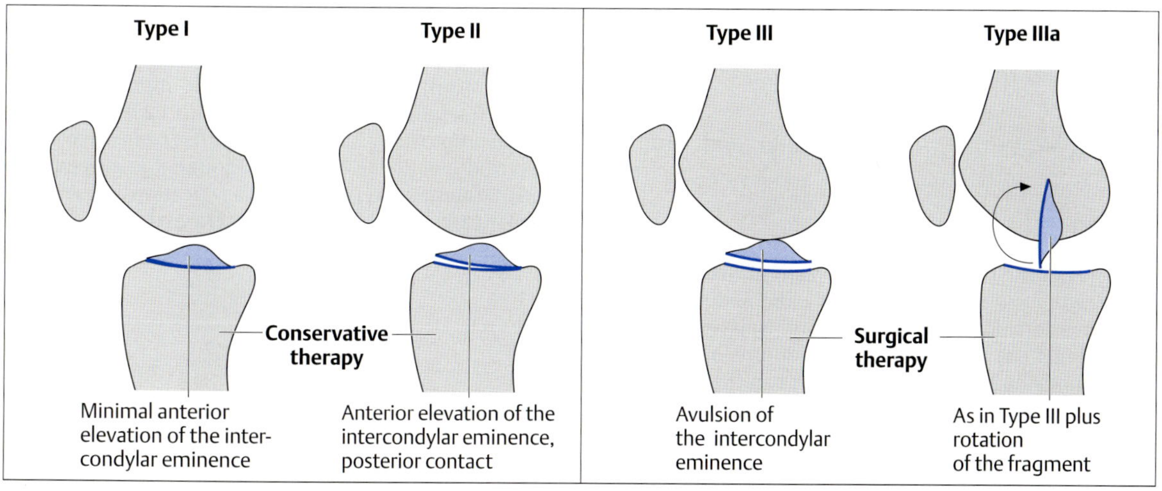

Fig. 1.**235** Avulsion fractures of the intercondylar eminence (according to Meyers and McKeever).

MRI Radiographically questionable or negative findings should be investigated with MRI. In addition, MRI might disclose relevant concomitant injuries.

Avulsion of the Tibial Tuberosity

The avulsion fracture of the tibial tuberosity also occurs most often in the growing skeleton. Dislocated avulsed fragments (relatively frequent) have to be reattached surgically. Undisplaced or only minimally displaced fractures can be treated conservatively.

! A secondary ossification center of the tibial tuberosity or fragmentation seen with Osgood-Schlatter disease should not be mistaken for an avulsion fracture (Fig. 1.**236**). It is important to include clinical findings and history in the diagnostic assessment.

Glossary: Typical **epiphyseal fractures** and **epiphysiolysis** of the proximal tibia are very rare injuries. Nondisplaced epiphysiolysis is particularly easily overlooked, especially if the metaphysis is uninvolved and the typical clinical findings (swelling, point tenderness) are ignored. An isolated fracture of the proximal fibula can be an indirect indication of nondisplaced epiphysiolysis. The presumptive diagnosis can be confirmed when follow-up radiographs show a periosteal reaction around the growth plate.

Fractures of the Fibular Head

The fragments of a fibular head fracture (direct trauma or osseous avulsion of the conjoined tendon or biceps femoris muscle) can be mistaken for an avulsion fracture of the lateral tibial condyle. A slightly oblique or lateral radiographic view (Fig. 1.**237 b**) is most suitable to locate the site of origin of these fragments. It is important to consider a possible concomitant ligamentous injury of the knee whenever this injury is encountered.

Fractures of the Tibia and Fibula

■ Fractures involving both tibial and fibular shafts are often referred to as fractures of the lower leg. ■

Fractures of the **tibia** with involvement of the **fibula** can be caused by direct injury (blow) and indirect injury (shearing, torsion, axial compression). Isolated fractures of the fibula can be caused by direct injury, but are rare. In addition, fibular fractures can occur together with fractures of the tibial plafond and tibial plateau.

Isolated fractures of the fibula must be distinguished from **ankle fractures (Weber Type C)** because of their different treatment. Weber Type C ankle fractures should be suspected from the history of the typical traumatic mechanism (pronation and external rotation) as well as signs of rupture of the interosseous membrane (swelling, pain and point tenderness over the interosseous membrane, widened mortise and subluxation of the talus).

X-RAY Radiographic views in two 90° projections, which must include the proximal and distal joints, are adequate.

Special Manifestation: Metaphyseal Fractures of the Tibia in the Growth Period Caused by Axial Forces

Axial forces acting on the lower leg cause trabecular impaction and compression of the thin cortex of the proximal or distal metaphysis. These therapeutically inconsequential fractures may be visible radiographically only as subtle band-like, transversely oriented trabecular interruptions with minimal irregularity of the cortical contour (torus fracture) (Fig. 1.**238**).

! If the radiographic findings are subtle, examining the child can help pinpoint the exact anatomic location of the injury. Furthermore, sonography can be used to show contour irregularities. MRI is the method of choice if the findings remain inconclusive and accurate diagnosis will result in a change in therapy.

Plafond or Pilon Fractures of the Tibia

■ Fractures of the distal metaphysis with involvement of the ankle joint are referred to as pilon or plafond fractures. ■

In contrast to ankle fractures, tibial plafond fractures result from **axial compression** (e.g., fall from height). The talus is driven into the distal tibial articular surface, also referred to as the pilon or plafond. This is always a severe injury with a high association of post-traumatic osteoarthritis and often needing treatment by arthrodesis.

Classification: The major characteristic findings of typical plafond fractures are summarized in Fig. 1.**239**. The classification proposed by Rüedi-Allgöwer has been selected for the purpose of illustration, even though it is infrequently used in trauma surgery. The AO classification also refers to the plafond or pilon fractures as **extra-articular** fractures of the distal tibial metaphysis.

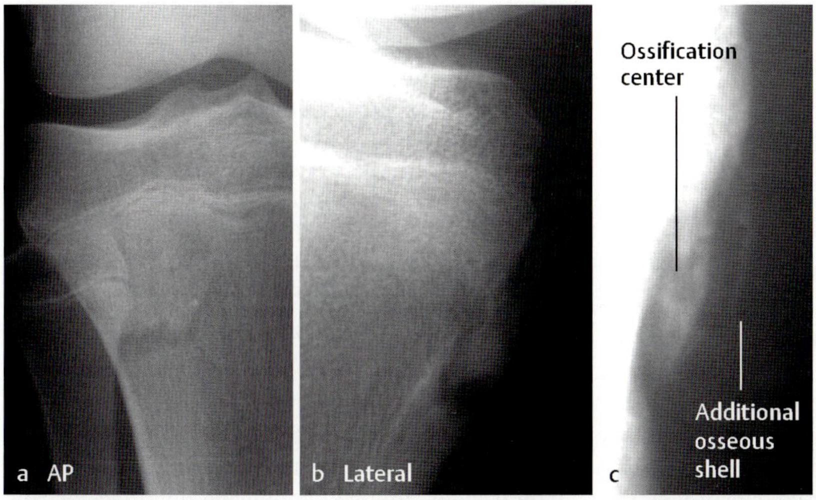

Fig. 1.**236** Conditions resembling an avulsion fracture.
a, b Secondary ossification center of the tibial tuberosity. In Osgood-Schlatter disease (**c**) an additional osseous shell is seen anterior to the ossification center.

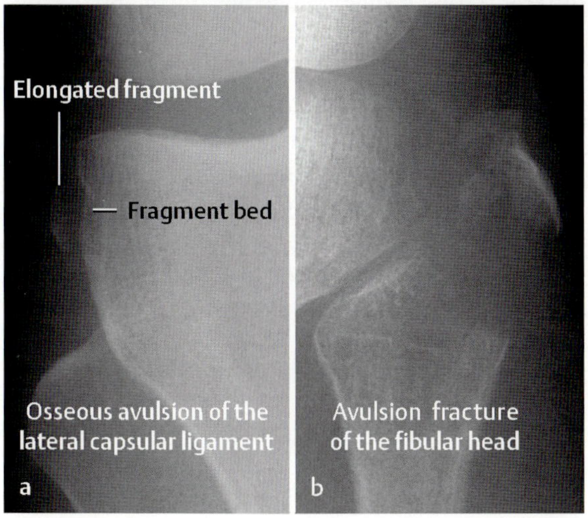

Fig. 1.**237** Fragments at the lateral tibial plateau. **a** The Segond fracture.

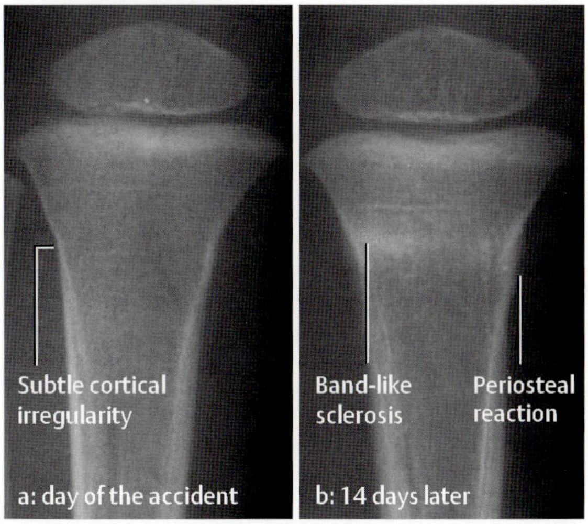

Fig. 1.**238** Impacted fracture of the proximal tibial metaphysis (1-year-old girl).

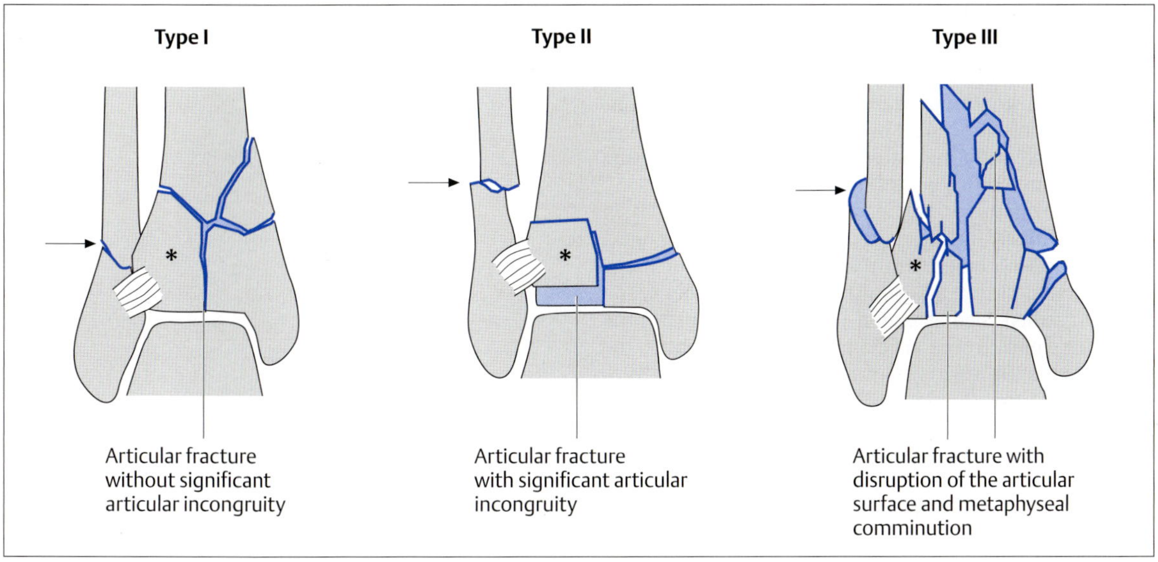

Fig. 1.**239** Fractures of the distal tibial metaphysis (according to Rüedi-Allgöwer). Arrow shows frequently associated distal fibular fracture. * Osseous avulsion of the anterior interosseous membrane (tubercle De Chaput).

Distal Fractures of the Tibia in the Growth Period

1. Epiphysiolysis of the distal tibia

The distal tibia is the most frequent location of epiphysiolysis.

2. Fractures of the medial malleolus

Epiphyseal fractures of the distal tibia before closure of the growth plate invariably involve the medial malleolus (with or without metaphyseal involvement). They occur along the line extending from the medial border of the trochlea of the talus (Fig. 1.**240**). It is critical to recognize these fractures and any displacement, since dislocated fractures are at risk for premature partial closure of the growth plate and resultant varus deformity. Surgical intervention can lower the risk of this outcome. Nondisplaced fractures present no risk of growth disturbance and are treated conservatively.

! In certain circumstances, the fracture might not be visible on the initial AP radiograph. In cases where a medial malleolar fracture is clinically suspected, MRI should be obtained to exclude any possible fracture and to determine the degree of displacement if a fracture is identified.

3. Transitional Fractures of the Distal Tibial Epiphysis

■ Transitional fractures of the distal tibial epiphysis refer to fractures occurring at the age between adolescence and adulthood when the growth plate is partially fused. ■

PATH The mineralization of the distal tibial epiphyseal growth plate proceeds eccentrically, beginning at the anterior aspect of the medial malleolus, progressing posteriorly and laterally and eventually fusing the lateral anterior aspects of the growth plates.

The same trauma that leads to an epiphysiolysis in childhood merely induces loosening of the partially fused lateral aspect of the growth plate at the transitional age between adolescence and adulthood. At the border of the already-ossified medial region of the growth plate, the fracture extends to the articular surface (exception: the intramalleolar fracture is extra-articular). The medially located fused growth plate remains intact (Fig. 1.**241 a**). Such a fracture is also referred to as a 'two plane fracture,' since the fracture extends along two planes (transverse and sagittal). With an associated posterior metaphyseal avulsion, it is a so-called 'tri-plane fracture' (additional fracture along the frontal plane, Fig. 1.**242**). Such tri-plane fractures are further divided into Type 1 and Type 2. In Type 2, the posterior fracture extends into the epiphysis, in contrast to Type 1.

X-RAY The transitional fracture can be diagnosed by the characteristic finding of obliquely oriented epiphyseal fractures seen on the AP view. The fracture type is determined from the lateral view (Fig. 1.**241 b**).

! An absent epiphyseal fracture cleft on the AP view excludes a transitional fracture.

The lateral view usually fails to show the fracture lines of the two-plane fractures but displays the metaphyseal avulsion of the tri-plane fractures. Differentiating a tri-plane fracture of Type 1 from a fracture of Type 2 is not always possible from the lateral view, and MRI should be obtained for this differentiation if therapy will be affected by the distinction.

All undisplaced fractures and extra-articular fractures can be treated conservatively. Intramalleolar fractures must be assessed further to distinguish between a two-plane fracture (extra-articular), a tri-plane fracture Type 1 (extra-articular), or a tri-plane fracture Type 2 (intra-articular). Growth disturbances are no longer to be expected in this age group.

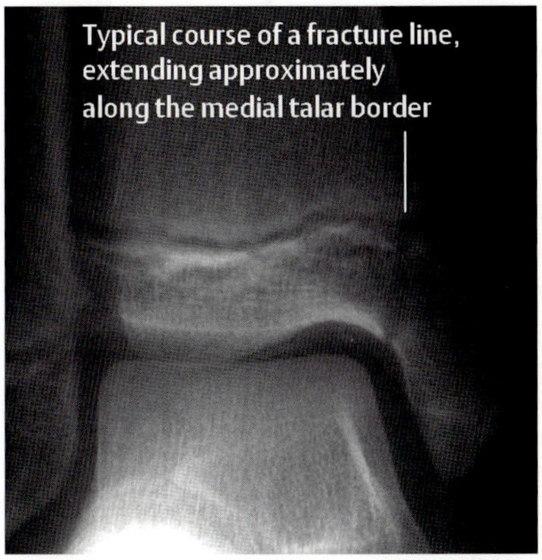

Fig. 1.**240** Fracture of the medial malleolus, typical epiphyseal fracture of the distal tibia with patent growth plate (Aitken Type II fracture in a 12-year-old boy).

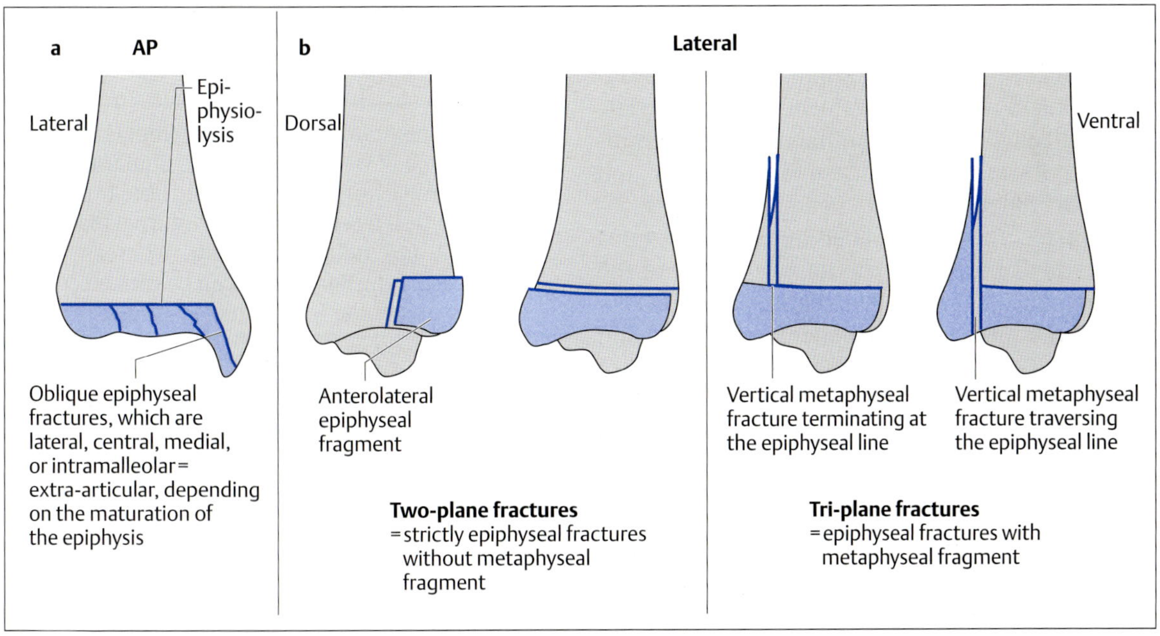

Fig. 1.**241** Fractures of the distal tibial epiphysis. **a** Possible fracture lines as seen on the AP radiograph. **b** Classification of the fractures on the basis of the **lateral view.**

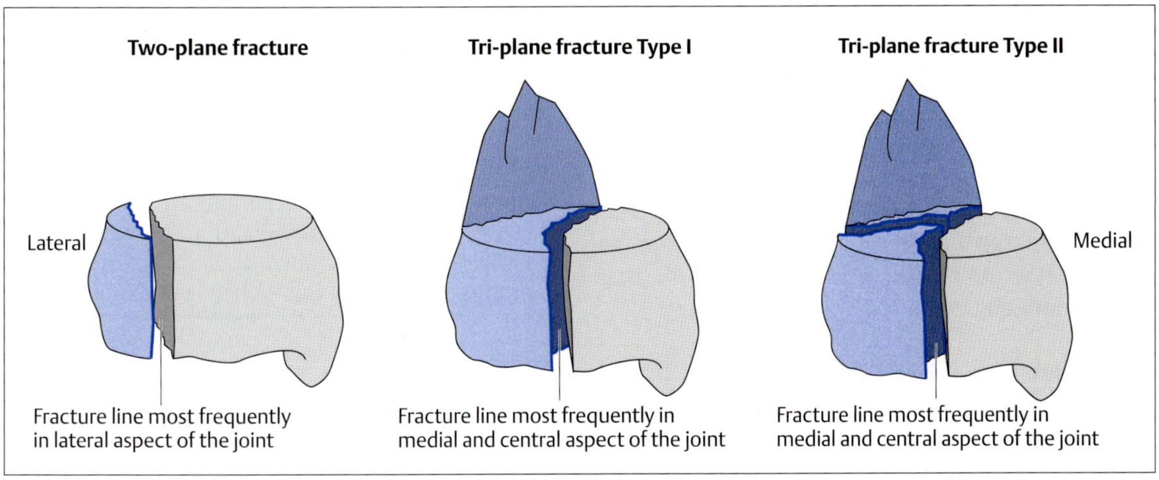

Fig. 1.**242** Characteristic fragments of the various fractures of the distal tibial epiphysis.

Fractures of the Ankle

■ Ankle fractures are the most frequent type of fractures. ■

Fractures of the ankle are caused by rotation (external rotation relative to the transverse plane) or tilting of the talus (abduction and adduction in the coronal plane) relative to the ankle mortise. The **Danis-Weber** classification of the ankle fractures is pathologic-anatomic, consisting of three types that are divided by the level of the fibular fracture relative to the interosseous membrane (Figs. 1.**243** – 1.**245**).

The **Weber Type A fracture** is caused by adduction of the talus with the foot in supination (Fig. 1.**243**).

The pull of the lateral ligaments avulses the lateral malleolus laterally. The fracture line is infrasyndesmotic, and the syndesmotic (anterior and posterior tibiofibular) ligaments themselves remain intact. The force applied by the tilting talus on the medial aspect of the tibia can fracture the medial malleolus or, less frequently, the medial aspect of the posterior articular margin (Volkmann triangle). If the forces of the same mechanism of trauma are weak, the fibular injury can become manifest as avulsion of the lateral ligament at the malleolar tip or as a partial or complete rupture of the lateral ligament.

The **Weber Type B fracture** is caused either by external rotation of the talus with the foot in supination (producing an oblique fracture that rises from inferoanterior to superoposterior, best seen on the lateral view) or by abduction of the talus with the foot in pronation (transverse fracture) (Fig. 1.**244**).

The fracture line lies at the level of the syndesmotic ligaments. It is possible that an osseous avulsion of the tibia occurs at the posterior insertion ('Volkmann triangle') or anterior insertion ('tuberosity of Tillaux-Chaput'). In general, the interosseous membrane remains intact. The mechanism of trauma acting on the medial aspect of the tibiotalar articulation can cause a concomitant transverse avulsion fracture of the medial malleolus or a tear of the deltoid ligament.

The **Weber Type C fracture** is caused by external rotation of the talus with the foot in pronation (Fig. 1.**245**).

In contrast to the Weber Type B fracture, the fibular fracture is suprasyndesmotic. The syndesmotic ligaments are ruptured and the interosseous membrane above the ligaments is torn to the level of the fibular fracture, with loss of the normal ankle mortise formed by the tibia and fibula. The retractile forces acting on the medial malleolus cause the deltoid ligament or the medial malleolus to rupture. An avulsion of the posterior Volkmann triangle or the tuberosity of Tillaux-Chaput is also possible.

The **Maisonneuve fracture** is a special form of the Weber Type C fracture. The same mechanism dislodges the fibula from the fibular groove of the tibia and fractures the fibula proximal to the level of its midpoint (Fig. 1.**245**). In rare cases, the tibiofibular articulation dislocates instead.

Another relatively rare injury is the isolated syndesmotic rupture, or the avulsion of the Volkmann triangle.

! Weber Type A: infrasyndesmotic fibular fracture,
Weber Type B: transsyndesmotic fibular fracture,
Weber Type C: suprasyndesmotic fibular fracture.
Weber Type C fractures require internal fixation to maintain acceptable alignment, whereas Weber Type A and Type B fractures can be treated conservatively unless the fragments are displaced.

X-RAY Technical considerations: It is very important to obtain the AP view with 20° internal rotation of the ankle for an unobstructed projection of the talus and malleolar relationships.
Findings:

1. On the correctly obtained AP view, all segments of the joint are approximately equal in width (Fig. 1.**246a**).
2. Even minimal elevation of the lateral malleolus is evident radiographically (Fig. **246b**).

If a Maisonneuve fracture is suspected clinically (point tenderness over the proximal fibula), the entire lower leg must be imaged.

All ankle injuries must be scrutinized for osteochondral fractures of the talus.

! Because of different therapeutic ramifications (short period of immobilization instead of internal fixation), the isolated fibular fracture must be distinguished from the Weber Type C fracture.

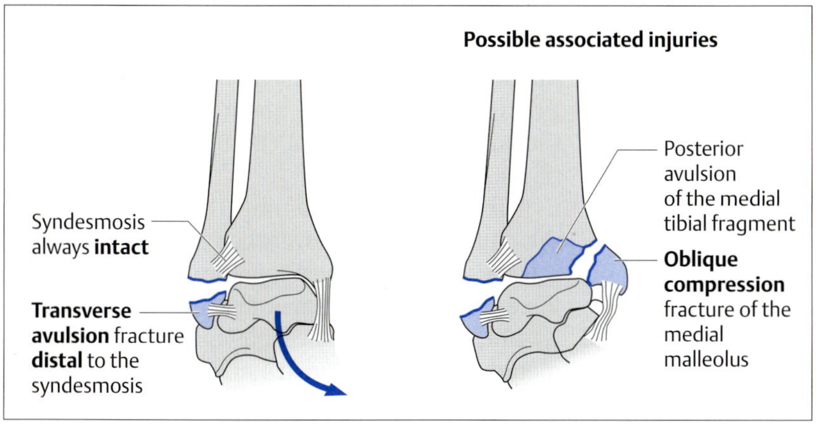

Fig. 1.243 Weber Type A fracture. Adduction of the talus with the foot in supination.

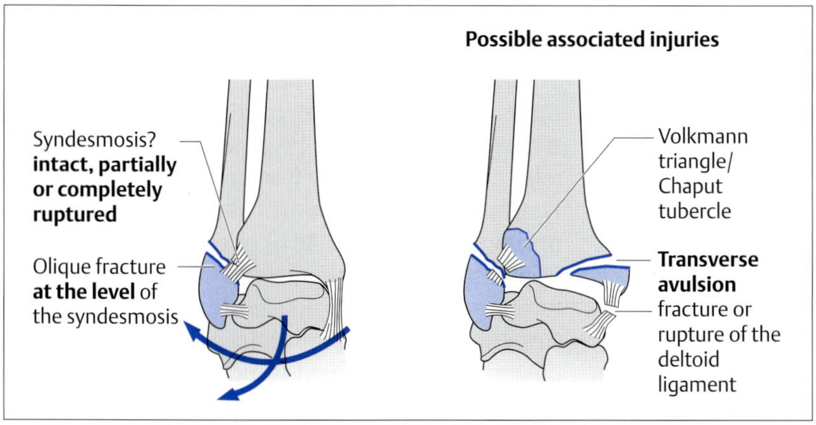

Fig. 1.244 Weber Type B fracture. External rotation of the talus with the foot in supination, or abduction of the talus with the foot in pronation.

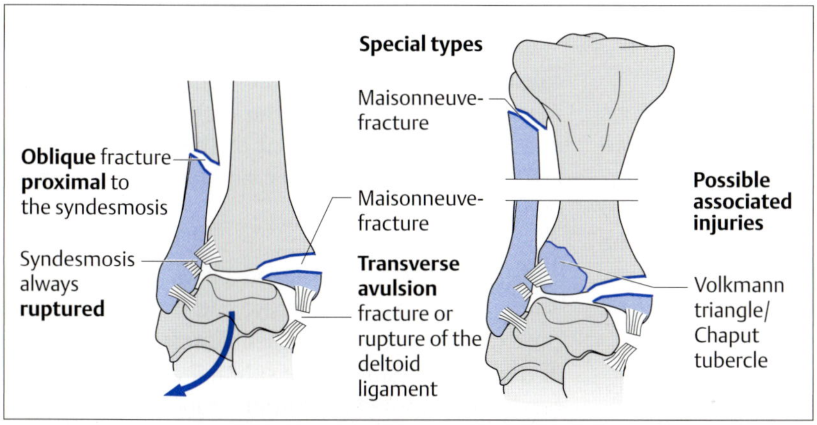

Fig. 1.245 Weber Type C fracture. External rotation of the talus with the foot in pronation.

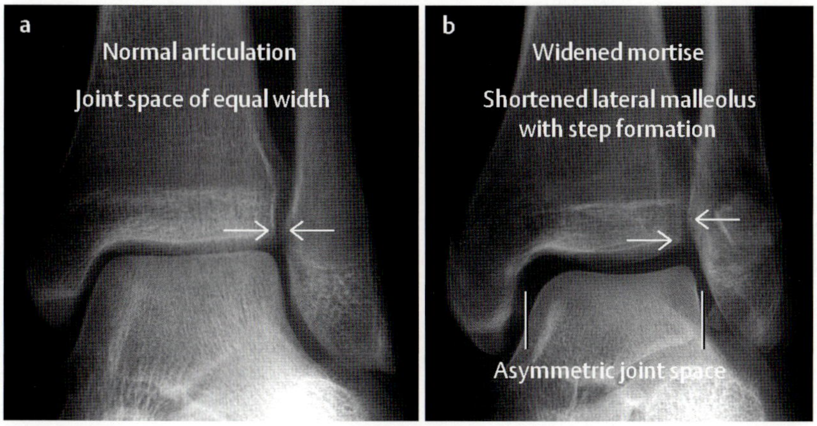

Fig. 1.246 Articular planes of the ankle as seen in the AP projection with 20° internal rotation.

Tarsal and Metatarsal Bones

Talar Fractures

CLINIC The most frequent fracture location here is the talar neck, and it is usually caused by axial loading, e.g., a fall from a height or a motor vehicle accident with the foot dorsiflexed on the pedal. This mechanism pinches the talar neck between the calcaneus and the anterior border of the tibia. The osteochondral fractures of the talar dome are caused by shearing forces.

Anatomic Peculiarities

The nutrient vessels enter the talus at two sites: at the dorsum of the talar neck and at the plantar surface above the sinus tarsi (Fig. 1.**250**). Following a displaced fracture of the talar neck or a talar dislocation, the talus is at risk for necrosis because of vascular compromise.

Classification of Talar Fractures

On the basis of their anatomic location, talar fractures are divided into fractures of the head, neck, and body. Fractures of the talar body include the osteochondral fractures of the talar dome and the fractures of the lateral and posterior processes. The classification system proposed by Hawkins, which considers the degree of the displacement of the tibiotalar and subtalar articulation, is used for fractures of the talar neck. It also has prognostic implications (Fig. 1.**247**).

X-RAY Radiographic views in two 90° projections are standard (AP and lateral). Undisplaced osteochondral fractures of the lateral or medial surface of the talar dome might only be diagnosed by dislocated fragments seen on stress views of the ankle joint. If the standard views are inconclusive, spot films under fluoroscopic guidance or CT should be obtained for further evaluation.

MRI MRI is a very sensitive method and can detect radiographically occult subchondral fractures and bone bruises as manifestation of trabecular fractures.

Calcaneal Fractures

CLINIC The typical mechanism of a calcaneal fracture is the axial load such as a vertical fall from a height. An exception is the rare beak fracture, representing an osseous avulsion caused by the pull of the Achilles tendon on the calcaneal tuberosity (Fig. 1.**248**).

Classification of Calcaneal Fractures

About one-third of calcaneal fractures are extra-articular (Fig. 1.**248**), and about two-thirds involve the subtalar articulation (posterior compartment) (Fig. 1.**249**).

In **intra-articular** fractures, the lateral process of the talus, which rests over the central region of the calcaneal body, is driven into the calcaneus by axial force. The resulting **primary** fracture line (Fig. 1.**249a**) breaks the calcaneus into two main fragments, the anteromedial (sustentacular) and the posterolateral (tuberosity) fragments. An additional sustentacular fragment frequently avulses from the anterior process (Fig. 1.**249a**). With a stronger axial force, an additional **secondary** fracture line separates the posterior facet from the tuberal fragment (Figs. 1.**249b,c**). According to Essex-Lopresti, two fracture types can be generated, depending on whether the secondary fracture line curves cranially around the subtalar articular surface (**joint depression type,** Fig. 1.**249b**) or extends horizontally in a posterior direction to the tuberosity with the formation of a tongue-like posterior facet fragment (**tongue type,** Fig. 1.**249c**). In either situation, the posterior facet fragment is rotated and pushed into the tuberal fragment and can be fractured in itself. The calcaneus increases in width and decreases in height.

The primary surgical therapy for intra-articular calcaneal fractures is to restore the anatomic alignment and the integrity of the subtalar joint as nearly as possible. Involvement of the calcaneocuboid articulation generally has no therapeutic consequence.

X-RAY From the lateral and axial views of the calcaneus, the fracture can be classified and the extent of the displacement assessed. The degree of the compression of the subtalar articular surface can be determined by **Böhler's** tuberosity-joint angle (Fig. 1.**252**).

! The condition of the subtalar articular surface (degree of articular step deformity; size, number, and position of the fragments) determines the therapy planning and can be assessed with the necessary accuracy only by CT (Fig. 1.**251**).

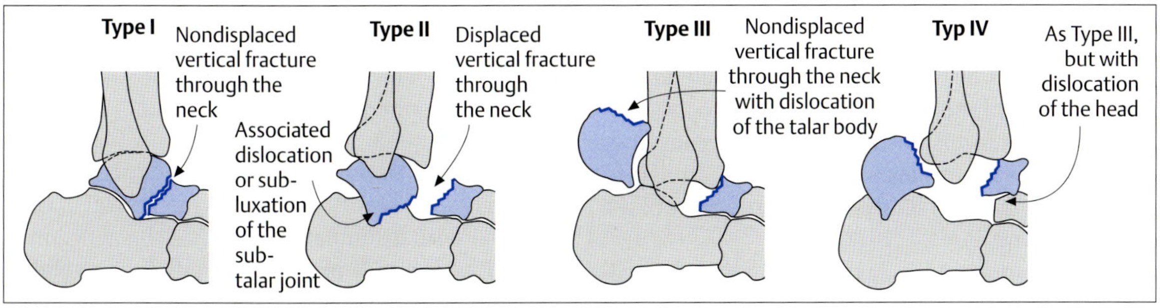

Fig. 1.**247** Classification of talar neck fractures according to Hawkins.

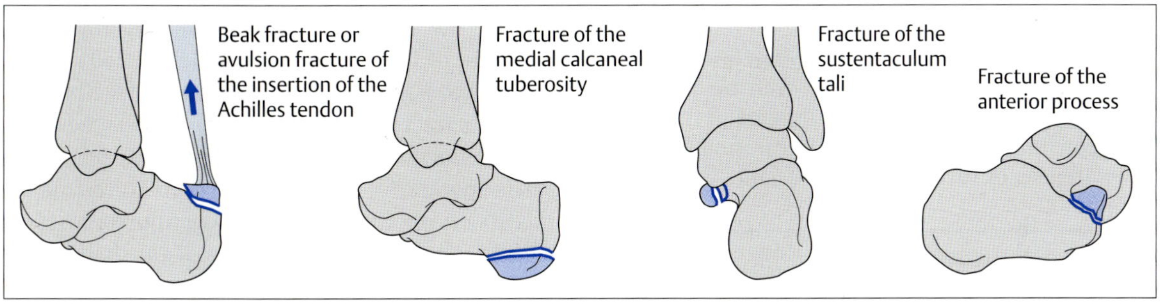

Fig. 1.**248** Extra-articular calcaneal fractures – without involvement of the subtalar articular surface.

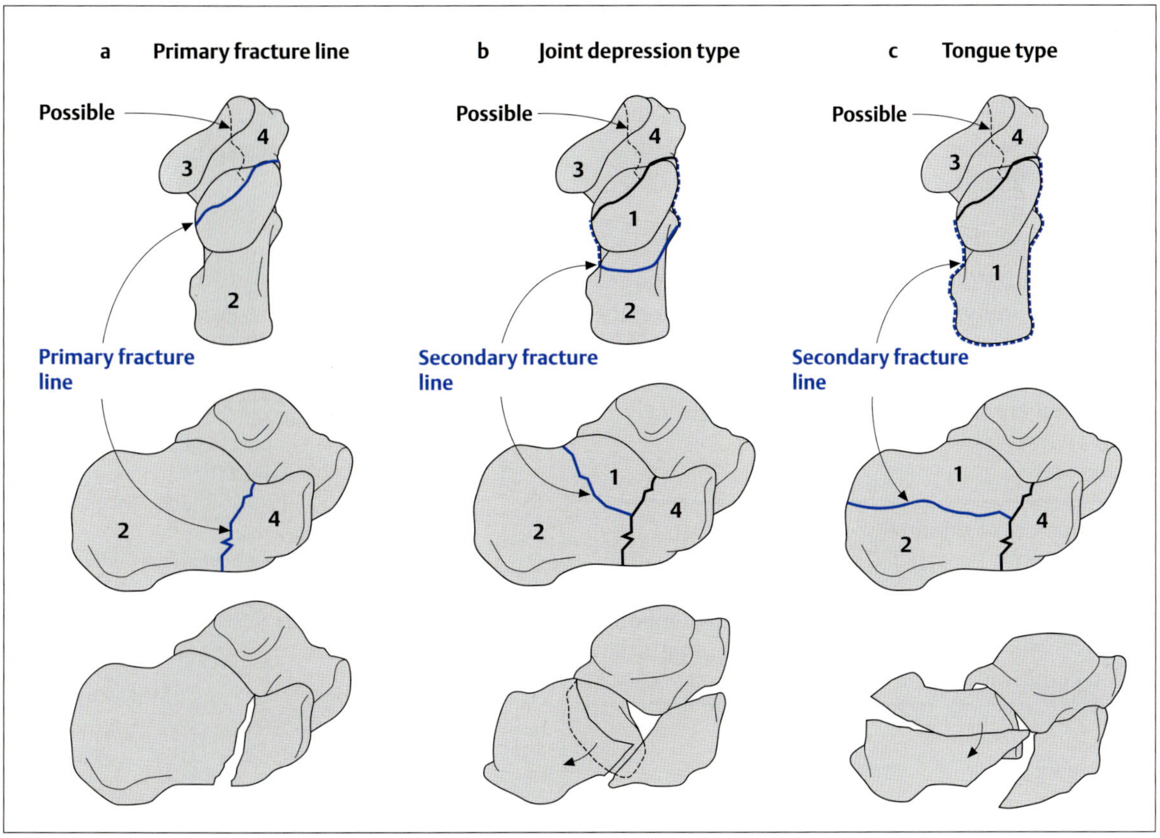

Fig. 1.**249** Intra-articular calcaneal fracture – with involvement of the subtalar articular surface. Major fragments: (1) posterior facet fragment, (2) tuberosity fragment, (3) sustentacular fragment, (4) anterior process fragment.

Fractures of the Remaining Tarsal Bones

Typical injuries of the navicular bone include osseous avulsion of the dorsal surface close to the talonavicular joint, avulsion at the tuberosity caused by the pull of the posterior tibial tendon as part of pronation trauma, and fracture through the body of the navicular bone.

Aside from fractures associated with dislocations of the Lisfranc articulation (see below), the cuneiform bones and cuboid frequently have small avulsions caused by direct trauma which are often difficult to detect.

> **!** Secondary ossification centers can be mistaken for traumatic avulsions at many sites in the tarsal region. Correlation with physical findings and awareness of various normal variants are important.

Dislocations of the Foot

Classification of the foot dislocations: All the joints of the foot can dislocate. If the ankle is counted as part of the foot, the tibiotalar articulation and the Lisfranc articulation are most frequently dislocated (Fig. 1.**250**). Dislocations of the subtalar joint and Chopart joint, as well as talar dislocation with the talus dislocated at the tibiotalar joint or subtalar joint are also encountered.

X-RAY Depending on the trauma, dislocation of the Lisfranc joint involves all the metatarsals or each individually. Fractures of the metatarsal bases – in particular of the second metatarsal base – as well as fractures of the cuneiform bones and cuboid are frequent accompanying injuries.

> **!** Overlooking a minimally dislocated Lisfranc articulation can be avoided by thorough evaluation of the alignment of the metatarsal bases relative to the distal tarsal row on PA, lateral and oblique PA (40–45°) views. Some dislocations might be detectable only on CT.

Fractures of the Metatarsals

X-RAY PA, lateral, and oblique PA (40–45°) views are standard.

A special metatarsal fracture is the **avulsion fracture** of the tuberosity of the fifth metatarsal in conjunction with a supination trauma. The avulsion is caused by the pull of the peroneus brevis tendon together with the pull of a long extension of the plantar aponeurosis and the plantar longum tendon (Fig. 1.**253**).

The so-called **Jones fracture** is a transverse fracture of the proximal metadiaphyseal transition (isthmus) of the fifth metatarsal (Fig. 1.**253**). It can be an acute fracture or a stress fracture (see below). The Jones fracture has a tendency for delayed healing, pseudarthrosis, and refracture.

The metatarsal fatigue (stress) fracture (march fracture), is another special type of injury, most frequently involving the middle or distal shaft of the second and third metatarsals. The osseous reaction is radiographically seen as a transverse, indistinctly outlined, broad sclerotic band. With continuing abnormal stress, this lesion can progress to a complete fracture. Metatarsal stress fractures can heal rather slowly (over several weeks) (Fig. 1.**254**). Osteomyelitis must be considered in the differential diagnosis but is characterized by more irregularities in the osseous structures and the development of osteolytic areas.

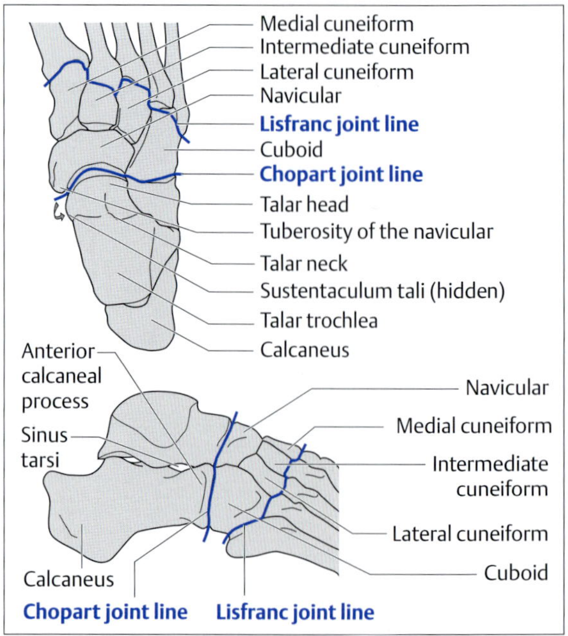

Fig. 1.**250** Anatomy of the tarsal bones.

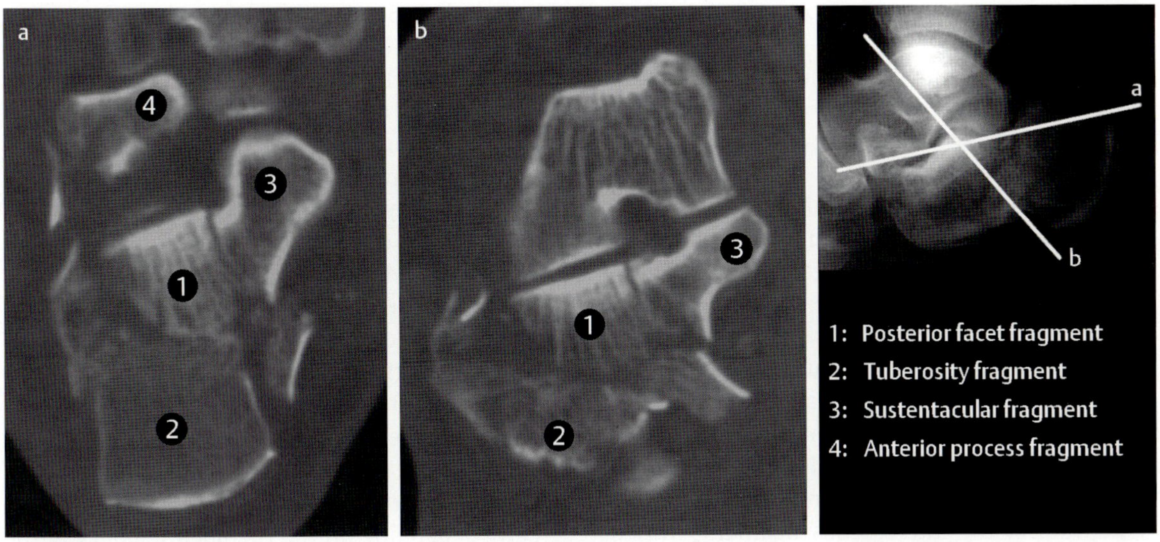

Fig. 1.**251** Calcaneal-axial (**a**) and semi-coronal (**b**) CT section of an intra-articular calcaneal fracture (joint depression type).

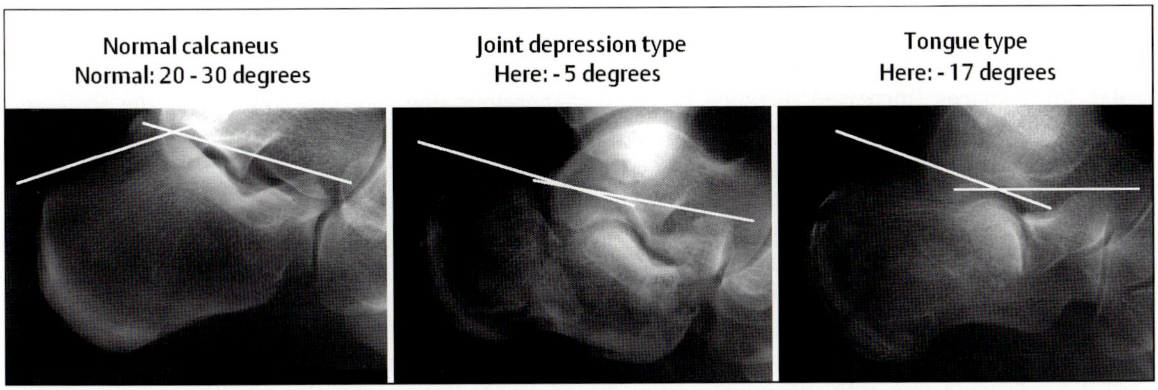

Fig. 1.**252** Tuberosity-joint angle according to Böhler. The angle is formed by line **a,** which connects the highest point of the calcaneal tuberosity with the posterior border of the subtalar articular surface, and line **b,** which connects this point with the highest point of the anterior process. It should measure 20–40°.

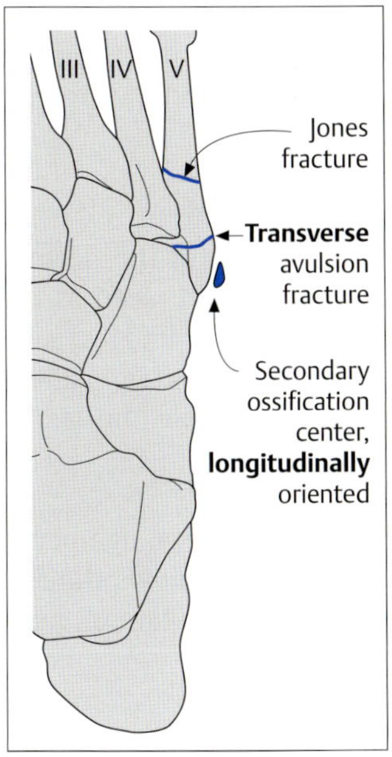

Fig. 1.**253** Avulsion and Jones fracture of the fifth metatarsal. The fracture line of the avulsion fracture traverses the metatarsal base perpendicular to its long axis and can extend into the cuboideometatarsal articulation. In contrast, the radiolucent line separating the secondary ossification center is longitudinally oriented and without articular extension.

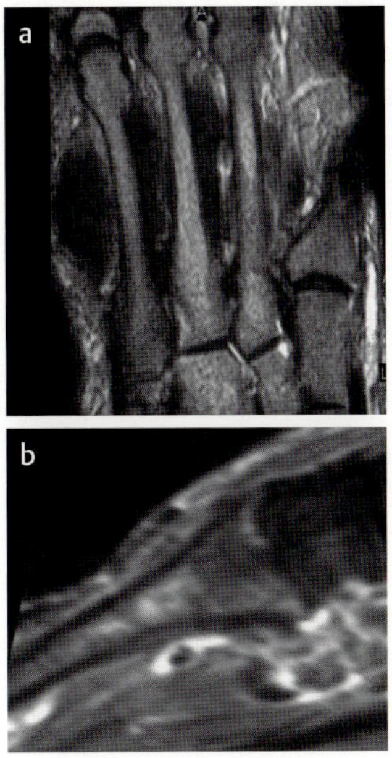

Fig. 1.**254** MRI of a stress fracture. The T2-weighted image (**a**) does not visualize the fracture and only suggests an edema. In contrast, the STIR image (**b**) clearly exhibits the extensive bone bruise.

Ligamentous Injuries of the Ankle

The ligamentous support of the ankle consists of three units (Fig. 1.**255**):

- distal interosseous ligament: anterior and posterior tibiofibular ligaments
- lateral ligament: anterior and posterior talofibular ligaments, calcaneofibular ligaments
- medial ligaments: deltoid ligament

Distal Interosseous Ligaments

Injury of the distal interosseous ligaments is frequently associated with a fibular fracture. In these cases, the interosseous ligaments are repaired and the fracture is internally fixed. Isolated tears of the distal interosseous ligaments are relatively rare.

Rupture of the interosseous ligaments widens the ankle mortise; however, the width of the ankle mortise is extremely projection-dependent on the AP view, and only a marked **widening of the mortise** is diagnostically relevant. A more reliable radiographic finding is **asymmetry of the talomalleolar joint spaces** (increased distance between medial malleolus and talus, Fig. 1.**256**). Inconclusive findings can be further evaluated by side-to-side comparison and possibly also by early post-traumatic conventional arthrography. Contrast medium extending upward from the tibiotalar articulation between the tibia and fibula indicates a tear. MRI can be considered a reliable method to evaluate the distal interosseous ligament because of its direct visualization of the ligament.

Injury of the Lateral or Tibiofibular Collateral Ligaments

Injuries of the tibiofibular ligaments following supination trauma are the most frequent of all ligamentous injuries. The tear primarily affects the anterior talofibular ligament, with two or three ligaments involved in 60% of the injuries.

Therapy: Definitive surgical indications are not established. Some authors recommend surgery only in special cases (professional athletes) while others consider a talar tilt of more than 20° an indication for surgery.

X-RAY **Stress views of the ankle:** After a fracture is excluded by conventional radiographs in two projections, stress views are obtained with the hindfoot angled manually or in a device with a defined force (in general 150 N) (Fig. 1.**257**). A tilt up to 5° is normal and more than 10° abnormal. A tilt between 5° and 10° requires comparison views of the contralateral side, with a side to side difference of more than 5° considered pathologic (some authors consider a higher tilt normal as long as it is symmetrical). This method does not allow exact determination of extent, degree, and location of the ligamentous injury. A tilt of more than 20°, however, generally is a manifestation of ligamentous injuries involving two to three ligaments.

The rupture of the anterior talofibular ligament can be assessed by a second stress view, with the foot pushed anteriorly relative to the ankle mortise ('talar translation'). The distance between the posterior tibial articulating surface and talus is measured on the lateral view. Measured values exceeding 10 mm are pathologic, and between 5 and 10 mm require comparison views. The benefit of this stress examination is judged rather differently, greatly depending on the therapeutic policy of the particular institution.

SONO The hematoma found with acutely injured ligaments precludes any adequate sonographic evaluation of acute trauma. Sonography, therefore, does not play any role in the acute setting.

MRI MRI can visualize the small ligaments and their injuries by examining the foot in a defined position in any preselected imaging plane. Like all ligamentous structures, the ligaments are of low signal intensity in all sequences, with a smooth contour and high contrast relative to the periligamentous fat (Fig. 1.**258**). An exception is the posterior talofibular ligament, which is triangular in configuration and is found to have linear fatty deposits. The signs of a ligamentous injury, up to a complete a tear, are:

- increased signal intensity within the ligament (on T1-weighted and, especially, on T2-weighted images)
- ligamentous thickening
- elongation with undulating contour
- thinning or complete disruption of the normal contour with visualization of fluid (seen as increased intensity on T2-weighted images) surrounding the ligamentous remnants (Fig. 1.**259**).

MRI is also helpful in evaluating remote injuries.

Medial or Tibial Collateral Ligaments

An isolated injury of the tibial collateral ligaments is rare. The evaluation by imaging follows the approach described for the fibular collateral ligaments.

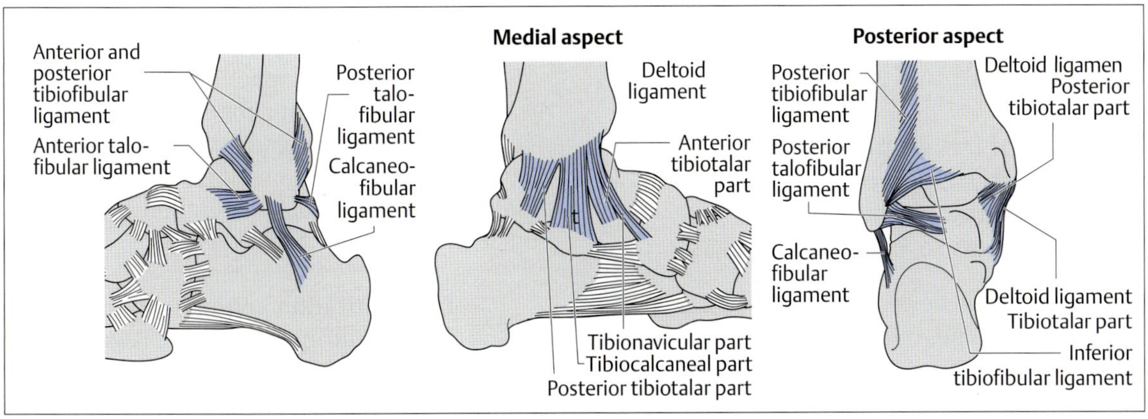

Fig. 1.**255** Schematic representation of the ligaments of the ankle and the tibiofibular syndesmosis.

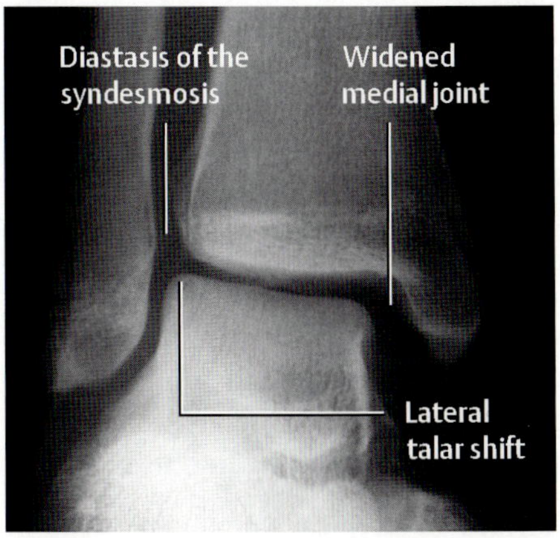

Fig. 1.**256** Signs suggestive of ruptured syndesmosis as seen on the AP radiograph. Widened ankle mortise with asymmetrical joint space.

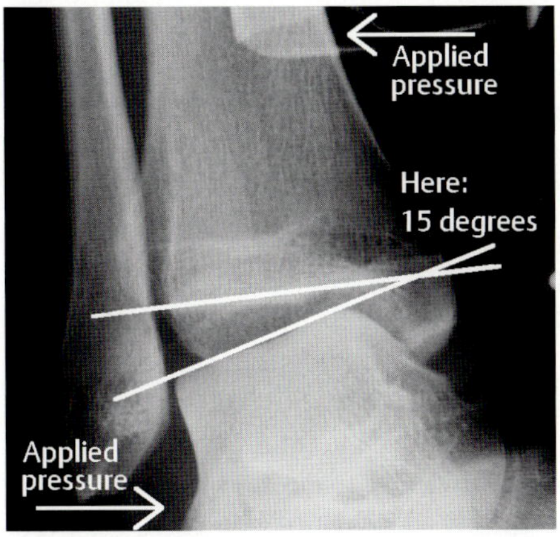

Fig. 1.**257** Stress view. To measure the stress-induced talar tilt, tangents to the tibial plafond and talar dome are drawn.

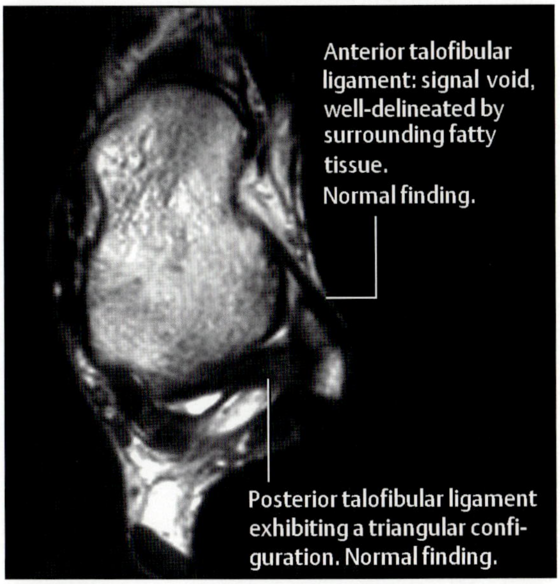

Fig. 1.**258** Axial MRI (T2-weighted image) of the lateral ankle ligaments. Normal findings of the dorsiflexed foot. Compare with Fig. 1.**259**.

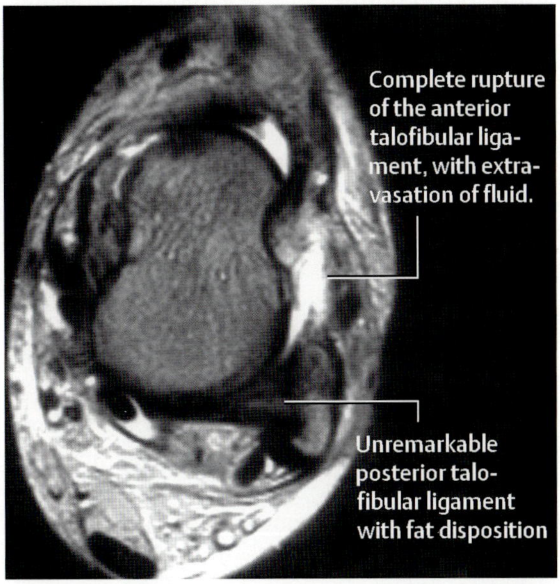

Fig. 1.**259** Axial MRI (T2-weighted image), lateral ankle ligaments. Complete rupture of the anterior talofibular ligament with extravasation of fluid.

Special Problems Encountered in Children

The Normal Development of the Epiphyseal Growth Zone, Developmental Variations, and Transition to Pathologic Cases

Postnatal skeletal development follows a predetermined course and consists of three ossification phases interposed between periods of longitudinal growth:

- development of ossification centers in the preformed cartilage epiphyses of the short and longitudinal bones, as well as in the carpal and tarsal bones,
- development of the ossification centers in the apophyses,
- osseous closure of the epiphyseal plates.

Only two epiphyseal ossification centers can be observed in the mature newborn: the distal femoral epiphysis and, less frequently, the proximal tibial epiphysis. Additional ossification centers appear with increasing age. After the appearance of an ossification center, the ossification progresses to the edges of the epiphyseal cartilage (Fig. 1.**260**). At the time of the epiphyseal closure, the cartilage plate between osseous epiphysis and shaft involutes with a thin cartilage layer remaining and forming the articular cartilage.

The apophyseal ossification centers appear later, just before or during puberty. Fusion of the apophysis to bone begins after puberty and generally is completed at the age of 25 years.

The schedule for the appearance and growth of the ossification centers and for the fusion of the ossified epiphysis and apophysis with the bone is fairly constant within a certain range, allowing the determination of the skeletal maturation and deriving from it an estimation of skeletal age.

X-RAY The **ossification centers** within the epiphyseal and apophyseal cartilage are subject to numerous anatomic variants during skeletal growth, such as the formation of two or more ossification centers, which later fuse to a single ossification center. During this phase, the ossification centers exhibit an irregular border and are fragmented and irregularly mineralized (Fig. 1.**261**). Epiphyseal and apophyseal variants are frequently encountered:

Cone-shaped epiphyses, often associated with an endochondral growth disturbance of the affected phalanges, are observed in the skeleton of the hands in about 4% of otherwise normal children (Fig. 1.**262**), but are also frequently found in children with chromosomal anomalies and skeletal dysplasias. Errors can be made by under- and overinterpretation of the radiographic findings.

Pseudoepiphyses or atypical epiphyses occur in healthy children at the proximal second through fourth metacarpals and at the distal first metacarpal and are without clinical significance. They are more frequently seen with systemic skeletal growth disturbances.

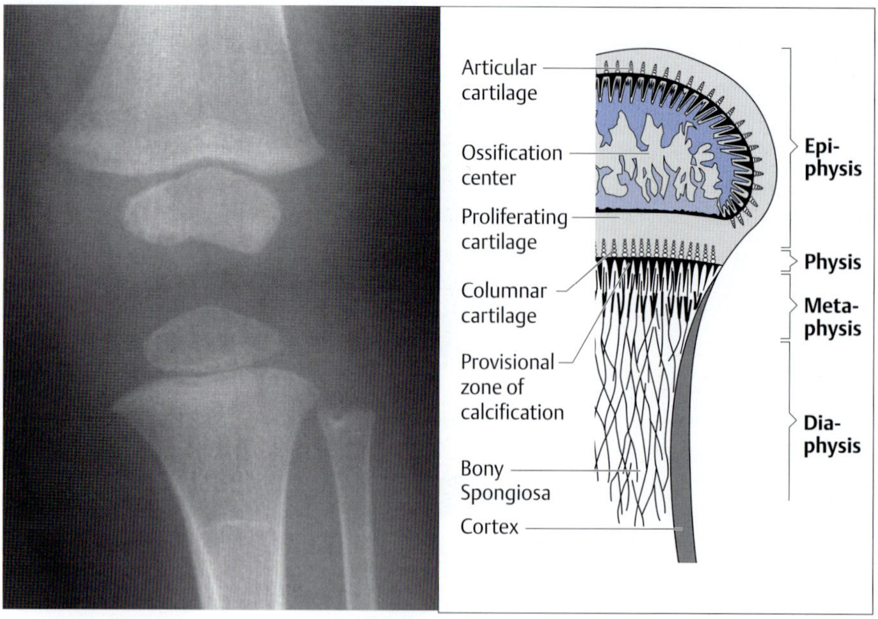

Fig. 1.**260** Anatomy of the epi-/metaphyseal growth plate of a long bone and the corresponding radiographic findings.

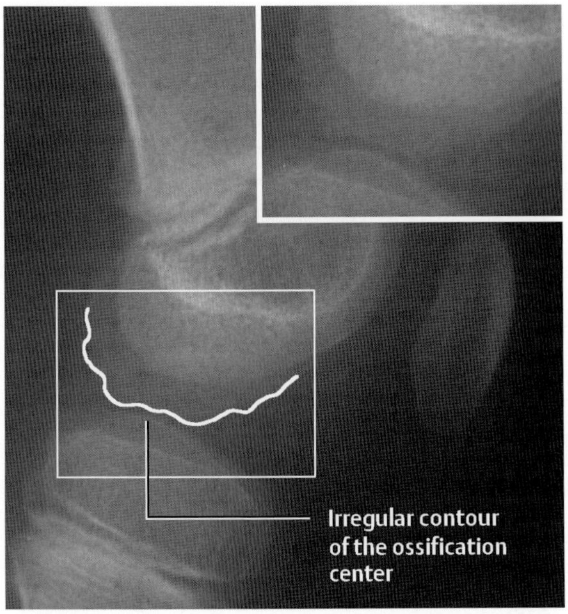

Fig. 1.261 Physiologic irregular contour of the ossification center of the epiphyseal condyle (6½-year-old girl). Normal variant.

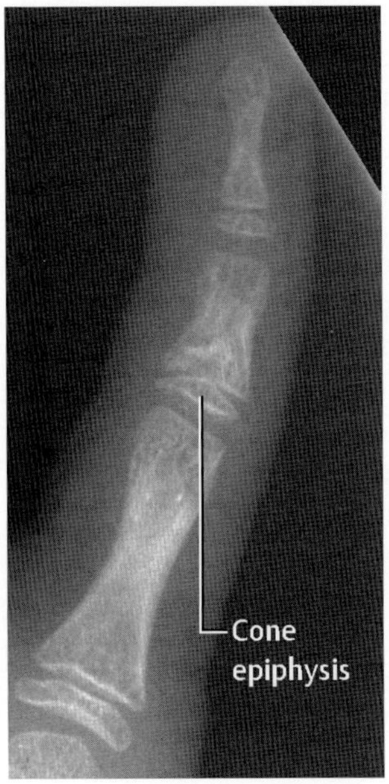

Fig. 1.262 Cone-shaped epiphysis with brachymesophalangia in a 9-year-old girl: **Normal variant** with minor enchondral growth disturbance.

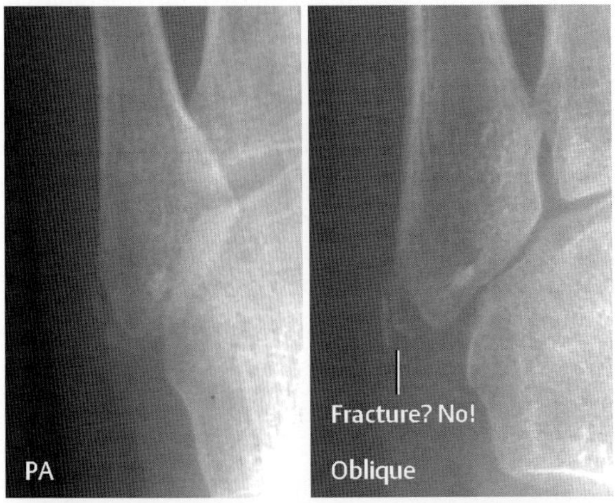

Fig. 1.263 Normal variant versus fracture: two shell-like apophyseal ossification centers at the proximal fifth metatarsal (13-year-old boy). No known trauma, no local tenderness. **Normal variant!**

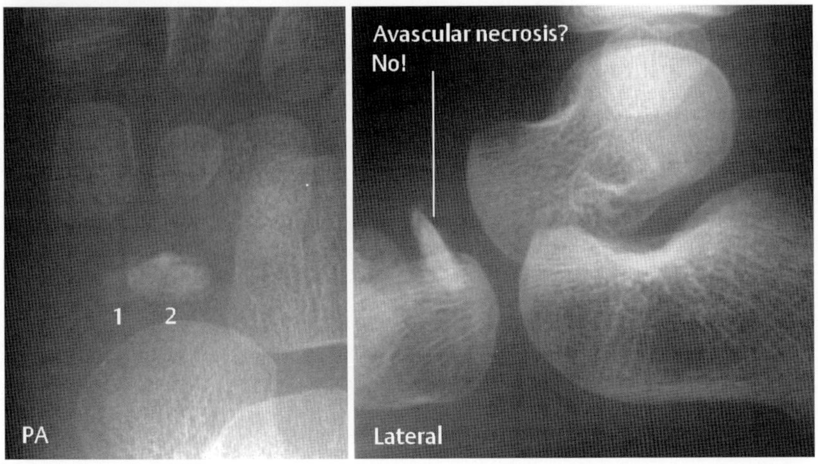

Fig. 1.264 Normal variant versus Köhler's disease: 5-year-old boy, without complaints. Two ossification centers of the navicular mimic avascular necrosis with fragmentation. **Normal variant!**

Increased mineralization of the epiphyseal ossification centers can occasionally be observed in healthy children, predominately seen in the distal phalanges as so-called ivory or marble bone epiphyses.

Apophyseal variants present not only as capricious configuration of the ossification centers and their prolonged persistence due to delayed osseous fusion, but also as accessory ossification centers.

The **carpal and tarsal bones** are particularly prone to radiographic variation:
- different temporal appearance of the ossification centers,
- irregular mineralization,
- fusion with adjacent ossification centers,
- occasional appearance of accessory ossification centers.

Separating a growth variant from a skeletal alteration of clinical significance can be difficult, especially in the presence of local pain with joint effusion. This clinical situation mandates the confirmation of a developmental variant or the exclusion of a pathologic finding. The differential diagnostic considerations of an epiphyseal or apophyseal variant can be narrowed to:
- epiphyseal or apophyseal fracture with supernumerary atypical ossification centers (Fig. 1.**263**),
- avascular osteonecrosis with irregular sclerosis and diminution of the ossification centers (Fig. 1.**264**),
- osteochondritis dissecans or osteochondral fracture if the articular contour is irregular (Fig. 1.**265**),
- congenital skeletal anomaly with atypical epiphysis (Fig. 1.**266**).

SONO Identifying the ossification center within the epiphyseal cartilage in the neonatal age group and demonstrating its relationship to the already-ossified metaphysis allows the sonographic differentiation of a normal finding from a traumatic epiphyseal dislocation and joint effusion. If subchondral fracture, osteochondritis dissecans, or avascular osteonecrosis is suspected in infants and children, the sonographically demonstrated joint effusion should prompt a more extensive diagnostic evaluation. Failure to find a joint effusion sonographically makes acute trauma unlikely.

NUC Bone scintigraphy can differentiate between a developmental variant (no asymmetric tracer uptake) and a traumatic epiphyseal or apophyseal lesion or avascular necrosis. Its disadvantage is the low resolution with limited anatomic detail.

MRI Morphologic findings and signal pattern almost always allow a distinction between trauma and variant or disturbed ossification. MRI is well suited to supplement inconclusive sonographic findings.

The cases of several epiphyseal and apophyseal developmental variants shown here illustrate the problem of differentiating variants from true pathologic changes.

Many more anatomic variants of the radiographic appearance of the epiphyses and apophyses can be encountered in all growth areas of the skeleton, with detailed information of a specific variant best searched for in the appropriate reference literature.

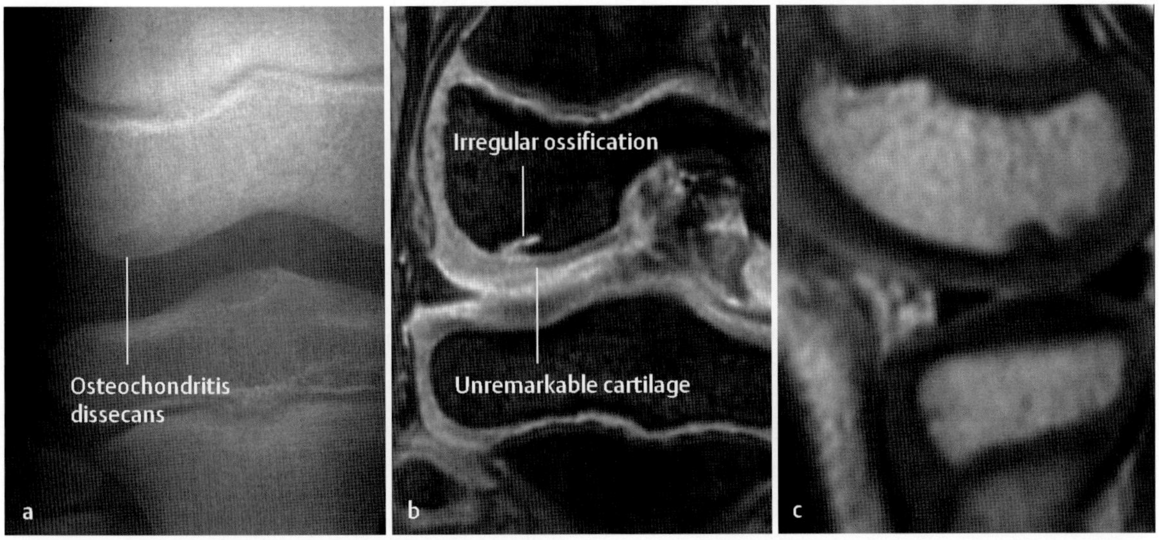

Fig. 1.265 Normal variant versus osteochondritis dissecans: 7-year-old boy with knee pain for 4 weeks. **a** Subtle contour irregularity along the lateral condylar epiphysis. MRI: Coronal GRE (**b**) and sagittal T1-weighted (**c**) images show irregular ossification but an unremarkable articular cartilage. **Normal variant!**

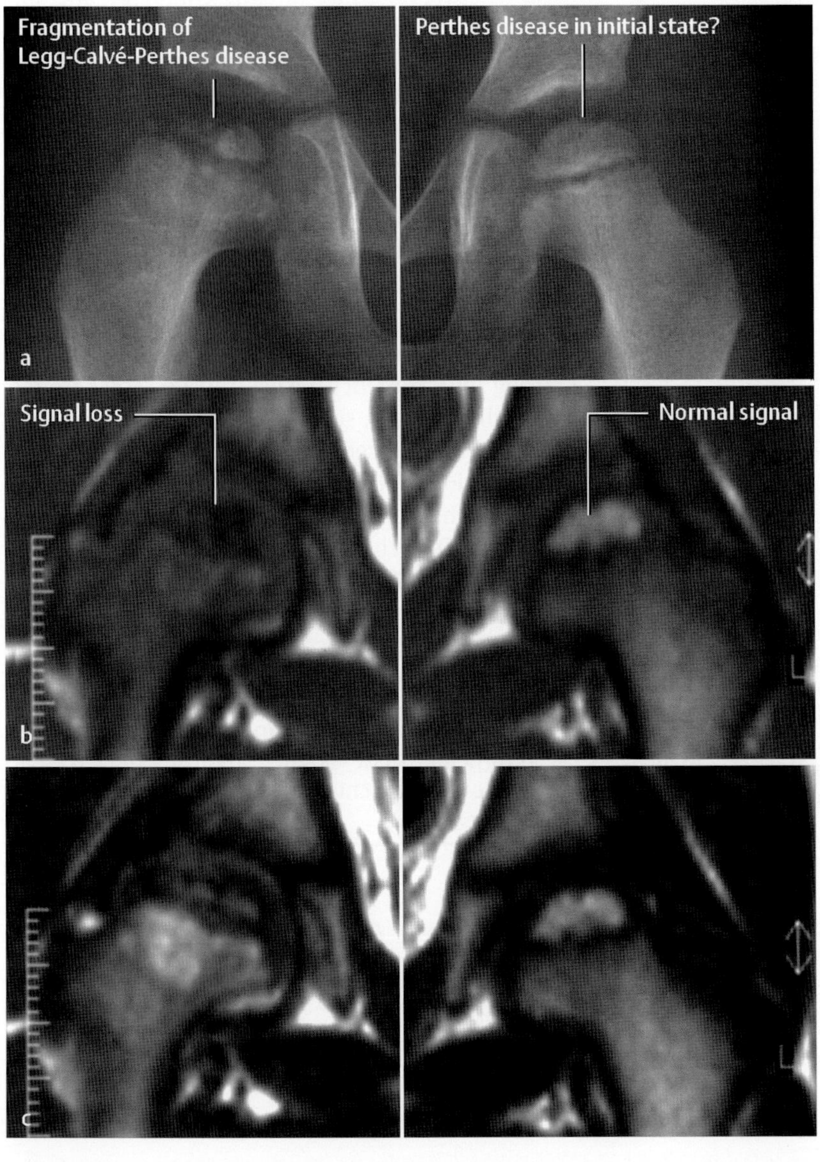

Fig. 1.266 Normal variant (Meyer's dysplasia) versus Legg-Calvé-Perthes disease. Known Legg-Calvé-Perthes disease with fragmentation (Catterall IV) on the right. Left: Irregularly outlined epiphysis composed of several fragments. MRI: T1-weighted (**b**) and T2-weighted (**c**) images show a loss of signal intensity as seen with Legg-Calvé-Perthes disease on the right and a normal signal in an irregularly outlined epiphysis composed of several ossification centers on the left: Meyer's dysplasia. **Normal variant!**

Battered Child Syndrome

Synonym: child abuse.

Battered child syndrome encompasses all injuries in children ranging from physical or psychic trauma to neglect and sexual abuse. The term 'battered child' refers to the physically abused child.

Most cases of child abuse involve the **newborn and infants.** The number of unreported cases is high and the percentage of prosecuted cases low. Radiology plays a decisive role in diagnosing abusively inflicted skeletal injuries, and in some cases might even be lifesaving.

CLINIC The suspicious findings are summarized in Table 1.**21**.

Table 1.**21** Findings suspicious for child abuse

- Hematomas, abrasions, and burns of various ages and unusual locations
- Inadequate explanation of the nature of any trauma and delay in seeing a physician
- Skeletal injuries at different stages of healing as well as at sites 'pathognomonic' for an abused infant (e.g., ribs, scapula, sternum)
- Subdural hematomas, cerebral contusions with or without skull fracture
- Under the age of 2 years

Skeletal injuries of a battered child may be solitary or multiple and usually are at various stages of healing with marked periosteal reaction and callus formation. Older fractures have become asymptomatic. Extremity fractures are equally distributed between metaphyseal and diaphyseal lesions.

Cerebral injuries are caused by direct trauma or indirect trauma induced by whiplash injury, with or without skull fracture, subdural hematomas, and cerebral contusion. Furthermore, forceful shaking can tear the bridging veins and lead to subdural hematomas. Associated retinal hemorrhages can also be identified. Cerebral CT or MRI and, within the first year of life, sonography are the diagnostic modalities of choice.

X-RAY **Metaphyseal lesions** are a strong indicator of infant abuse. The classic radiographic findings are corner fractures, partially with peripheral extension of the fracture as a delicate thin cortical fragment along the proliferative zone of the metaphysis (Figs. 1.**267**, 1.**268**).

Explanation: These injuries are caused by violently pulling or twisting the extremities. The metaphyseal corner fracture represents a metaphyseal fragment avulsed together with the epiphysis due to the strong attachment of periosteum and inserting joint capsule in the region of the metaphyseal ossification zone.

! Subtle metaphyseal avulsions, so-called corner fractures, are pathognomonic of an abused child. Generally, they imply a concomitant epiphysiolysis.

Rib fractures are rare in early childhood and, like fractures of the **scapula, sternum,** and **spinous processes,** are a strong radiologic hallmark of abusive injuries (Fig. 1.**270**).

Periosteal bone formation without fracture is frequently found as well. In early childhood, the periosteum is only loosely attached to the diaphyseal cortex. Consequently, trauma easily induces a subperiosteal hematoma (Fig. 1.**269**).

Osseous lesions at different stages of healing are strong indicators of abusive injuries. They are forensically relevant, since the age of the inflicted injury can be deduced from the radiographic appearance. Periosteal bone formation is usually not seen radiographically before the sixth day but is often present after the eighth day following trauma (Figs. 1.**271**, 1.**272**).

! Conventional radiographs are generally the first imaging studies. The severity of the inflicted injury, especially of the metaphyseal corner fractures, is difficult to assess radiographically since the epiphyses in early childhood are still cartilaginous to a large extent.

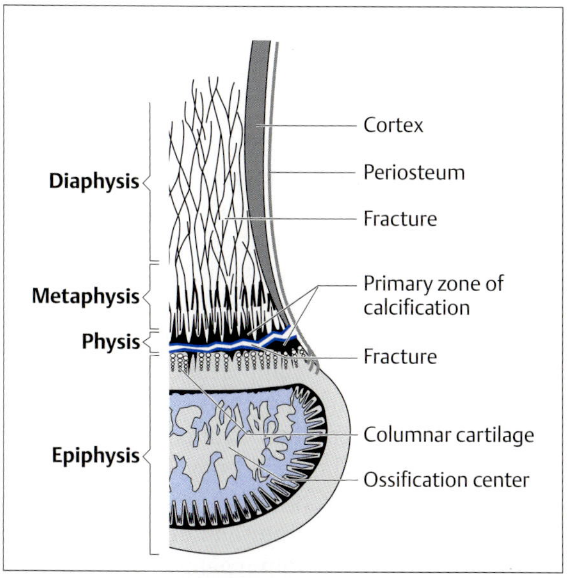

Fig. 1.**267** Fracture line with marginal metaphyseal avulsion (corner fracture).

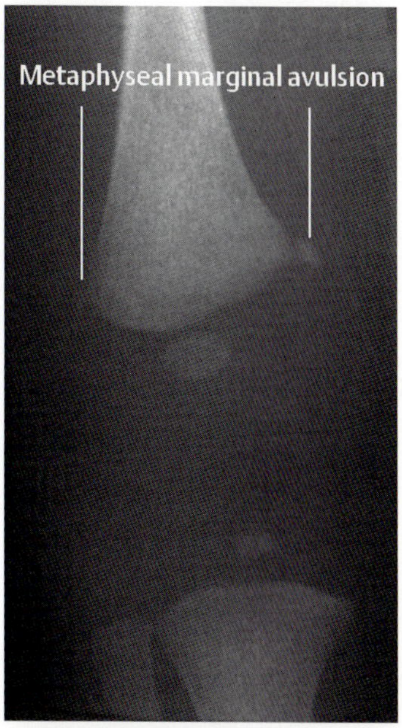

Fig. 1.**268** Battered child: 9-day-old newborn. The metaphyseal corner fractures are radiographic evidence of a complete epiphyseal separation.

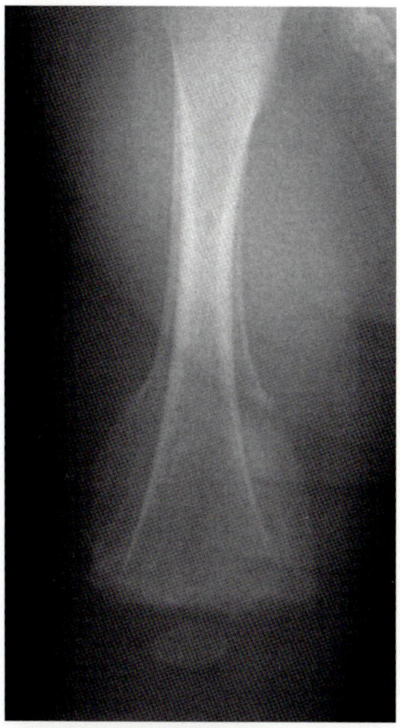

Fig. 1.**269** Battered child: Distal metaphyseal fracture with periosteal bone collar around the metaphysis.

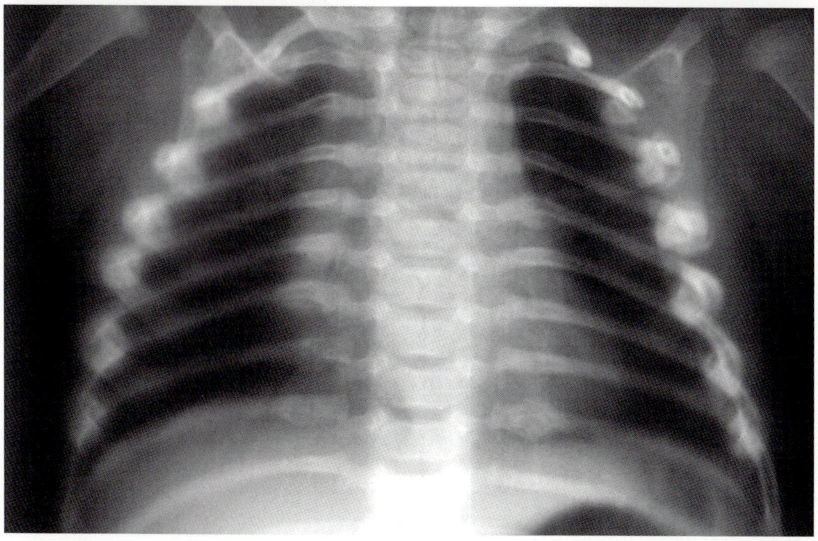

Fig. 1.**270** Multiple rib fractures of a battered child. **Caution:** Rib fractures may also be a manifestation of osteogenesis imperfecta!

! Sonography can delineate the special relationship between the already-ossified metaphysis and the cartilaginous epiphysis. Consequently, it can determine the extent of the traumatic damage and the epiphysiolysis (Fig. 1.**273**). Any joint effusion is easily shown. Subperiosteal hematomas can be detected early, even before any radiographically visible periosteal bone formation.

NUC Bone scintigraphy is a reliable screening method to detect clinically silent osseous lesions. Skull fractures and extremity fractures older than 3–5 months might not show any increased uptake and, if old abusive injuries are suspected, a complete radiographic evaluation in one plane is indispensable.

! Skeletal scintigraphy is a sensitive screening method to detect occult osseous lesions if child abuse is suspected.

MRI In individual cases, MRI can provide a better differentiation between Salter-Harris Type II and Type IV fractures involving complex joints, such as the elbow joint. Its larger field of view in comparison to sonography is advantageous for preoperative planning. The major disadvantage is that sedation is required.

DD If infant abuse is suspected, the diagnostic approach illustrated in Fig. 1.**274** is recommended.

The classic spectrum of radiologic findings is a strong indicator of inflicted injuries. The legal ramifications, however, require the exclusion of disorders with similar radiographic patterns before the diagnosis of an abused infant is assigned to the particular case (Table 1.**22**).

Table 1.**22** Differential diagnosis of the skeletal changes seen in abused infants

- Birth trauma as well as traumatic fracture from rough play
- Fractures in newborns with neurologic deficits, e.g., meningomyelocele, caused by vigorous physical therapy
- Osteogenesis imperfecta
- Metabolic bone diseases
  - Rickets
  - Menke syndrome
- Prostaglandin therapy
- Infantile cortical hyperostosis

Birth-related and **accidental fractures** must be excluded as causative traumatic mechanisms by reviewing the child's clinical history. The same applies to fractures observed in children with cerebral palsy, who underwent forceful physical therapy. Diagnosing **osteogenesis imperfecta** should be easy as long as blue sclerae and opalescent blue-gray teeth are present and a positive family history can be obtained, though the differentiation can be difficult in an individual presenting with multiple fractures of various ages. Strong indicators of child abuse are the classic metaphyseal corner fractures. Metabolic abnormalities, such as **rickets** or **Menke syndrome,** can produce similar metaphyseal changes and should be excluded on the basis of laboratory parameters. Periosteal new bone formation after **prostaglandin therapy** and **infantile cortical hyperostosis** differs from changes seen in the abused infant by the absence of fractures and suspicion of any abuse, and by the clinical course and laboratory findings.

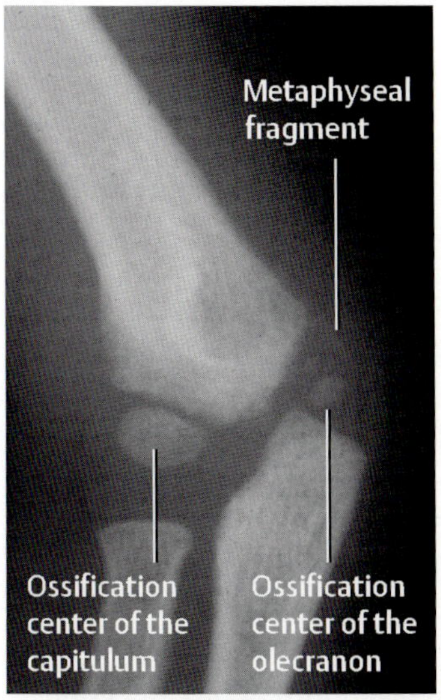

Fig. 1.**271** Abused infant: 6-month-old newborn. Elbow in neutral position, with evidence of acute metaphyseal corner fractures of the distal humerus.

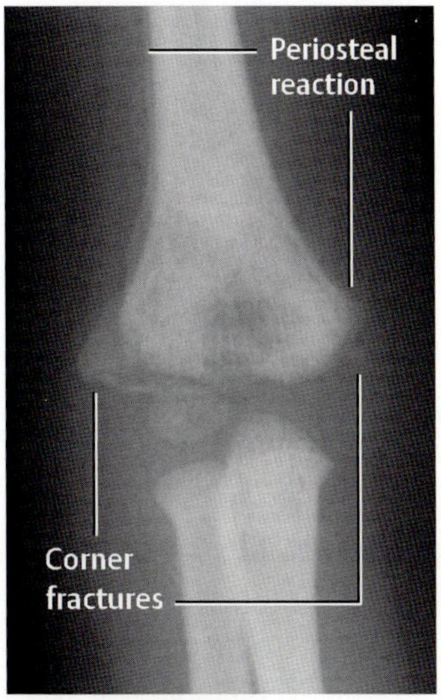

Fig. 1.**272** The same child as in Fig. 1.**271**, 3 weeks later. Subtle periosteal bone formation with now discernible bilateral metaphyseal corner fractures.

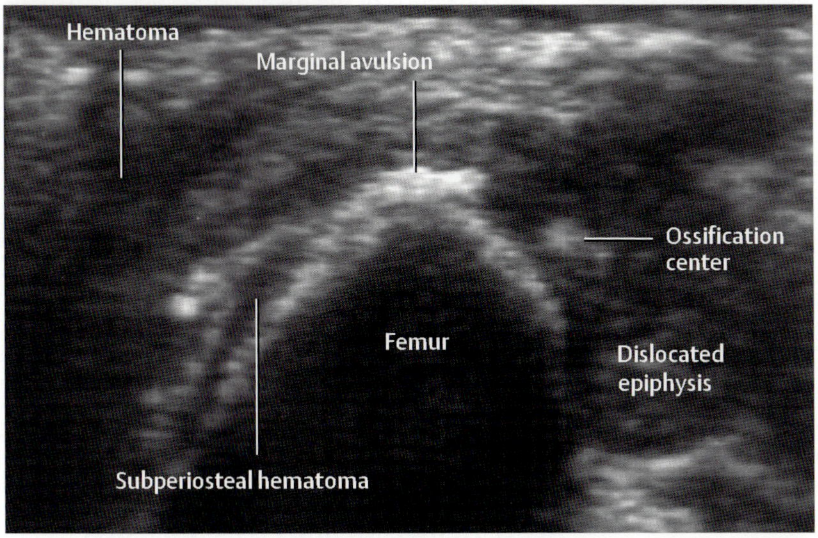

Fig. 1.**273** Battered child with epiphyseal displacement, metaphyseal corner fractures, and subperiosteal hematoma.

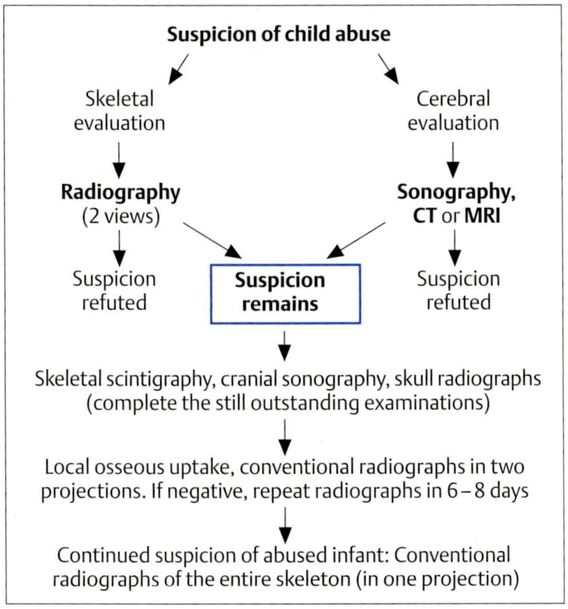

Fig. 1.**274** Diagnostic approach to suspected child abuse.

2 Bone and Soft-tissue Infections

Osteomyelitis

■ Osseous infection primarily confined to the bone marrow is a local manifestation of a systemic infection and referred to as hematogenous osteomyelitis. It must be differentiated from secondary osteomyelitis, an osseous infection following trauma or surgery, which might present as osteitis without bone marrow involvement (Table 2.**1**). ■

Septic arthritis and spondylitis/diskitis are discussed in Chapter 9 (pages 331 – 337).

Organisms:
- Staphylococcus aureus in 80 – 90% of cases.
- Streptococcus B and pneumococci in the newborn.
- Pseudomonas, which is more frequent in drug addicts than in the general population.
- Salmonella typhi in patients with diabetes mellitus and sickle cell anemia.
- Mycobacterium tuberculosis. With the return of tuberculosis, skeletal tuberculosis can be expected to increase.
- Treponema pallidum (syphilis). A rare cause of neonatal osteomyelitis in the Western world.
- Fungi.
- Viruses.

! Osteomyelitis is diagnosed by integrating clinical, laboratory, and imaging findings. Isolating the responsible organism is desirable for testing antibiotic sensitivity, but succeeds in only a portion of cases. Establishing the diagnosis 'osteomyelitis' by open or percutaneous biopsy is rarely necessary today.

Route of infection:
- Direct spread to the bone through a penetrating wound.
- Direct spread from surrounding soft tissues. This route is likely after soft-tissue trauma, as well as in diabetic patients with plantar ulcers or bedridden patients with decubitus ulcers (Fig. 2.**1**). Overall, the most common osseous infection is osteomyelitis of the mandible secondary to dental granulomas.
- Hematogenous spread. This type most commonly follows a bacteremia caused by urogenital infections, enteritis, cholangitis, or endocarditis.

PATH The infection arises as the organisms spread into the perivascular interstitial structures, leading to a leukocytic infiltration that permeates the bone marrow. The dissemination progresses along the Volkmann's canals and through the Haversian canals. The infiltration leads to vascular compression, compromises the nutrition of the bone marrow and, together with the bacterial toxins, ultimately causes **'necrosis'.**

The necrotic tissue can be resorbed and replaced with new bone. If this fails, purulent cavities (abscesses) or sequestra form.

Acute Hematogenous Osteomyelitis

■ Acute hematogenous osteomyelitis occurs primarily in the pediatric age group, but its incidence also increases after 50 years of age. Depending on the age of manifestation, a distinction between newborn osteomyelitis, juvenile hematogenous osteomyelitis, and adult osteomyelitis is usually made. ■

Acute osteomyelitis is treated with high doses of antibiotics. The major role of imaging is to identify abscesses or sequestra since they are not adequately treated by antibiotics and often require decompression or surgical intervention.

Newborn Osteomyelitis

Newborn osteomyelitis is generally an acute disease and has a predilection of the proximal and dis-

Table 2.1 Classification of osteomyelitis

Nonspecific osteomyelitis Acute types	 Chronic types	**Specific osteomyelitis**
Hematogenous osteomyelitis (newborn, child, adult)	Primary (endogenous) – Chronic hematogenous osteomyelitis – Brodie abscess – Chronic recurrent multifocal osteomyelitis – Plasma cellular osteomyelitis Secondary (exogenous)	*Mycobacterium tuberculosis* *Salmonella* *Treponema pallidum* Fungi and others

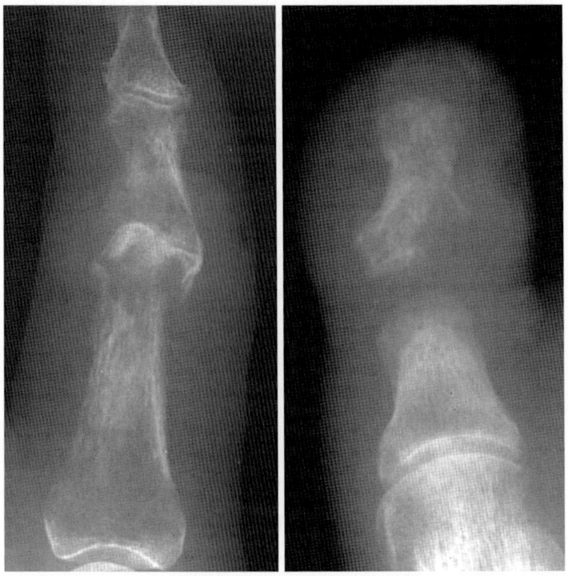

Fig. 2.1 Two different examples of osteomyelitis spread from contiguous soft-tissue infection.

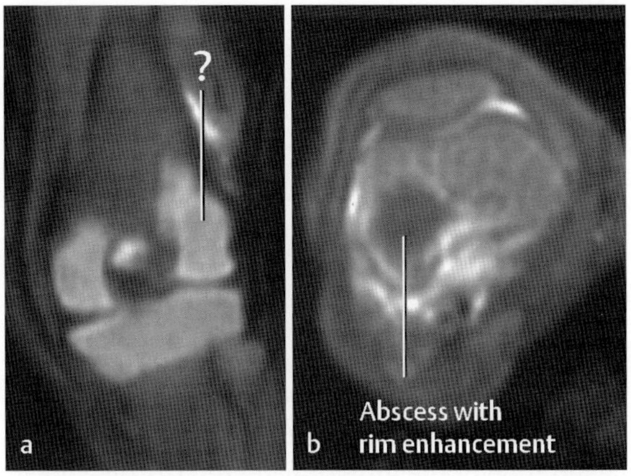

Fig. 2.2 Osteomyelitis in an 18-day-old newborn with abscess in the femoral epiphysis. The coronal T1-weighted sequence (**a**) fails to delineate the abscess clearly. The abscess, however, is distinctly displayed after enhancement on the axial T1-weighted image with fat suppression (**b**).

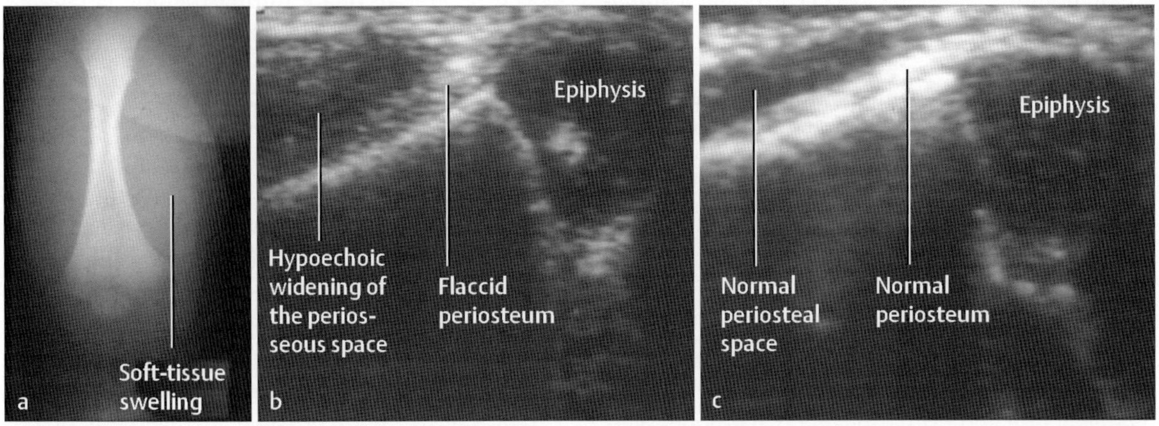

Fig. 2.3 Acute osteomyelitis in an 11-day-old newborn with extension along the subperiosteal space. There is considerable soft-tissue swelling (**a**). Sonography (**b**) shows periosteal and parosteal changes, more readily appreciated by comparing the findings with the normal contralateral site (**c**).

tal femoral metaphyses. Predisposing conditions include infections of the umbilicus, ear, nose, and throat, and the most common organisms are streptococci. If untreated, the infection spreads rapidly through the Haversian canals into the subperiosteal space or across the still patent meta-epiphyseal vessels to the epiphysis (Figs. 2.**2**, 2.**3**). The result is a septic arthritis with capsular empyema, destruction of the epiphyseal cartilage, and epiphyseal separation, ultimately causing severe joint deformity if not aggressively treated.

CLINIC The typical acute clinical course consists of fever, restriction of motion often due to pain, severe point tenderness, and elevated inflammatory parameters. Soft-tissue swelling, erythema, and increased skin temperature develop relatively late in the clinical course.

Juvenile Hematogenous Osteomyelitis

Beginning in the second year of life, metaphyseal vessels no longer penetrate the growth plate and form dilated loops in the metaphysis. This vascular change provides favorable conditions for infective organisms and explains the development of metaphyseal inflammatory foci. This absence of vascular penetration of the growth plate retards the spread of infection to the epiphysis (epiphyseal barrier). At this time the suppurative process generally penetrates the thin cortex rapidly and spreads along the subperiosteal space, elevating the periosteum. The infection then spreads into the joint only if the metaphysis is intra-articular, as in the hip and knee.

The organisms causing juvenile osteomyelitis are predominantly staphylococci, especially *Staphylococcus aureus*.

CLINIC In this condition the patient generally presents with sudden onset of fever, chills, severe pain, and extreme local tenderness. The major clinical findings are restriction of motion of the affected extremity usually due to pain, local swelling, erythema, and hyperthermia with elevation of inflammatory parameters.

Acute Hematogenous Osteomyelitis in the Adult

Acute hematogenous osteomyelitis in the adult is relatively rare and primarily affects flat bones, vertebral bodies, and the diaphysis of the tubular bones. The suppurative process can involve the entire medullary space (medullary phlegmon).

Vascular connections between the metaphysis and epiphysis are restored after closure of the growth plate, and there is subchondral extension of the vessels. This modification of vascular flow allows spread of the infection into the joint capsule more frequently. Since the metaphyseal cortex is thick and the overlying periosteum fibrosed and firmly attached, subperiosteal abscesses rarely develop. In the rare cases of cortical penetration, the suppurative process breaks through the rather rigid periosteum and spreads into the soft tissues, resulting in the formation of fistulous tracts. Sequestration is rare.

CLINIC The local findings (swelling, pain, tenderness) are associated with occasionally severe systemic findings (fever, weakness). The inflammatory parameters (complement fixation tests, sedimentation rate, leukocytes) are generally elevated.

Imaging Features of Acute Hematogenous Osteomyelitis (All Ages)

X-RAY Numerous radiographic findings have to be considered:

- The types and extent of **medullary destruction** are variable. The entire destructive spectrum can be encountered, including a solitary radiolucency (Fig. 2.**4**), irregular, multiple radiolucencies ('mottling' or permeative pattern), and homogeneous bone loss.
- The lesions are generally indistinct and irregular in outline.
- In contrast to those in newborns and infants, the **soft-tissue findings** in adults are rarely diagnostically helpful.
- Lamellated **periosteal reactions** are invariably present (Fig. 2.**5**).
- The reparative phase during therapy is characterized by endosteal and periosteal new bone formation, development of a surrounding sclerosis, and even large osteosclerotic areas.
- In the newborn and infants, the loss of normal fat planes on conventional radiographs might be an early sign of soft-tissue swelling (within days of the onset of clinical findings). It takes about 7 to 10 days for the osseous findings to become radiographically visible, whereby the lamellated periosteal changes are generally discernible before any bone destruction. A late manifestation in this age group is the 'ballooned metaphysis', with possible involvement of the epiphysis. Late in the disease, a strong periosteal reaction can appear as periosteal ossification.

NUC The radionuclides used for diagnosing osteomyelitis can be divided into bone-seeking tracers (e.g., Tc 99 m diphosphonate) and inflammation-avid tracers (e.g., Tc 99 m-labeled leukocytes).

Three-phase Bone Scan with Tc 99 m diphosphonate

Tc 99 m can be considered an ideal diagnostic radionuclide because of its short half-life of 6 hours, its photon energy of 140 keV, and negligible β emission, rendering images of a relatively high photon flux while delivering a low radiation burden to the body.

The osseous accumulation of diphosphonate depends on:
- regional blood flow,
- regional distribution of sympathetic innervation,
- osseous turnover at the site of the inflammation.

The three phases of the examination are:
- vascular phase, representing the initial passage of the tracer, of about 1 minute,
- blood pool phase, corresponding to the first 2–4 minutes after the injection of tracer,
- static or bone phase, about 2–4 hours after the injection of tracer.

Acute osteomyelitis produces intense focal radionuclide accumulation in **all three phases.** Increased blood pool activity without osseous uptake on the static images suggests an inflammation confined to the soft tissues (Fig. 2.**6**).

Cautionary Note: In the newborn, acute osteomyelitis can lead to a decreased uptake, resulting in a false-negative bone scan or a 'photon-deficient' lesion. This has been attributed to increased intramedullary pressure. Another false-negative finding can be caused by the inability to discern increased radionuclide uptake of inflammation because of the accentuated activity of the growth plates.

Tc 99 m-labeled WBC Scan

Two labeling techniques can be used:
1. HMPAO to label a suspension of autologous leukocytes with Tc 99 m *in vitro.*
2. Murine monoclonal antibodies for *in vivo* labeling of granulocytes, with the antibodies not only binding to the granulocytes but also diffusing through the capillary walls into the inflammatory tissue.

Any tracer accumulation outside the expected physiologic pattern suggests an osteomyelitis. Whether alone or combined, the WBC scan will increase the specificity but not affect the sensitivity of detecting inflammation. Since nonspecific WBC accumulation can occur in tumors and fractures, correlation with current conventional radiographs is necessary.

Ga 67 scanning no longer plays a major role in diagnosing infection because of its high radiation dose and low specificity. Nanocolloid scanning has been abandoned because of its low sensitivity.

SONO The acoustic properties of the neonatal anatomy are especially suitable for sonography. The first sonographic sign, seen even **before** any periosteal reaction, is deep soft-tissue edema and swelling. This is followed by sonographic detection of a thin hypoechoic fluid layer, which elevates the periosteum and may progress to a space-occupying abscess if the infection is not adequately treated. Sonography, however, should not be overrated since these ultrasonographic findings are not always detectable. Depending on the site examined, the false negative rate can be as high as 40%.

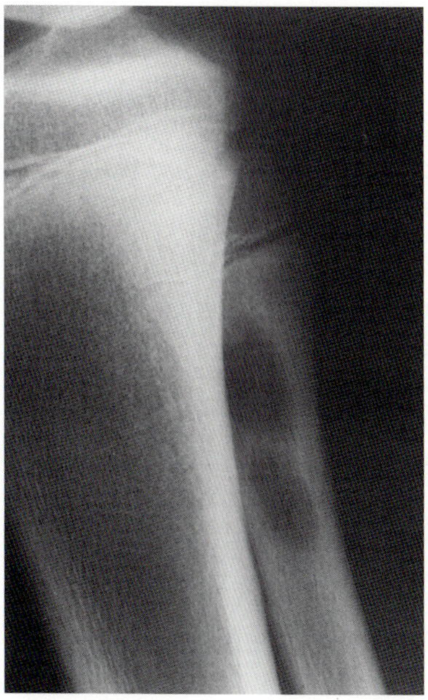

Fig. 2.**4** Acute osteomyelitis of the proximal fibula, manifested as multiple radiolucencies.

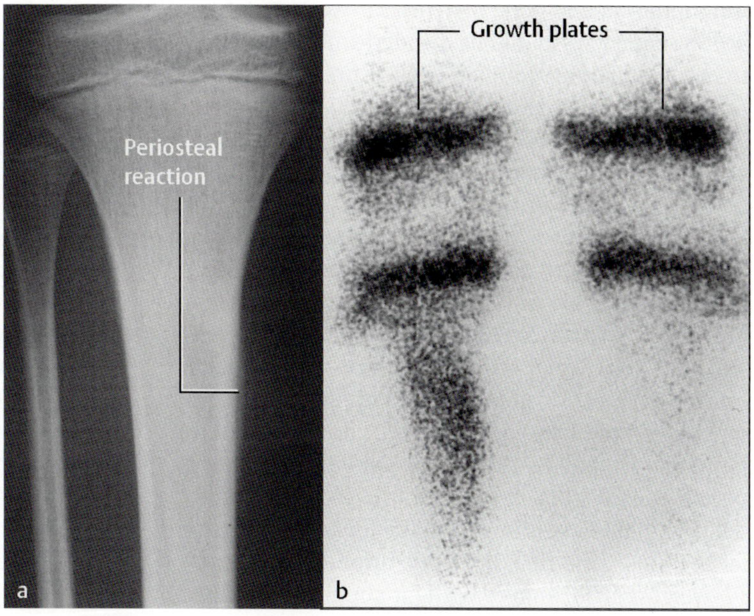

Fig. 2.**5** Acute osteomyelitis of the right tibia. The slightly underexposed radiograph (**a**) reveals periosteal reaction. The static image (osseous phase) of the bone scan (**b**) shows increased uptake in the proximal right tibia compared to the contralateral side.

Moreover, sonographic findings are often nonspecific and can be falsely interpreted as evidence of osteomyelitis.

In the older child and adult, sonography is an examination that supplements the evaluation of the soft tissues adjacent to bone. Soft-tissue abscesses, subperiostal abscesses, cysts, and hematomas are excellently demonstrated on ultrasound as hypoechoic or anechoic lesions and as such are suitable for sonographically guided aspiration. Any associated cortical destruction may also be shown if the sonographic conditions are optimal. Diffuse soft-tissue infection and abscess can confidently be differentiated by sonography. Any diffuse soft-tissue swelling is characterized by echogenic thickening of the subcutaneous tissue.

Furthermore, sonography can detect a joint effusion that might explain the pain and restriction of motion. This finding frequently prompts a diagnostic joint aspiration in this clinical setting.

MRI

Examination Technique: The most suitable sequences for screening are the STIR (short time inversion recovery) sequences because of excellent visualization of the inflammatory edema, attained by combining T1 and T2 weighting with fat signal suppression. The STIR images are supplemented by T1-weighted SE or fast-spin-echo images, which provide excellent anatomic detail. The echo times of the T2-weighted images should exceed 100 msec for an excellent contrast between inflammation and bone marrow. T2-weighted 'turbo' SE sequences should be avoided since they tend to mask any intramedullary edema, unless the contrast can be augmented by frequency-selected fat suppression. Unless contraindicated, intravenous gadolinium-based contrast medium should always be administered since only enhancement can differentiate abscesses or necrotic areas (sequestra) from inflammatory edema. Furthermore, enhancement may exclude a neoplastic process.

Morphology and Signal Pattern: The affected areas are low signal intensity on the T1-weighted images with a corresponding area of high signal intensity on the STIR sequence. These areas are often large and irregularly outlined. As a general rule, a periosseous edema is consistently present, and a delicate high-signal rim should be looked for on axial sections. This rule, however, applies to STIR or T2-weighted TSE images with fat suppression only. As long as high-resolution coils are used, STIR and T2-weighted images invariably reveal intracortical areas of increased signal intensity.

Intraosseous **abscesses** generally are sharply demarcated and display a low-signal rim on the T2-weighted fast-spin-echo and STIR images. A strong peripheral contrast enhancement without any central contrast enhancement supports the presence of an abscess (Fig. 2.**7**). Necrotic **sequestra** also fail to show contrast enhancement, but can be differentiated on the T2-weighted or STIR image. In contrast to an abscess, the sequestrum shows a signal void on these images.

As with other imaging methods, differentiating osteomyelitis from septic arthritis can be difficult. Septic arthritis can induce edematous changes in the epiphysis and metaphysis, without evidence of an underlying osteomyelitis. In our experience, the reverse applies as well. No imaging modality has so far solved this dilemma, and image-guided joint aspiration remains unsurpassed in the diagnostic evaluation. In contrast, MRI is generally quite successful in differentiating between osteomyelitis and primary soft-tissue inflammation.

Evidence of Healing of Acute Osteomyelitis

Radiographically, the first sign of healing is progressive sclerosis beginning at the periphery. Scintigraphically, the intensity of osseous uptake decreases with healing. MRI shows resolving edematous changes and soft-tissue swelling as well as a progressing fibrovascular rim with contrast enhancement. Ideally, the affected bone returns to its original state, but in most instances a persistent defect remains. Radiographically, this 'scar' is often seen as localized sclerosis or periosteal thickening.

Complications of Acute Hematogenous Osteomyelitis (All Age Groups)

- Osteonecrosis and sequestration.
- Recurrence: can occur even years later at the site of a previous osteomyelitis.
- Multifocal osteomyelitis: multifocality is most frequent in neonates. Altogether, it occurs in about 10% of all cases of hematogenous osteomyelitis.
- Ankylosis: results from a septic arthritis induced by intra-articular extension of an adjacent osteomyelitis.
- Extension of the osteomyelitis to the surrounding soft tissues and formation of a soft-tissue phlegmon (Fig. 2.**9**).
- Penetration of the cortex with development of a periostitis and formation of periosteal abscesses.

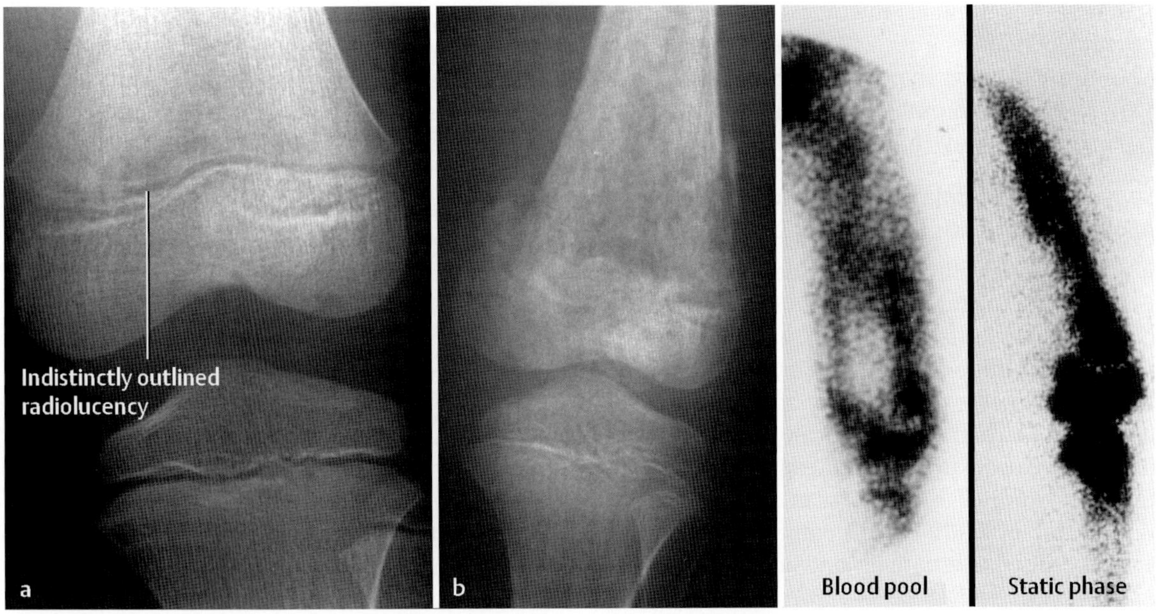

Fig. 2.**6** Acute osteomyelitis. The radiograph (**a**) was obtained because of severe pain and falsely interpreted as unremarkable. The pain was attributed to a presumed trauma and a cast was applied. The radiograph obtained 3 weeks later (**b**) shows extensive bone destruction caused by osteomyelitis. The bone scan shows increased activity in the blood pool phase (**c**) and in the static (osseous) phase (**d**).

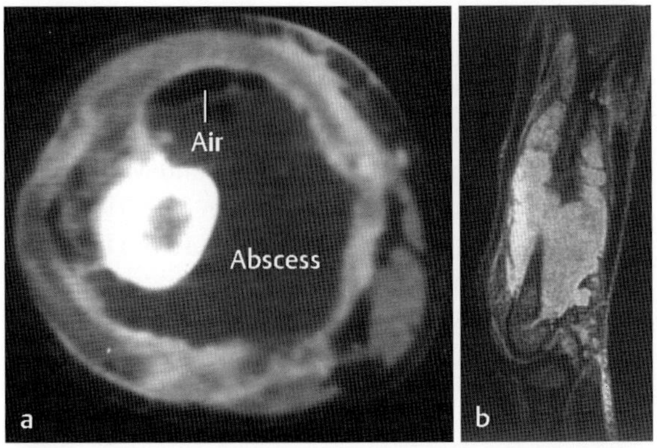

Fig. 2.**7** The same patient as in Fig. 2.**6**. CT (**a**) and MRI, T2-weighted sequence (**b**), demonstrate the extent of the associated soft-tissue abscess.

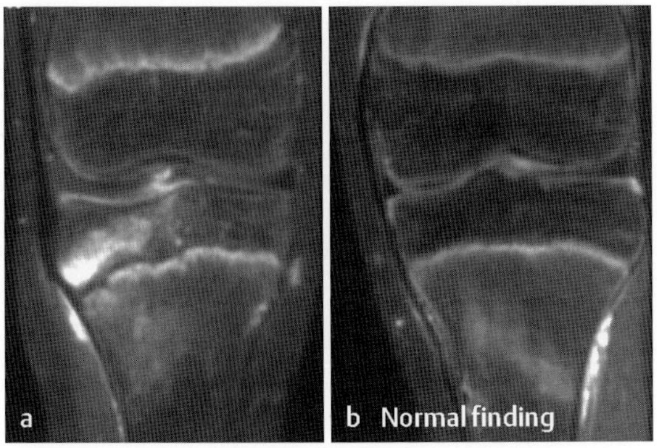

Fig. 2.**8** Acute osteomyelitis involving the **epiphysis** of the knee, T1-weighted image with fat suppression and enhancement (**a**). Healthy contralateral knee for comparison (**b**).

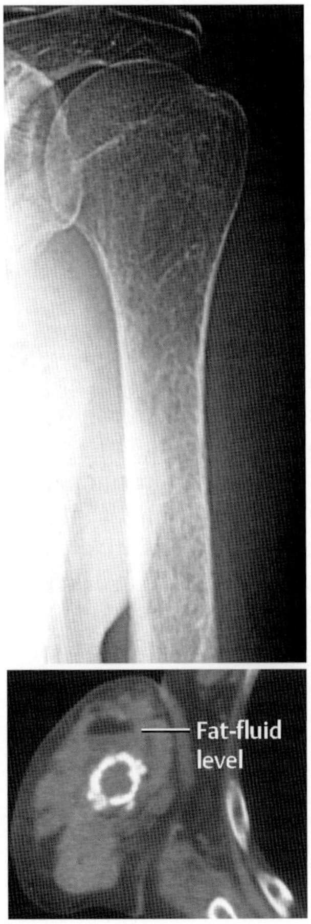

Fig. 2.**9** Salmonella osteomyelitis of the humerus. CT shows a soft-tissue abscess with a fat-fluid level.

– Altered longitudinal growth: extension of the osteomyelitis to the growth plate often leads to limb shortening. Hyperemia, however, can also induce cartilage proliferation and accelerate the longitudinal growth.

Summary of the Role of Imaging in Diagnosing Acute Osteomyelitis (see Table 2.2)

If acute osteomyelitis is suspected clinically, conventional radiography remains the method of choice for the initial evaluation. It should be supplemented routinely by sonography in the newborn and infants unless the clinically affected area cannot be approached sonographically. If clinically indicated, the evaluation should continue with scintigraphy (three-phase bone scan, Tc 99 m-labeled WBC scan) or MRI. These competing modalities should be used alternatively and not additively.

The spine (see pages 334–337) and other skeletal regions of complex anatomy (e.g., SI joints, facial bones) are often best evaluated by MRI, which therefore should be applied early in the evaluation of these structures.

In some pediatric centers, the three-phase bone scan is preferentially used for neonates and infants suspected of having an acute osteomyelitis, since it has superior detection of early and multiple lesions.

MRI should always be performed if an abscess is suspected. Ultrasound is an alternative but is less sensitive and specific.

CT no longer plays a role in the early detection of acute osteomyelitis, but remains indicated in the search for sequestra.

DD **Primary and Secondary Bone Tumors:** Ewing sarcoma and, less frequently, osteosarcoma must be considered in children and adolescents since their clinical presentation and laboratory findings often suggest an inflammatory process. Conventional radiography and scintigraphy generally do not allow a differentiation, in contrast to MRI, which provides valuable discriminating information. After intravenous gadolinium-based contrast medium, a tumor shows a difference in the enhancement of the solid (tumorous) lesion and peritumorous edema. Osteomyelitis shows diffuse or heterogeneous ('mottled') enhancement.

The clinical differentiation between tumor and inflammation is less difficult in adults. The differentiating imaging criteria are the same in children and adolescents.

On MRI, ring enhancement around fluid-filled cavities can also represent **cysts, necrotic tumors,** or **post-traumatic seromas** (see also chronic osteomyelitis). The diagnostic possibilities can be narrowed down by the width of the enhancement and by any possible concomitant edema. An abscess, for instance, is invariably surrounded by edema. Most necrotic tumors also penetrate the cortex due to their size alone since, unless treated, tumors do not undergo necrotizing cavitation before they have reached a certain size. Any differentiation between necrotic tumors and abscesses in the peripheral soft tissues is futile, and only needle aspiration can settle the issue.

Chronic Hematogenous Osteomyelitis

The distinctions between acute, subacute, and chronic osteomyelitis are fleeting. An incompletely treated acute infection proceeds to a subacute or, after months and years, to a chronic osteomyelitis. This happens more often in adults than in children.

Primary chronic hematogenous osteomyelitis can be observed, skipping the clinically overt acute infection. It is assumed that this course indicates an impaired immune response.

The radiographic features are dominated by reparative processes as characterized by irregular sclerosis with loss of the trabecular structure, in addition to osteolytic destruction and solid periosteal reactions. Sequestration is also possible.

Imaging, especially scintigraphy and MRI, is crucial for detecting or excluding new infectious foci and excluding sequestration (Figs. 2.**10**, 2.**11**).

Therapy is largely surgical, often open drainage and irrigation with antibiotic solutions.

Table 2.2 Key points in the radiologic diagnosis of **acute** osteomyelitis

1. Radiographic findings of acute osteomyelitis are not detectable within 10 days after the onset of clinical symptoms (exception: neonatal period).
2. The first radiographic finding is the obliteration of fat planes because of soft- tissue edema (especially in the pediatric age group).
3. Trabecular destruction is seen before cortical destruction.
4. Epiphysiolysis and growth disturbance can complicate osteomyelitis in children.
5. Ewing sarcoma is the most frequently considered differential diagnosis in children and adolescents.
6. A **sequestrum** is a necrotic osseous fragment completely surrounded by the infectious process (= radiolucent rim). It is dense radiographically and fails to enhance on MRI or CT.
7. An **involucrum** is the periosteal bone formation that appears as parosteal ossification. It is frequent in children since the cortex and periosteum are not yet firmly connected.
8. The most sensitive methods to detect an acute osteomyelitis are bone scintigraphy and MRI.
9. In the newborn and infants, sonography is an important method for early diagnosis and follow-up.

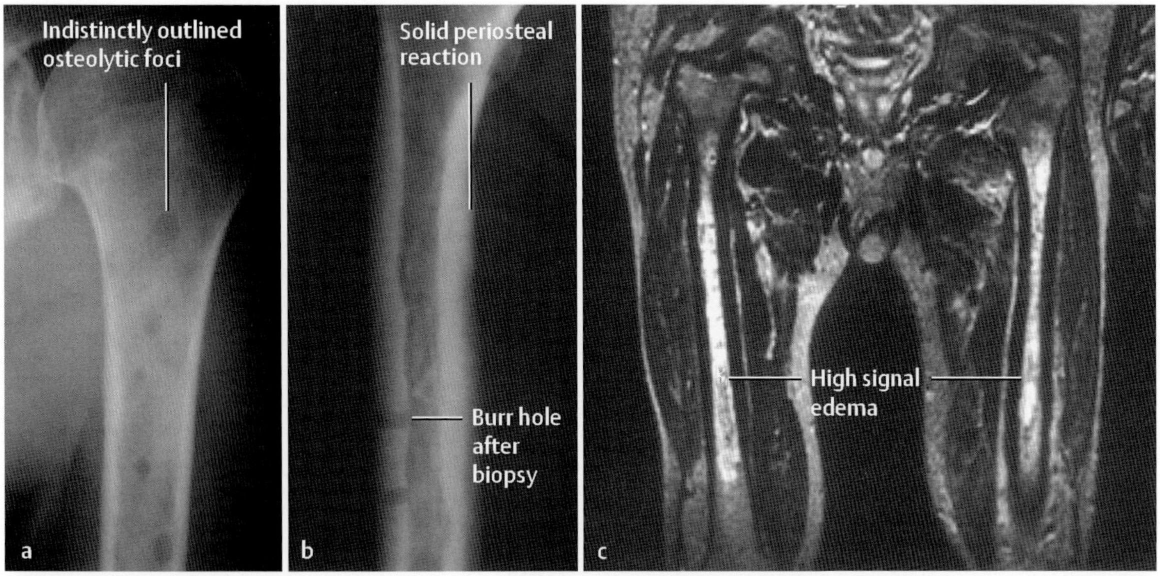

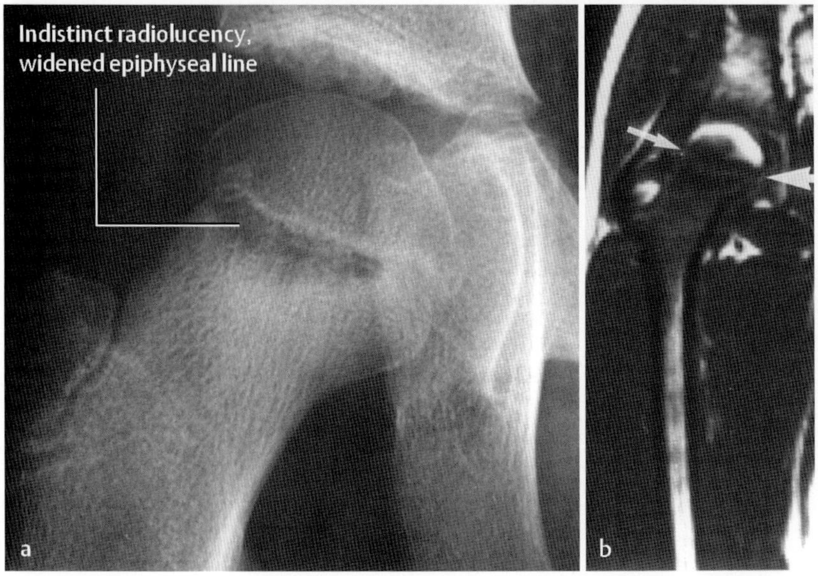

Above:
Fig. 2.**10** Chronic hematogenous osteomyelitis involving all extremities.
a, b Radiographs of the affected humerus and femur as representative bones.
c T2-weighted image.

Left:
Fig. 2.**11** 'Subacute' osteomyelitis of the femoral growth plate in a 14-year-old boy. MRI shows involvement of the epiphysis (T1-weighted SE sequence).

Brodie Abscess

The Brodie abscess is a primary chronic pyogenic infection, usually producing a round abscess cavity 1–4 cm in diameter. Patients with this lesion do not often develop fistulous tracts. It involves primarily the distal femoral metaphysis or tibial plateau. The clinical findings are minimal and patients may not be seen by a physician for many years (Figs. 2.**12**–2.**15**).

X-RAY The Brodie abscess always presents as a round to ovoid **radiolucency** with a thick **sclerotic rim.**

MRI The Brodie abscess generally appears as a defect without contrast enhancement. However, the defect can enhance if the abscess cavity is filled with infectious granulation tissue rather than pus (rare). The lesion has high signal intensity on STIR and T2-weighted images. The sclerotic rim is of low signal intensity, but may faintly enhance with contrast.

DD **Cysts** and, above all, **fibrous dysplasia,** can be distinguished by MRI (especially on STIR sequences): the Brodie abscess is surrounded by a delicate edematous rim, rarely seen with these lesions.

The **osteoblastoma** can usually be distinguished radiologically by its calcific nidus.

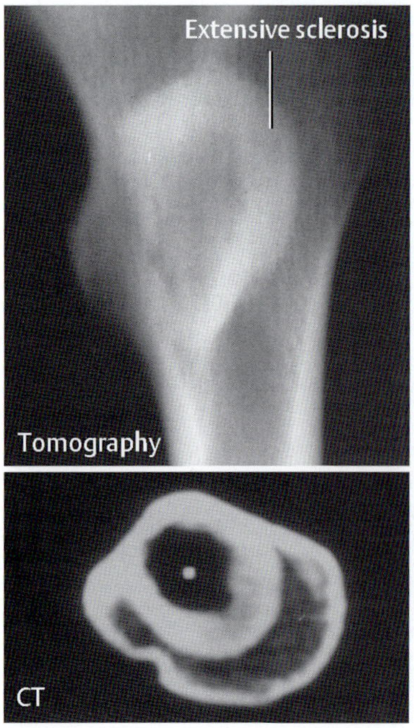

Fig. 2.**12** Brodie abscess in the proximal femur with marked sclerotic rim.

Chronic Recurrent Multifocal Osteomyelitis (CRMO)

CRMO is a rare but clinically well-defined type of osteomyelitis affecting children and adolescents. The disease begins as a synchronous or sequential development of multifocal circumscribed osseous lesions and follows a chronic course over a period of up to 15 years. This entity is characterized by remissions, local recurrences, and new lesions. The etiology of this disease is still unclear, since neither biopsy of the lesions nor blood cultures commonly isolate any organisms. An underlying immunologic deficit has been contemplated, and CRMO seems to be related to pustulosis palmoplantaris (Figs. 2.**16**, 2.**17**).

X-RAY The radiographic features of CRMO depend on the time from the appearance of the clinical findings to the radiographic examination. If the interval is short (less than 3 weeks) or the lesion has induced no symptoms, the dominating finding is osteolytic destruction similar to acute osteomyelitis. The radiographic findings vary if the clinical findings have been present for a longer time; osteolytic lesions with sclerotic rims, mixed osteolytic and osteoblastic lesions, and purely osteosclerotic processes can be found. Involvement of the sacro-iliac and sternoclavicular joints is rare. The radiographic evolution of the lesion, even without therapy, ranges from progressive sclerosis to complete restoration of the normal osseous structures over several years.

NUC The three-phase bone scan with Tc 99 m diphosphonate is crucial for diagnosing and following the disease since CRMO might only be detectable scintigraphically (Fig. 2.**17**).

MRI The early stages are identical to those of acute osteomyelitis. The osteosclerotic areas seen in the later stages are also imaged with MRI.

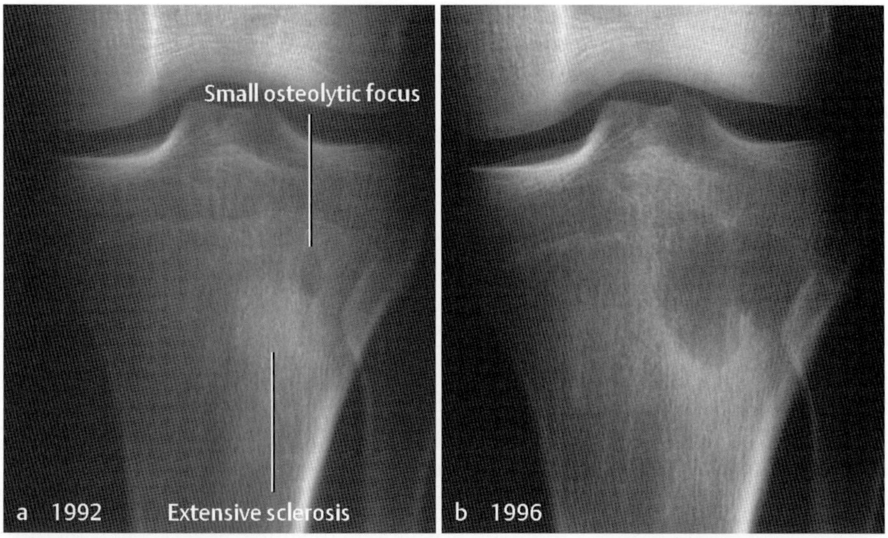

Fig. 2.**13** Evolution of a Brodie abscess in the proximal tibia. The sclerosis around the osteolysis is attributed to slow growth.
The patient declined further diagnostic evaluation in 1992 because of spontaneous resolution of pain.

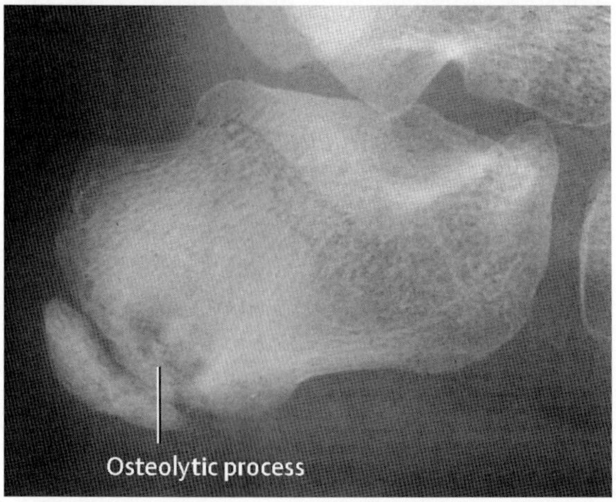

Fig. 2.**14** Brodie abscess in the calcaneus.

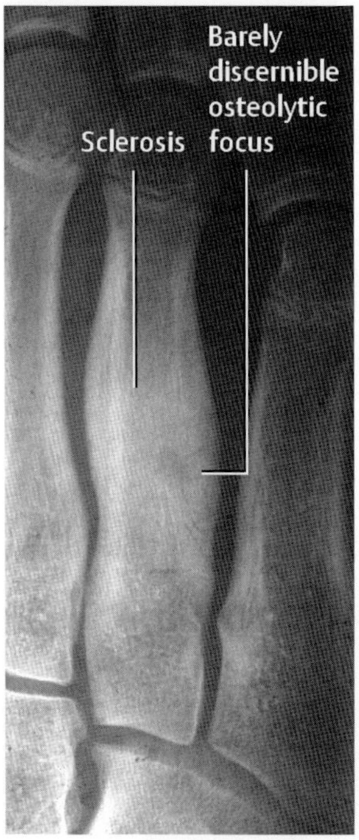

Fig. 2.**15** Brodie abscess in a metatarsal bone.

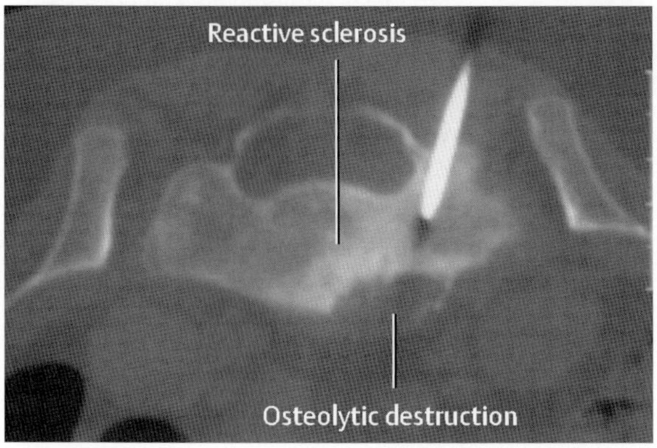

Fig. 2.**16** Chronic recurrent multifocal osteomyelitis (CRMO) involving the sacrum, CT guided biopsy to establish the diagnosis.

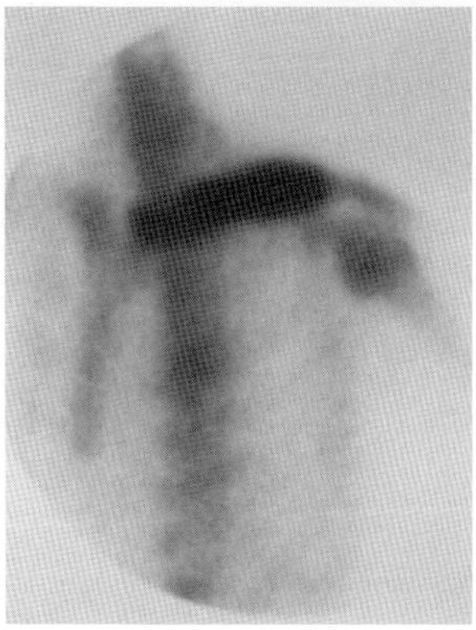

Fig. 2.**17** Bone scan with intense uptake in the clavicles representing chronic recurrent multifocal osteomyelitis (CRMO).

Post-traumatic Osteomyelitis

The exogenous post-traumatic or postsurgical infection is mostly a local infection of the bone (osteitis). The spread of the infection depends not only on the number and virulence of the organisms and resistance of the patient, but also on the local conditions, such as the extent of soft-tissue damage, the nutrient blood supply, the stage of bone healing, and the type of foreign material introduced. Despite speedier trauma care and improved surgical techniques, the infection rate of compound fractures still remains between 5 and 10%.

Impaired vascularization and altered stability of the traumatized soft tissues and bones are predisposing factors to the insidious development of chronic osteomyelitis.

CLINIC **Acute** post-traumatic osteomyelitis must be suspected whenever inflammatory changes (pain, erythema, swelling, fever, laboratory parameters) develop and fracture healing does not occur or is delayed. The infection can become a **chronic** osteomyelitis and follows a protracted course with patients presenting with local pain, erythema, and draining sinus tracts. An **acute attack** of a chronic osteomyelitis occurs with an aggravation of the infection after months or years (Fig. 2.**18**).

X-RAY The radiographic findings of postsurgical infection after a compound fracture may be delayed for a long time. Comparison with the immediate postsurgical radiographs is critical for making the diagnosis (relatively) early. The osseous structures appear rarefied at a time when signs of callus formation and osseous bridging should already be present, and a radiolucent halo may develop around any hardware present. Furthermore, a (re-)infection can elicit a new delicate linear periosteal reaction. Careful analysis of the inserted screws and plates may reveal an indistinct osseous interface of the surrounding halo, in contrast to the sclerotic border of the halo caused by loosening.

The generally protracted course of the infection induces an endosteal and periosteal reaction. In the true sense of its meaning, a 'variegated picture' develops, whereby later in the process the new bone formation largely dominates over the destructive changes (Figs. 2.**18**–2.**22**). Finding a sequestrum confirms the diagnosis and has therapeutic ramifications since it must be surgically resected. The sinogram performed by instilling contrast medium into the fistulous tract often documents the communication between the fistulous tract and the sequestrum (Fig. 2.**20**).

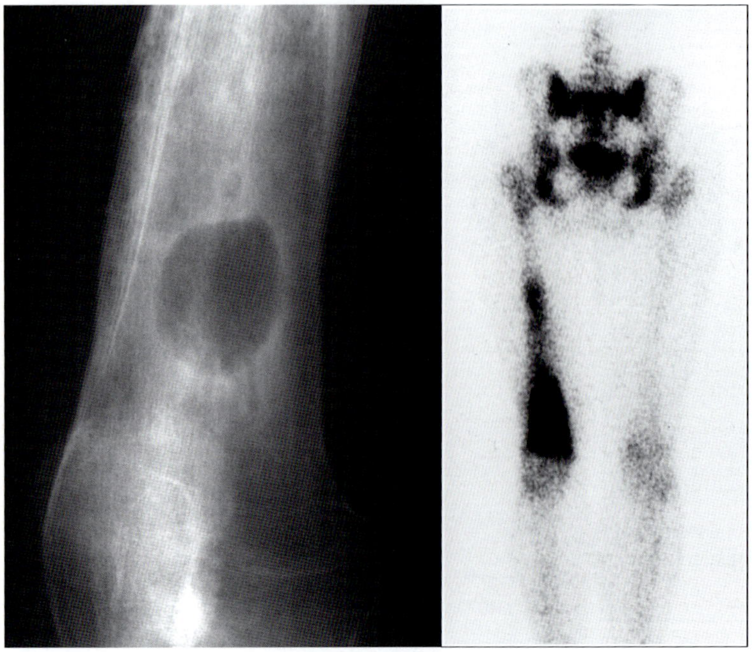

Fig. 2.**18** Exacerbation of chronic post-traumatic osteomyelitis of the femur with a well-demarcated osteolytic lesion, surrounding sclerosis and periosteal thickening. The bone scan shows intense uptake.

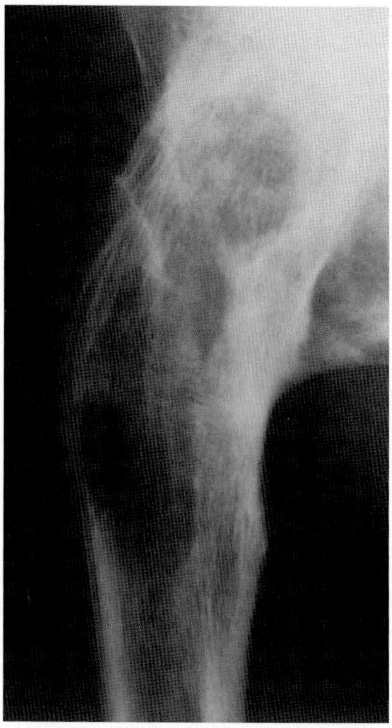

Fig. 2.19 Chronic post-traumatic osteomyelitis. The large osteolytic destruction is strongly suspicious for an abscess.

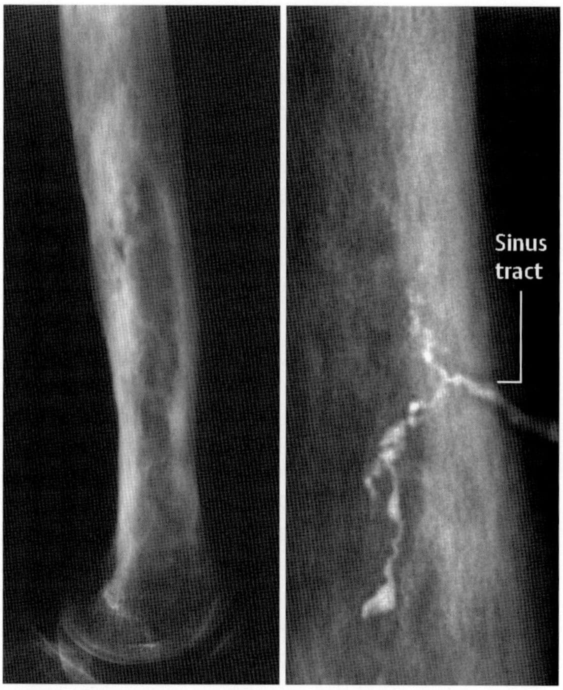

Fig. 2.20 Chronic osteomyelitis with sinus tract.

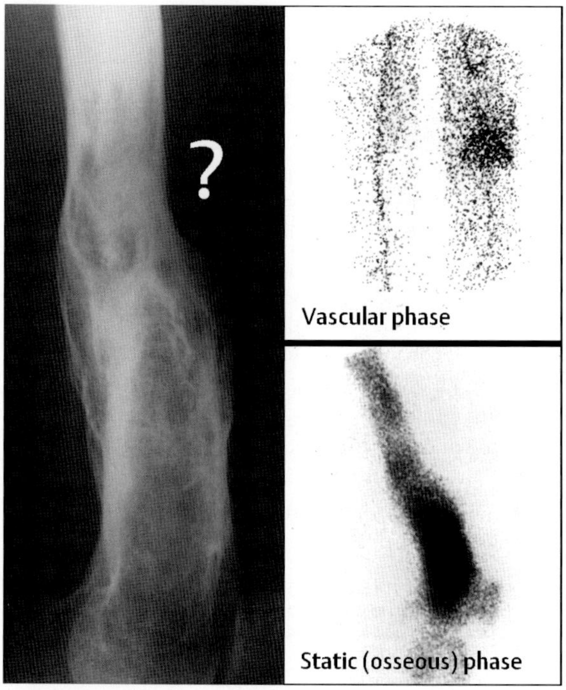

Fig. 2.21 Chronic post-traumatic osteomyelitis of the femur with inconclusive radiographic findings. There is localized hyperperfusion on the vascular phase of the bone scan and diffuse osseous uptake on the static (osseous) phase.

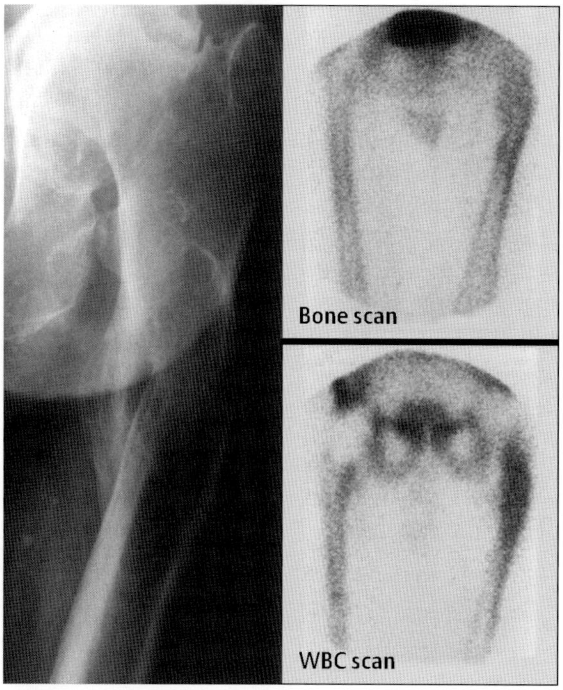

Fig. 2.22 Remote post-traumatic osteomyelitis and renewed pain. The bone scan (static phase) shows only slightly increased cortical uptake, but the WBC scan exhibits striking increased accumulation. The suspected exacerbation could not be confirmed clinically, and the WBC scan finding most likely reflects regenerated bone marrow.

CT Except for the detection of sequestra, CT is rarely indicated in chronic osteomyelitis. The sequestrum is an avascular osseous fragment of high density and entirely surrounded by fluid or soft tissues (Fig. 2.**25**).

NUC Secondary chronic osteomyelitis generally shows persistent increased uptake as a manifestation of increased bone turnover. Though the intensity of the vascular and blood pool activity of the three-phase bone scan can be used as an indication of a reactivation, the WBC scan with labeled autologous leukocytes is superior in determining the activity of the inflammatory changes.

MRI The MRI findings of exogenous chronic osteomyelitis are basically the same as those observed with acute hematogenous osteomyelitis, though the lesions may be more irregular in outline due to the endosteal and periosteal new bone formation and the surgical alterations. The inflammatory edema is seen as areas of increased signal intensity on the STIR and T2-weighted images with fat suppression. Both sequences invariably show the associated edema of the soft tissues. Identifying an acute attack of a chronic osteomyelitis is always difficult within the first 6 months after trauma or surgery and can remain so for up to 12 months in some cases. In this relatively early phase, edema and fluid accumulation of high signal intensity can be present, and biopsy or aspiration may not yield a positive bacteriologic culture. Cystic accumulations of sterile fluid can be observed even years after a fracture or surgical intervention and, even without inflammatory changes, are seen as high-signal intensity areas on the appropriate sequences. These cystic areas, which are found in both the medullary space and the soft tissues, are **sharply** demarcated and **not** surrounded by peripheral edema. This finding helps distinguish these cystic areas from a reinfection (Figs. 2.**23** – 2.**26**).

DD The history and clinical findings and laboratory findings virtually exclude any other diagnostic possibility.

Summary of the Role of Imaging in Diagnosing Chronic Post-traumatic Osteomyelitis

Conventional radiography provides information on the condition of the bone and, most importantly, discloses the post-traumatic and postoperative changes that must be incorporated into the general assessment. In contrast to acute osteomyelitis, the diagnostic evaluation generally must be supplemented by determining the extent of osseous involvement, since accurate preoperative assessment is the basis for adequate surgical therapy and an important prerequisite for improving the final outcome. MRI is the best imaging study to determine the extent of disease and frequently reveals unanticipated findings. Scintigraphy, especially the WBC scan with labeled autologous white blood cells, provides information that is comparable in establishing the status of osteomyelitic reactivation. Frequently, the clinical findings alone attest to an active infection, especially when a draining sinus tract is present. CT is indicated only if a sequestrum cannot be excluded or confirmed by conventional radiography or MRI. Sonography, which can be performed at the bedside, can sometimes be helpful in expeditiously assessing the soft tissues and excluding or confirming a soft-tissue abscess.

Table 2.**3** Key points in the radiologic diagnosis of **chronic** osteomyelitis

1. Chronic osteomyelitis produces a 'variegated radiographic picture' of cortical thickening, irregular osteosclerosis, and osteolytic destruction.
2. The radiographic changes induced by a reactivated chronic osteomyelitis are vague. Changes suggestive of reactivation are new radiolucencies, lamellated periosteal reaction, sinus tracts, and sequestration.
3. Interpreting WBC scintigraphy and MRI in conjunction with the radiographic findings is the most dependable method of determining reactivation of a chronic post-traumatic osteomyelitis.
4. CT is the best imaging method for detecting or excluding a sequestrum.
5. MRI is the best imaging method for the preoperative assessment of the extent of chronic osteomyelitis.

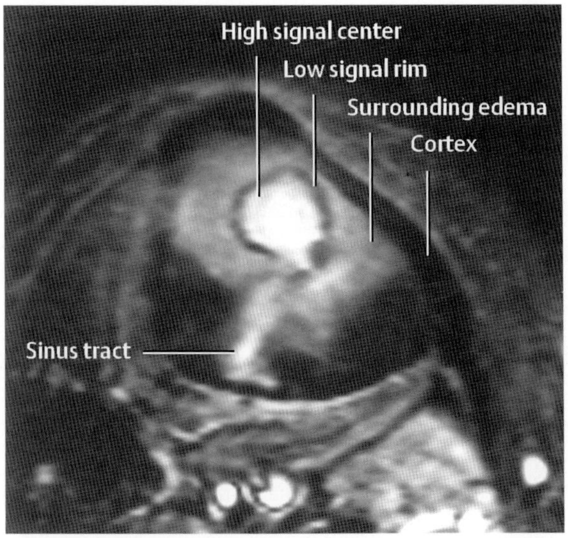

Fig. 2.**23** Intraosseous abscess in chronic post-traumatic osteomyelitis of the proximal tibia with sinus tract (STIR image).

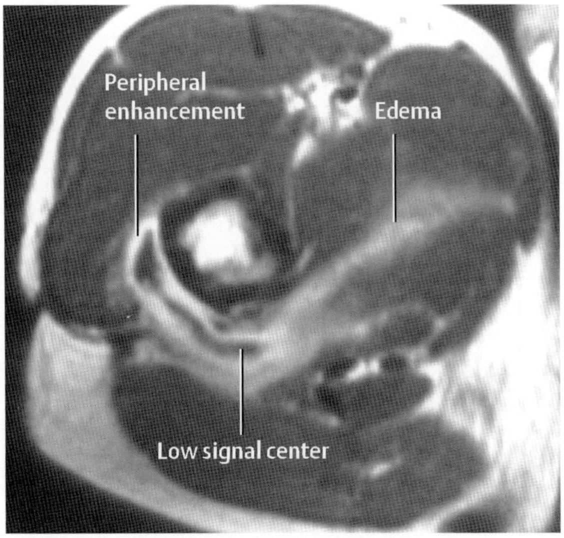

Fig. 2.**24** Chronic osteomyelitis with soft-tissue abscess. Enhanced T1-weighted image.

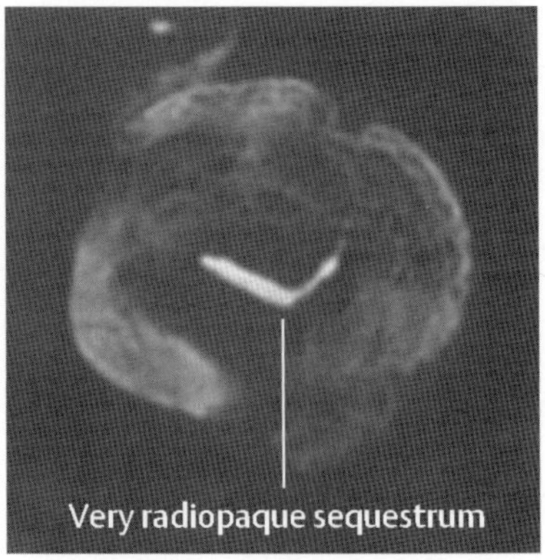

Fig. 2.**25** CT of chronic osteomyelitis with sequestrum.

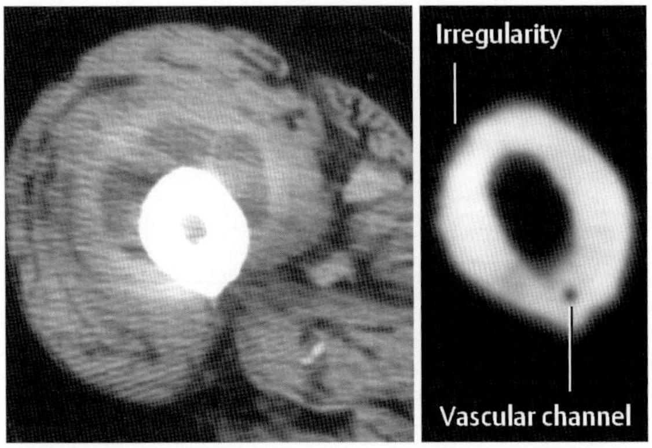

Fig. 2.**26** Soft-tissue abscess with subtle external cortical erosion.

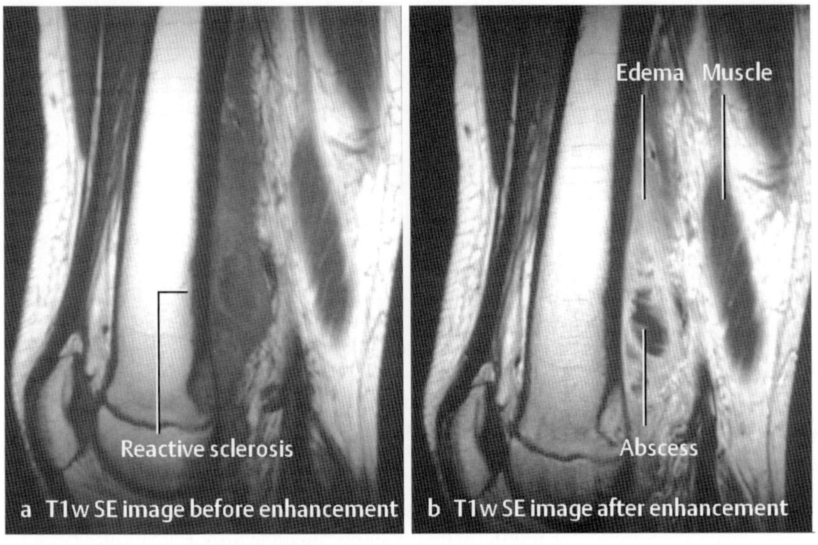

Fig. 2.**27** Soft-tissue abscess in the thigh with minimal secondary osseous involvement. T1-weighted image before (**a**) and after (**b**) administration of contrast medium.

Tuberculosis

Historically, skeletal tuberculosis has been rare in industrialized countries, but it has become more common in recent years, especially in drug users, alcoholics, and immunosuppressed patients. In these patients tuberculosis is by no means a rare diagnosis.

The most common infecting organism is *Mycobacterium tuberculosis*, but *Mycobacterium bovis* can also be encountered. The skeletal involvement is preceded by primary asymptomatic complex involvement of the lungs, urogenital tract, or intestines.

PATH Tuberculous infection begins in the marrow space with infiltration and trabecular destruction. Caseating necrosis surrounds the trabeculae, which become necrotic themselves and, as observed in suppurative osteomyelitis, form sequestra. Based on the morphologic appearance, the predominantly **productive** type with tuberculous granulation and osseous resorption is distinguished from the predominantly **exudative** type characterized by caseating necrosis and necrotic trabeculae. The histologic findings in bone are identical to those found in tuberculous infection of other organs and, depending on the manifestation, varying degrees of caseous necrosis with granulomas of epithelioid macrophages and giant cells of the Langerhans type are seen.

CLINIC An insidious course is characteristic of tuberculous infection. The patient generally is in poor general health and has weight loss and a low-grade fever. Local pain and swelling without erythema are common. Laboratory inflammatory parameters are elevated.
Location: Vertebral body (more than 50%, see pages 334–337), epiphyses of the long tubular bones, and in the hands and feet.

X-RAY
- Characteristically there is osteolytic destruction without sclerotic reaction, but a subtle, slowly progressing sclerosis can develop. In rare cases (most commonly in the spine) a sclerotic pattern dominates (Figs. 2.**28**–2.**32**).
- The severity of the periosteal reaction is quite variable.
- In children, a destructive pattern of 'punched-out' lesions is not uncommon (Fig. 2.**28**).
- In the newborn and infants, today, the so-called dactylitis of the phalanges of the hand and foot is rarely seen. This causes a periosteal reaction with diffuse phalangeal expansion ('spina ventosa', Fig. 2.**29**).
- The permeative pattern without periosteal reaction is rare (Fig. 2.**31**).

DD In the individual case, it can be difficult to distinguish tuberculous osteomyelitis from other chronic nonspecific types of osteomyelitis.

Tuberculosis can produce a 'cystic' pattern on conventional radiographs, and tuberculosis mimicking a solid tumor on MRI has been described. In most cases, tuberculosis cannot be diagnosed without a biopsy.

Glossary: Rare Skeletal Infections

Plasma cellular osteomyelitis: This is a rare chronic osteomyelitis, almost exclusively containing plasma cells. It is defined as a primarily chronic hematogenous osteomyelitis that, contrary to earlier views, is bacterial in origin and caused by staphylococci or streptococci. Plasma cellular osteomyelitis is primarily diagnosed histologically with the help of immunohistologic stains. The lesion is almost always unifocal and primarily affects adolescents and young adults. The healing is markedly accelerated after surgical removal of the inflammatory process. Since plasma cells are also seen in the reparative phase of the CRMO, it can be difficult to distinguish both types of osteomyelitis histologically, and the diagnosis must rest on the clinical and microbiologic findings.

Radiologically, lamellated periosteal reaction dominates, and the areas of cortical destruction may have partially indistinct outlines or have partially sclerotic borders. Sequestra are rare.

Since this condition is so rare, experience with MRI is limited.

Syphilis: Syphilis is rarely seen in the newborn but can occur in infants or adults, and can even be acquired in adults.

The radiographic findings include:
- Transverse radiolucent bands across the metaphyses of the long tubular bones. Occasionally, irregular destruction is seen at the metaphyseal-epiphyseal junction.
- Symmetric erosion along the medial contour of the tibial shaft ('Wimberger sign') is a characteristic finding.
- The involvement of the diaphysis of the tubular bones is dominated by osteolytic lesions with surrounding sclerosis and periosteal reaction.
- The periosteal reaction can be so striking that it produces a 'bone-within-a-bone' appearance.

Skeletal Echinococcosis
Skeletal echinococcus occurs in approximately 2% of cases of echinococcal infestation. The route is by hematogenous seeding, and the iliac wings and sacrum are most commonly affected.

Radiographically, multiple expansile 'cystic' osteolytic lesions, occasionally traversed by trabeculae, are characteristic. The cortex can be destroyed.

Sclerotic Nonpurulent Osteomyelitis of Garré
This rare condition, dominated by diffuse sclerosis, has a predilection for the mandible and long tubular bones (Fig. 2.**33**).

Another reasonable differential diagnosis is osteoid osteoma, which can be diagnosed by scintigraphy, CT, or MRI.

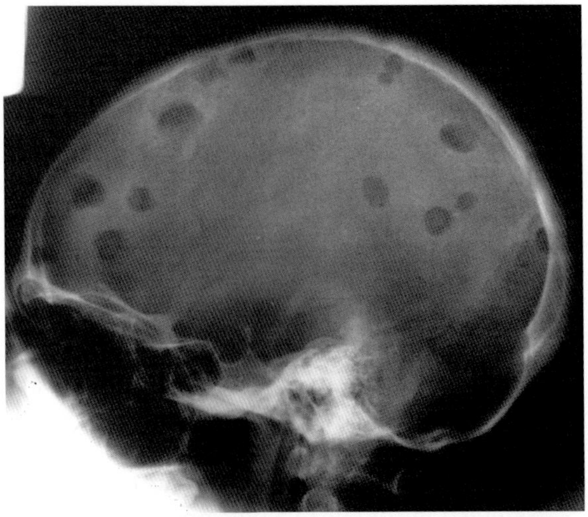

Fig. 2.**28** Skeletal tuberculosis with involvement of the skull in a 13-year-old boy. Punched-out osteolytic lesions.

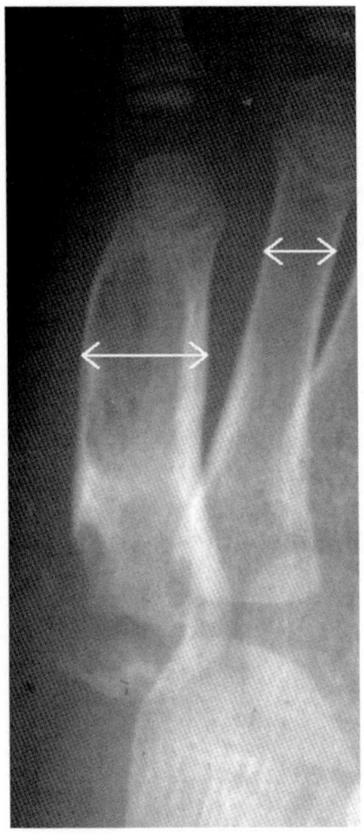

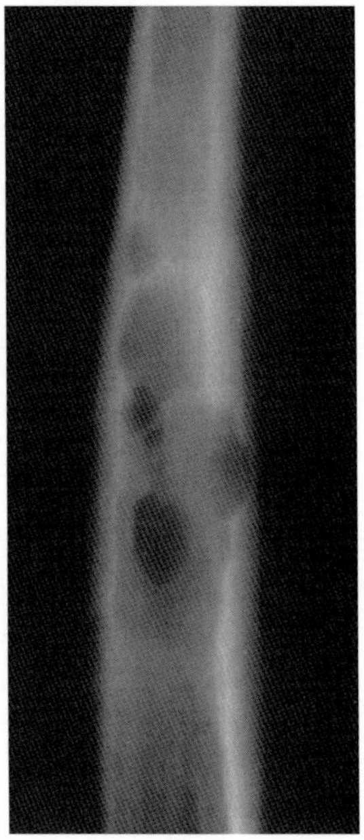

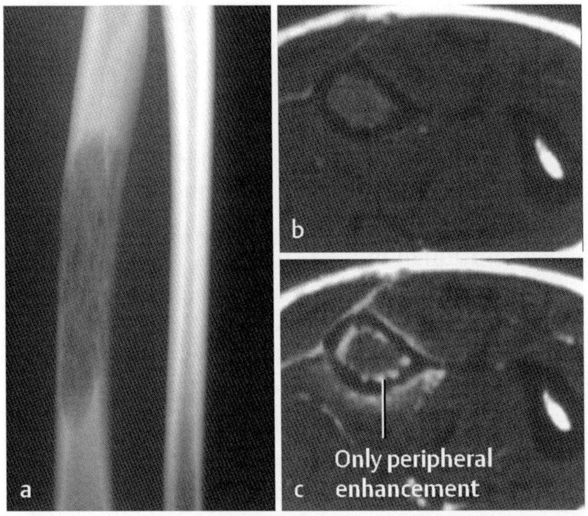

Top, left:
Fig. 2.**29** 'Spinal ventosa': tuberculous osteomyelitis in the fifth metatarsal. Same child as in Fig. 2.**28**.

Top, right:
Fig. 2.**30** Tuberculous osteomyelitis of the femur with osteolytic destruction surrounded by a relatively subtle sclerosis.

Left:
Fig. 2.**31** Tuberculous osteomyelitis of the radius with permeative destruction (**a**). Unenhanced (**b**) and enhanced (**c**) T1-weighted images, with only peripheral enhancement. This finding could just represent central caseation.

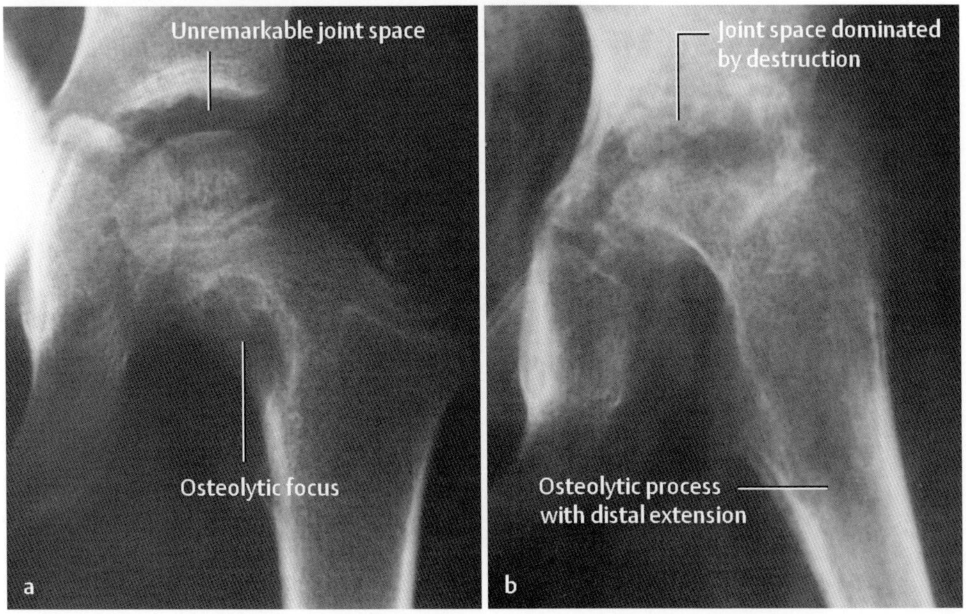

Fig. 2.**32** The natural evolution of tuberculosis in the proximal femur in a 4-year-old child. The extensive articular destruction found a year later suggests a primary tuberculous arthritis at the time of the initial radiograph.

Soft-tissue Infections

The soft tissues can become infected by hematogenous seeding during bacteremia, but direct infection from adjacent soft-tissue injury is far more common. The infection usually enters the soft tissues at the site of injury and spreads contiguously or through lymphatic channels.

The following conditions should be distinguished:

Erysipelas: This is an infection that spreads proximally from a distal site of broken skin (lacerations, abrasions, ulcerations) along the path of lymphatic drainage and causes a cutaneous and subcutaneous cellulitis. *Streptococcus pyogenes* is the commonest organism involved.

Phlegmonous Cellulitis: In contrast to erysipelas, this type of infection does not spread lymphatically but invades the soft-tissue spaces diffusely. Most cases are also caused by *Streptococcus pyogenes.* A special manifestation is the palmar phlegmonous cellulitis, which usually starts from the fingers and spreads beneath the palmar aponeurosis along the flexor tendons. The most serious complication is progression to the forearm, with involvement of the tendon sheaths, and then to the wrist.

Abscess: As in other sites of the body, an abscess is a circumscribed collection of pus. Staphylococci are the most frequent causative agents.

The soft tissues are examined best by sonography, with any additional evaluation by MRI and nuclear medicine reserved for unclear cases. CT is inferior to MRI because of its limited differentiation of soft-tissue structures, but it may still demonstrate an abscess if it is present. CT also has the advantage of being available in the acute setting.

SONO The sonographic findings of soft-tissue infections can be classified into three categories:

- Diffuse hyperechogenicity: This reflects soft-tissue edema, but its etiology (e.g., erysipelas versus congestion) cannot be determined sonographically.
- Localized hypoechoic to anechoic areas: These findings correspond to different degrees of tissue liquefaction. The presence of an abscess can only be established sonographically if a capsule is unequivocally delineated, and this is not always possible (Fig. 2.**34**).
- Hypoechoic to anechoic linear bands or areas of a burrow-like configuration: These correspond to collections of pus in a phlegmonous infection (Fig. 2.**35**).

CT Diffuse infections show generalized edematous infiltration of the subcutaneous fatty tissue (increased density). An abscess appears as ring-like enhancement around a hypodense center.

MRI Infectious edema is seen as increased signal intensity on STIR images or on T2-weighted SE images with fat suppression, without any alteration in muscle structure.

These sequences show an abscess as a lesion of high signal intensity surrounded by a rim of low signal intensity. Following injection of contrast medium, enhancement of variable width is seen around the abscess (Fig. 2.**36**).

MRI is used to determine whether the infectious process has spread to the adjacent bones. Bone marrow edema and periosteal reaction (which should be compared with the radiographic findings) suggest osseous involvement (compare with Fig. 2.**27**).

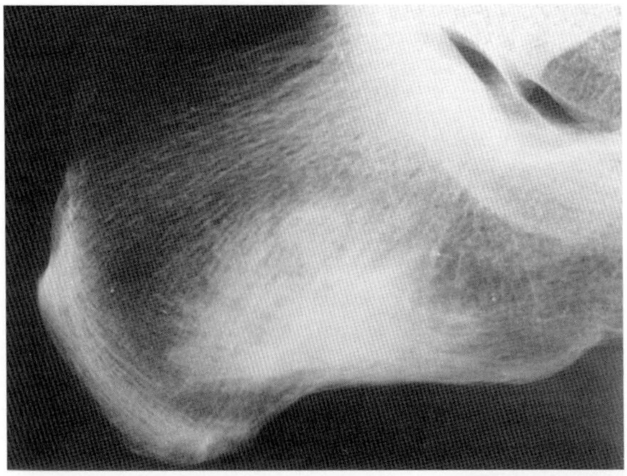

Fig. 2.**33** Chronic sclerosing osteomyelitis of Garré. It is difficult to distinguish this finding from osteoid osteoma.

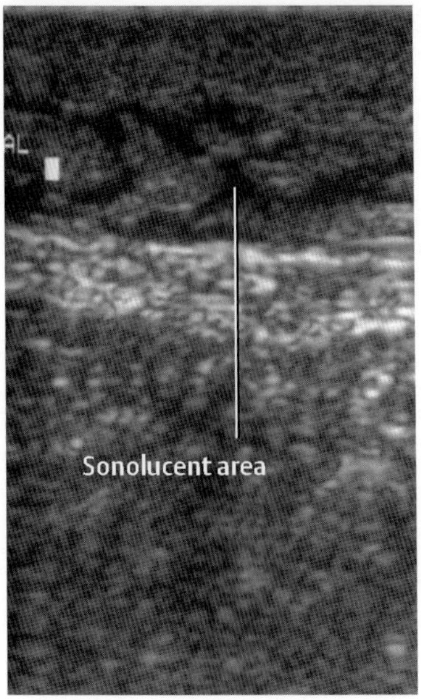

Fig. 2.**34** Sonographic features of phlegmonous inflammation of the dorsum of the foot. The burrow-like anechoic and hypoechoic areas are characteristic.

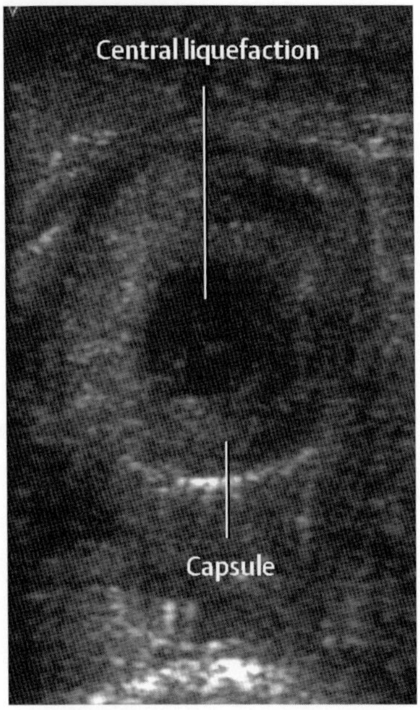

Fig. 2.**35** Sonogram of an abscess in the soft tissues of the forearm with central, almost anechoic liquefaction, surrounded by a thick capsule. *Staphylococcus aureus* was the causative organism.

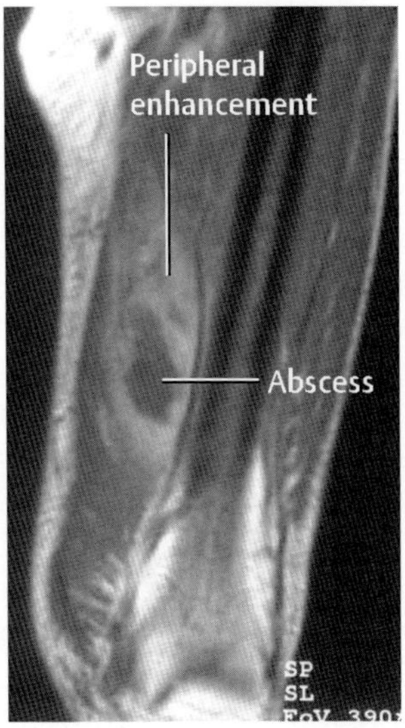

Fig. 2.**36** Abscess in the soft tissues of the thigh, as seen on an enhanced T1-weighted image. Differentiation from a tumor with central necrosis can be difficult.

3 Tumors and Tumorlike Lesions of the Skeleton and Soft Tissues

General Considerations in Diagnosing Skeletal Tumors

Primary bone tumors are rare compared to metastases (secondary bone tumors) and hematologic conditions which include plasmocytomas and malignant lymphomas (Chapter 4). Tumorlike lesions are distinctly different from primary bone tumors but are customarily discussed with them. Tumorlike lesions can spontaneously regress or cease to grow and never metastasize. They are relatively common, they often defy any radiologic classification, and only a few of them require therapy.

Bone tumors must be distinguished from primary soft-tissue tumors (pages 200–203).

The classification of bone tumors according to the World Health Organization (WHO) is summarized in Table 3.**1**, and rare conditions are deliberately excluded. This classification is based on the dominant matrix produced by the primary tumor. Since this approach is not universally applicable, the site of tumor origin is also embodied in the classification.

! The matrix is the intercellular substance produced by mesenchymal cells and includes osteoid, cartilage, myxoid ground substance, and (fibrous) collagenous fibers.

There are many tumorlike lesions that mimic primary and secondary bone tumors. These lesions resemble a tumor radiographically (localized osteolytic destruction or sclerosis), but fail to fulfill the pathologic criteria for a tumor (Table 3.**2**).

! The clinically most important tumorlike lesion is osteomyelitis, which is dealt with separately under Infections in Chapter 2.

Table 3.**1** Summary of the primary bone tumors

Benign tumors	Malignant tumors
1. Bone-producing tumors	
Osteoid osteoma	Osteosarcoma
Osteoblastoma	(subclassifications)
2. Cartilage-producing tumors	
Chondroma	Chondrosarcoma
Osteochondroma	
Chondroblastoma	
Chondromyxoid fibroma	
3. Giant cell tumor	
4. Tumors arising from the bone marrow	
	Ewing sarcoma
	Hematologic tumors (Lymphoma, plasmocytoma, see Chapter 4)
5. Vascular tumors	
Hemangioma	Hemangiopericytoma
Lymphangioma	Hemangioendothelioma
Glomus tumor	Angiosarcoma
6. Connective tissue tumors	
Lipoma	Fibrosarcoma
Desmoplastic fibroma	Malignant fibrous
Benign fibrous histiocytoma	histiocytoma
7. Other tumors	
	Chordoma
	Adamantinoma of the long tubular bones

Table 3.**2** Summary of the tumorlike lesions

- Bone island/osteoma
- Non-ossifying fibroma (= fibrous cortical defect)
- Periosteal desmoid
- Simple ('juvenile') bone cyst
- Aneurysmal bone cyst
- Eosinophilic granuloma
- Fibrous dysplasia
- Brown tumor of hyperparathyroidism (see page 244)
- Myositis ossificans (see page 286)
- Intraosseous ganglion (see page 374)

The Role of the Radiologist in Evaluating Skeletal Lesions Suspicious for Tumors

1. After a lesion has been detected, distinguished from a normal variant, and categorized as pathological, a reasonable differential diagnosis of three most likely possibilities should be offered. In many cases, the lesion can only be classified as 'probably benign' or 'probably malignant.' If a lesion is judged by the examiner on the basis of his or her experience as unequivocally benign, this should be stated as such to avoid unnecessary biopsy or surgical therapy.
2. The location of the lesion should be described to help plan the safest approach for biopsy or surgical excision. Depending on the presumptive nature of the lesion (benign versus malignant), either biopsy or primary excision should be considered in consultation with the surgeon. The radiologist should be conversant with the staging of primary bone tumors and with the imaging modalities most suitable for staging the individual case. A biopsy should be obtained only after a thorough imaging evaluation. It should be remembered that an open biopsy alters the MRI signal. Therefore, definitive diagnosis in patients who have had biopsies becomes more difficult.
3. The radiologist should know the imaging modality suitable for monitoring any therapy and be familiar with the practical intervals of follow-up examinations.
4. A correct diagnosis and rational therapeutic strategy for primary bone tumors can only be accomplished by the close cooperation of the radiologist, the surgeon, and the pathologist.

The Role of Diagnostic Imaging

All imaging methods play a role in diagnosing and staging primary and secondary bone tumors (metastases).

After radiographic or scintigraphic detection of an osseous lesion that could be a tumor, its radiographic features should be analyzed. These include:
- type of destruction,
- margin of the lesion,
- cortical changes,
- periosteal reaction,
- soft-tissue infiltration or mass.

This analysis generally determines the biologic activity (inactive, active, aggressive). This information coupled with the type of matrix production can often provide a definitive diagnosis.

The following lesions should be recognized and distinguished from other conditions:
- Inactive and benign 'leave-me-alone' lesions not requiring any therapy. Typical examples are bone infarcts, non ossifying fibromas, and bone islands.
- Bone lesions highly likely to be benign, which do not need immediate histologic evaluation and can be observed. Examples are fibrous dysplasia and post-traumatic myositis ossificans. Histologic confirmation is needed in individual cases only if an aggressive clinical course ensues after the lesion is discovered.
- Lesions that are probably benign and are unresectable for anatomic reasons regardless of the histologic finding. Examples are enchondromas and osteochondromas.
- All lesions of undetermined biologic activity or categorized as aggressive (perhaps malignant). These lesions must be biopsied after further diagnostic imaging and staging. Going straight to surgical resection is justified only if malignancy could be excluded by imaging.

! A suspected primary bone tumor or, less frequently, a tumorlike lesion of unknown nature should undergo an open surgical biopsy since a percutaneous biopsy may fail to obtain enough material for histologic evaluation. This does not apply to lesions suspected to be metastases, plasmocytoma, malignant lymphoma, or an inflammatory process. In these instances, percutaneous biopsy is more reasonable and less invasive.

Ten Rules for Classifying Skeletal Lesions Suspicious for Tumors (according to Manaster)

Analysis of unknown skeletal lesions using the following ten determinants should lead to a definitive diagnosis, suggest a presumptive diagnosis or, at least, offer a limited and reasonable differential diagnosis.

1. **Age of the patient:** Many tumors have a typical age distribution. This applies to Ewing sarcoma (childhood and adolescence), aneurysmal bone cyst (adolescence and young adulthood), osteosarcoma (childhood to young adulthood), and several sarcomas, such as chondrosarcoma and malignant fibrous histiocytoma (after the age of 30 years). Metastases and plasmocytomas usually do not occur before the fourth decade, with the notable exception of breast cancer metastases, which can occur at a younger age.
2. **Soft-tissue involvement:** Cortical destruction with tumor extension into the soft tissue generally indicates a more aggressive growth and suggests a malignant lesion.
   Caution: Aneurysmal bone cyst and eosinophilic granuloma are notable exceptions. Lesions with pathologic fractures may also present diagnostic problems.
   A primary soft-tissue tumor is best demonstrated by MRI. Except for very aggressively infiltrating tumors, soft-tissue tumors respect the fascias for quite some time (in contrast to soft-tissue infection).
3. **Growth pattern:** Analyzing the bone lesion (pattern of bone destruction, cortical involvement, periosteal reaction, etc.) usually allows categorization into three groups of biologic activity:
   a) slow growth ('inactive'),
   b) intermediate growth ('active'),
   c) fast growth ('aggressive').
4. **Size of the lesion:** The size of the lesion coupled with the pattern of bone destruction frequently reveals additional information about the biologic nature of the lesion. **Large** lesions with cortical destruction and little periosteal reaction should, for all intents and purposes, be assumed to be malignant.
5. **Location of the lesion:** Some tumors commonly involve particular bones; for example the adamantinoma almost exclusively occurs in the tibia. Other lesions occur predominately in a preferred location in a tubular bone; for example chondroblastoma, is always an epiphyseal tumor. Some tumors occur more frequently in the axial than in the appendicular skeleton. Furthermore, the location within the bone (central versus eccentric, epiphyseal versus diaphyseal) can suggest the diagnosis. This will be discussed in more detail in the appropriate sections.
6. **Zone of transition:** The transition from abnormal, pathologic bone to normal bone provides an additional indication of the nature of the lesion. A wide and indistinct zone of transition invariably indicates an aggressive and rapidly growing lesion, while a narrow zone of transition, in particular one with a sclerotic rim, can be assumed to be slow growing.
7. **Margin of the lesion:** Though the margin is included in the preceding rule (6, Zone of transition), it can be seen as a different entity. Despite a very thin and well-demarcated zone of transition, a lesion can still be malignant or aggressive. This is seen in plasmocytomas and giant cell tumors.
8. **Tumor matrix:** A categorization of bone and cartilage-forming tumors is possible by analyzing the visible tumor matrix. Furthermore, MRI can distinguish between myxoid substances and water-containing components (cysts).
9. **Host response:** The response of the host bone to the tumor is reflected by cortical reaction (cortical thickening, formation of a neocortex, destruction, infiltration) and by periosteal reaction.
10. **Monostotic, oligostotic,** or **polyostotic lesions:** Benign polyostotic lesions may include fibrous dysplasia, Paget disease, eosinophilic granuloma, and enchondromas. Malignant polyostotic lesions include metastases, plasmocytoma, and lymphoma.

! By incorporating these analytical characteristics into the clinical findings, the correct histologic diagnosis can often be established. At least the growth pattern of the lesion (least aggressive, more aggressive, highly aggressive) should be determined. It should also be remembered that aggressive growth does not invariably imply malignancy; this is characterized by aggressively growing benign lesions such as infection, eosinophilic granuloma, and aneurysmal bone cyst.

Staging (Determining the Extent of the Lesion)

The Enneking method is the generally accepted staging systems for primary bone tumors, especially malignant tumors.

This method is based on the histologic grading of the tumor (benign, low-grade malignant, high-grade malignant), its anatomic extent (mostly as determined by imaging), and the presence of metastases (in the skeleton or, above all, in the lung). These three factors are combined to plan the treatment strategy for a particular bone or soft-tissue tumor. The major role of the imager is to determine the local extent of the tumor and to search for skeletal metastases by scintigraphy and pulmonary metastases by chest CT.

A distinction should also be made between the intra- and extracompartmental locations of the tumor.

Intracompartmental lesions are defined as follows:

- All lesions confined to the subcutaneous fat (soft-tissue tumors).
- All lesions confined to the parosteal soft tissues. These tumors displace the muscles without infiltrating either muscle or osseous cortex.
- All bone tumors that are intracortical, i.e., the cortex or a surrounding neocortex is still visible.
- All soft-tissue tumors confined to a muscle compartment. The fascial planes enclosing these compartments are not violated. Examples of recognized muscle compartments are the posterior compartment of the calf, the anterior compartment of the calf, and the dorsal compartment of the forearm.

Extracompartmental lesions are defined as follows:

All tumors that violate any of the above-mentioned compartments or that abut or invade major neurovascular bundles. In addition, tumors are considered primary extracompartmental if located at a site without natural barriers.

These anatomic sites include mid-hand, mid-foot, hind foot, popliteal fossa, femoral triangle, and axilla. Any tumor (bone or soft-tissue tumor) with articular extension is also considered extracompartmental.

Relative Values of the Different Imaging Modalities for Tissue Diagnosis, Assessing Biologic Activity, and Staging

Conventional Radiography

Radiography remains in the forefront of detecting skeletal lesions. Furthermore, it is the primary imaging modality to suggest the tissue diagnosis and to judge the biologic nature of tumorous lesions. For tumorlike or benign lesions, it can determine their extent.

Scintigraphy

Tc 99 m diphosphonate scintigraphy of the skeleton is used primarily to establish multifocality such as that seen with osseous metastases, and to monitor osseous lesions following therapy. Only a few entities, such as Paget disease and osteoid osteoma, exhibit a diagnostic pattern of bone uptake. The intensity of uptake within a lesion is not a reliable differentiating imaging finding.

CT

Although the role of CT for staging malignant tumors has decreased with the growth of MRI, it remains the standard method of evaluating uncertain radiographic and scintigraphic findings in the spine and pelvis. Some comparison studies could demonstrate that CT has the same accuracy as MRI for staging lesions as intra- versus extracompartmental in location. Because of its sensitivity in detecting calcifications and ossifications, CT is superior to conventional radiography in determining the tumor matrix and can add to the differential diagnostic assessment.

Sonography

Sonography is an acceptable bedside method for the detection and further evaluation of an undetermined swelling of the peripheral soft tissues, and supplements palpation and inspection. Ultrasonography is also suitable to guide percutaneous biopsies, especially of lesions in the peripheral soft tissues. Color Doppler duplex sonography can also provide differential diagnostic criteria, distinguishing, for instance, a solid tumor from a hematoma.

Angiography

Angiography has become obsolete for detecting and staging tumors and for offering differential diagnostic information. Even establishing the relationship between the neurovascular compartments and tumors has been taken over by MRI. Angiography still plays a role if embolization is contemplated (e.g., preoperative embolization of metastases or embolization of soft-tissue hemangiomas).

MRI

MRI is considered the gold standard for staging malignant and benign tumors. This applies to the entire skeleton, but above all to the extremities. Furthermore, MRI can provide a variety of differential diagnostic criteria by means of the different signal intensities and contrast enhancement. This application has increased significantly in recent years, showing a definite change from the initial verdict that MRI, like scintigraphy, provided only 'non-specific' data.

Technical Considerations: Differential diagnostic criteria are furnished by the signal intensities of the T1-weighted and T2-weighted SE sequences. The STIR sequence is a very good screening sequence. After intravenous administration of contrast medium, the T1-weighted sequences, preferably with fat suppression, generally add useful clues. Depending on the size of the tumor, large body coils or special surface coils, adapted to the anatomy, are applied. MRI has the advantage of multiplanar imaging, providing a comprehensive assessment of the transitional zone between tumor and healthy tissue.

Caution: If a bone tumor is suspected, the MRI findings must be correlated with those from conventional radiography.

! MRI is frequently unable to distinguish between benign and malignant bone or soft-tissue tumors. It is, however, quite reliable in distinguishing tumors from inflammatory and ischemic lesions. This is especially true in differentiating between tumor, osteomyelitis, and bone infarct, which is of profound clinical importance.

Table 3.**3** Suspected tumors or tumorlike conditions that can be diagnosed with MRI

- Lipoma
- Hemangioma
- Pigmented villonodular synovitis (joint tumor)
- Cyst
- Aneurysmal bone cyst
- Enchondroma

Table 3.**4** Bone and soft-tissue lesions with high signal intensities on T1-weighted SE images

- Lipoma
- Hematoma (within the first 14 days to 3 weeks)
- Pigmented melanoma

Table 3.**5** Structures with low proton density: dark or black on all sequences

- Cortical bone
- Calcifications
- Air
- Foreign material
- Fibrous tissue with high collagen content (ligaments/tendons, fibrosis, scar, hypocellular fibrous tumors)
- Vascular structures with flow void
- Iron deposits

The detection of peritumoral edema, within or outside the bone, is a non-specific finding, but can aid in detecting tumors and arriving at a tissue diagnosis:

- Peritumoral edema is more frequent with malignant tumors than with benign ones, but it is not a reliably distinguishing finding.
- Edema can occur with infections and trauma and, rarely, with acute bone infarcts. A space-occupying lesion (tumor) can generally be identified against the surrounding edema. In many cases, this finding can help in the tentative differentiation between tumor, inflammation, and infarct.
- It should be kept in mind that clusters of tumor cells (only microscopically detectable) can be embedded in the edema surrounding the tumor. This is important when determining the margins of resection, which should generally include the edematous zone.

- The most sensitive detection for a peritumoral edema is rendered by the STIR sequence and the T1-weighted SE sequence with fat suppression, together with the administration of contrast medium. Remember that edema does not enhance.

Staging and MRI

The most elemental question in staging is whether the lesion is intracompartmental or extracompartmental, and this is determined by MRI in the majority of cases. The multiplanar capability of MRI also makes it the modality of choice for determining the osseous and soft-tissue extent of the tumor and the relationship of the tumor to fascia and adjacent articular structures. Furthermore, MRI can reliably delineate the relationship of the tumor to the major neurovascular compartments.

The **intraosseous extent** of a lesion is best determined on the T1-weighted SE images. The imaging plane should be determined by the anatomy (e.g., coronal or sagittal planes for tubular bones). The T2-weighted images, especially the so-called turbo SE sequences, are **not** suitable for determining the osseous extent of the lesion. The administration of contrast medium is only meaningful if the T1-weighted sequences can be combined with fat suppression.

The **soft-tissue extent** is best assessed on STIR sequences because these sequences achieve a high contrast between tumor, muscle, and fat. The T1-weighted SE sequences, excellent for anatomic detail, are most helpful when obtained with fat suppression and after administration of contrast medium.

When assessing the relationship between the tumor and the adjacent joints as part of the staging, the following questions must be addressed:
- Is the joint involved?
- Do the tumor margins abut the joint, producing a sympathetic effusion? Remember, however, that the effusion may not be induced by the tumor itself. A tumor-induced effusion occurs only after direct tumorous invasion of the capsule.
- Is the tumor intracapsular?
- Is the tumor growth transarticular?

Tumors can extend directly to the subchondral interface, as is the situation with aneurysmal bone cysts, giant cell tumors, or chondroblastoma. This is relevant for planning the surgical approach since the articular surface might not be preserved in many of these cases, and it might be necessary to modify the surgical technique, possibly resorting to an endoprosthesis.

Therapeutic Strategies of Bone and Soft-tissue Tumors

The different therapeutic strategies, primarily surgical, are determined by the tissue diagnosis and the extent of the lesion. Intralesional excision (curettage) is to be distinguished from marginal excision. An additional surgical strategy is the wide excision (4 cm beyond the tumor margin) or radical resection (resection of the tumor, including the entire surrounding musculature and surrounding bone). Malignant bone and soft-tissue tumors generally undergo preoperative and often also postoperative chemotherapy. This is especially true in tumors such as Ewing sarcoma and osteosarcoma. Radiotherapy of primary bone and soft-tissue tumors is less commonly performed today. However, palliative radiation remains effective for certain bone and soft-tissue metastases.

Primary Bone Tumors

Bone-Producing Tumors

Osteoid Osteoma

■ This is a benign, painful osseous lesion that is characterized by small size (less than 2 cm) and sharp demarcation, frequently surrounded by a sclerotic reaction. ■

PATH The tumor consists of highly vascularized stroma with osteoid and immature bone.

CLINIC Severe pain (especially at night), relieved by aspirin (less than 50% of cases).
Age: First through third decade.
Location: The femur (30%) and tibia (25%) are most frequently involved. The lesion is eccentric, frequently intracortical (80–90%).
Therapy: Surgical excision (immediate pain relief indicates successful removal). Percutaneous excision or alcohol ablation can be used in selected cases.

! Clinically relevant locations are intracapsular osteoid osteomas (joint pain) and the spine (reactive scoliosis).

X-RAY The tumor causes focal bone destruction (nidus) that is surrounded by varying degrees of sclerosis (Figs. 3.**1**–3.**3**). The osteoid produced by the tumor can ossify, leading to diffuse or punctate areas of increased density within the osteolytic destruction. A severely ossified nidus can merge with the surrounding sclerosis. The following are possible locations for the nidus:

1. **Intracortical,** surrounded by severe reactive ovoid or biconvex new bone formation and occurring in the cortex with possible bone marrow extension (Fig. 3.**2**).
2. **Medullary,** (e.g., in the hands or feet), generally with less severe surrounding sclerosis and frequently demarcated as a sclerotic structure (Fig. 3.**3**).
3. **Intraspinal,** (often in the vertebral arch) where the nidus and sclerosis are barely separable.
4. **Intra-articular,** (e.g., hip joint), often seen as a relatively subtle, subarticular, round to ovoid radiolucency. The lesion can also bulge into the joint and be surrounded solely by a subtle sclerotic rim.

NUC Localized, frequently eccentric uptake of severe intensity, coupled with radiography, usually allows a definitive diagnosis to be rendered.

CT Same as the radiographic findings, with the advantage that the lesion is delineated without superimposed osseous structures.

MRI The nidus is of low signal intensity on T1-weighted images, but of variable signal intensities on T2-weighted images (depending on the extent of the calcifications) (Fig. 3.**4**).
Caution: Extensive edema surrounding the lesion with soft-tissue involvement can cause confusion with a more aggressive lesion.

DD **Brodie's abscess:** small abscesses appear identical to those of osteoid osteoma.
Bone island: osteoid osteoma almost always induces an osseous reaction, whereas the bone island does not.
Osteoblastic metastases: especially in the spine, when randomly distributed multiple lesions are shown on the bone scan.
Chronic osteomyelitis and fractures: Diffuse, indistinctly demarcated osteoid osteomas of the foot and hand skeleton can mimic these lesions.

Osteoblastoma

■ This is a benign bone-forming tumor larger than 2 cm (the so-called 'big brother' of the osteoid osteoma). It can be difficult to distinguish the aggressive type of this osteoblastoma from an osteosarcoma (rare). ■

CLINIC The pain is less severe than that experienced with osteoid osteoma.
Location: About 40% of osteoblastomas are in the spine; the rest are found in the tubular bones, skull, and other bones.
Therapy: Curettage.

X-RAY Relevant findings:

1. Osteolytic destruction, usually sharply demarcated. Intralesional calcifications are frequent (Fig. 3.**5**).
2. Surrounding sclerosis is induced less frequently than with the osteoid osteoma.
3. Cup-like cortical defect if extrinsically located.
4. Osseous extension is frequent.

CT Important for the assessment of the tumor margin and the method of choice for the spine (Fig. 3.**6**).

DD **Osteosarcoma:** Individual cases can be radiographically identical. **Brown tumors of hyperparathyroidism:** Differentiation by clinical findings and laboratory parameters. **Aneurysmal bone cyst:** Cystic cavities, trabeculated.
Caution: Osteoblastoma and aneurysmal bone cysts can co-exist.

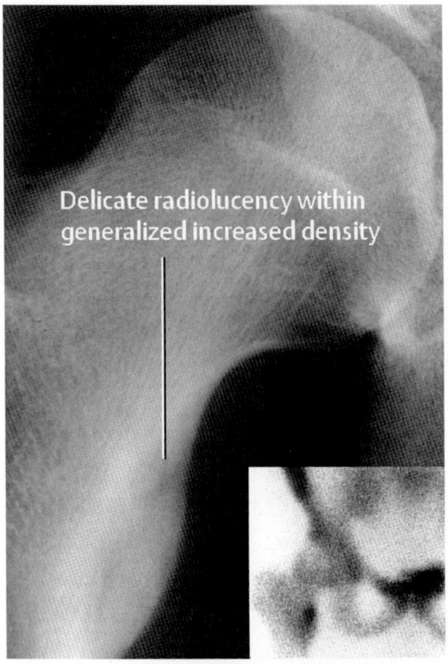

Fig. 3.1 Osteoid osteoma in the lesser trochanter of the femur.

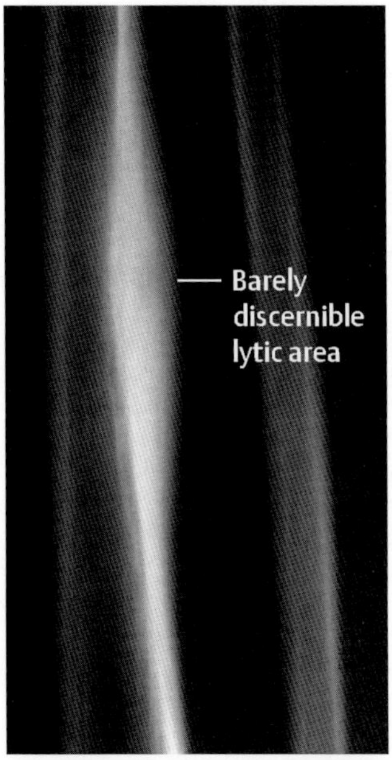

Fig. 3.2 Osteoid osteoma of the tibia with typical fusiform periosteal reaction.

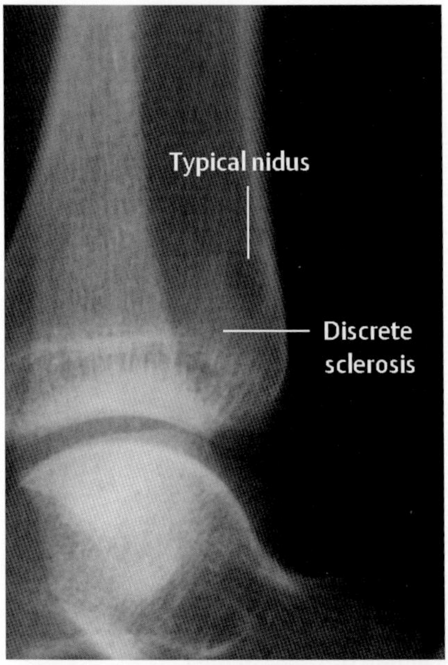

Fig. 3.3 Osteoid osteoma of the distal tibia surrounded by only a minimal reaction.

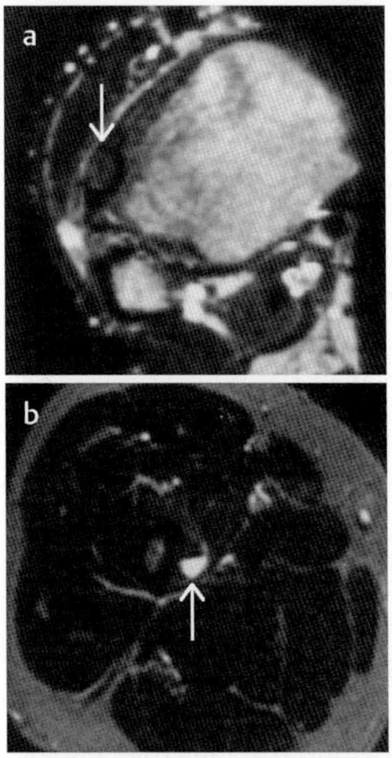

Fig. 3.4 MRI of osteoid osteoma, T2-weighted images.
a Lesion of relatively low signal intensity corresponding to delicate calcifications not yet visible radiologically.
b Lesion of high signal intensity in the cortex.

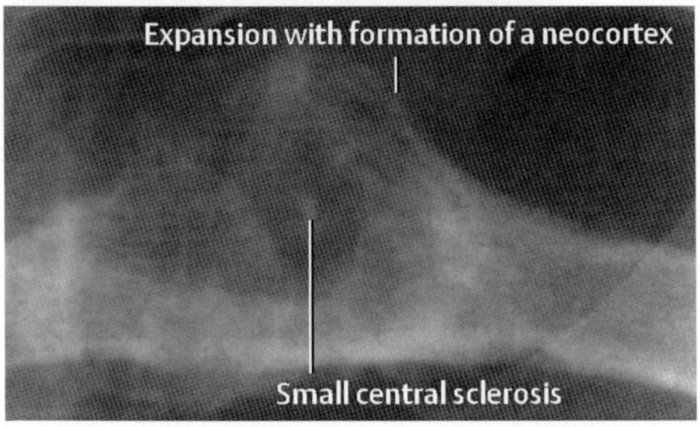

Fig. 3.5 Osteoblastoma of the rib. The margin is not completely discernible (→ CT).

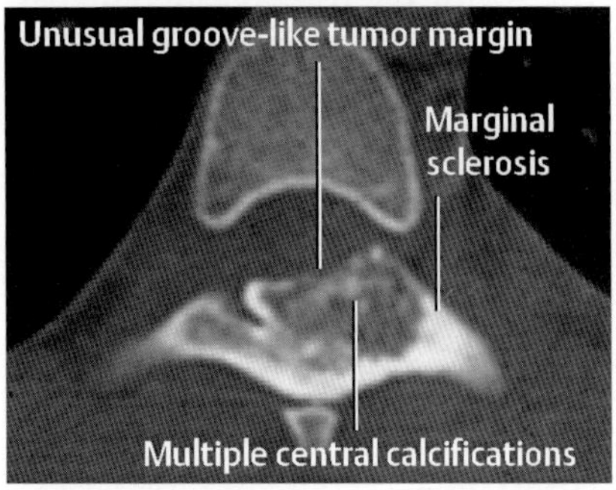

Fig. 3.6 Osteoblastoma of the vertebral arch.

Osteosarcoma

Synonym: Osteogenic sarcoma

Osteosarcoma is the most common malignant primary bone tumor, most frequently occurring in children and adolescents.

PATH The tumor cells form osteoid. Histologically, subclassifications are made on the basis of the dominating tissue differentiation (osteoblastic, chondroblastic, fibroblastic, etc.). Numerous variants exist:
- 'conventional' osteosarcoma (about 75%, see below),
- periosteal osteosarcoma (see below),
- parosteal osteosarcoma (see below),
- telangiectatic osteosarcoma (highly malignant, purely lytic osteosarcoma),
- 'low-grade' osteosarcoma (prognostically favorable, slow-growing osteosarcoma),
- osteosarcoma of older patients (above 60 years of age, e.g., associated with Paget disease, post-radiotherapy),
- soft-tissue osteosarcoma (beginning after the age of 40 years).

CLINIC Slowly worsening local pain.
Age: Two incidence peaks: age 10–25 years and age 60–80 years, but can occur at any age.
Location: The tumor can arise in any bone but over 80% occur in the long tubular bones (femur, tibia) and involve the metaphysis in the majority of cases.
Prognosis and therapy: The five-year survival rate depends on the type of tumor and on the time of the diagnosis, ranging between 30 and 80%. Preoperative chemotherapy is followed by amputation or wide resection. The surgical approach depends on the local tumor stage, best shown by MRI, and on the presence of metastases shown by bone scintigraphy and chest CT.

'Conventional' Osteosarcoma

X-RAY The radiographic findings are variable.
Mixed osteolytic/osteoblastic morphology: This is the most frequent manifestation. Radiographically, osteolytic and osteoblastic changes are found together, with the osteoblastic changes corresponding to mineralized osteoid. The degree of osteolytic and osteoblastic changes varies from case to case. The tumor margins are indistinct and periosteal new bone formation, characteristically spiculated, is invariably present. The Codman triangle, a manifestation of periosteal elevation, is often observed. Furthermore, lamellated, intermittently disrupted periosteal bone formation is consistently observed (Fig. 3.**7 b**).
Osteolytic osteosarcoma (about 10% of cases): moth-eaten pattern of destruction, almost always with periosteal reaction (Fig. 3.**7 a**).
Osteoblastic osteosarcoma (about 10% of cases): characterized by ivory or dense cloudlike sclerotic tumor mass (Fig. 3.**8**). The tumor can be confined to the outline of the affected bone and sharply demarcated from the surrounding spongiosa. Any extension of the tumor into the soft tissues induces a periosteal reaction.

NUC This is important to exclude metastases and to monitor the tumor's response to therapy.

CT This is superior to conventional radiography in differentiating reactive changes (e.g., periosteal response) from the tumor itself.

MRI The signal pattern is determined by the degree of ossification of the matrix. MRI is the method of choice for staging lesions in tubular bones (intramedullary extension, soft-tissue infiltration, intracompartmental versus extracompartmental tumor component, joint involvement) (Fig. 3.**9**).

DD **Ewing sarcoma:** No differentiation if there is no matrix produced by the osteosarcoma or if it is only faintly ossified.
Cortical desmoid: The eccentric location at the distal femoral metaphysis is the key to the diagnosis of a cortical desmoid.
Chronic osteomyelitis: Usually differentiated by MRI by showing a solid tumor that is absent in osteomyelitis.
Chondrosarcoma: The considerable amount of cartilage produced by some osteosarcomas might preclude the differentiation between a so-called 'chondroblastic osteosarcoma' and a chondrosarcoma.

Glossary

Parosteal osteosarcoma (juxtacortical osteosarcoma, parosseous osteosarcoma):
This well-differentiated osteosarcoma has its epicenter adjacent to the periosteum and has a much better prognosis than the 'conventional' osteosarcoma.
Parosteal osteosarcoma appears as a lobulated density along the surface of the metaphyseal cortex of the tubular bone and leads to thickening and deformity of the cortex. Only 10% of the tumors extend into the bone marrow space (Fig. 3.**10**).
The differential diagnosis includes myositis ossificans, juxtacortical osteoma, and other osseous sarcomas.

Periosteal Osteosarcoma: Like the parosteal osteosarcoma, this is a surface lesion, preferentially involving the tibial and femoral diaphyses. It is dominated by a soft-tissue mass with a tumor matrix that is less mineralized than the parosteal osteosarcoma. MRI is essential for tumor staging.

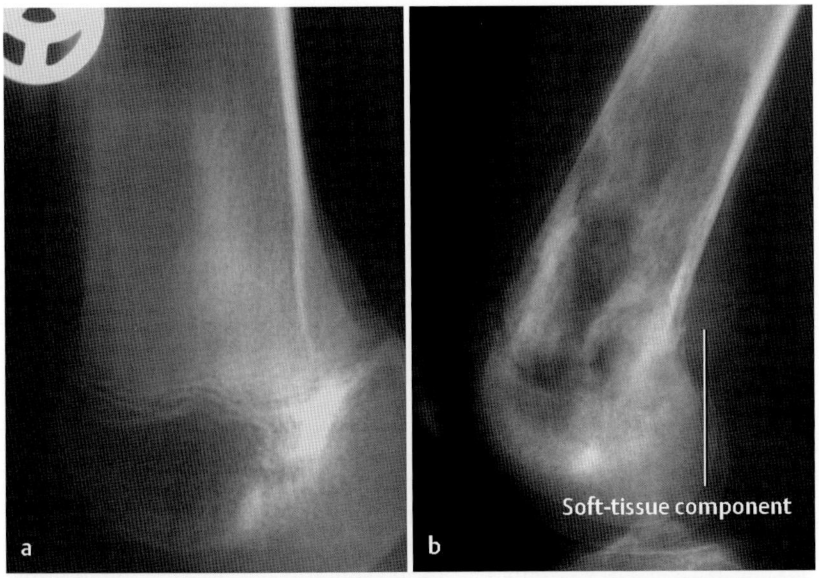

Fig. 3.7 Osteosarcoma, initially lytic (**a**) was misinterpreted as Brodie abscess at the time of presentation). Typical mixed osteolytic/osteoblastic osteosarcoma (**b**) 7 months later.

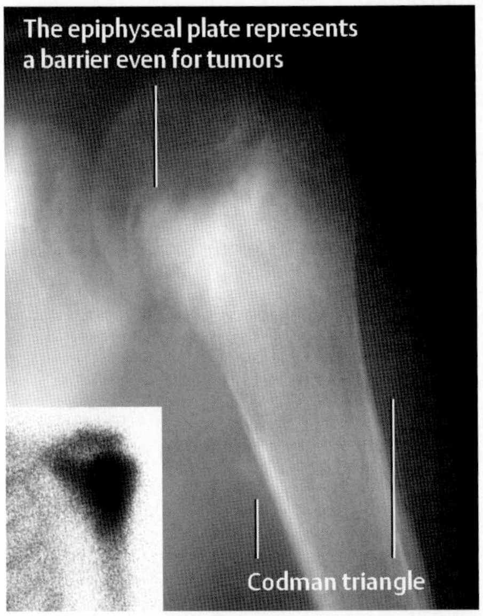

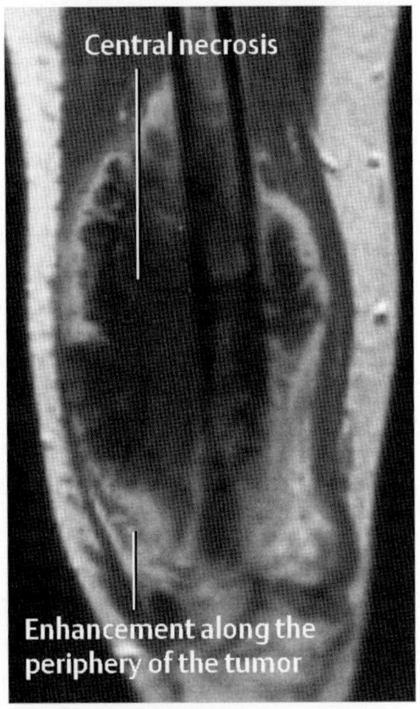

Far left:
Fig. 3.**8** Predominately osteoblastic osteosarcoma.

Near left:
Fig. 3.**9** MRI of an osteosarcoma.

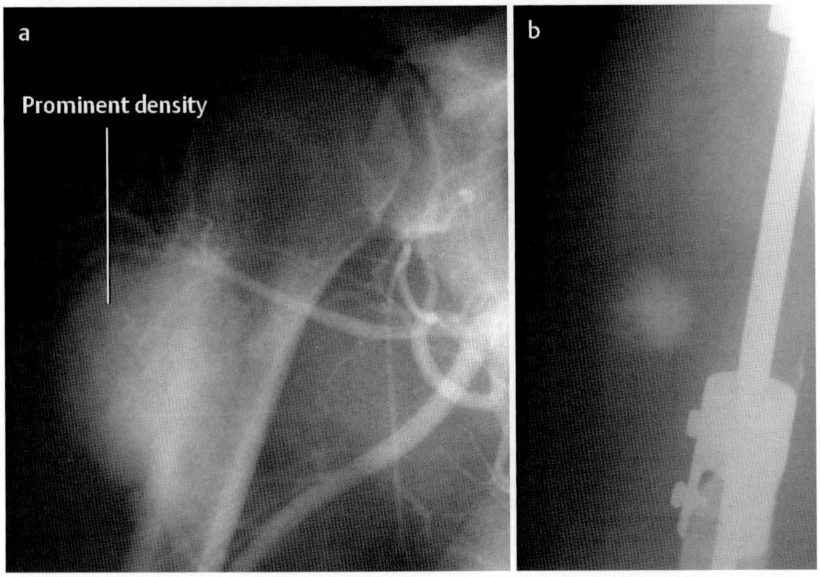

Fig. 3.**10**
- **a** Parosteal osteosarcoma (frame from an angiographic series).
- **b** Local soft-tissue metastasis after tumor excision and insertion of a prosthesis.

Cartilage-Producing Tumors

Osteochondroma

Synonym: Cartilaginous exostosis

■ This is a very common benign osseous neoplasm that extends from the underlying bone. ■

PATH The cartilaginous center ossifies with the outer layer, remaining as a non-ossified layer of cartilage of varying thickness forming a cartilaginous cap. Because of its self-limiting growth, it is more appropriately characterized as a tumorlike lesion.

CLINIC No pain, usually an incidental finding, unless there is mechanical pressure on a neurovascular bundle or formation of a 'pseudobursa'.
Age: First to third decade of life.
Location: Metaphyseal region of the tubular bones.
Therapy: None, or simple excision, depending on clinical symptoms and location.

X-RAY The osteochondroma can be pedunculated, arising by a stalk from the cortex (cauliflower-type, Fig. 3.**11**), or sessile, with its broad base incorporated in the bone and associated with loss of a discernible cortex (see 'localized bone thickening', Fig. 3.**12**). Large osteochondromas can deform the bone (Fig. 3.**13**). Calcifications (linear, geographic, coarse, irregular) are always detectable, unless the osseous chondroma has matured and is completely incorporated into the osseous structures (Fig. 3.**14**).
- It is clearly demarcated from the surrounding soft tissues, but frequently irregularly outlined.
- No sclerotic margins.

CT To delineate the radiographic findings without superimposed structures and, especially in the central skeleton, to determine the site of origin to better advantage (superior to MRI). The delineation of the cartilaginous cap is poor.

SONO The cartilaginous cap of superficial osteochondromas can be superbly visualized.

MRI Like CT, it confirms the diagnosis by showing the continuity of the bone marrow with the marrow-filled internal space of the mature osteochondroma. MRI is the optimal method for determining the thickness of the cartilaginous cap (Fig. 3.**16**).

! A cartilaginous cap measuring more than 2 cm suggests sarcomatous degeneration. Sarcomatous degeneration can be expected to occur in approximately 1% of solitary and 10–15% of multiple osteochondromas.
The multiple osteochondromas associated with multiple hereditary exostosis, an autosomal dominant disorder, are more often sessile than pedunculated.

DD **Pedunculated cauliflower exostoses:**
- **parosteal osteosarcoma:** broader base, thick matrix,
- **juxtacortical (parosteal) osteoma:** homogeneous osseous matrix (Fig. 3.**15**),
- **chondrosarcoma:** thicker cartilaginous cap!
- **myositis ossificans:** ossification in the soft tissues that is separated from the cortex. This is best shown by CT or MRI.

Broad-based exostoses:
- **fibrous dysplasia:** no fatty marrow within the lesion.

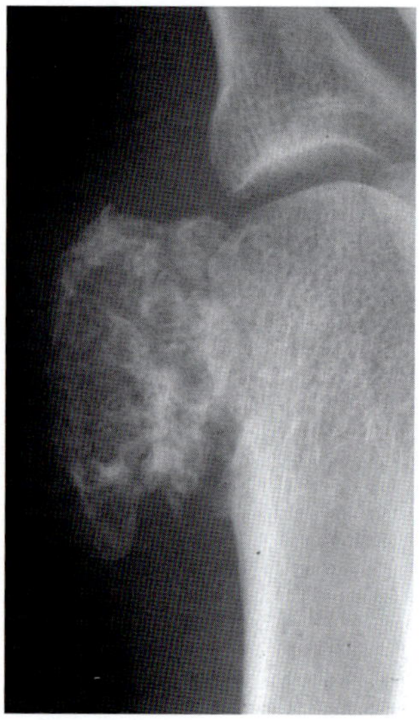

Fig. 3.**11** Osteochondroma. Cauliflower exostosis arising from the first metatarsal bone.

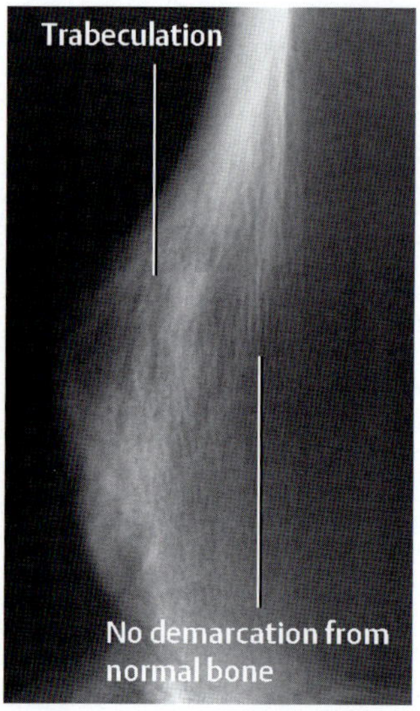

Fig. 3.**12** Osteochondroma. Broad-based excrescence arising from the underlying bone. The cartilage matrix has been transformed into trabecular bone through ossification.

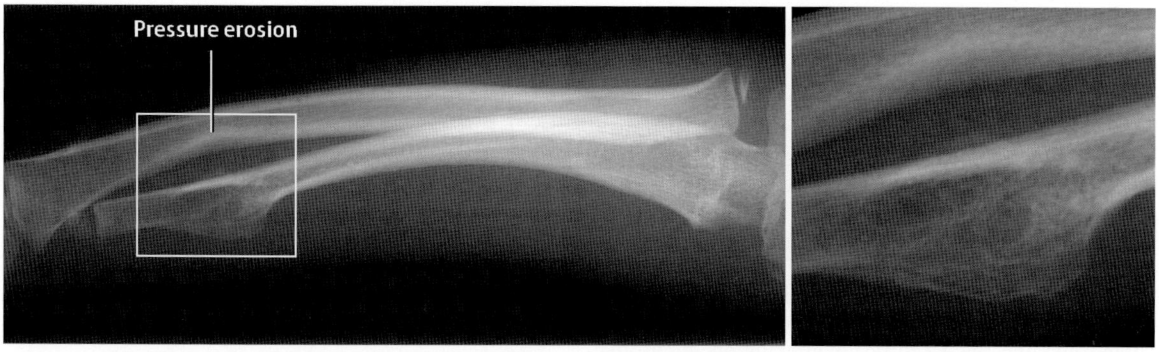

Fig. 3.**13** Osteochondroma of the ulna. Its broad base is incorporated into the shaft. The cartilage cap (not visible) is only indirectly visualized as a pressure erosion on the radius. There is also an ulnar minus variant and curvature deformity of the ulna.

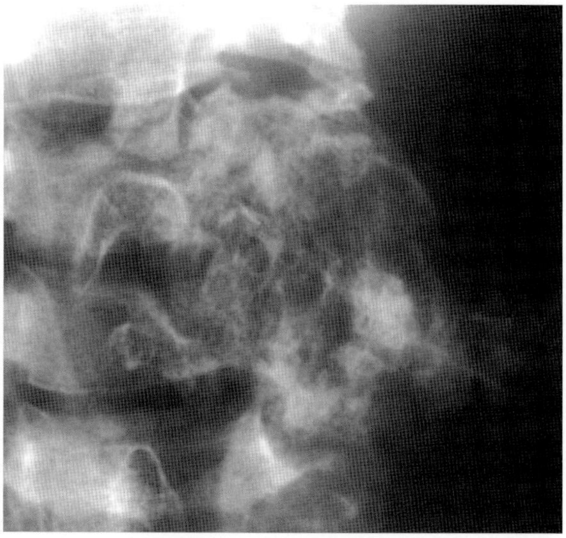

Fig. 3.**14** Osteochondroma of the cervical spine. The point of origin of the tumor can no longer be determined. Coarsened trabecular pattern, stippled calcifications, and slow expansile growth permit the diagnosis.

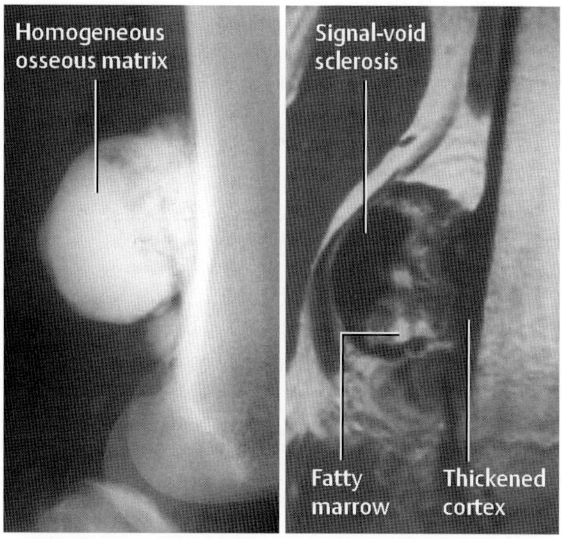

Fig. 3.**15** Parosteal **osteoma**. It can be differentiated from an **osteochondroma** by the underlying cortex. The fatty marrow within the internal tumor space is noteworthy (MRI: T1-weighted image).

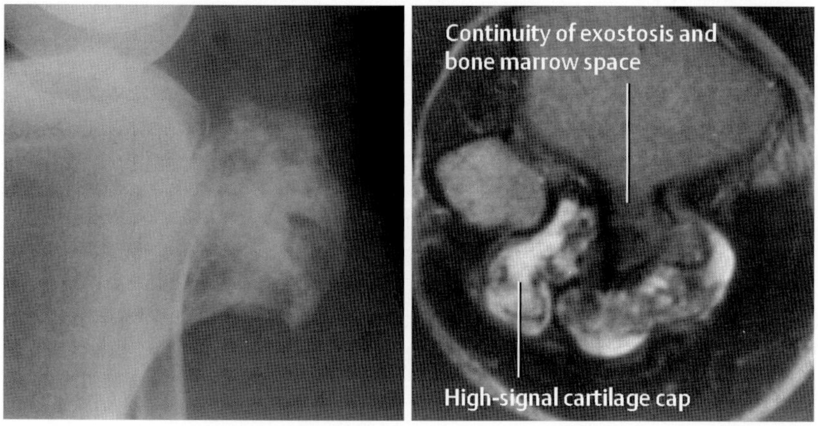

Fig. 3.**16** Osteochondroma with coarsened trabeculation (compare with Fig. 3.**15**). The exostosis is well demarcated from the soft tissues. Only MRI (T2-weighted image) shows the entire 1 cm thick bright cartilage cap. Notice that the cortex and osteochondroma are directly connected.

Enchondroma

Synonym: Chondroma

This is a benign cartilage-forming tumor, which may, in certain instances, be difficult to differentiate histologically from a low-grade chondrosarcoma.

PATH The tumor consists of mature cartilage. A distinction can be made between the central enchondroma and the eccentrically growing enchondroma with cortical destruction and formation of a 'subperiosteal enchondroma'.

CLINIC **No** pain (a feature distinguishing it from chondrosarcoma).
Age: Usually discovered before age 40 years.
Location: All bones with enchondral ossification can be affected. The tumor has a predilection for the tubular bones of the hands and feet. In the long bones, the enchondroma is characteristically located in the metadiaphyseal region.
Therapy: Lesions of the tubular bones should be left alone. Curettage should pe performed only if the lesion is painful or if it is located in the axial skeleton.

X-RAY Round or ovoid radiolucencies, often with a scalloped border, or a lesion with a matrix of mixed coarse, ringlike, or confluent calcifications. A sclerotic margin is not always detectable. The lesion may thin and scallop the cortex because of endosteal erosion. Periosteal reaction and bone expansion are possible (Figs. 3.**17**, 3.**18**).

CT Superior visualization of the calcifications shows the same diagnostic information as that of conventional radiography and demonstrates calcification to better advantage.

MRI Hypointense signal on T1-weighted images. The signal intensity on T2-weighted images depends on the degree of calcification. Noncalcified enchondromas can be so bright that the differentiation from a cyst can be difficult. IV administration of contrast medium can be helpful by disclosing the typical image of a lobulated lesion with septation (Fig. 3.**19**).

DD **Hands and feet:**
- **Giant cell tumor** of the tendon sheath (soft-tissue tumor with extrinsic bone erosion).
- **Aneurysmal bone cyst, juvenile bone cyst** (MRI can be helpful in the differentiation).

Other locations:
- **Bone infarct:** The calcifications are more peripheral than central ('encasing the lesion'). MRI may be helpful in some cases.
- **Chondrosarcoma:** A diagnostic dilemma! (See chondrosarcoma). Differentiation from a low-grade chondrosarcoma is often very difficult.

! Remember: Multiple enchondromatosis = Ollier disease. Multiple enchondromatosis with soft-tissue hemangiomas = Maffucci syndrome.

Chondroblastoma

Synonym: Codman tumor

Chondroblastoma is found almost exclusively in the epiphyses of the tubular bones of adolescents before closure of the growth plate.

PATH Benign tumor consisting of chondroblasts and numerous giant cells.

CLINIC Mild, increasing pain. Possible joint effusion.
Age: About 75% of cases occur between 10 and 25 years of age.
Location: All bones with enchondral calcification can be affected (especially the humerus). Characteristically, the lesion is centrally located within the epiphysis and may have metaphyseal extension.
Therapy: Curettage. There is a recurrence rate of 15%.

X-RAY
1. Round, solitary radiolucency 1–4 cm in diameter with sharp demarcation and sclerotic rim (Fig. 3.**20**).
2. Intralesional calcifications in about 50% of cases.
3. Osseous expansion in flat bones. This occurs less frequently in tubular bones.
4. Periosteal reaction in about 40% of cases.

CT Delineation of the radiographic changes where there is superimposition of other structures (Fig. 3.**21**).

MRI Findings similar to those of enchondroma, but the lesion may be surrounded by edema that can penetrate the cortex.

DD
1. Giant cell tumor (no calcification).
2. Chondrosarcoma (soft-tissue extension).

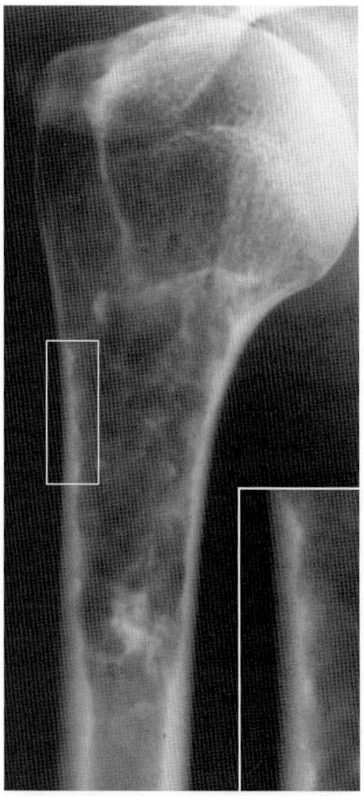

Fig. 3.**17** Classic enchondroma with scalloping of the cortex (see magnified view).

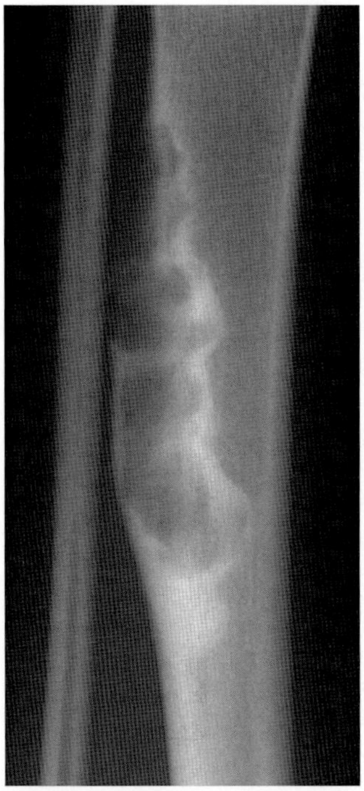

Fig. 3.**18** Periosteal chondroma. This eccentric lobulated tumor has a thick sclerotic rim which is somewhat atypical.

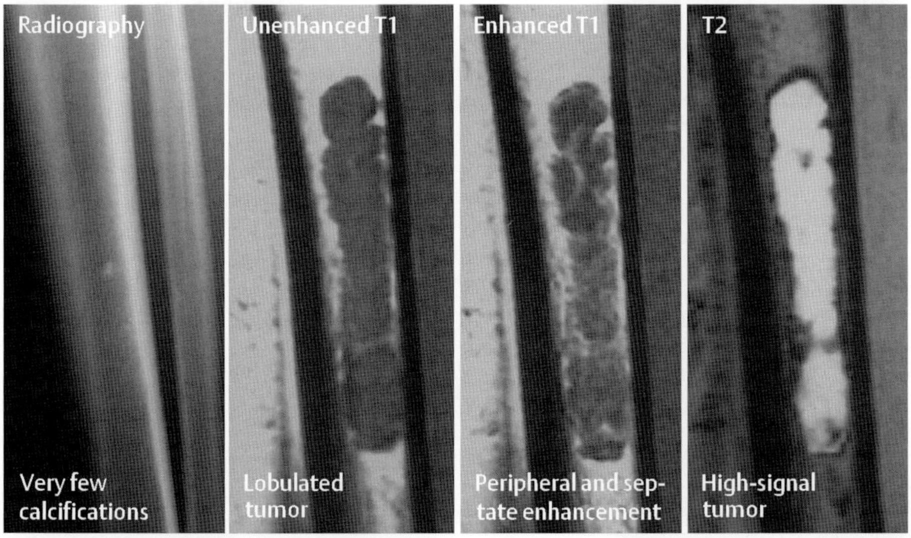

Fig. 3.**19** Enchondroma. The differentiation from a cyst on MRI can be difficult. Conventional radiography provides the definitive findings of calcifications and absent marginal sclerosis.

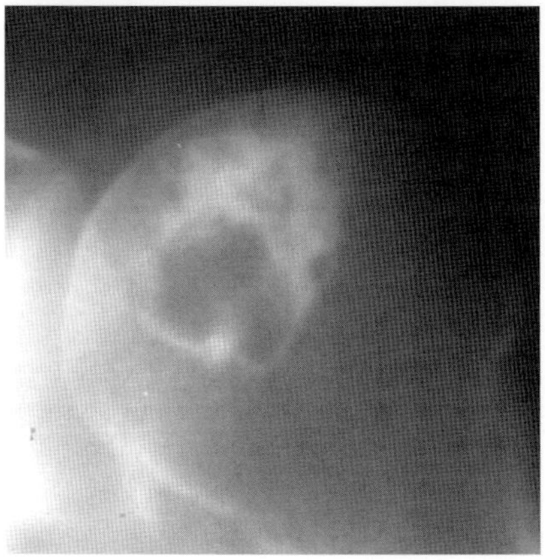

Fig. 3.**20** Chondroblastoma. Classic location and thick sclerotic rim.

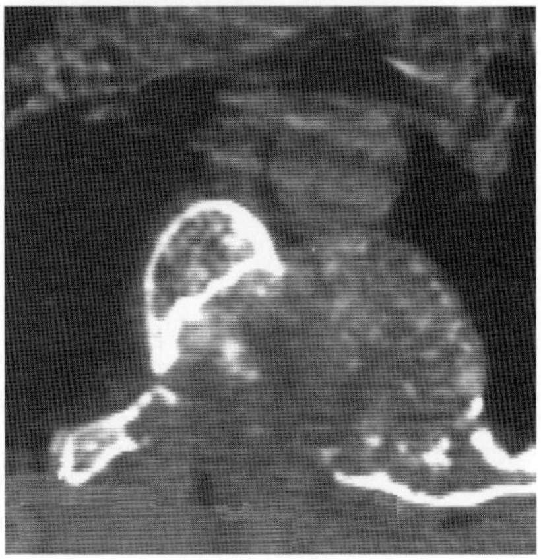

Fig. 3.**21** Chondroblastoma of the posterior vertebral arch with intralesional calcification (axial CT).

Chondromyxoid Fibroma

This is a very rare benign cartilaginous tumor, characterized by an abundance of myxoid or chondroid intracellular substance. It occurs almost exclusively in the proximal tibia and usually presents radiographically as a sharply demarcated solitary radiolucency that rarely calcifies.

Chondrosarcoma

■ This lesion is a malignant cartilage-forming tumor of adulthood. It may be primary or may occur secondarily to a pre-existing lesion. It may also arise from soft tissues. ■

PATH In contrast to the chondroma, the chondrosarcoma demonstrates marked hypercellularity and pleomorphic cells, as well as plump cells, with large nuclear or binucleated cells. Mitotic activity is infrequently seen. Histologically different grades of malignancy can be determined (low grade, intermediate grade, or high grade). A distinction is usually made between primary (without pre-existing lesion) and secondary (malignant degeneration of a pre-existing lesion, Fig. 3.**23**) chondrosarcomas. Central, eccentric, and subperiosteal chondrosarcomas are distinguished by the site of origin. Finally, subgroups such as clear-cell chondrosarcoma and undifferentiated chondrosarcoma can be identified histologically.

CLINIC The central chondrosarcoma can cause insidious, dull pain.
Age: Predominately in the fourth to sixth decade of life.
Location: All bones, as well as other structures containing cartilaginous tissue, can be affected. The most frequent location is in the metaphyseal ends of the long bones, ribs, and pelvis.
Therapy: Wide excision.

! The more centrally a cartilage-producing tumor is located, the more likely it is that it represents a chondrosarcoma. The reverse also applies (e.g., cartilaginous tumors of the hands are almost never malignant).

X-RAY **Central chondrosarcoma:**
1. Localized radiolucency, which often demonstrates a permeative pattern (Fig. 3.**22**).
2. The tumor margins may be variably well delineated or indistinctly outlined. A sclerotic margin is rare.
3. Periosteal reaction and osseous extension are often present.
4. The tumors can calcify (like enchondromas) or can be purely lytic.

Eccentric chondrosarcoma:
Radiographically, this lesion resembles an osteochondroma, but frequently has areas of permeative lytic destruction. In addition, large tumors produce destruction of cortex and periosteal reaction.

NUC In general, there is intense uptake compared to endochondromas (Fig. 3.**24**).

CT Demonstrates osseous expansion and destruction better than conventional radiography.

MRI Very helpful for assessing the cartilage cap of eccentric chondrosarcomas. Less informative for the differentiation between low-grade chondrosarcoma and enchondroma (Fig. 3.**25**).

DD The most challenging problem is the clinical, histologic, and radiographic distinction between low-grade chondrosarcoma and enchondroma. Both imaging and histology often fail here and are invariably followed by excessive or inadequate therapy. The age of the patient, location of the tumor, and pain pattern are often more relevant than the imaging findings.

! In cases that remain unclear, radiologists and pathologists with special expertise in bone pathology should be consulted.

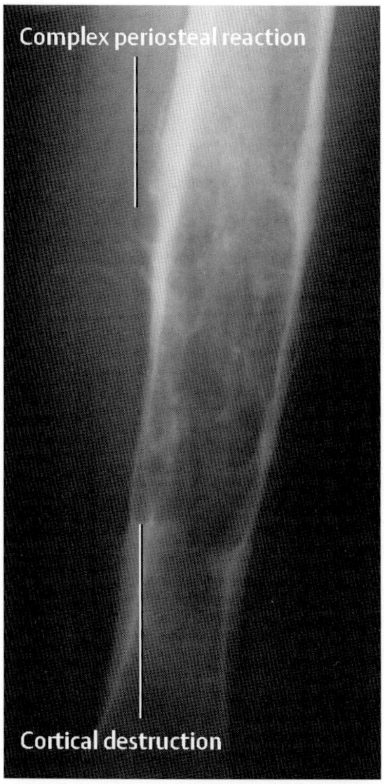

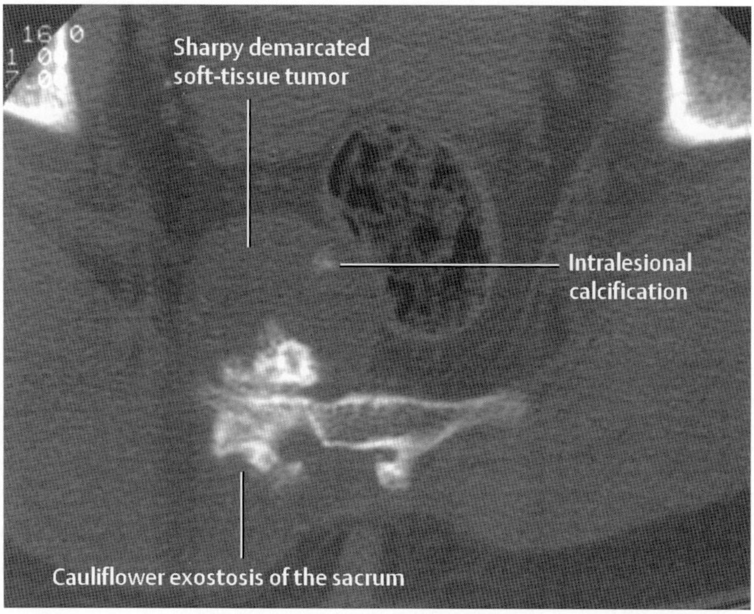

Fig. 3.**23** Secondary chondrosarcoma of the sacrum arising from a pre-existing exostosis.

Left:
Fig. 3.**22** Chondrosarcoma. The signs of malignant transformation are clearly apparent, and the cartilage matrix is only barely visible.

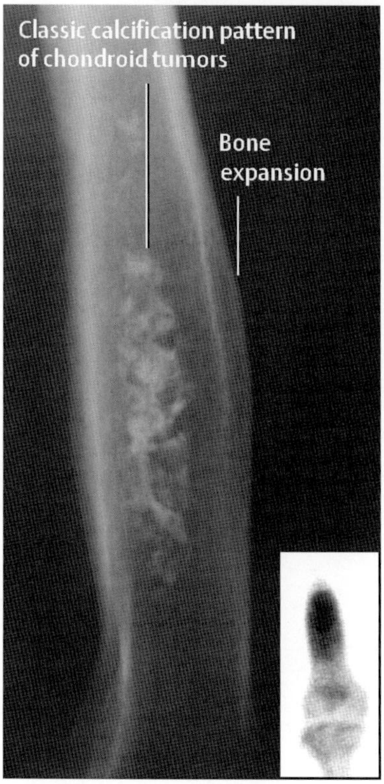

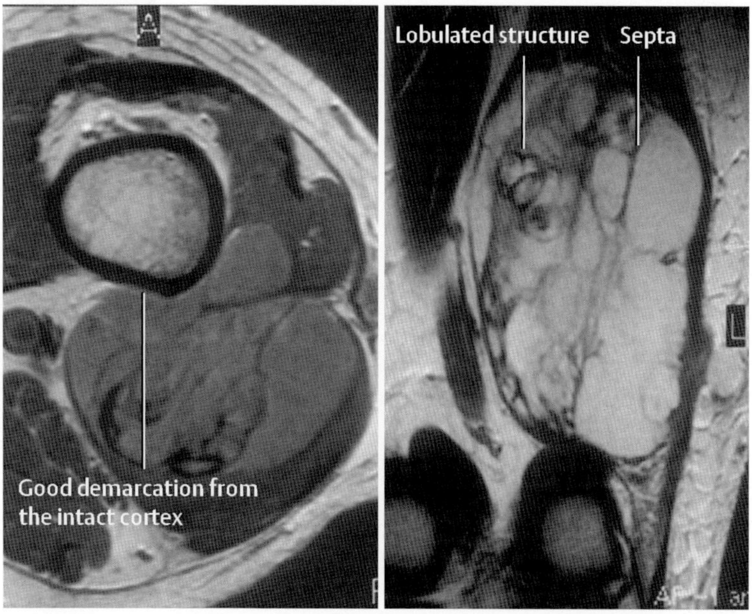

Fig. 3.**25** Chondrosarcoma of the soft tissues. MRI with proton density and T2-weighted sequences shows high signal intensity due to extensive myxoid components.

Left:
Fig. 3.**24** Chondrosarcoma Grade I. Differentiating this lesion from an enchondroma may be difficult. Bone pain and a positive bone scan (insert) support the diagnosis of chondrosarcoma.

Giant Cell Tumor

■ This bone tumor of unknown etiology is characterized by hypervascular tissue and multinucleate giant cells. It is locally aggressive and has a high recurrence rate. ■

PATH The tumor consists of giant cells that are evenly distributed throughout the tumor. Giant cells also occur in a variety of other skeletal lesions (e.g., aneurysmal bone cyst), often leading to histologic misinterpretations.

CLINIC The main complaint is local pain, increasing over months. Metastases (primarily to the lungs) can be expected in about 5% of cases.

Age: Giant cell tumor has a definite predilection for the third decade of life, when 40% of the lesions are detected. About 25% of the lesions occur in the fourth decade, and 15 to 16% of tumors occur in the second and fifth decades.

Location: Half of the giant cell tumors occur around the knee, and other common locations are the distal radial epiphysis and the proximal humeral epiphysis. Other sites are rare. Giant cell tumor is frequently extrinsically located in the metaphyseal end of the tubular bone and extends towards the epiphysis, which is almost always involved at the time of diagnosis.

Therapy: Wide resection or curettage. (**Caution:** high recurrence rate.)

X-RAY – Giant cell tumor is characterized by an eccentrically located epiphyseal lesion with osteolytic destruction and no matrix ossification.

- About half of the cases exhibit delicate or coarse septum-like internal densities.
- The lesion is usually smoothly marginated and uniform, and the zone of transition to normal tissue is relatively narrow (Figs. 3.**26**–3.**28**).
- Rapidly growing tumors can have indistinct and irregular margins and can be very aggressive (Fig. 3.**29**).
- Giant cell tumor has a tendency to grow outside the bone producing either complete cortical destruction or periosteal reaction and the formation of a neocortex (osseous shell).
- Lamellated or complex periosteal reactions rarely occur. In thin bones, the tumor frequently shows concentric rather then eccentric growth, expanding the entire bone and breaking out into the surrounding soft tissues.

CT The classic tumor lacks matrix production (Figs. 3.**27**, 3.**28**). Occasional reactive calcifications (septa) should not be mistaken for calcium-producing matrix.

MRI Classic tumor signs (hypointense signal on T1-weighted images and hyperintense signal on T2-weighted images) and strong enhancement make it difficult to establish the diagnosis of a giant cell tumor. The tumor is generally homogeneous but rarely may be heterogeneous because of necrosis and hemorrhage.

DD **Chondroblastoma:** In contrast to giant cell tumor, chondroblastoma usually has calcifications and generally exhibits a thick sclerotic margin.

Plasmacytoma/metastases: Age of the patient and additional lesions (multiple sites of giant cell tumors are extremely rare) are often the only differentiating criteria.

Aneurysmal bone cyst: As a general rule, there are no differentiating radiographic signs. MRI may be diagnostic when fluid and blood, which are characteristically observed in aneurysmal bone cysts, are detected.

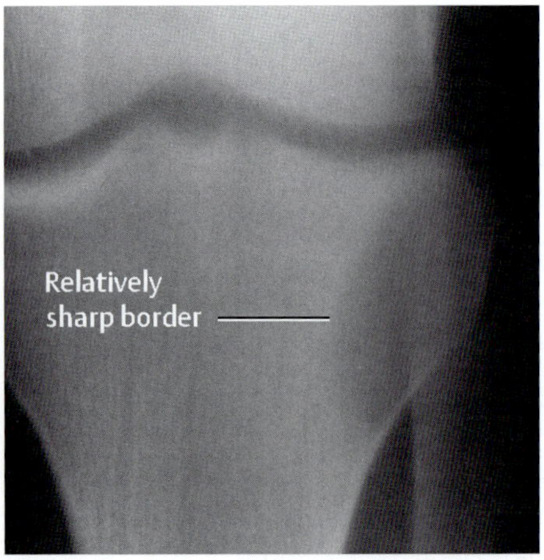

Fig. 3.**26** Giant cell tumor, early stage.

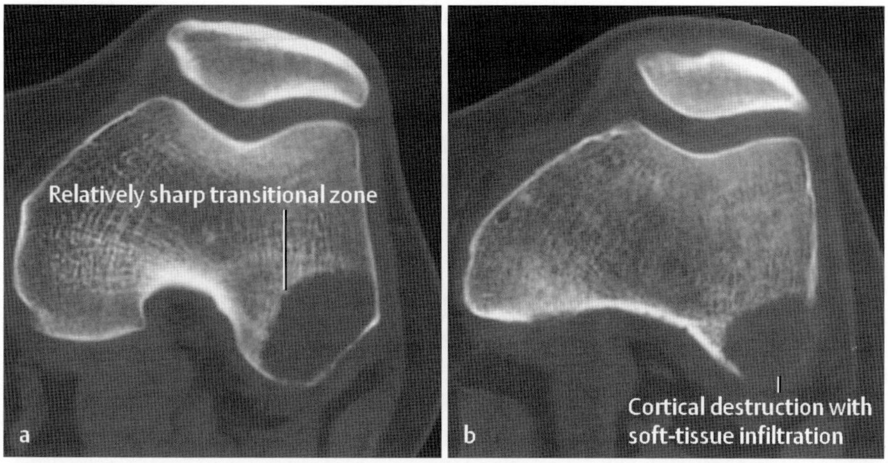

Fig. 3.**27** Giant cell tumor. Different axial CT sections from the same patient.

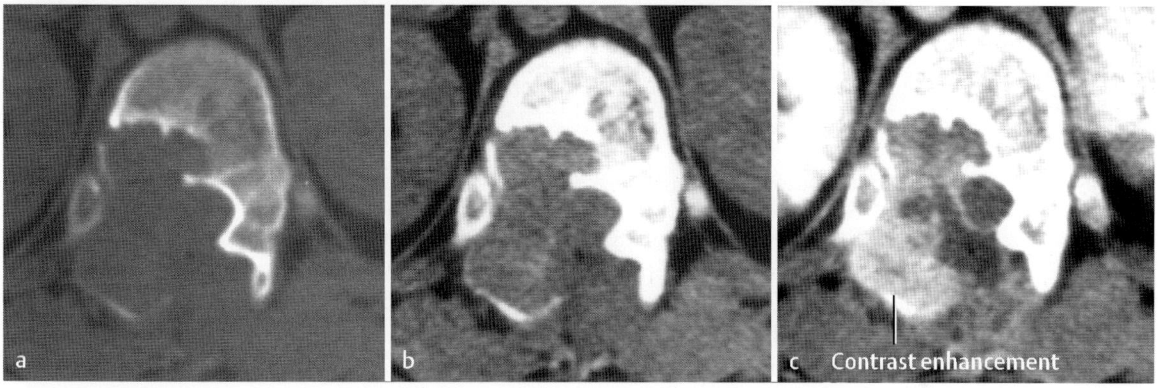

Fig. 3.**28** Giant cell tumor of the vertebral body. Axial CT with bone (**a**) and soft-tissue window (**b, c**). There is marked tumor enhancement (**c**).

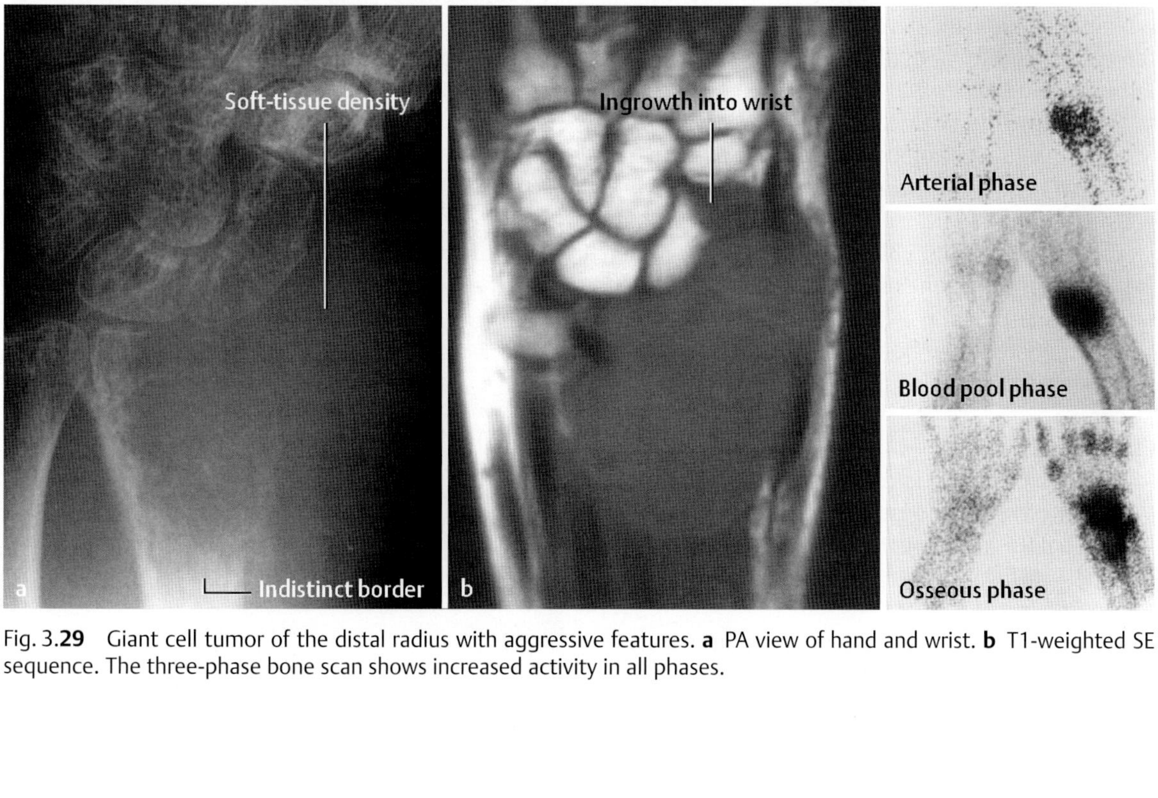

Fig. 3.**29** Giant cell tumor of the distal radius with aggressive features. **a** PA view of hand and wrist. **b** T1-weighted SE sequence. The three-phase bone scan shows increased activity in all phases.

Tumors Arising from Bone Marrow

Ewing Sarcoma

This is a highly aggressive, malignant, round-cell tumor of childhood and adolescence.

PATH It is characterized by the uniform appearance of crowded small cells with round nuclei that do not produce a matrix.

CLINIC In contrast to patients with bone tumors, patients with Ewing sarcoma can present with fever, anemia, leukocytosis, and accelerated erythrocyte sedimentation rate. Soft-tissue swelling, local pain, and erythema are also frequently encountered.

Age: Most Ewing sarcomas occur between 9 and 18 years of age.

Location: Although Ewing sarcoma can occur in any bone, about 25% of tumors occur in the femur. In the tubular bones, the lesion generally involves the metadiaphyseal region.

Therapy: Preoperative chemotherapy to reduce the tumor size, followed by resection. Postoperative chemotherapy is often necessary, especially after limb-preserving resection.

X-RAY The radiographic findings of Ewing sarcoma are quite variable, and the lesion may be misinterpreted as a benign lesion (e.g., infection or osteomyelitis). In the majority of cases, however, the aggressive nature of the tumor can be deduced from its radiographic appearance. Generally there is a large soft-tissue component to the tumor, which also helps in differentiating it from other differential diagnostic possibilities.

Tubular bones:

- Predominately permeative destruction, ranging from a solitary radiolucency with a moth-eaten appearance to multicentric osteolytic foci.
- The permeative destruction causes the cortex to appear frayed (Fig. 3.**30**).
- There is a wide zone of transition.
- Periosteal reaction with interrupted fine linear or lamellated new bone formation is frequently present and complex periosteal reaction can occur.

Flat bones:

- There is generally irregular and indistinctly demarcated osseous destruction, or the lesion may be strictly permeative with patchy sclerotic zones diffusely interposed. Osteolytic lesions rarely occur (Fig. 3.**31**).
- Strictly sclerotic Ewing sarcomas occur mainly in the flat bones and are caused by necrosis or exuberant reactive endosteal and periosteal new bone formation (Fig. 3.**32**).

NUC Most cases show intense tracer uptake. The bone scan can be used to exclude skeletal metastasis and monitor therapy.

CT CT is most effective in evaluating tumors of the axial skeleton. It confirms the absence of matrix production. However, the distinction between osseous remnants, reactive changes, and tumor matrix can be challenging.

MRI The tumor shows a signal pattern characteristic of most tumors with hypointensity on T1-weighted and hyperintensity on T2-weighted SE images and strong contrast enhancement. A large soft-tissue mass around the involved tubular bones is highly characteristic and invariably observed at the time of diagnosis (Fig. 3.**33**).

DD **Acute hematogenous osteomyelitis:** Clinical and radiographic differentiation is often impossible. However, MRI can often distinguish the edema or abscess of an osteomyelitis from the solid space-occupying Ewing sarcoma, especially after development of the sarcomatous soft-tissue mass. The enhancement pattern after administration of contrast medium enables a relatively reliable differentiation between tumor and peritumoral edema. In the rare Ewing sarcomas confined to the bone and containing a non-enhancing necrosis, differentiation can be especially difficult (Fig. 3.**34**).

Eosinophilic granuloma: If found in tubular bones, differentiation by imaging can be formidable, particularly in the presence of lamellated periosteal reaction, which can be found in both entities. A biopsy is inevitable.

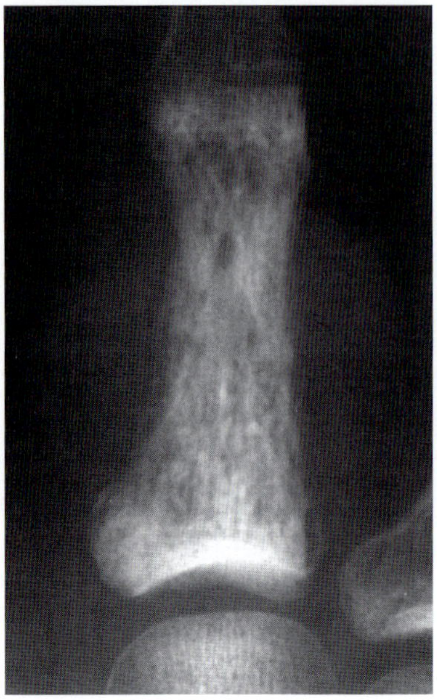

Fig. 3.**30** Ewing sarcoma of the phalanx with predominately permeative destruction but only mild sclerosis. Note the large soft-tissue mass.

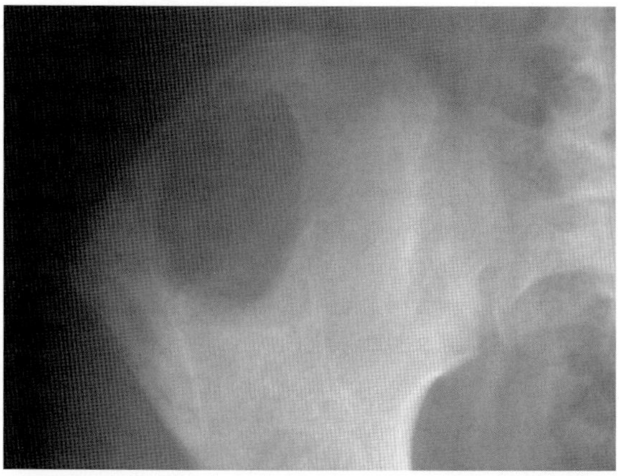

Fig. 3.**31** Ewing sarcoma of the ilium manifested as a predominately osteolytic lesion with a relatively sharp border. This appearance is unusual.

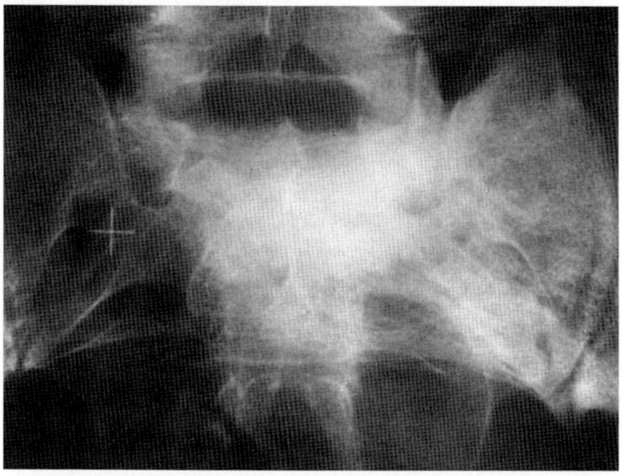

Fig. 3.**32** Sclerotic type of Ewing sarcoma. A more typical presentation in the pelvis.

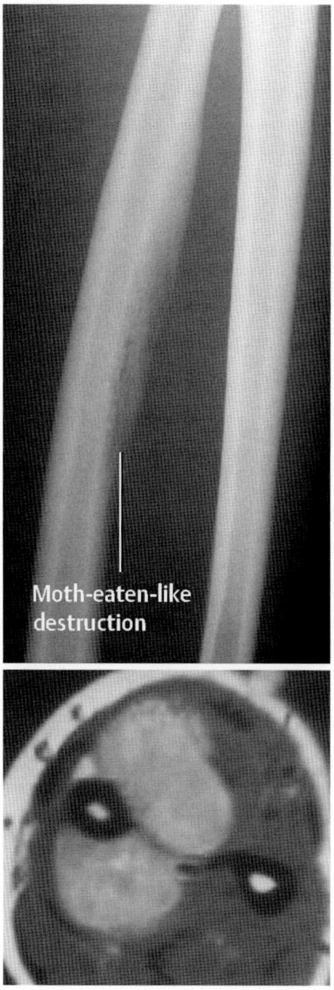

Fig. 3.**33** Ewing sarcoma with moth-eaten cortical destruction in the distal third of the ulna of a 33-year-old woman. MRI (T1-weighted SE sequence after enhancement) shows the large soft-tissue component of the tumor.

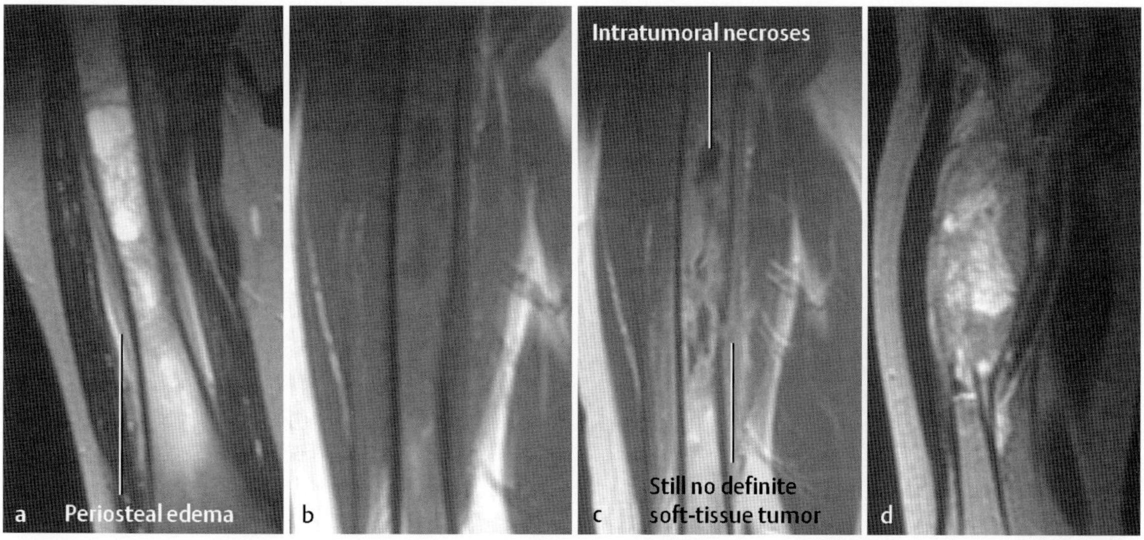

Fig. 3.**34** Ewing sarcoma of the femur. **a–c** Initial MRI: **a** T2-weighted SE sequence. **b, c** T1-weighted SE sequence before (**b**) and after (**c**) administration of contrast medium. The differentiation from an osteomyelitis was difficult in this case. The medullary extension of the findings and the presence of only minor periosteal edema is atypical of osteomyelitis. The enhanced image shows evidence of necrosis. **d** Follow-up examination after 2 months (T2-weighted image) reveals development of a large soft-tissue component.

Vascular Tumors

Hemangiomas

The hemangioma is the most frequent osseous tumor and represents a benign tumorlike lesion consisting of capillary and cavernous blood vessels. It is found primarily in the spine and is almost always asymptomatic. Its etiology is unknown.

PATH It is now generally accepted that this is a tumorlike lesion rather than a genuine tumor. It has traditionally been categorized as a tumor because a small subgroup found in the vertebral bodies has a propensity to grow with an evolving soft-tissue component. In this case the term 'tumor' is justified.

Hemangiomas are distinguished by their structure: capillary hemangiomas consist of lobules of capillaries with several large supplying vessels, whereas cavernous hemangiomas are composed of numerous thin-walled cavities. Hemangiomas characteristically contain a relatively large amount of fat.

CLINIC Generally asymptomatic. In some vertebral hemangiomas, neurological symptoms can develop because of the close proximity of the spinal canal.
Age: Predominately in the second to fifth decades of life, but any age group may be affected.
Location: Hemangiomas have a predilection for the vertebral bodies (more than 70%) and in this site may be multiple. Other sites are the pelvis, calvaria, mandible, ribs, and long tubular bones.
Therapy: No therapy for asymptomatic patients. In cases with cord compression, resection is indicated, conceivably following preoperative embolization. Radiotherapy of hemangiomas is no longer recommended.

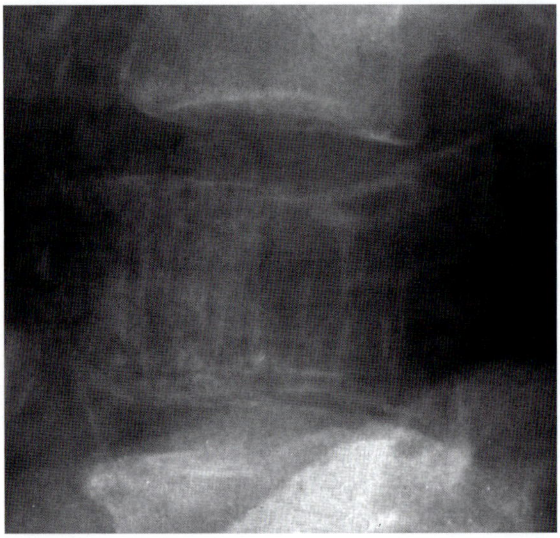

Fig. 3.**35** Typical vertebral hemangioma. Note the vertical striations (corduroy appearance).

X-RAY
- Vertebral hemangiomas can cause pressure on the horizontal trabecula and a compensatory enforcement of the vertical trabecula, resulting in a coarse vertical trabecular pattern (corduroy appearance) (Figs. 3.**35**, 3.**39**).
- In the vertebral bodies, hemangiomas may also show diffusely distributed coarse osteosclerotic areas (Fig. 3.**37**).
- Hemangiomas in flat bones appear radiographically as round, sharply demarcated, osteolytic lesions surrounded by a thin sclerotic rim (Fig. 3.**36**). There may be internal striation. Tangential views may show a complex periosteal reaction (sunburst), caused by the internal structures seen on the orthogonal view.
- In tubular bones, hemangiomas may also present as sharply demarcated osteolytic foci, partially surrounded by a sclerotic rim. In this site periosteal reaction and osseous expansion are rare.
- Soft-tissue hemangiomas can erode adjacent bones.

CT Hemangiomas are frequently incidental findings in examinations performed for other reasons. The entire vertebral body or portions of it show a honeycomb or patchy sclerotic appearance. Density measurements can detect fatty tissues in selected areas, and this finding is pathognomonic. In rare cases (less than 5%), the hemangioma expands paravertebrally and causes a soft-tissue tumor (Fig. 3.**38a**).

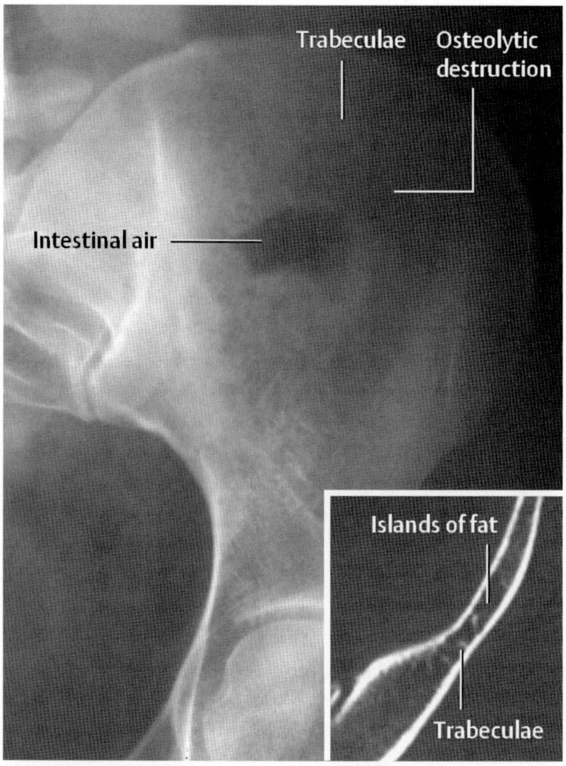

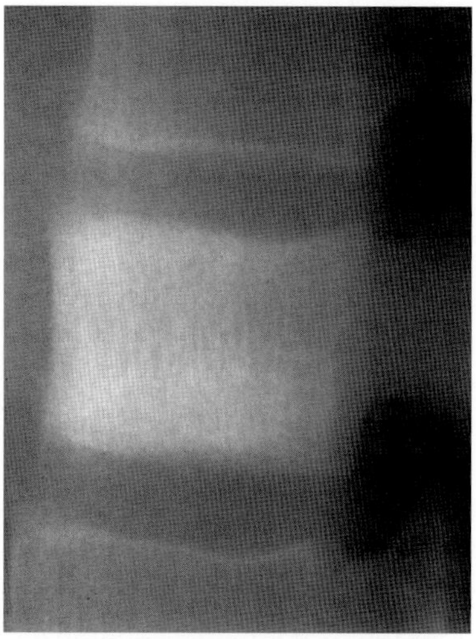

Fig. 3.**37** Osteosclerotic vertebral hemangioma in the lumbar spine.

Left:
Fig. 3.**36** Lytic lesion with striations caused by a hemangioma in the ilium.

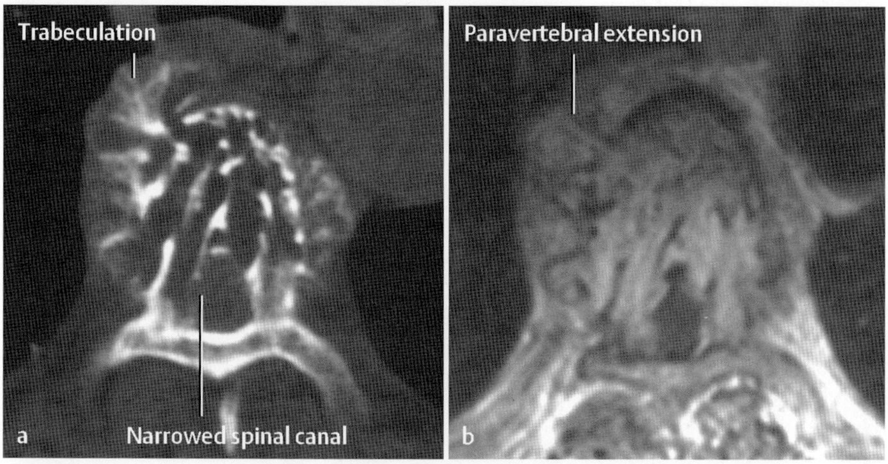

Fig. 3.**38** Hemangioma with paravertebral extension.
a axial CT,
b T1-weighted SE sequence.

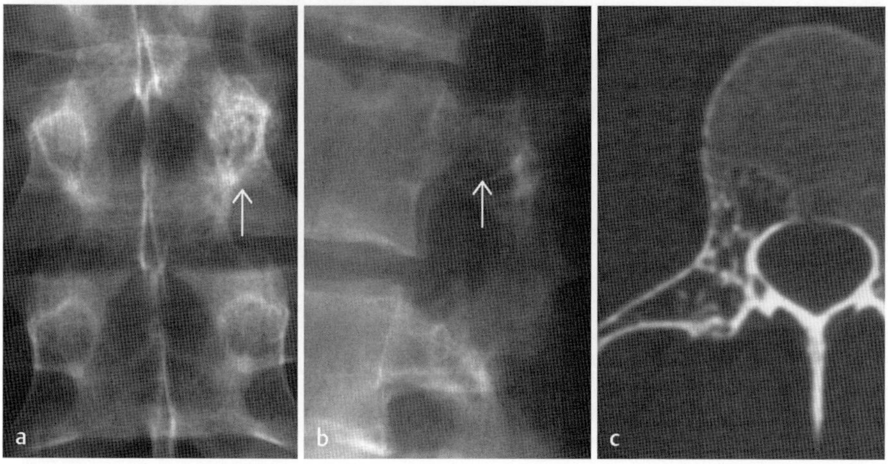

Fig. 3.**39** Hemangioma of the vertebral arch. It should be noted that the honeycomb pattern is already visible on the conventional radiographs.

MRI Frequently an incidental finding. MRI shows a characteristic signal pattern of high signal intensity on T1-weighted and T2-weighted SE images (caused by the fatty component, Fig. 3.**38b**). Classic hemangiomas have minute stroma and barely enhance. The vascularity is more pronounced in hemangiomas with a soft-tissue component.

DD **Spine:**

- **Plasmacytoma/metastases:** These tumors rarely induce radiographically visible, thickened, striated trabecula. Unclear cases can be reliably categorized with MRI or CT.
- **Paget disease:** Condensation of bone along the contours of the vertebral body and generalized enlargement of the vertebral outline indicate Paget disease. Since fatty remnants can be seen in the vertebral bodies with Paget disease, MRI and CT are only of limited value in the differential diagnosis.

Flat bones:

Fibrous dysplasia, solitary plasmocytoma, eosinophilic granuloma, and metastases. These diagnoses should be considered whenever the trabecular pattern does not follow the classic hemangiomatous manifestation. In these cases, MRI can be helpful: the absence of any soft-tissue component and, above all, the detection of a fatty component corroborate the diagnosis of a hemangioma. The differentiation from lipoma is difficult, but clinically irrelevant.

Glossary

Lymphangioma: Extremely rare finding consisting of dilated lymphatic vessels in bone, seen in children, adolescents, and young adults. Radiographically, the bone shows multiple, sharply demarcated radiolucencies.

Massive osteolysis (Gorham-Stout disease): This is an angiomatosis with regional bone loss. The bone disappears without reaction. The disease can arrest suddenly or progress to become fatal.

Cystic angiomatosis: Rare, multicentric hemangiomatosis or lymphangiomatosis, usually associated with visceral findings. It presents as regions of mottled destruction with variable sclerotic reaction.

Glomus tumor: A rare benign tumor located in the dorsal aspect of the distal phalanx of the fingers and toes. Clinically, it is very painful. The tumor is really of soft tissues, not bone in origin. Osteolytic destruction and variable sclerosis around the lesion are the major radiographic features.

Malignant vascular tumors (hemangioendothelioma, hemangiothelial sarcoma, angiosarcoma, hemangiopericytoma): Classifying the aggressiveness of the various vascular tumors of bone (and soft tissue) is controversial, inconsistent, and difficult to do by imaging alone. Of all the vascular tumors, the hemangioendothelioma has the best prognosis, despite its potential to metastasize (Figs. 3.**40**, 3.**41**). Except for hemangiopericytoma, these tumors can also be polyostotic.

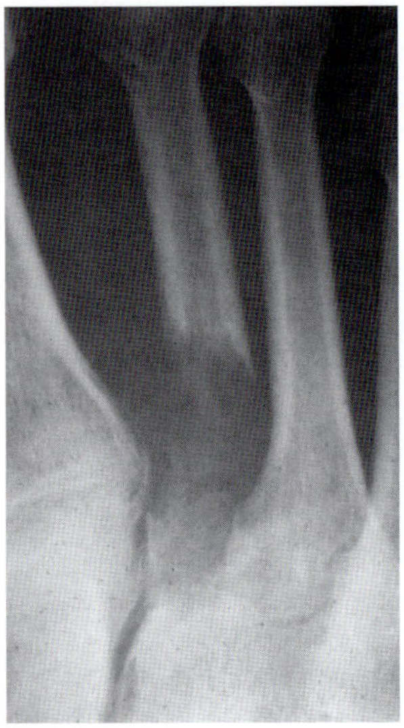

Fig. 3.**40** Hemangioendothelioma of the base of the second metatarsal.

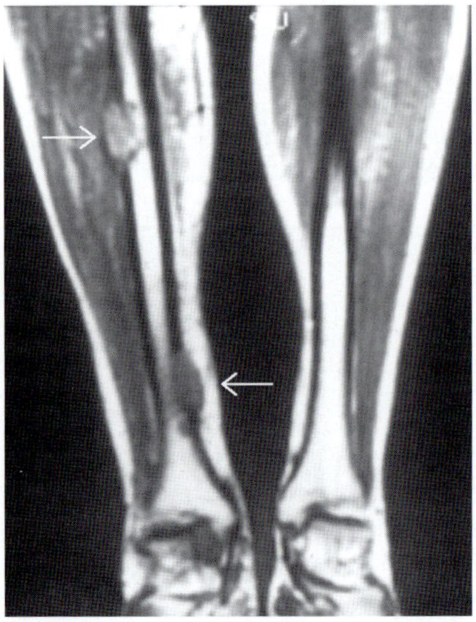

Fig. 3.**41** Multilobular hemangioendothelioma of the tibia, T2-weighted SE image.

Tumors Arising from Connective Tissue

Lipoma

■ This is a benign fatty tumor. ■

! There are three main types of lipomas:
1. Lipomas without central necrosis
2. Lipomas with central, frequently calcified necrosis
3. Lipomas with advanced necrosis and cystic transformation.

X-RAY Osteolytic destruction with a sclerotic rim and occasional bony expansion (Figs. 3.**42**, 3.**43**).

CT The lipomatous tissue can be directly visualized. Central calcifications or cysts corroborate the diagnosis.

MRI The lesion shows the expected signal pattern of fat, i.e., high signal intensity on T1-weighted and intermediate to high signal on T2-weighted images (Fig. 3.**44**). The tumor signal also suppresses with fat saturation.

DD **Bone infarcts** resemble lipomas, and some authors believe lipomas represent remote areas of bone infarction. Bone infarcts, however, frequently contain cystic, fibrous, or calcified components.

In flat bones, the differentiation between lipoma and **hemangioma** can be difficult if the hemangioma fails to show the corduroy pattern. **Cysts** can be differentiated from lipomas on MRI and CT, as they will show intralesional fluid and not fat.

Liposarcomas of bones are distinctly rare and problematic to diagnose preoperatively.

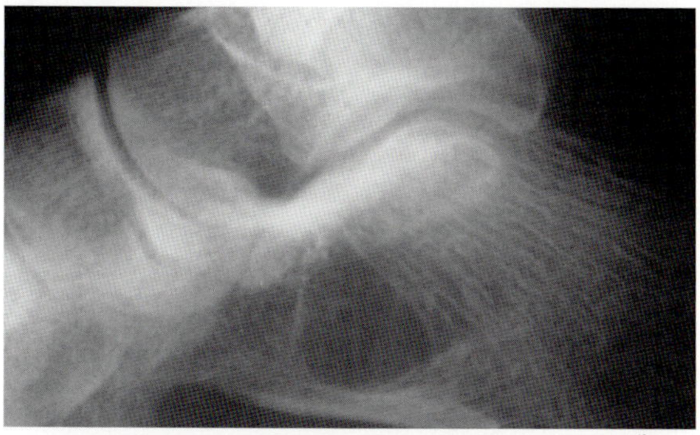

Fig. 3.**42** Lipoma of the calcaneus. Since in this case a central calcification is absent, differentiation from a cyst cannot be made radiographically. Compare with the lipoma in Fig. 8.**19** with typical dystrophic calcification.

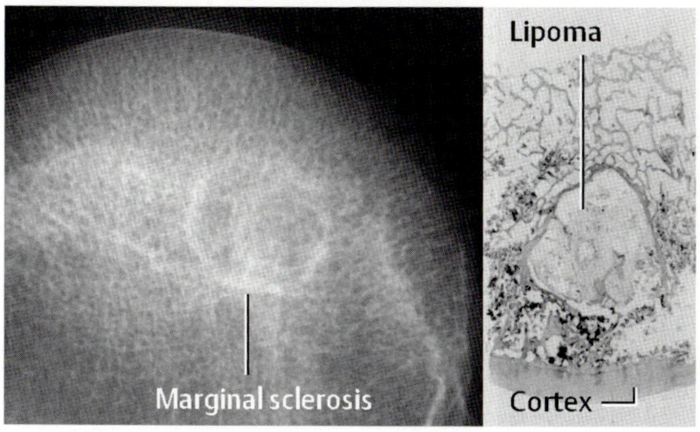

Fig. 3.**43** Specimen radiograph and corresponding histologic specimen of a lipoma in the humeral head.

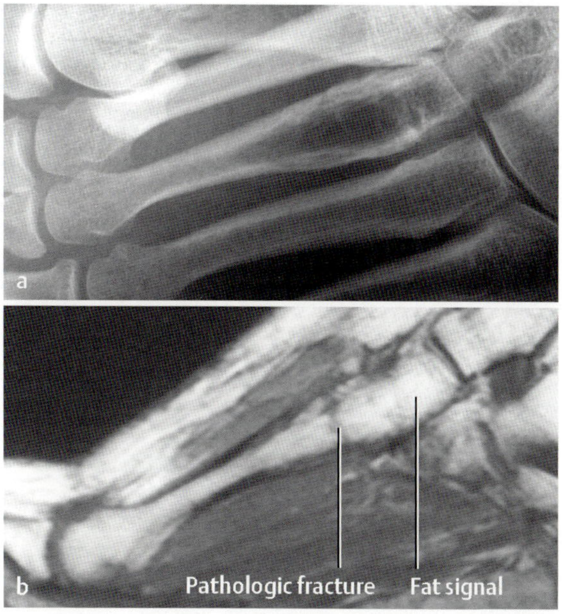

Fig. 3.**44** Lipoma of the base of the third metatarsal with pathologic fracture. MRI (T1-weighted SE sequence) confirms the diagnosis by showing pure fat within the lesion.

Glossary

Desmoplastic fibroma: This is the intraosseous equivalent of the aggressive fibromatosis (desmoid) of the soft tissues. It occurs in young adults, tends to have a locally infiltrative growth pattern, and does not metastasize. Radiographically, the lesion shows nonspecific osteolytic destruction.

Benign (fibrous) histiocytoma: This is a variant of the more frequent malignant fibrous histiocytoma. The histologic differentiation from nonossifying fibroma is difficult. Unlike nonossifying fibroma, which mainly affects the tubular bones, benign fibrous histiocytoma also involves the ribs, pelvis, and spine. Radiographically, it is characterized by a well-demarcated osteolytic destructive lesion that is partially surrounded by a sclerotic rim (Figs. 3.**45**, 3.**46**).

Malignant fibrous histiocytoma and fibrosarcoma: These malignant fibrous tumors occur mostly in the soft tissues and rarely in bones and histologically are not easily distinguished (Fig. 3.**48**, 3.**49**).

! Malignant fibrous histiocytoma can arise from a pre-existing bone infarct, and in some cases is identified initially by conventional radiography or MRI. This association should be taken into consideration when planning biopsy. Tissue should be obtained from the most aggressive-appearing area, as biopsy of the 'bone infarct' may unduly delay the correct diagnosis and appropriate therapy (Fig. 3.**47**).
The tumors are most frequently in the tubular bones and tend to be diametaphyseal in location. The classic signs of neoplastic bone destruction, especially the moth-eaten pattern, are the cardinal findings.

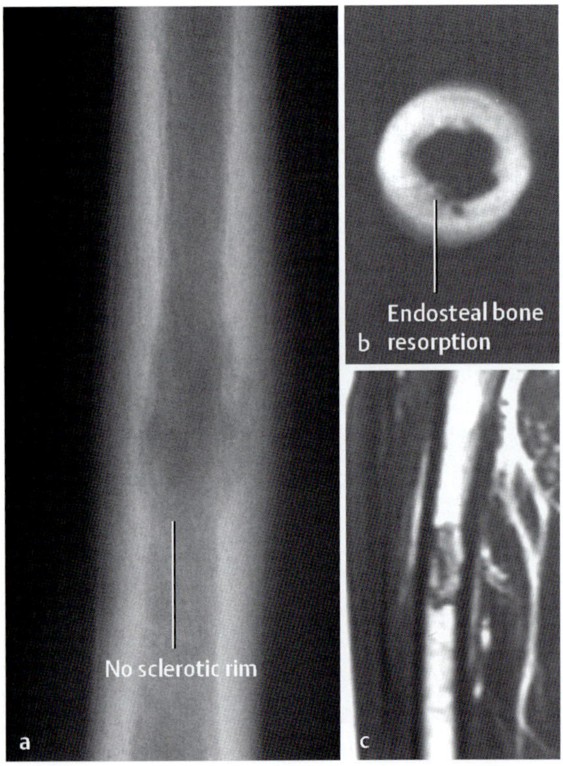

Fig. 3.**45** Benign fibrous histiocytoma in a tubular bone (femur). The axial CT section (**b**) shows endosteal resorption. **c** Corresponding coronal T2-weighted SE image.

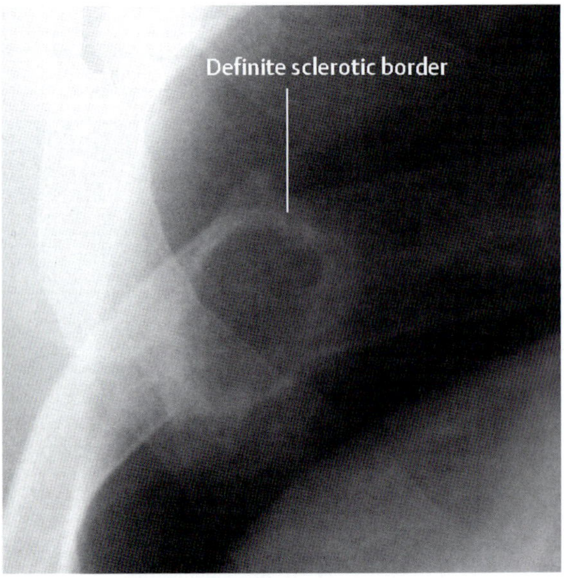

Fig. 3.**46** Benign fibrous histiocytoma in a rib.

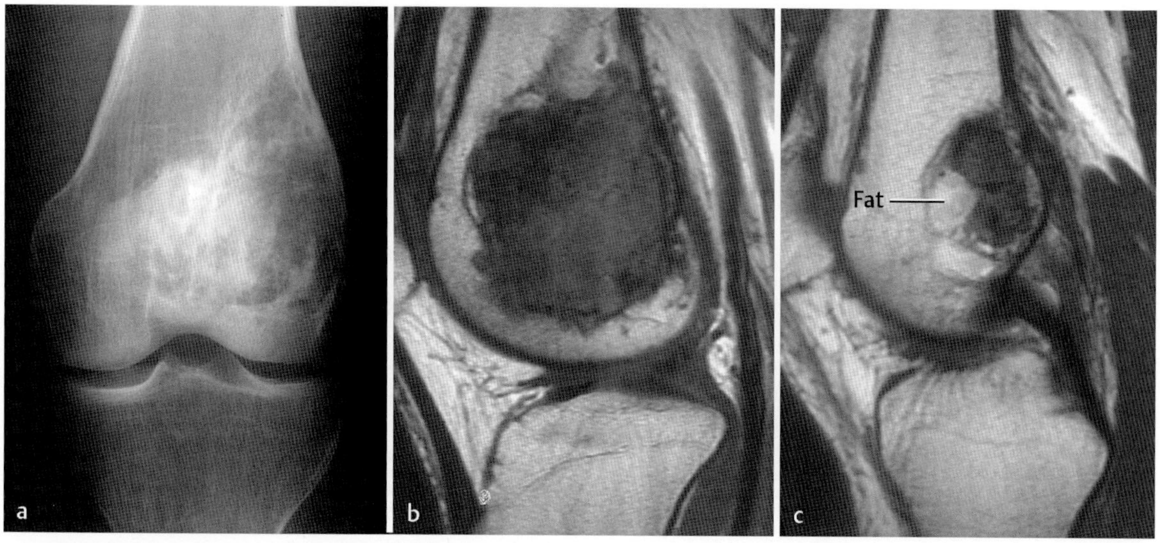

Fig. 3.**47** Malignant fibrous histiocytoma. The fat indicates likely evolution of the tumor from a bone infarct (**b, c** differential sagittal sections of T1-weighted SE sequences).

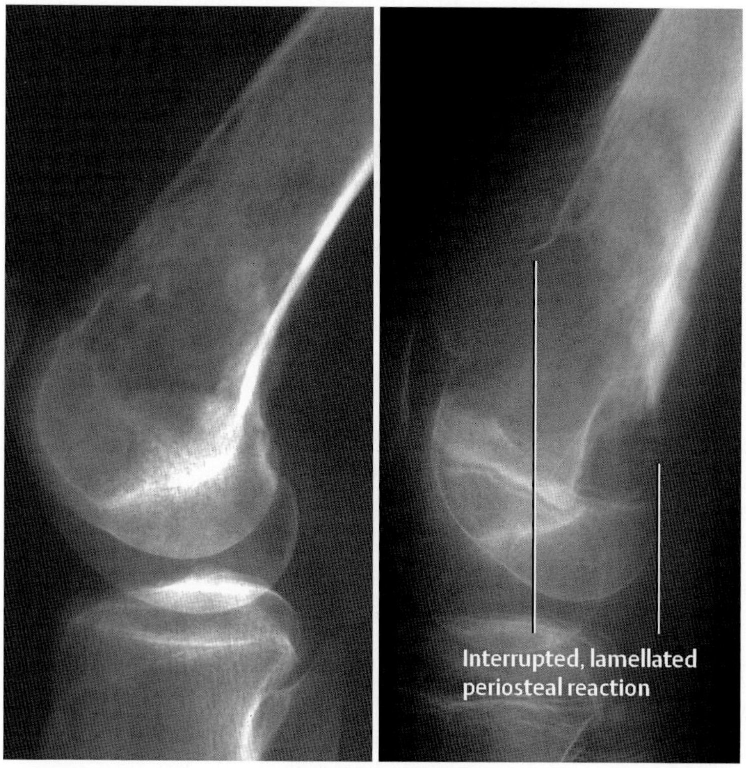

Fig. 3.**48** Malignant fibrous histiocytoma. Different patients with different degrees of bone destruction and periosteal reaction.

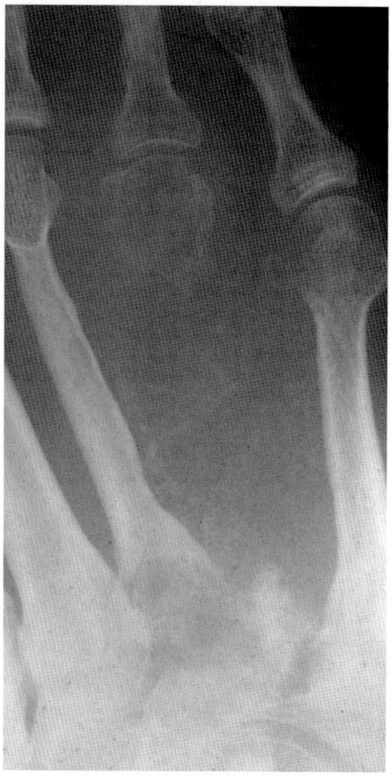

Fig. 3.**49** Fibrosarcoma with complete destruction of the fourth metatarsal.

Other Tumors

Chordoma

■ This is a malignant tumor of notochordal origin. It is observed in the axial skeleton only and has a high recurrence rate. ■

PATH The tumor has a lobular structure and usually consists of highly vacuolated (physaliphorous) cells and intercellular substance (WHO classification).

CLINIC Clinically, the symptoms of chordoma can mimic disk herniation. A cervical location with anterior tumor extension can cause dysphagia or stridor secondary to displacement of the esophagus or trachea. Sacrococcygeal chordomas are usually palpable on digital rectal examination anterior to the sacrum, and beyond a certain size can lead to dysfunction of the bladder and rectum. Intracranial chordomas cause headaches, impaired visual fields, and double vision.
Age: The tumor can occur at any age, but has a predilection for the fifth and sixth decades of life.
Location: The tumor has a predilection for the spheno-occipital and sacrococcygeal region.
Therapy: Wide resection. Frequent recurrence since the surgical goal of wide resection is not always achieved.

X-RAY An osteolytic defect, perhaps surrounded by a scalloped sclerotic rim, and a soft-tissue mass. There is no tumor matrix, but calcifications representing osseous remnants or reactive changes are often detectable.

CT Helpful for determining the size and extraosseous extent of the tumor.

MRI The method of choice because of the multiplanar display, especially since the relationship of the tumor to the spinal cord and brain stem superiorly is easily visualized on the sagittal plane (Figs. 3.**50**, 3.**51**).

DD **Sacrum:**
Giant cell tumors, chondrosarcomas, plasmocytomas, and metastases are all more common than chordomas. A distinction between these and chordoma cannot be definitely accomplished.
Clivus/Cervical Spine:
Metastases and chondrosarcoma are the important differential diagnostic considerations in this region, although there is no reliable way to differentiate them from chordoma. Craniopharyngiomas, another differential diagnosis, lacks calcifications, and this can be a helpful diagnostic clue.

Adamantinoma of the Long Tubular Bones

■ This tumor affects only the tibia and fibula and occurs in children, adolescents, and young adults. It grows relatively slowly, and individual cases can metastasize. ■

PATH This is a malignant tumor characterized by localized accumulation of epithelial cells, surrounded by spindle-cell tissue (WHO classification).

! The term 'adamantinoma' is used because the histology of this lesion is similar to adamantinomas (ameloblastomas) of the mandible. It is, however, a separate and distinct entity.

CLINIC The chief complaint of patients with adamantinoma is local pain.
Age: The peak incidence is in the second to third decades of life.
Location: More than 95% of all adamantinomas occur in the tibia and are diametaphyseal. Other locations are rare.
Therapy: Wide surgical resection.

X-RAY
- Multicentric confluent radiolucencies with marginal sclerosis (Fig. 3.**52**).
- Bubbly osteolytic destruction with a distinct rim.
- Formation of a neocortex due to solid periosteal reaction.
- Two or three disconnected osteolytic foci.

MRI Limited experience reported in the literature thus far.

DD **Fibrous dysplasia** should be considered but is rarely multicentric in any location, especially in the tibia.

Osteofibrous dysplasia is a separate entity first described by **Campanacci** and is a variant of fibrous dysplasia, see page 192. This lesion is characterized histologically by the components of both adamantinoma of the tubular bones and fibrous dysplasia. Osteofibrous dysplasia is a benign tumor with a tendency to recur. The recurrences have identical radiographic findings (Fig. 3.**53**).

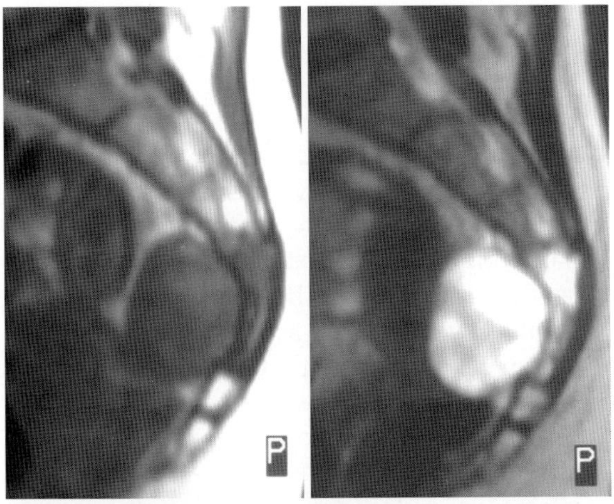

Fig. 3.**50** Sacrococcygeal chordoma, T1-weighted (**a**) and T2-weighted (**b**) image.

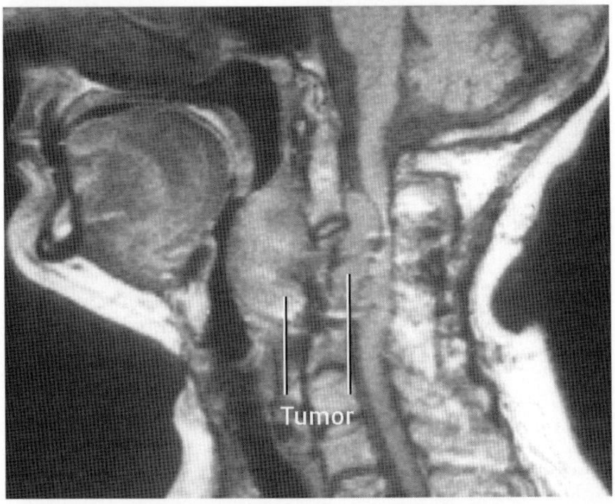

Fig. 3.**51** Recurrent chordoma of the cervical spine following surgical resection. Sagittal T1-weighted image.

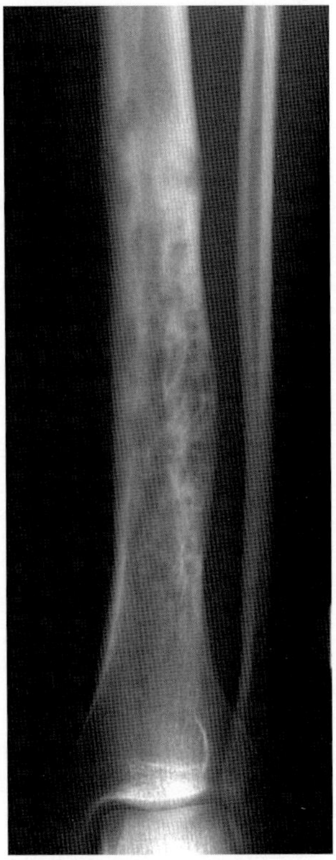

Fig. 3.**52** Adamantinoma of the tibia. Multicentric radiolucencies with reactive sclerosis.

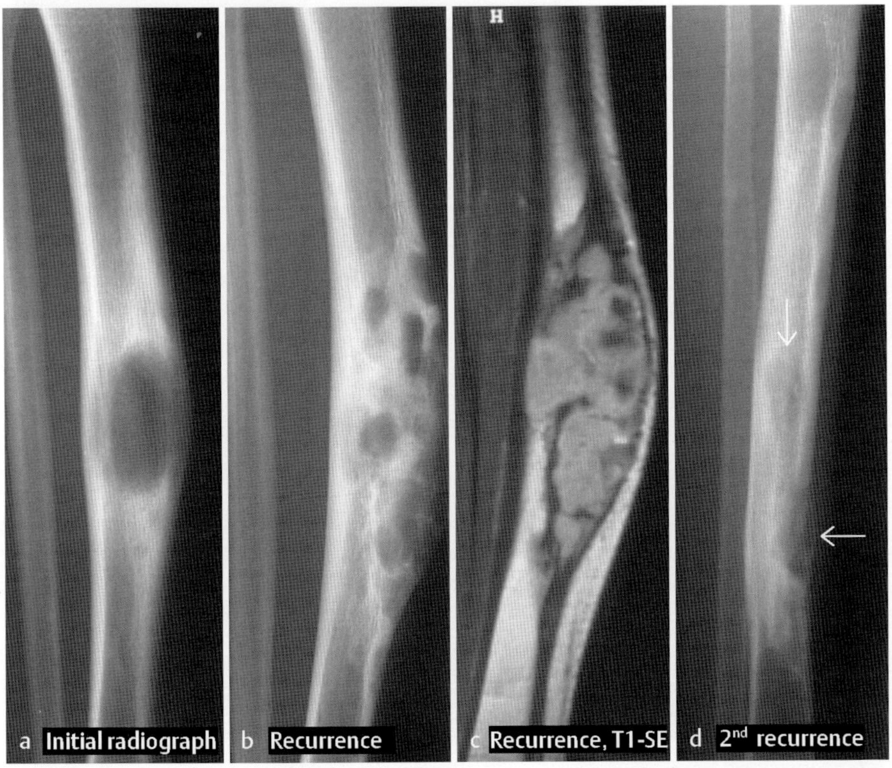

Fig. 3.**53** Osteofibrous dysplasia of Campanacci. **a** At the time of diagnosis the tumor was resected. **b, c** At 5 years there was extensive recurrence. **d** After tibial resection with maternal fibular implantation, a second tumor recurrence was seen in the transplanted bone.

Tumorlike Lesions

Osteoma, Bone Islands, Osteopoikilosis

■ Osteomas and bone islands, benign bone-forming lesions, can be monostotic or polyostotic. They are frequently incidental radiographic findings that must be distinguished from osteoblastic metastases. ■

PATH These lesions consist of well-differentiated mature osseous tissue of a predominantly lamellar structure and very slow growth (WHO classification). Most authors today regard osteomas as hamartomas and not tumors.

There are three types of osteomas:

1. **'Classic Osteoma.'** This is almost exclusively found in bones derived from condensed mesenchymal tissue, such as the calvaria, frontal sinus, and facial bones. It is observed after the second decade of life and does not cause symptoms. It represents a distinct radiologic entity, consisting of an extremely dense, sharply demarcated lesion of round, globular, or ovoid configuration (Figs. 3.**57**, 3.**58**). On the bone scan classic osteomas show no, or only faint, uptake.

! The association of classic osteomas, intestinal polyps, and soft-tissue fibromas is called Gardner syndrome.

2. **Parosteal Osteoma.** This consists of dense appositions in the tubular bones (mainly the femur) (Fig. 3.**15**) but also occurring in the facial bones. The clinically immaterial differentiation from melorheostoses can be difficult. Calcified osteochondromas can resemble parosteal osteomas, but are more heterogenous and are surrounded by a cartilaginous rim (see MRI).
3. **Medullary Osteoma** (enostoma, solitary enostosis, bone island, Figs. 3.**54** – 3.**56**). This is a lesion of polymorphic density reaching up to 3 cm in size. It frequently adapts to the anatomy of the harboring bone and exhibits a round to ovoid configuration only in the tubular bones. Radiographically, it appears as a sharply demarcated lesion that on close inspection (particularly with a magnifying glass) discloses characteristic pediculate extensions. Bone islands are observed after the second decade of life. All bones can be affected, and slow growth over several years is not uncommon. The bone scan shows only slight radionuclide uptake, and the intensity increases with increasing size of the lesions.

The critical exclusion of osteoblastic metastases, especially of osteoblastic metastases from carcinoma of the prostate, rests on correlating the clinical history, laboratory parameters, and clinical findings with the scintigraphic findings. Radiographic criteria, such as distinct versus indistinct outline of the bone lesion, are not helpful. Elevated serum alkaline phosphatase, bone tenderness, and markedly increased radionuclide accumulation generally indicate metastases.

! **Osteopoikilosis** is an inherited, autosomal dominant, osseous dysplasia consisting of multiple osteosclerotic foci. They aggregate in the epiphysis and metaphysis of the tubular bones. Patients with this condition have no symptoms from it (Fig. 3.**59**).

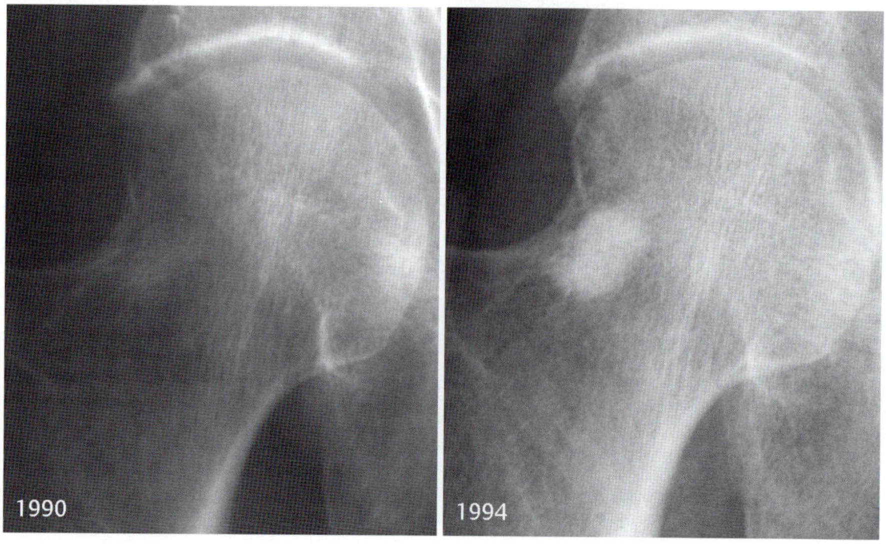

Fig. 3.**54** Evolving osteoma in the femoral neck. Four-year interval.

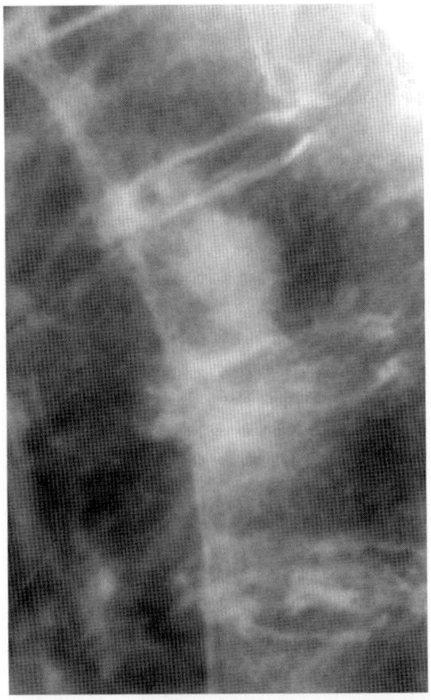

Fig. 3.55 Osteoma in a vertebral body.

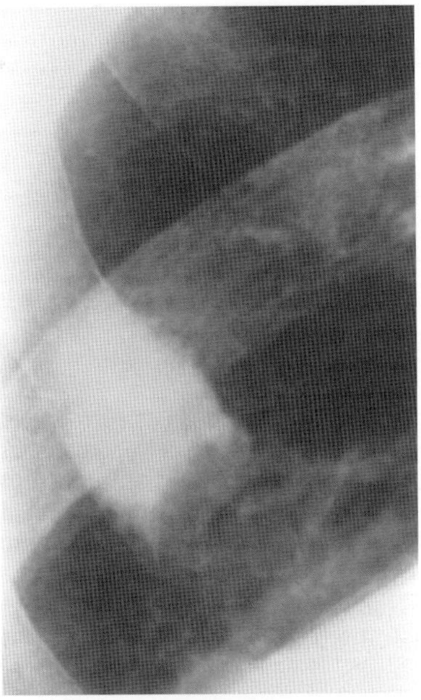

Fig. 3.56 Osteoma in an anterior rib segment with subtle osseous expansion.

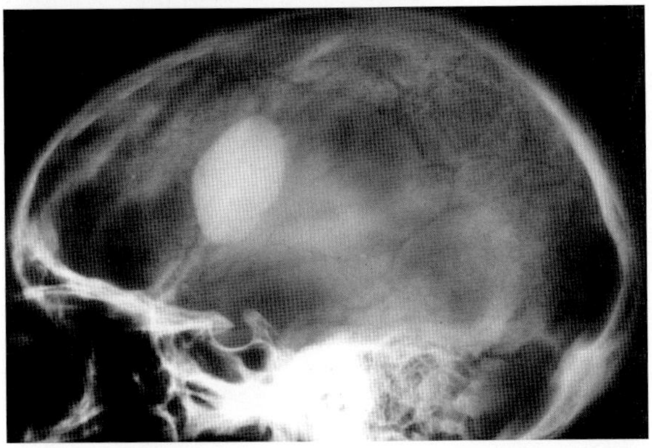

Fig. 3.57 Classic osteoma of the skull.

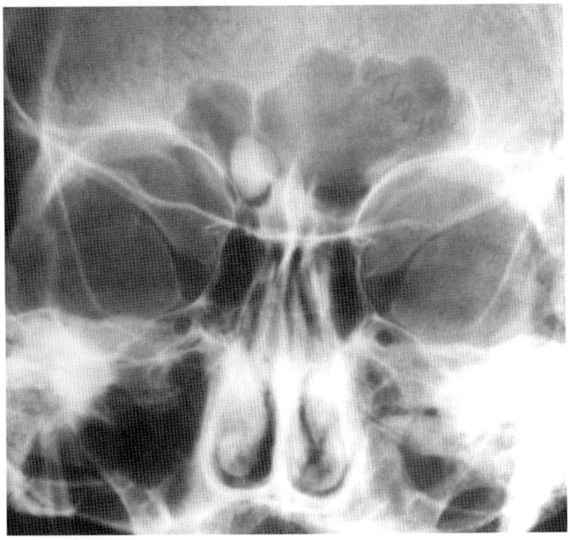

Fig. 3.58 Osteoma in the frontal sinus.

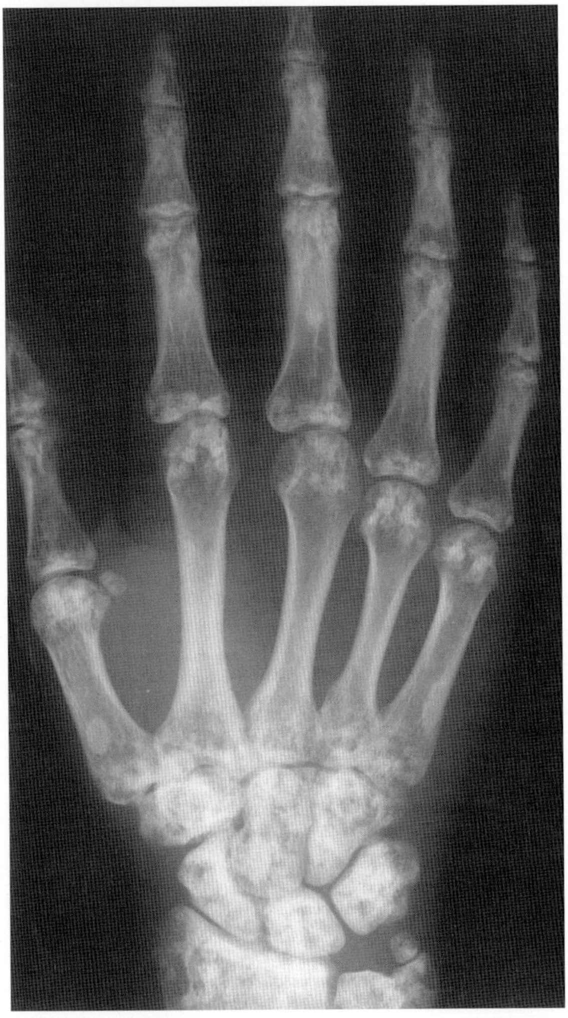

Fig. 3.59 Osteopoikilosis with characteristic epiphyseal clustering of the bone islands.

Fibrous Cortical Defect/ Nonossifying Fibroma

Synonym: fibrous metaphyseal defect.

■ This is a frequent, eccentrically located, metaphyseal lesion that generally regresses spontaneously during bone growth. The fibrous cortical defect is a classic tumorlike lesion and generally an incidental radiographic finding. ■

PATH The lesion is filled with fibroblasts surrounded by multinucleate giant cells or macrophages and connects to the overlying periosteum. The 'nonossifying fibroma' can be seen as nonphysiologic progression of a 'fibrous cortical defect,' justifying the placement of both entities under the heading 'fibrous metaphyseal defect.'

According to Ritschel, the fibrous cortical defect can be considered as disturbed development at tendinous insertions.

CLINIC Symptomless, usually incidental finding. Spontaneous fractures are very rare (Fig. 3.**64**).
Age: The nonossifying fibroma is observed in the first and second decades of life.
Location: The lesion develops in the metaphyseal region of the long tubular bones, with a predilection for the lower extremities (90%).
Therapy: None.

X-RAY
- The fibrous cortical defect is characterized by a well-demarcated, solitary ovoid radiolucency, with its long axis oriented along the cortex of the tubular bone. It is separated from the normal bone by a thin sclerotic rim and generally demarcated from the adjacent soft tissues by neocortex (Fig. 3.**60**).
- Larger lesions (up to 7 cm in longitudinal diameter) can extend into the adjacent trabecular space. These lesions develop thicker (1–2 mm) sclerotic margins, occasionally scalloped in appearance (Fig. 3.**61**).
- During regression or physiologic remodeling as part of bone growth, the lesion can become completely sclerotic (Figs. 3.**62**, 3.**63**).

CT The CT generally confirms the radiographic findings (Figs. 3.**61**, 3.**62**).

MRI MRI adds no further information of clinical relevance. This technique can occasionally show fat and cystic areas in addition to connective tissue within the lesion.

DD The classic picture is unambiguous.
In elderly patients complaining of pain at the site of the lesion and found to have a positive bone scan, the histologically similar diagnosis of a **benign fibrous histiocytoma** should be considered.

A 'large' nonossifying fibroma might resemble an aneurysmal bone cyst in selected cases (differentiation by fluid levels detected on MRI).

Glossary

The nonossifying fibroma is the counterpart of the **ossifying fibroma.** The latter is a benign bone tumor found in the facial bones and rarely in the tibia and fibula. The tumor exhibits an osseous matrix or ground glass phenomenon.

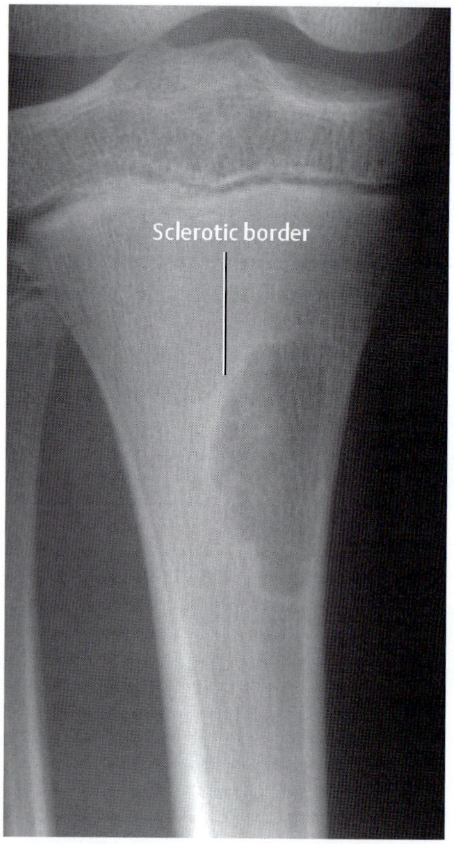

Fig. 3.**60** Typical fibrous cortical defect in the tibia of an 11-year-old boy.

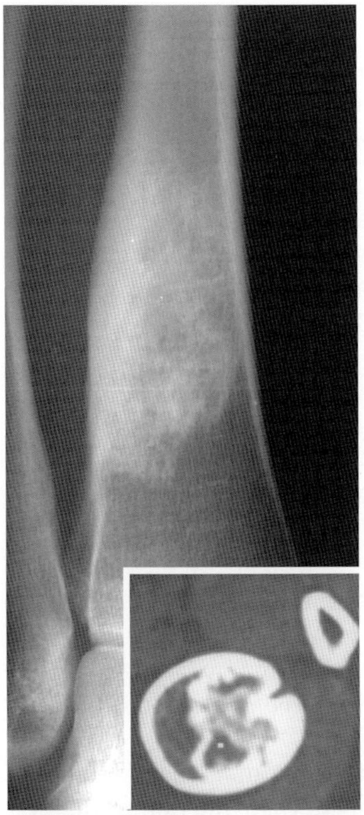

Fig. 3.**61** 23-year-old woman with nonossifying fibroma of the distal tibia. Note thick periosteal reaction and sclerosis. CT confirms the strong **marginal** sclerosis.

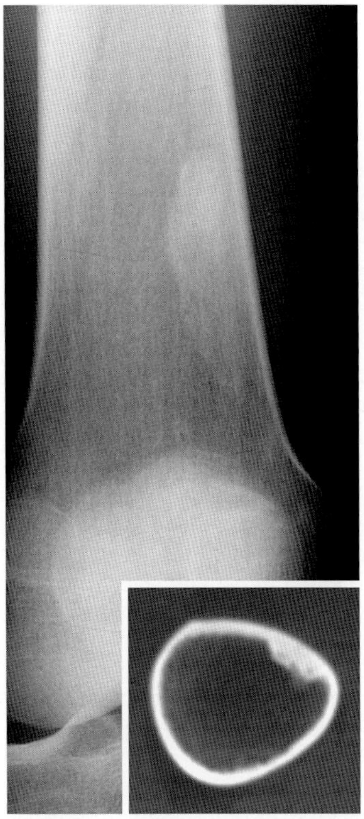

Fig. 3.**62** Fibrous cortical defect in the femur of a 22-year-old man. Note the different extent of this lesion compared to Fig. 3.**61**.

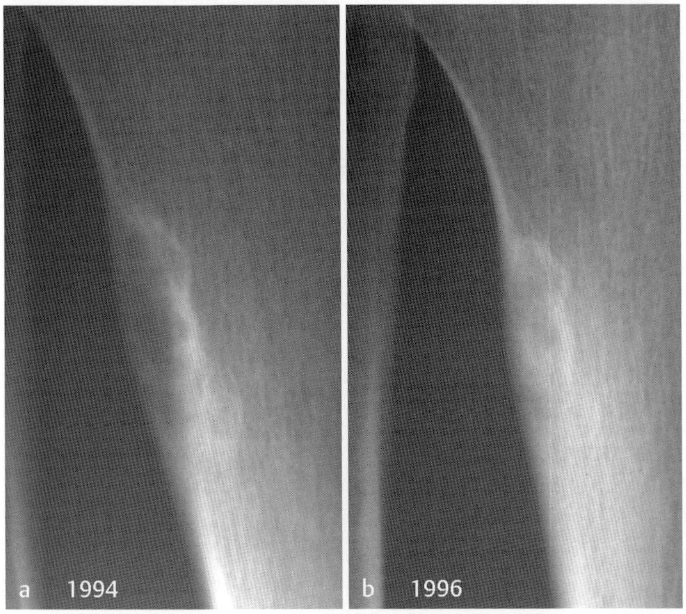

Fig. 3.**63** Spontaneous regression of a fibrous cortical defect that was detected in a 15-year-old child (**a**). Marked regression of the lesion after 2 years (**b**).

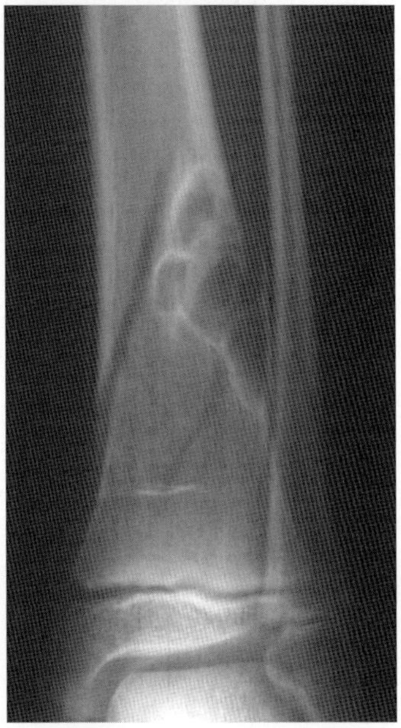

Fig. 3.**64** Pathologic fracture through a fibrous cortical defect. This 8-year-old girl fell from a vertical height of 1 m while playing.

Simple (Juvenile) Bone Cyst

Synonyms: solitary bone cyst, unicameral bone cyst.

■ The bone cyst is a benign, fluid-filled lesion with a peak incidence before 20 years of age. ■

PATH There is a unicameral cavity filled with clear or sanguineous fluid and lined with a fibrous membrane of variable thickness. The membrane is composed of loose vascular fibrous tissue that contains scattered osteoclastic giant cells and isolated zones of recent or old hemorrhages or cholesterol deposits (WHO classification).

CLINIC Simple bone cysts often become symptomatic only after spontaneous fractures.

Age: About 70–80% are found in patients aged under 20 years.

Location: Favored sites are the proximal humerus (40%) and proximal femur (30%). In older patients, however, bones formed by intramembranous ossification are more frequently involved. In tubular bones, simple bone cysts have a metadiaphyseal predilection.

Therapy: Corticosteroid injections. Surgical curettage, especially of multicameral cysts. Decompression drilling has been used as well. There are high recurrence rates regardless of the therapy used.

X-RAY The simple bone cyst appears as a centrally located, well-defined, solitary radiolucency (Fig. 3.**65**). A sclerotic rim is invariably present. Larger cysts elicit solid periosteal reactions with concentric expansion of the bone due to erosion of the original cortex (neocortex, Fig. 3.**66**). Intralesional fractures are frequent and might create the impression of a septated cyst.

! The 'fallen fragment sign', pathognomonic of unicameral bone cyst, is an osseous fragment of the pathologic fracture which has migrated to the dependent portion of the cyst.

CT Density measurements allow an unequivocal CT diagnosis. Whether the cyst is unicameral or multicameral can always be determined with certainty (Fig. 3.**70**).

MRI Detection of fluid allows the definitive diagnosis (high signal intensity on the T2-weighted SE image). The rim of the cyst and the membranous coverage along the septations enhance.

DD **Aneurysmal bone cyst:** This is more eccentrically located and extends into the soft tissues. The differentiation by MRI can be difficult since simple cysts can exhibit blood-fluid levels after fracture.

Giant cell tumor/osteosarcoma: This is a tumor of soft-tissue density in contradistinction to the cyst with its fluid density (see MRI and CT).

Fibrous dysplasia: Radiographically, fibrous dysplasia can resemble a simple bone cyst that contains areas of bone repair.

In the calcaneus, the radiographic differentiation between **cyst** and **lipoma** rests on the central calcification that characterizes the lipoma, but the differentiation is clinically inconsequential since both are 'leave-me-alone' lesions.

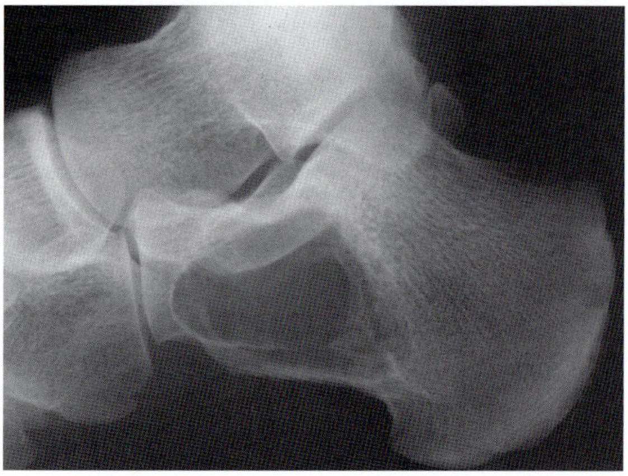

Fig. 3.**65** Simple bone cyst in the calcaneus.

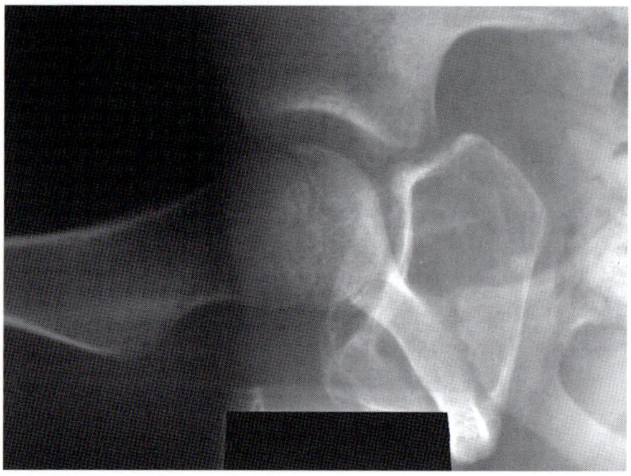

Fig. 3.**66** Extensive simple bone cyst of the pubic bone in a 9-year-old boy.

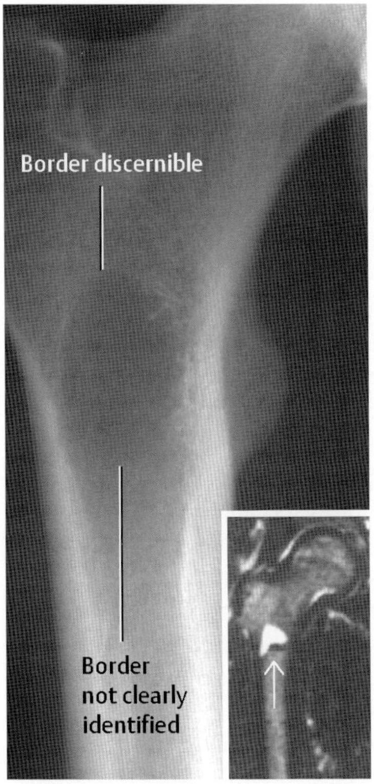

Fig. 3.**67** Small localized simple bone cyst in a 19-year-old man. MRI (T2-weighted sequence) confirms the fluid within the lesion.

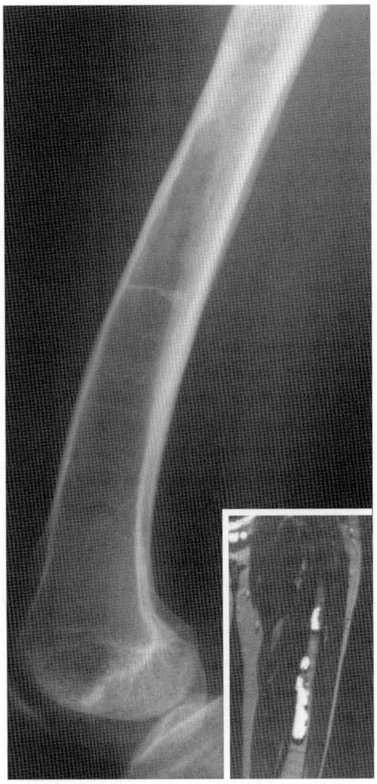

Fig. 3.**68** Extensive simple bone cyst in the femur of a 22-year-old man. The T2-weighted image again shows fluid within the lesion.

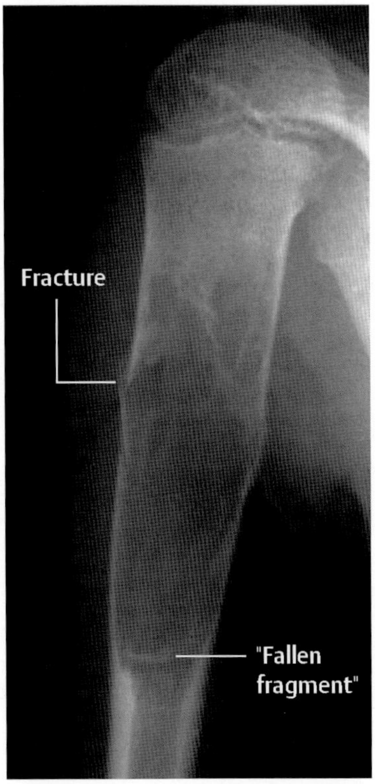

Fig. 3.**69** Pathologic fracture through a large simple bone cyst in the humerus of a 24-year-old woman.

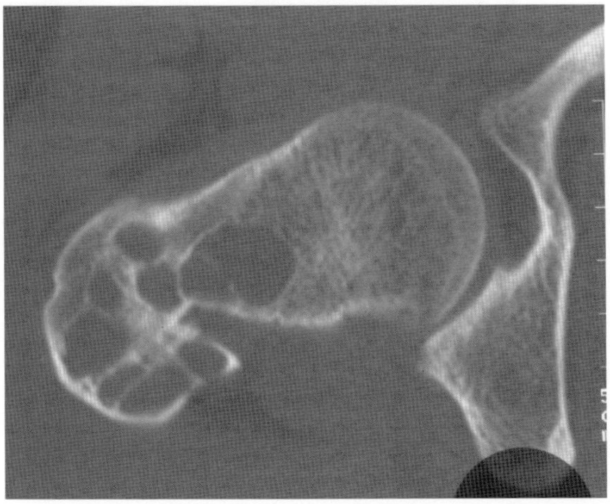

Fig. 3.**70** Impressive CT demonstration of the extension and septation of the simple bone cyst, with water equivalent densities measured within the lesion.

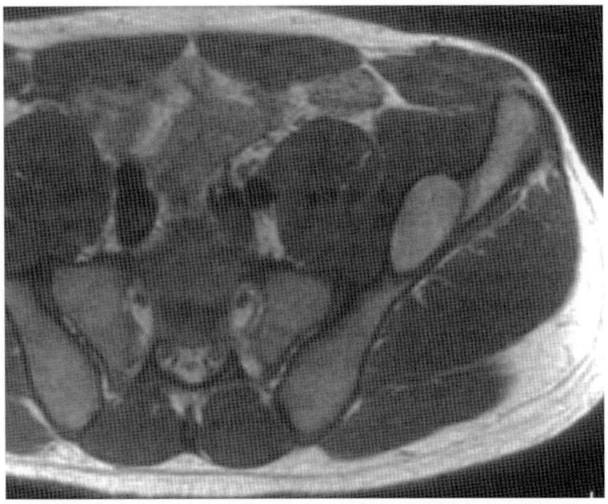

Fig. 3.**71** Simple bone cyst in the ilium of a 22-year-old man. T1-weighted sequence. The bright signal indicates the presence of blood products.

Aneurysmal Bone Cyst

The aneurysmal bone cyst is an expansile osteolytic lesion that can be secondary to other skeletal lesions (especially tumors).

PATH The lesion contains blood-filled cystic spaces of different sizes, separated by fibrous septa containing osseous or osteoid trabeculae and osteoblastic giant cells (WHO classification). The etiology and pathogenesis are unknown. A distinction is made between primary and secondary aneurysmal bone cysts, with the latter arising from benign or malignant bone tumors or after trauma.

CLINIC The findings are nonspecific and consist of swelling and bone pain. The lesion can grow rapidly and mimic a malignant tumor.
Age: Aneurysmal bone cysts (more than 80%) occur within the first and second decades of life.
Location: All bones can be affected, but there is a predilection for the spine, femur, tibia, and pelvis. In the long tubular bones, the lesions are located in the metaphysis and diaphysis.
Therapy: Curettage. Recurrence rate about 20–40%.

X-RAY The aneurysmal bone cyst generally appears as a solitary, large, eccentrically located, sharply demarcated radiolucency. It may be partially surrounded by a fine sclerotic rim (Figs. 3.**72**–3.**74**). Expansion into the surrounding soft tissues is frequent, with the extraosseous component either surrounded by an osseous shell (neocortex) or radiographically indistinguishable from the soft tissues (Figs. 3.**72**, 3.**76**).

Many aneurysmal bone cysts have a trabeculated or septated appearance (Fig. 3.**77**).

CT The neocortex can appear as a fine and radiographically invisible sclerotic rim. CT adds important information by demonstrating fluid levels in the multicameral cysts due to different intracystic densities (Fig. 3.**75**).

MRI Like CT, MRI can visualize the fluid-fluid levels best on T2-weighted SE sequences. Following injection of contrast medium, the cyst lining shows strong enhancement (Fig. 3.**77 c**). In addition, contrast enhancement can display the unevenly arranged solid structures (Fig. 3.**74 b**).

! Meticulous histologic examination of the curetted material is of utmost importance to detect associated small tumors (e.g., osteosarcomas, osteoblastomas, chondroblastomas).

DD **Giant cell tumor:** This generally can be distinguished from an aneurysmal bone cyst by CT or MRI. Usually a giant cell tumor is 'solid' and shows homogeneous enhancement (except with central necrosis) in contrast to the aneurysmal bone cyst, which enhances mainly in the periphery.
Simple bone cyst: The radiographic findings are indistinguishable, especially for multiple and septated cysts or for simple cysts following a spontaneous fracture. Simple bone cysts can, though rarely, contain fluid-fluid levels, but never show 'solid' enhancing areas.
Nonossifying fibroma: It has a thick sclerotic rim and appears more multiloculated or presents as elongated simple osteolysis. The nonossifying fibroma is always separated by a cortical rim from the soft tissues. Both MRI and CT can differentiate between fibrous tissues and fluid-containing cysts.

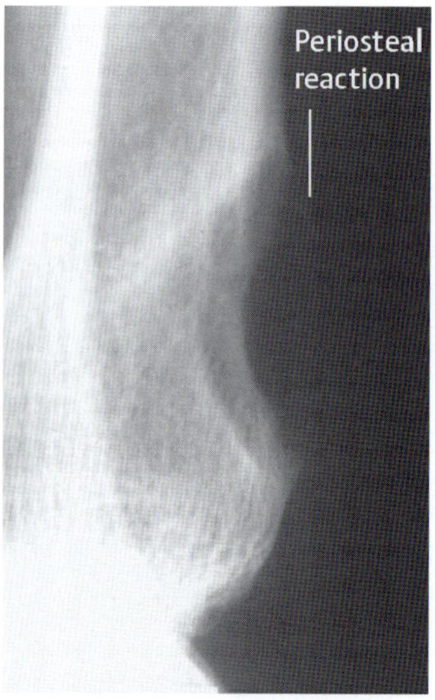

Fig. 3.**72** Eccentrically located aneurysmal bone cyst in the distal tibia in a 39-year-old woman. The thin periosteal reaction is discernible over only a short segment.

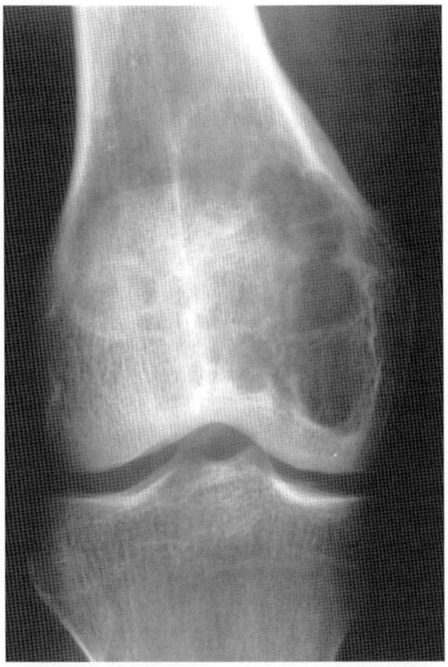

Fig. 3.73 Aneurysmal bone cyst in a 38-year-old man.

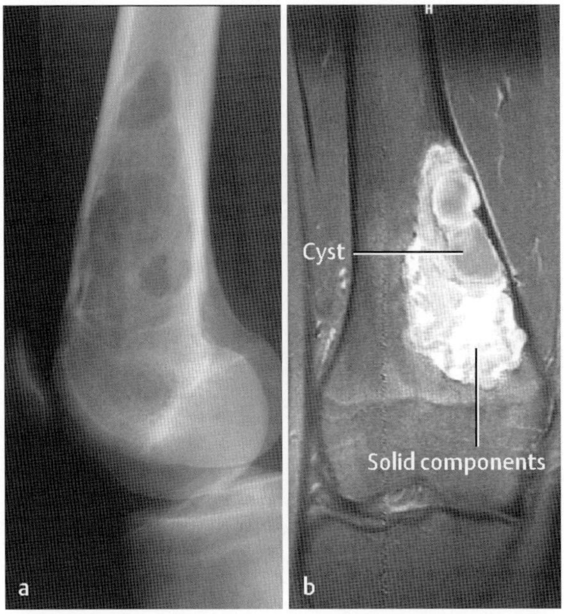

Fig. 3.74 Aneurysmal bone cyst in the distal femur of a 19-year-old female patient (**a**). **b** T1-weighted sequence with fat suppression and contrast enhancement.

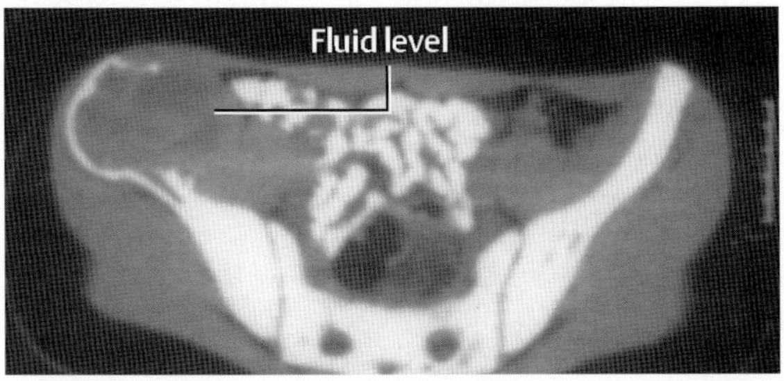

Fig. 3.75 CT of an aneurysmal bone cyst in the ilium, with fluid-fluid levels. The lesion lacks an osseous shell medially, making the differentiation from a malignant tumor difficult.

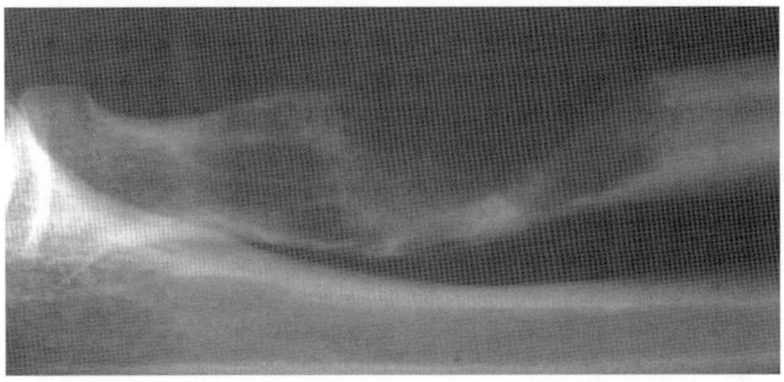

Fig. 3.76 Extensive destruction of the proximal ulna by an aneurysmal bone cyst.

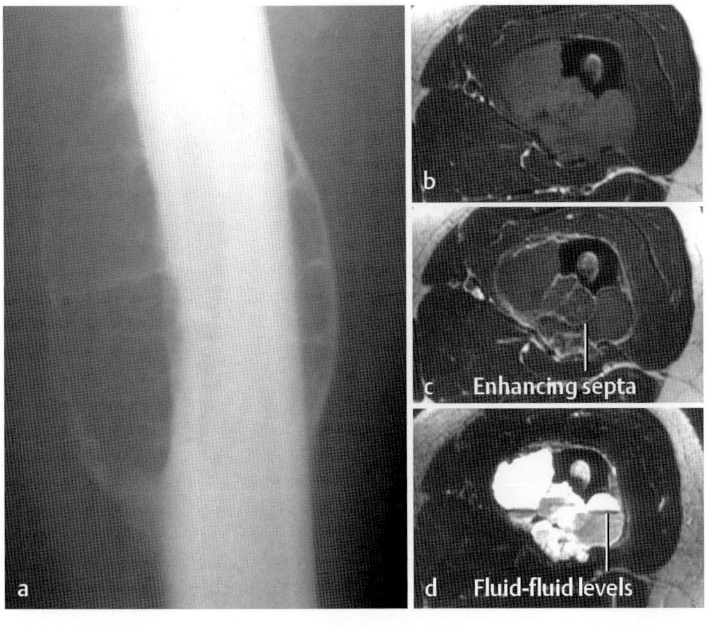

Fig. 3.77 Soap bubble-like aneurysmal bone cyst of the femur in a 20-year-old man (**a**). MRI with T1-weighted images before (**b**) and after (**c**) administration of contrast medium, and with a T2-weighted image (**d**). Note the fluid-fluid levels on the T2-weighted image.

Eosinophilic Granuloma and Histiocytosis X

Synonym for eosinophilic granuloma: Langerhans granulomatosis.

■ Histiocytosis X covers a range of disorders that are not confined to the skeleton. Eosinophilic granuloma is the commonest of these and is clinically the most indolent variant. Other manifestations are Hand-Schüller-Christian disease and Letterer-Siwe disease. All disorders show characteristic histiocytes (Langerhans cells). ■

Another classification of histiocytosis distinguishes a **chronic localized** type from an **acute disseminated** type. **Eosinophilic granuloma** belongs to the former and will be discussed here.

PATH Eosinophilic granuloma is a tumorlike lesion composed of proliferating histiocytes, which appear together with multinucleate giant cells, lymphocytes, and plasma cells.

CLINIC The eosinophilic granuloma often is an incidental radiologic finding, especially in the calvaria. Clinically, however, patients can present with soft-tissue swelling and localized bone pain.
Age: It most often occurs in the first and second decades of life, but can be detected in infancy and even up to the fifth decade of life.
Location: It has the tendency to involve the calvaria, ribs, spine, pelvis, and femur, but other skeletal sites can be involved. The disorder is usually monostotic, but multiple foci are observed in about 20% of cases.
Therapy: Spontaneous regression, especially of calvarial lesions, is common. Intralesional corticosteroid injections have been tried with variable success. Curettage is generally reserved for rapidly progressing lesions involving weight-bearing bones.

X-RAY Eosinophilic granulomas are characterized by great morphologic variety, and both aggressive and latent growth patterns have been described. The radiographic findings depend largely on the stage of the eosinophilic granuloma at the time of detection. The calvaria generally shows this lesion to be a round to ovoid lytic area measuring up to 3 cm in diameter ('punched-out lesion'). Bone remnants within the lesions resemble a sequestrum and are referred to as a 'button sequestrum' (Fig. 3.**84**). Despite its sharp margin, a sclerotic rim is usually absent in the early stages (Figs. 3.**79**, 3.**80**). Sometimes a geographic pattern of destruction can be observed.

Involved **vertebral bodies** can show osteolytic destruction, with the osteolytic areas traversed by trabeculae (Fig. 3.**81**). The vertebral body can collapse and become a dense vertebra, the so-called 'vertebra plana' (Fig. 3.**78**).

Tubular bones can have relatively sharply demarcated foci or a moth-eaten pattern of osteolytic destruction. Lamellar periosteal new bone formation can also be seen (Figs. 3.**79**, 3.**80**). **Caution:** Ewing sarcoma must be considered in the differential diagnosis.

Spontaneous regression of the lesion produces a sclerotic rim of increasing thickness, followed by sclerotic transformation (Fig. 3.**83**). Complete restitution of normal osseous appearance is not infrequent.

NUC This can make an important contribution by distinguishing between monostotic or polyostotic disease. The intensity of uptake depends on the activity of the lesion.

CT The 'punched-out' nature of the lesion is better appreciated on CT than on conventional radiography (Figs. 3.**81**, 3.**82**).

MRI The classic signal pattern seen with all tumors is present: low signal intensity on T1-weighted images and high signal intensity on T2-weighted images. The lesion shows variable degrees of contrast enhancement.

DD **Tubular bones:**
Osteomyelitis can mimic histiocytosis radiographically, although the latter often is identified by its relatively sharp demarcation from healthy bone. Despite limited experience, MRI should allow a reliable differentiation in many cases (edema with osteomyelitis versus 'tumor' with eosinophilic granuloma).
Ewing sarcoma: Imaging frequently cannot exclude a Ewing sarcoma, and excisional biopsy is necessary in these cases.
Skull: Multiple foci in infants can produce a pattern resembling tuberculosis.

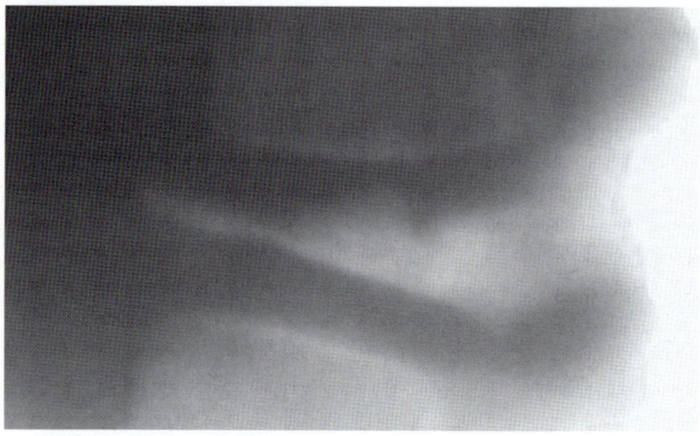

Fig. 3.**78** Vertebra plana in a 7-year-old boy.

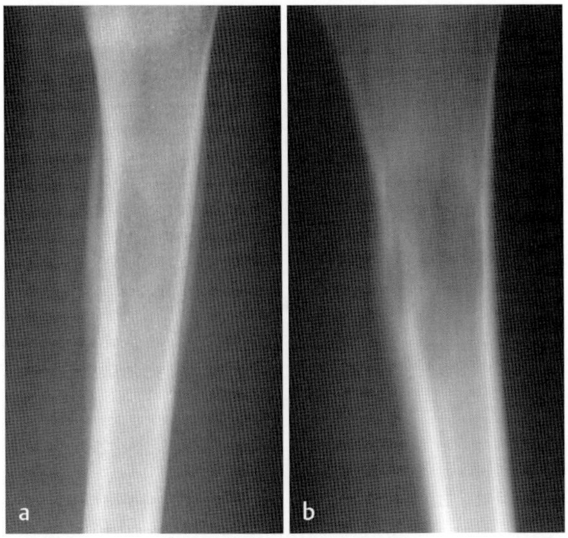

Fig. 3.**79** Eosinophilic granuloma of the tibia with permeative destruction and periosteal reaction in a 7-year-old boy. In this case differentiating this lesion from a malignancy, especially from Ewing sarcoma, is quite difficult.

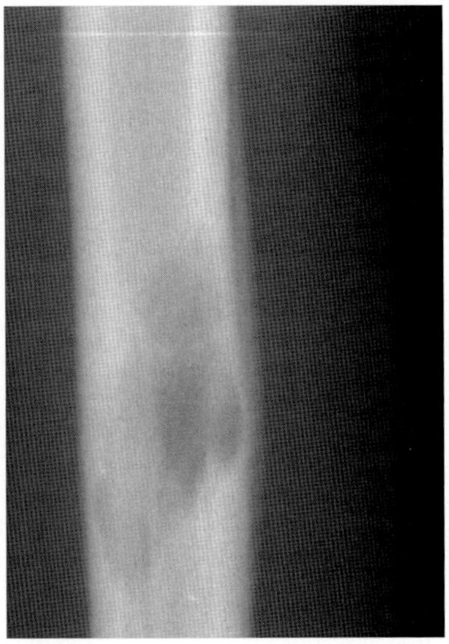

Fig. 3.**80** Eosinophilic granuloma in an 8-year-old child. In comparison to Fig. 3.**79** there is a relatively sharp demarcation of the lesion.

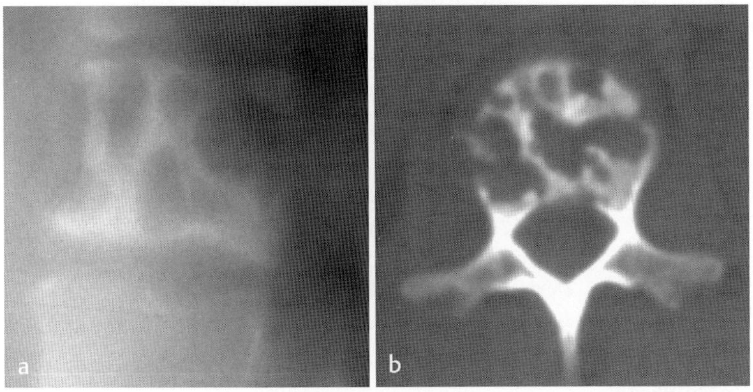

Fig. 3.**81** Conventional radiograph (**a**) and CT (**b**) of an eosinophilic granuloma of the vertebral body with confluent 'punched-out' lesions.

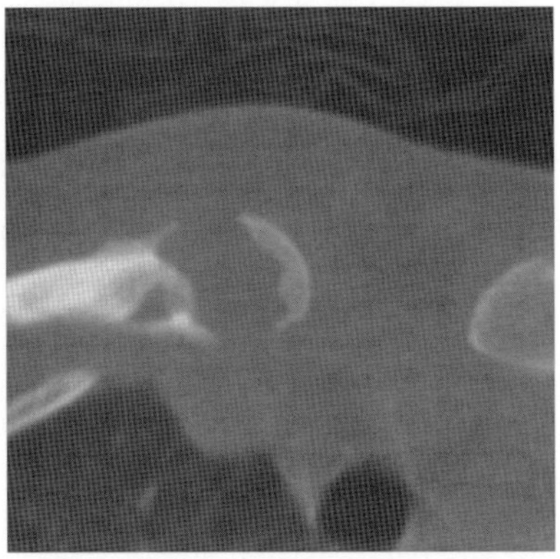

Fig. 3.**82** Eosinophilic granuloma of the clavicle with 'punched-out' lesion.

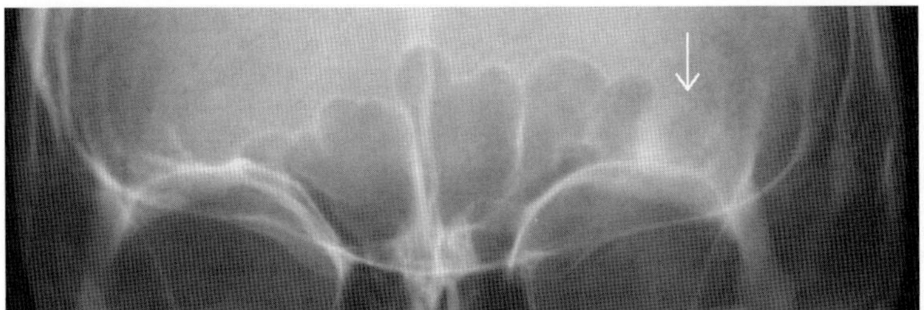

Fig. 3.**83** Old lesions with sclerotic rim in a 53-year-old man.

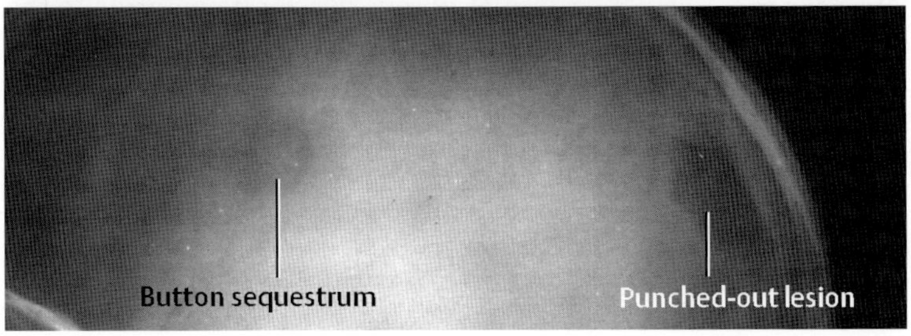

Fig. 3.**84** Two eosinophilic granulomas of the skull, one with the so-called 'button sequestrum' (= central osseous remnant).

Fibrous Dysplasia

Fibrous dysplasia is a common developmental disorder consisting of fibro-osseous tissue that displaces normal bone.

PATH This is a benign tumorlike process characterized by localized developmental arrest of the bone-forming mesenchyme. Instead of normal lamellar spongiosa, an isomorphic fibrous stroma is laid down and is subsequently transformed into a network of statically insufficient fibrous bone. The process is slowly progressive and usually arrests at the time of puberty. The etiology and pathogenesis are unknown although an enzyme defect has been proposed. The disorder is not inherited, and the chance of malignant degeneration is rare (0.5%).

Polyostotic fibrous dysplasia is frequently associated with other extradermal, mesodermal, and endodermal anomalies as well as with various developmental endocrinopathies. The most frequent association is the **Albright syndrome** (polyostotic fibrous dysplasia with *café-au-lait* skin pigmentation on the trunk and extremities and precocious puberty).

Age: Since the disease manifests itself during bone growth, it is usually diagnosed before the age of 20 years, but can be initially discovered well into adulthood.

CLINIC The monostotic type usually is an incidental radiologic finding. The polyostotic type can present with bone pain, spontaneous fracture, or osseous deformities. The cutaneous **café-au-lait** skin pigmentation can be found in up to 50% of patients. Craniofacial involvement can produce asymmetric facial features, bulbar protrusion, and cranial nerve compression and palsy.

Location: Fibrous dysplasia is predominately monostotic and less frequently oligo- and polyostotic. All bones can be affected, with involvement of vertebrae, shoulder girdle, and hand skeleton almost exclusively denoting the polyostotic type. Favored sites are the femur (invariably involved with polyostotic fibrous dysplasia), skull, and ribs. In the long tubular bones, the foci center within the metaphysis, with extension toward both the epiphysis and the diaphysis.

Therapy: Rarely indicated, but if needed, often surgical.

X-RAY The radiographic findings of fibrous dysplasia are highly diverse and depend on the age of the patient, location in the skeleton, and degree of ossification and calcium content of the fibrous stroma. Frequent findings are well-demarcated, cystlike areas of trabecular bone destruction with loss of normal texture. The concentric expansile growth induces a shell-like periosteal reaction, often with periosteal penetration, and a sclerotic rind of cortical thickening is often present (Fig. 3.**86**). A **'soap bubble' pattern** is highly typical, but only occasionally present. Likewise, the **'ground glass'** appearance, though a classic feature of fibrous dysplasia, is contingent on the condition of the matrix and its mineralization (Fig. 3.**85**). The lesion can also be cystic or diffusely sclerotic, or can contain irregular sclerotic areas (Figs. 3.**87** – 3.**89**). Curved shafts of the tubular bones and fractures with callus formation are frequent. Genuine cysts can develop following a necrosis and hemorrhage. Old foci are repaired by a coarse sclerotic trabecular pattern as an attempt of the bone to restore its stability.

Fibrous dysplasia of **ribs** characteristically produces a fusiform osseous expansion.

In **tubular bones,** the multicystic appearance predominates. Fractures and curvature of the shaft (shepherd's crook deformity of the proximal femur) are typical manifestations (Fig. 3.**90**).

In **flat bones,** fibrous dysplasia appears cystic with internal honeycombing and possibly a scalloped outline (Fig. 3.**88**).

Three types have been described in the **skull:**

Pagetoid type (Fig. 3.**89**):
- usually located in the vault,
- frequently a manifestation of polyostotic fibrous dysplasia,
- bubbly 'expansion' of the diploic space,
- cystic honeycomb radiolucency,
- patchy cloudy sclerosis.

Sclerosing type:
- usually located in the cranial base and maxilla,
- sclerosis dominates,
- practically no cystic components.

Cystic type:
- predominantly involving vault and mandible,
- multiple round or lobulated defects.

NUC The usually intense uptake enables the differentiation between monostotic and polyostotic fibrous dysplasia.

CT The 'ground glass' appearance is best appreciated on CT, often confirming the diagnosis of fibrous dysplasia and complementing the radiographic findings (Fig. 3.**89**).

MRI MRI generally does not play a role in diagnosing fibrous dysplasia but can contribute differential diagnostic information in cases with radiographically inconclusive findings. The signal pattern of fibrous dysplasia conforms to the universal pattern found with all tumors (low signal intensity on T1-weighted images and high signal intensity on T2-weighted images). The fibrous stroma enhances. Enhancement and T2-weighted images can be heterogeneous and variable because of signal alterations induced by blood, fat, and calcifications (Fig. 3.**91**).

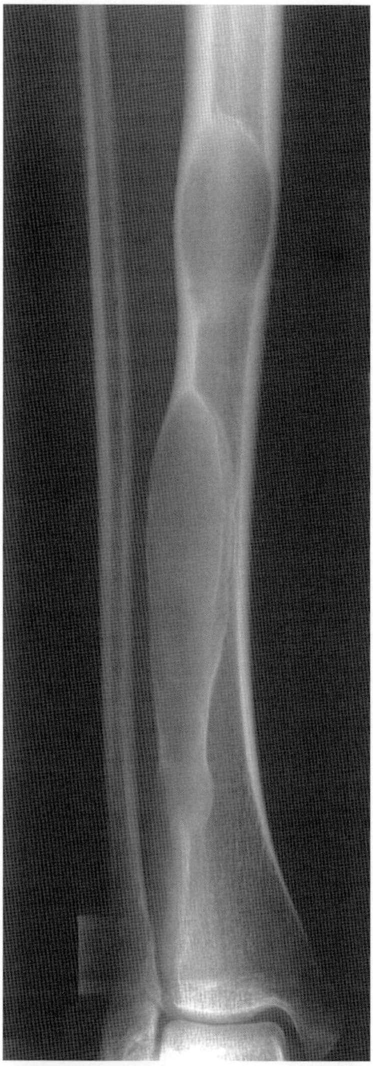

Fig. 3.**85** Fibrous dysplasia with the typical 'ground glass' appearance in a 17-year-old boy.

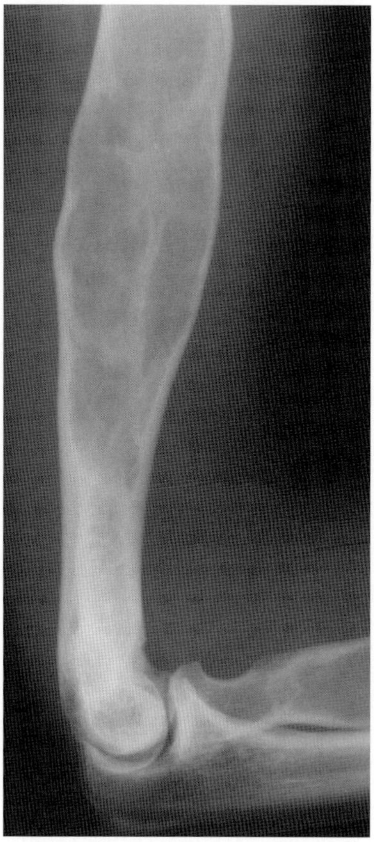

Fig. 3.**86** Marked bone expansion caused by fibrous dysplasia in a 50-year-old man.

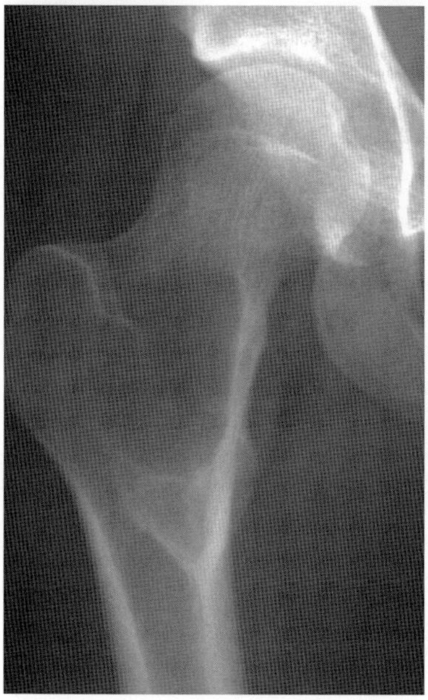

Fig. 3.**87** Round, solely osteolytic manifestation in fibrous dysplasia.

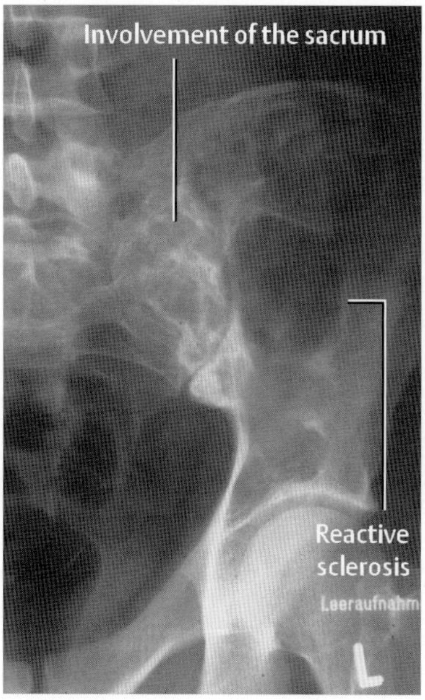

Fig. 3.**88** Fibrous dysplasia in a 32-year-old man. Multicentric radiolucencies with reactive sclerosis in the ilium, as well as in the sacrum.

DD

Tubular bones: Monostotic fibrous dysplasia must be distinguished from solitary or aneurysmal bone cysts if the dysplastic fibrous areas do not occupy large portions of the bone. Differentiation can usually be achieved by MRI.

Ribs: Since a rather aggressive-appearing growth pattern can be encountered in the ribs, differentiation from an eosinophilic granuloma can be difficult. CT can be helpful if it discloses the typical ground glass appearance seen with fibrous dysplasia.

Skull: Paget disease should be considered in the differential diagnosis in the elderly patient. The predominately sclerotic type of fibrous dysplasia should also be distinguished from meningioma (see CT and MRI).

Glossary

Periosteal (cortical) desmoid: This is a clinically irrelevant fibrous lesion of the cortex (perhaps as the result of previous trauma). The lesion occurs during the growth period in children and adolescents (3 to 17 years). It characteristically arises along the posteromedial aspect of the distal femoral metaphysis, but can involve the distal humeral, radial, and ulnar metaphysis, as well as the proximal tibial metaphysis.

Conventional radiography and CT reveal the periosteal desmoid as one or several shallow cortical erosions with a sclerotic base, about 3–4 mm deep and usually 1–2 cm long. The erosions are sharply demarcated and can be covered by a thin osseous shell due to periosteal reaction. The defect can also exhibit an irregular contour. Occasionally, the adjacent periosteum induces a severe cortical thickening (Fig. 3.**93**). Periosteal desmoids are generally 'cold' on radionuclide bone scan.

Epidermoid: This is an epithelial cyst beneath the periosteum producing a tumorlike osseous lesion. Although epidermoids of the skull cause no symptoms, involvement of other locations can cause bone pain. The lesions tend to involve the distal phalanx of the fingers and, less frequently, the skull. Radiographically, epidermoids cause a localized osseous 'expansion' with cortical thinning. The lesion generally lacks an internal structure. Active and severely painful epidermoids are often indistinctly outlined, whereas inactive lesions exhibit a sclerotic rim.

Giant cell reparative granuloma: This is a reactive tumorlike accumulation of giant cells with the propensity to involve the tubular bones of the hand and foot. Local bone pain generally prompts radiographic examination. The radiographic findings vary from lytic lesions with distinct or indistinct margins to cortical destruction, which can mimic an aggressively growing tumor. Simple bone 'expansion' with formation of a neocortex is also possible (Fig. 3.**94**).

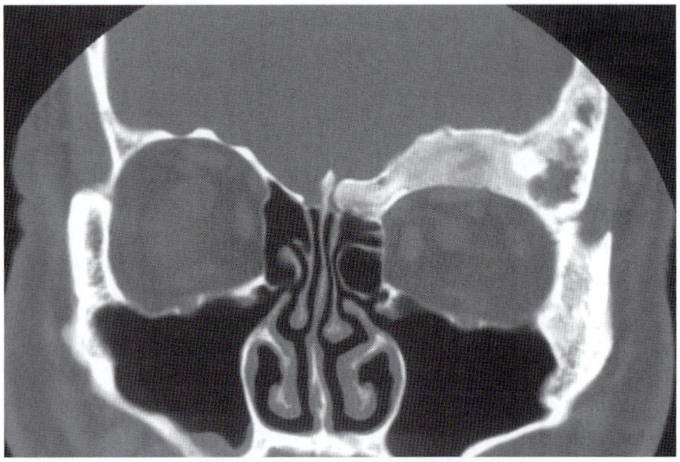

Fig. 3.**89** Pagetoid manifestation of fibrous dysplasia with 'ground glass' appearance in the skull of a 57-year-old man. Coronal CT.

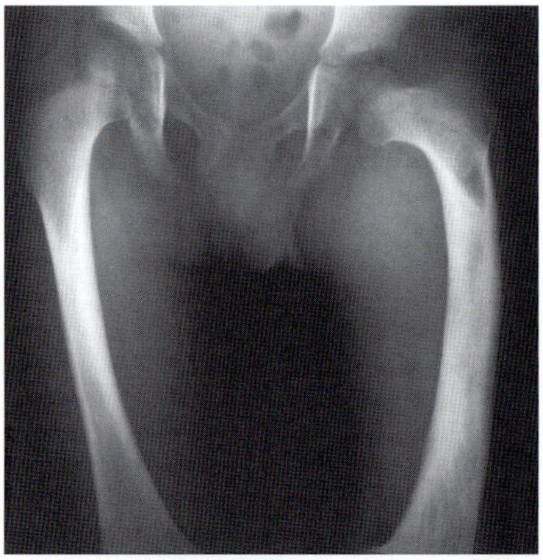

Fig. 3.**90** Polyostotic type of fibrous dysplasia. 'Shepherd's crook' deformity of both femora with diffuse osteosclerosis and enlargement of these bones.

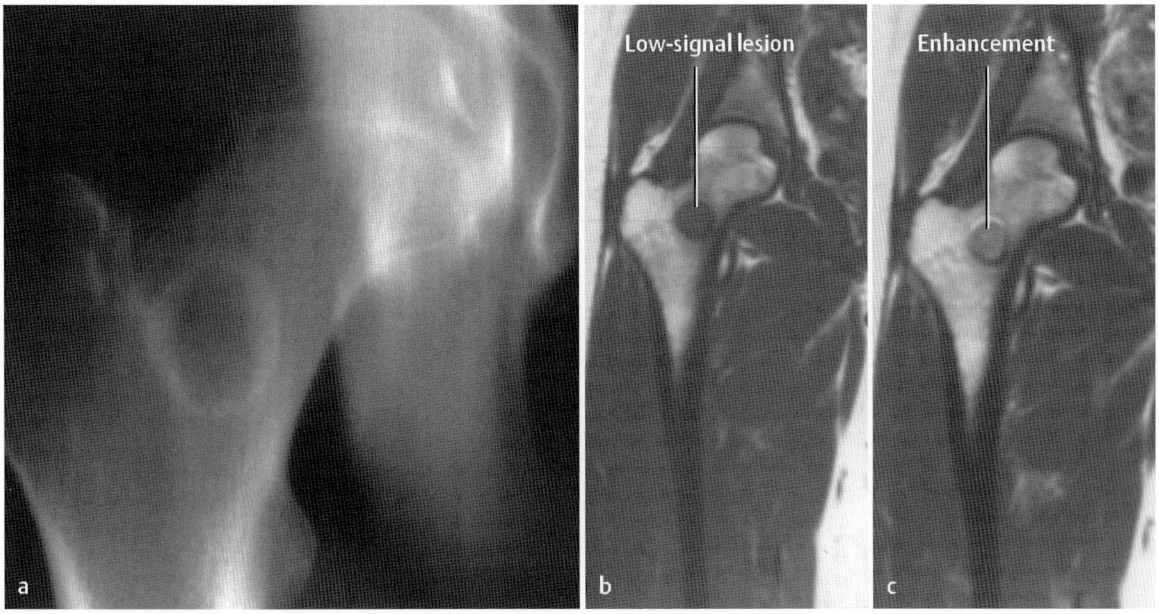

Fig. 3.**91** Fibrous dysplasia in a 17-year-old woman. MRI can assist in differentiating fibrous dysplasia from a cyst by showing diffuse contrast enhancement (T1-weighted sequence before (**a**) and after (**b**) administration of contrast medium).

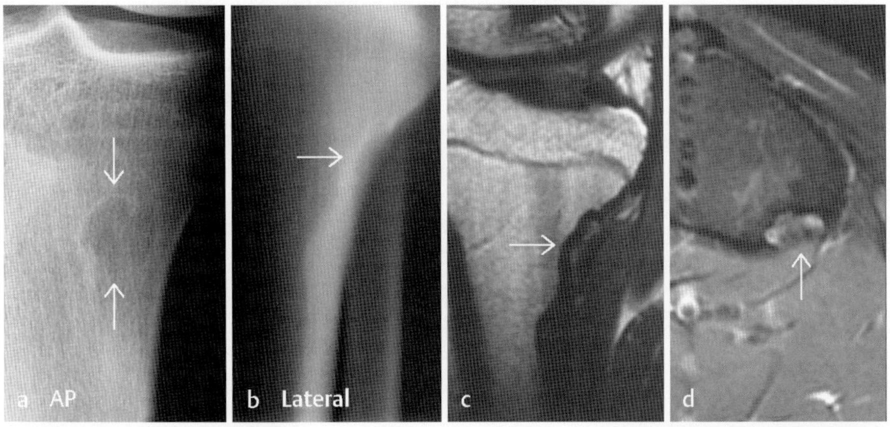

Fig. 3.**92** Cortical desmoid in the tibia of a 13-year-old child.
a AP view,
b lateral conventional tomogram,
c coronal T1-weighted SE image,
d axial T1-weighted SE image with frequency-selected fat suppression after administration of contrast medium showing an enhancement.

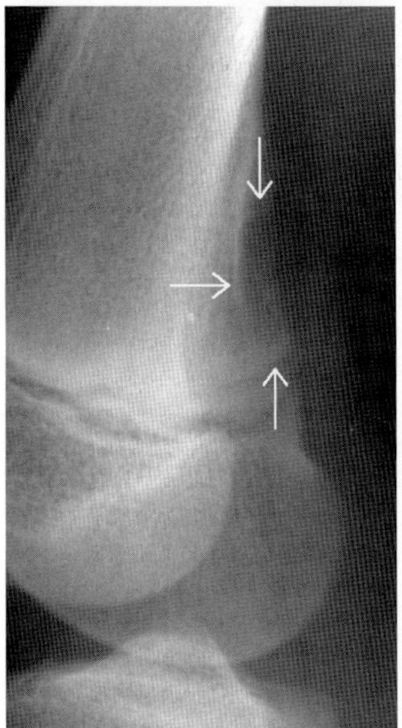

Fig. 3.**93** Periosteal desmoid of the dorsal aspect of the distal femur in a 13-year-old child, seen on a slightly oblique lateral projection.

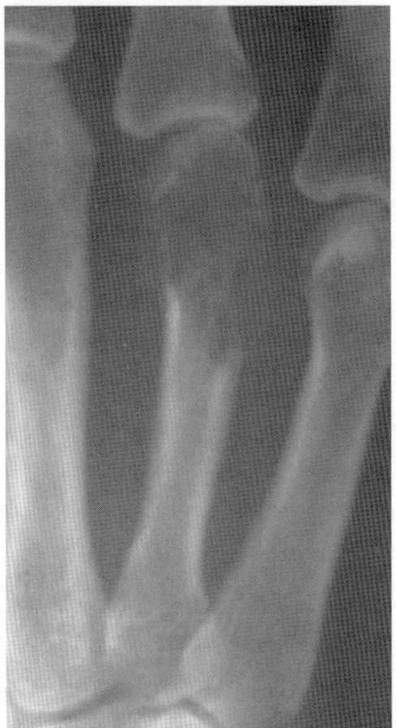

Fig. 3.**94** Reparative giant cell granuloma in the fourth metacarpal head in a 42-year-old man.

Metastases

■ Metastases are the most frequent tumors of bone. In patients over 40 years old, they are foremost in the differential diagnosis of an osteolytic or osteoblastic lesion. ■

PATH Bone destruction or formation induced by metastases is mediated by humoral factors such as hormones, lymphokines, and enzymes, which are probably secreted by the tumor cells. The detailed steps leading to the histologic and radiologic manifestation of metastatic cancer in bone are still under investigation.

CLINIC The chief complaint is an intermittent dull pain. Systemic findings such as weight loss, weakness, and fatigue suggest generalized involvement by the tumor. Inflammatory parameters can be elevated, and massive osteolytic destruction from metastases can induce hypercalcemia.

Age: Skeletal metastases are generally seen only after the age of 40 years. Notable exceptions include metastases from:

- neuroblastoma in children,
- breast carcinoma in young women, and
- seminoma in young men.

Table 3.**6** Primary tumors with predilection for skeletal metastases

– Breast carcinoma
– Prostate carcinoma
– Bronchial carcinoma
– Renal cell carcinoma
– Gastrointestinal carcinoma
– Thyroid carcinoma

Location: Metastases can involve **any** bone, but have a propensity to involve the axial skeleton and skull. As a general rule, the more peripheral bones are less likely to be affected, as exemplified by the rarity of the skeletal metastases involving the hands and feet.

! Only 10% of skeletal metastases present as solitary lesions.

X-RAY **1. Osteolytic** lesions with a pattern of destruction ranging from complete bone destruction to a moth-eaten infiltrative permeative destruction. There is generally an indistinct rim, but a sclerotic rim can be observed rarely. The periosteal reaction is variable. Conventional radiography can frequently reveal metastatic involvement of the soft tissues from cortical extension. This pattern is principally found in metastases from bronchial, renal, breast, and thyroid carcinomas (Figs. 3.**95**, 3.**96**).

2. Osteoblastic lesions of various sizes. The increased density ranges from small patchy areas to diffuse involvement of the entire bone (Figs. 3.**98**, 3.**99**). However, osteoblastic metastases can rarely destroy osseous borders.

This type of metastasis is primarily seen with carcinomas of the prostate and less frequently (about 20%) with breast and gastrointestinal tumors (e.g., colon, gastric, pancreatic carcinomas).

3. Mixed osteolytic-blastic lesions contain both osteolytic and osteoblastic foci. The most common primary tumors are breast, prostate, and gastrointestinal in origin (Figs. 3.**97**, 3.**99**).

Special manifestations:

Cystic expansile metastases: These reflect soft-tissue infiltration following widespread cortical destruction. The tumor components are surrounded by fine periosteal new bone formation, which can produce a 'soap bubble' appearance.

This type is rare and predominately seen with primary adenocarcinomas.

Cortical/periosteal metastases: These are areas of osteolytic destruction of the cortex that may be permeative or moth-eaten in appearance (Figs. 3.**96**, 3.**102**).

NUC Bone scintigraphy with Tc 99 m diphosphonate is the initial step to search for metastases. Positive findings of the initial bone scan should have conventional radiographic correlation to exclude false positive findings (degenerative, post-traumatic changes) or to detect potential complications (imminent pathologic fracture). If the problem cannot be solved clinically in scintigraphically positive but radiographically negative cases, other modalities (especially MRI) should be performed for possible clarification.

Small osteolytic metastases might not be discernible by bone scintigraphy because of inadequate spatial resolution or impaired osseous reaction to the osteolysis. In addition, the altered osseous response after chemotherapy can interfere with the assessment of the neoplastic activity for about 3 to 6 months. Finally, the 'superscan', a manifestation of generalized increased uptake due to diffuse or disseminated metastasis (frequently observed with carcinoma of the prostate), should not be misinterpreted as a normal scan.

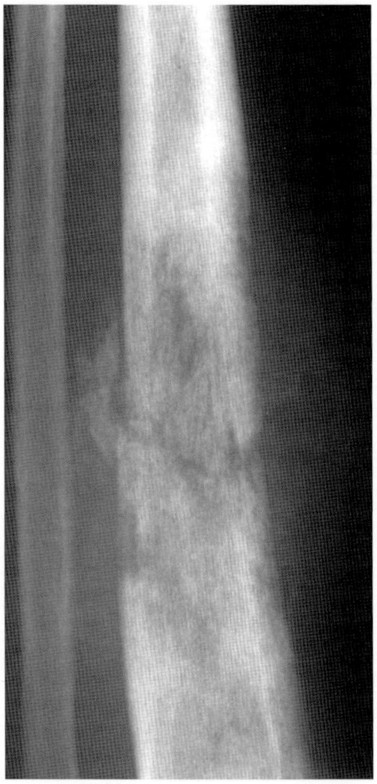

Fig. 3.**95** Colon metastasis causing moth-eaten-like destruction and pathologic fracture of the tibia. Note the soft-tissue infiltration.

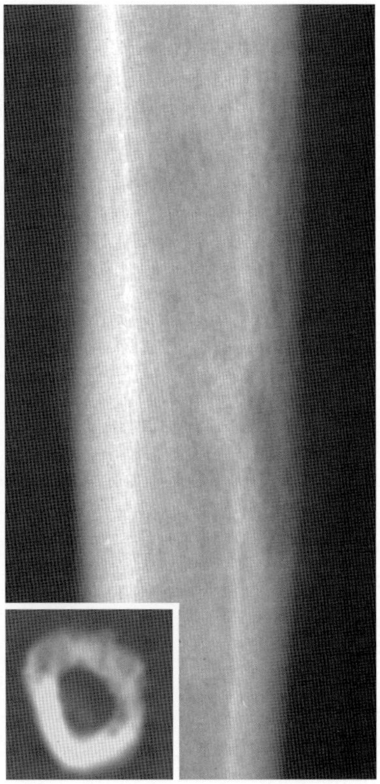

Fig. 3.**96** Cortical metastasis of a seminoma.

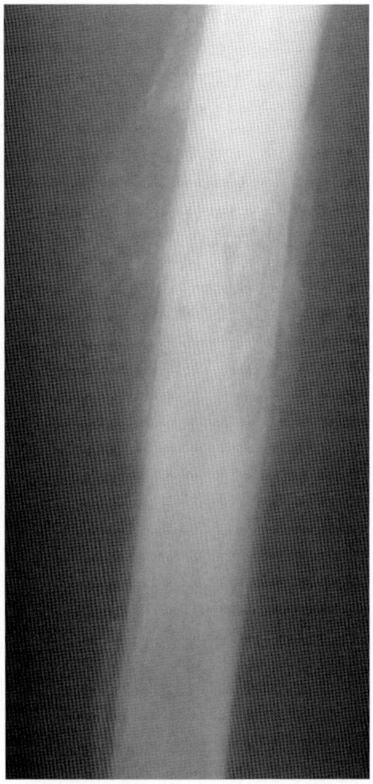

Fig. 3.**97** Metastasis from a rectal carcinoma with complex periosteal reaction.

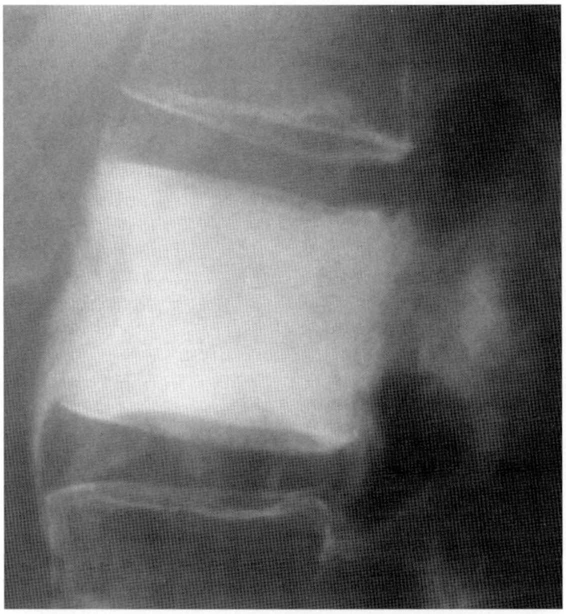

Fig. 3.**98** Osteoblastic metastasis ('ivory vertebra') from prostatic carcinoma.

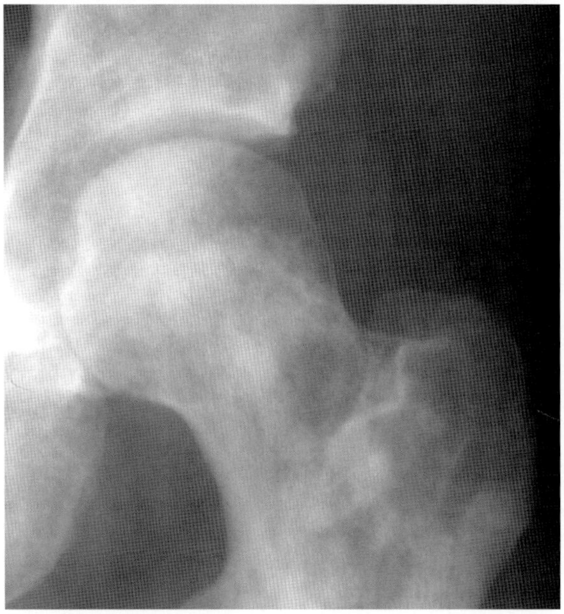

Fig. 3.**99** Diffuse osteoblastic and occasional osteolytic metastases from breast carcinoma.

SONO With experience, sonography can be used to evaluate superficially located bones (e.g., ribs), as it can easily delineate cortical disruption or interruption.

CT CT is far superior to conventional radiography in detecting bone destruction and is generally reserved for the spine (vertebral arch, articular processes) and the facial bones. CT is especially suitable for further evaluation of inconclusive findings suspicious for bone metastases at sites with complex skeletal anatomy.

MRI This is the most sensitive method for the detection of skeletal metastases. The signal alteration induced by metastases conforms to the classic tumor pattern (low signal intensity on T1-weighted images and high signal intensity, but also low signal intensity, on T2-weighted images) (Figs. 3.**100**, 3.**104**). The signal depends to a large extent on the degree of calcification of the metastases, and metastases invariably enhance.

Technical considerations: The most sensitive sequence is the STIR sequence since metastases will be easily shown as areas of high signal intensity. In adults above the age of 40, the T1-weighted sequence of marrow is usually uniformly bright from the fat within it. On this sequence, tumors are easily demarcated from fat (Fig. 3.**100**).

By displaying any tissue enhancement, the combination of the injection of contrast medium and T1-weighted images with fat suppression often provides valuable additional information on the enhancement pattern of the tumor.

Therapy: There are a variety of therapies for metastases. The osseous lesions may show considerable variability during any therapy (Figs. 3.**102** – 3.**104**).

DD Diagnosing skeletal metastases poses no problem in patients with known primary tumors and multiple randomly distributed foci on the bone scan that correspond to radiographs showing areas compatible with metastases. **Solitary** lesions require further assessment, which depends on the type of metastases expected:

Osteolytic lesions: Osteolytic malignant lymphomas and plasmocytomas cannot be differentiated from osteolytic metastases. Primary bone tumors (malignant fibrous histiocytoma, vascular malignant tumors, and others) are also difficult to exclude but fortunately are quite rare.

Osteosclerotic lesions: Solitary osteomas and bone islands may not be easily distinguished radiographically from osteoblastic metastases. However, metastatic lesions generally show intense uptake on the bone scan, whereas bone islands and osteomas show no or weak uptake.

Mixed osteolytic and osteoblastic lesions: This constellation always raises the possibility of a malignant lymphoma in addition to metastases.

The differential diagnosis of **vertebral** compression due to osteoporosis or underlying metastasis is discussed in Chapter 1 (page 52).

A metastasis diagnosed in a weight-bearing bone raises concerns about **'stability'.** If stability is deemed at risk, immobilization and local measures (e.g., radiotherapy) should be implemented. Two rules can provide some practical guidance:

Tubular bones: More than 50% cortical destruction.

Spine:

- destruction of the posterior border of the vertebral body,
- tumor-induced loss of height of the vertebral body,
- tumor replacement of the entire vertebral body by MRI, even without a break in the cortex.

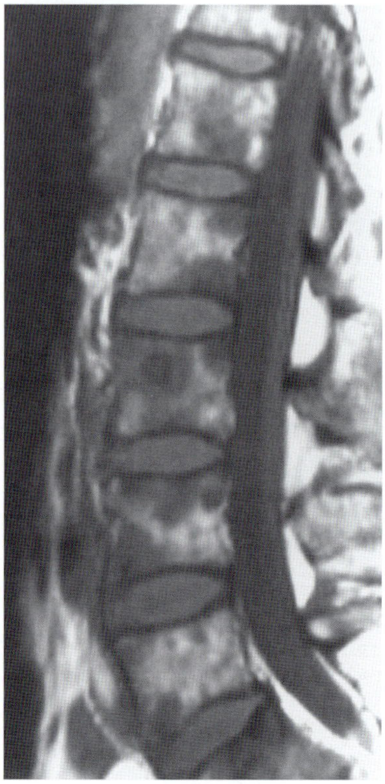

Fig. 3.**100** Typical pattern of widespread metastases on MRI (T1-weighted image). Randomly distributed low signal metastases from a breast carcinoma.

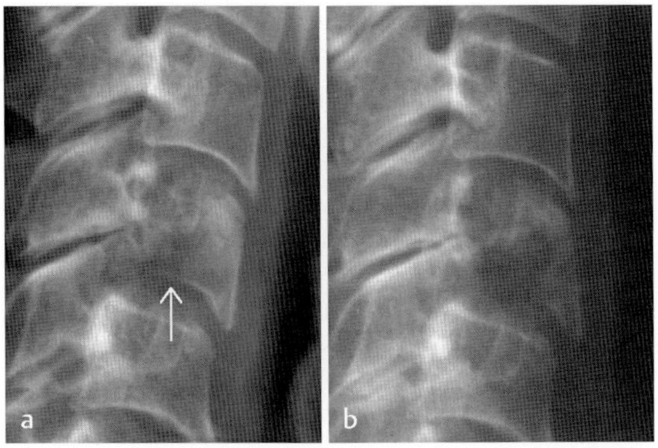

Fig. 3.**101** Careful observation is important! The osteolytic lesion with cortical destruction (**a**) was initially overlooked. The lesion is unequivocally visualized on the follow-up examination 3 months later (**b**).

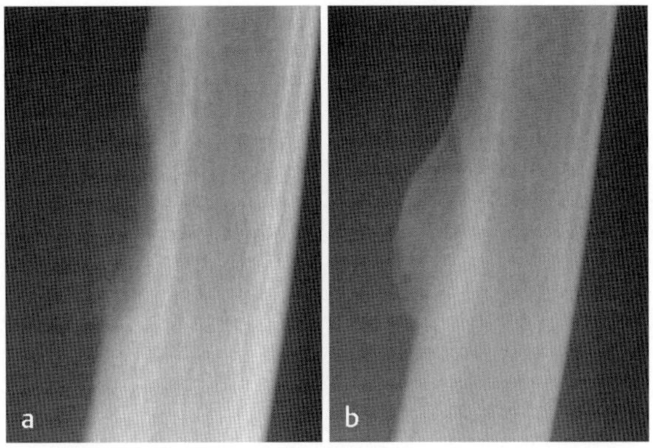

Fig. 3.**102** Follow-up of a cortical metastasis from a rectal carcinoma after chemotherapy.

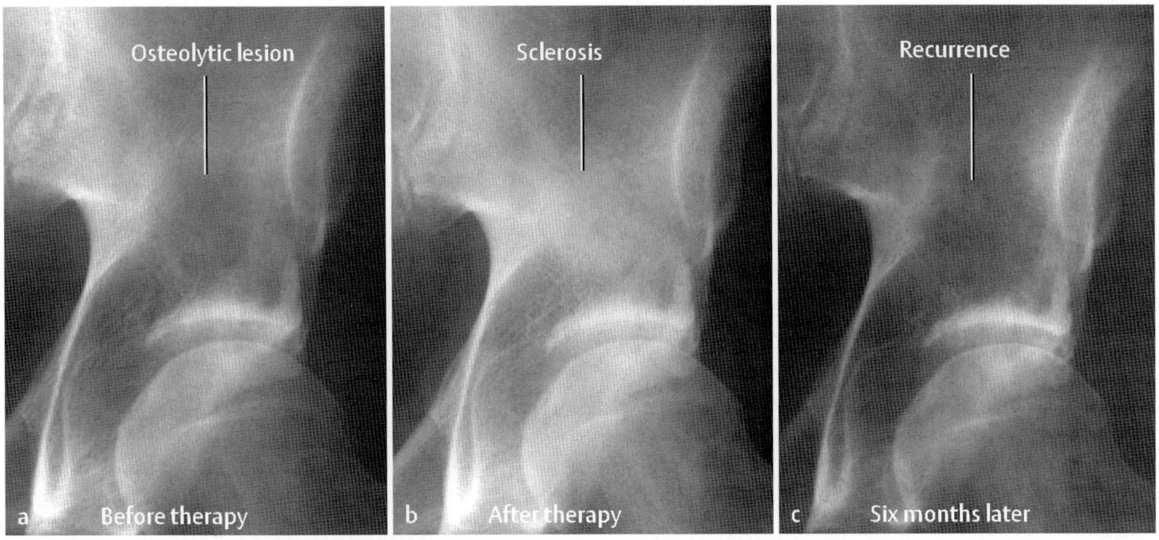

Fig. 3.**103** Course of a metastasis in the pelvis from a nasopharyngeal carcinoma. **a** Before chemotherapy, **b** after completion of chemotherapy, **c** recurrence 6 months later.

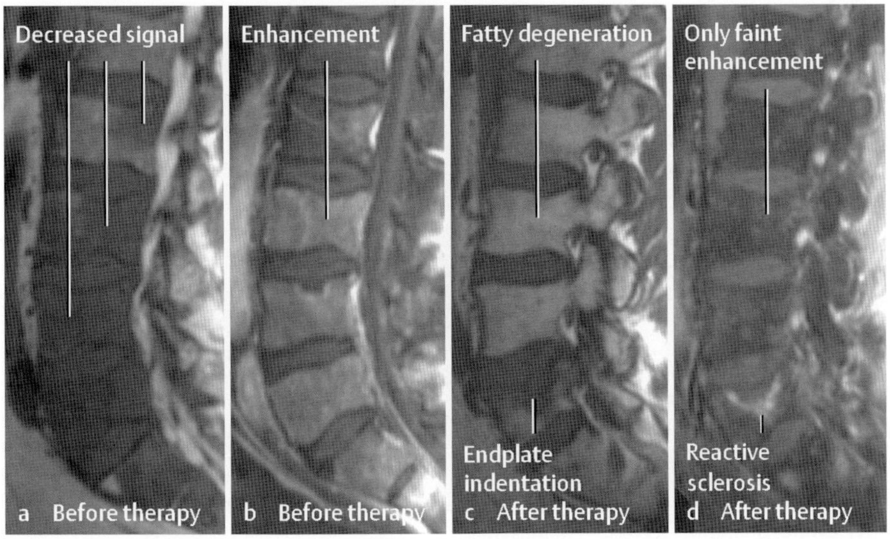

Fig. 3.**104** Course of a metastasis following radiation. **a, b** Before radiotherapy; **c, d** after radiotherapy. T1-weighted SE sequence before (**a, c**) and after (**b, d**) administration of contrast medium.

Soft-tissue Tumors

The WHO classification distinguishes between internal tumors (mediastinum, mesentery, retroperitoneum, orbits) and peripheral soft-tissue tumors. The latter group consists of tumors of the corium (skin), subcutaneous fatty tissue, fasciae, muscles, aponeurosis, periarticular tissues, and peripheral nerves. Despite the derivation from distinctively different tissues and the multitude of tumors (more than 100 histologic diagnoses), these tumors exhibit rather similar biologic behaviors.

Although benign soft-tissue tumors, such as lipomas and fibromas, are frequent, malignant soft-tissue tumors are rare, comprising about 1% of all malignant tumors.

Imaging of peripheral soft-tissue tumors is in the domain of sonography and MRI. CT has become less important, except in identifying calcification and ossification.

Most soft-tissue tumors are easily imaged but defy a reliable diagnostic classification. This applies particularly to the relatively frequent tumors such as neurinomas, neurofibromas, giant cell tumors of the tendon sheath, malignant fibrous histiocytomas, and rhabdomyosarcomas. (Open) biopsy is indicated in the majority of cases. Imaging is mainly used for tumor detection or exclusion and for staging and therapy planning.

X-RAY Conventional radiography can assess the osseous response to the soft-tissue tumor. The major findings are:
- erosions (Fig. 3.**108**),
- periosteal reaction.

Furthermore, conventional radiography can disclose any intratumorous
- radiolucency (see lipoma),
- calcific densities (phleboliths – see hemangiomas, (Fig. 3.**109**) and diffuse calcification (see fibromas, lipomas, lymph nodes, chondromas, Figs. 3.**106**, 3.**107**), sarcomas, and tumor metastases),
- ossification (see osteosarcomas).

Angiography plays only a secondary role today and is reserved for delineating the vascularization if needed for surgical planning and in conjunction with therapeutic embolization. Hemangiomas and AV malformations can angiographically be divided into high-flow and low-flow angiomas (Fig. 3.**110**). The extent of the vascularization, location of the supplying vessels, and flow rate determine the selection of the method of embolization.

SONO Lipomas are highly echogenic and are occasionally surrounded by a sonographically discernible capsule. Almost all other soft-tissue tumors appear heterogeneously hypoechoic (Fig. 3.**105**). Cystic tumor components, necrosis, or acute hemorrhage can be identified as sonolucent areas.

A histologic diagnosis is sonographically impossible.

MRI The majority of soft-tissue tumors are low signal intensity on T1-weighted and high signal intensity on T2-weighted images. Enhancement is variable.

MRI signs of malignancy:
- irregular border,
- heterogeneous signal pattern (T2-weighted image and after enhancement),
- peritumorous edema (the tumor is best demarcated from muscle after enhancement),
- fascial infiltration/permeation (especially of the fascia separating subcutaneous fatty tissue from musculature),
- involvement of several muscle groups or anatomic compartments.

Caution: On MRI, many tumors are enveloped by a low signal capsule that frequently is not conclusively verifiable histologically and therefore has also been referred to as a 'pseudocapsule.' A visualized capsule is no indication of benignity. Liposarcomas, especially, and malignant fibrous histiocytomas often exhibit such a capsule (Fig. 3.**113**).

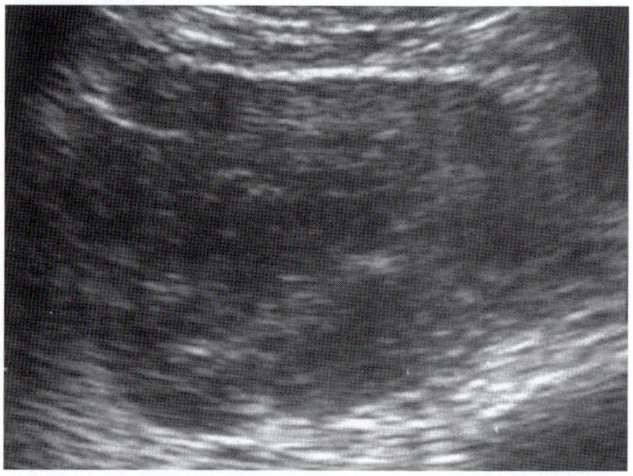

Fig. 3.**105** Sonography of a recurrent leiomyosarcoma. Space-occupying lesion of heterogeneous, decreased echogenicity.

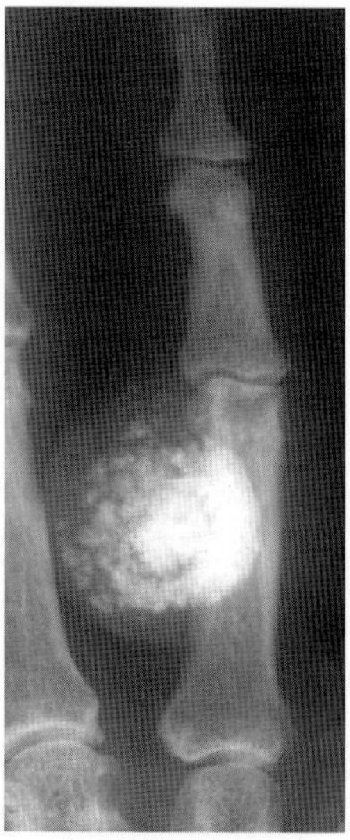

Fig. 3.**106** Tendon sheath chondroma with cartilage matrix.

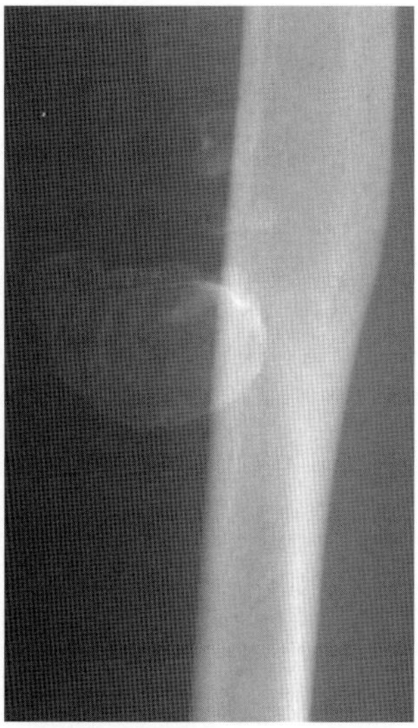

Fig. 3.**107** Lipoma of the upper arm with shell-like calcification.

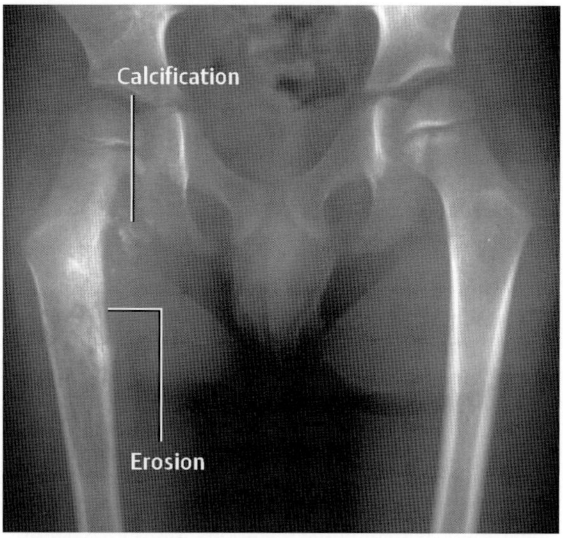

Fig. 3.**108** AP radiograph of a 5-year-old boy. Hemangiopericytoma with osseous erosions and tumor calcifications.

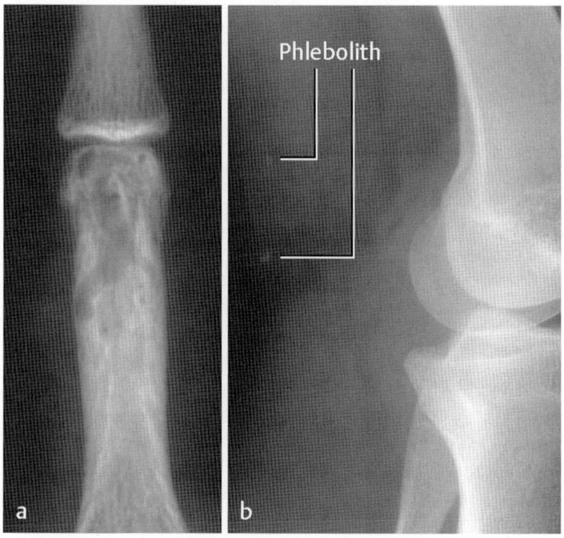

Fig. 3.**109**
a Hemangioma of the soft tissues with secondary bone involvement (18-year-old woman).
b Phleboliths with low-flow hemangioma (19-year-old woman). Pathognomonic finding.

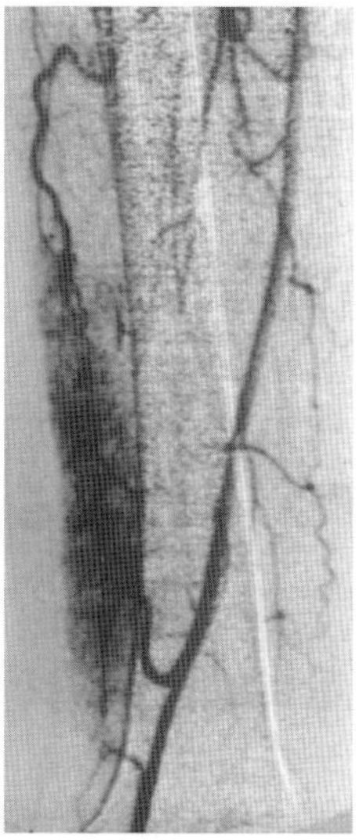

Fig. 3.**110** Angiography of a high-flow hemangioma in the lower leg.

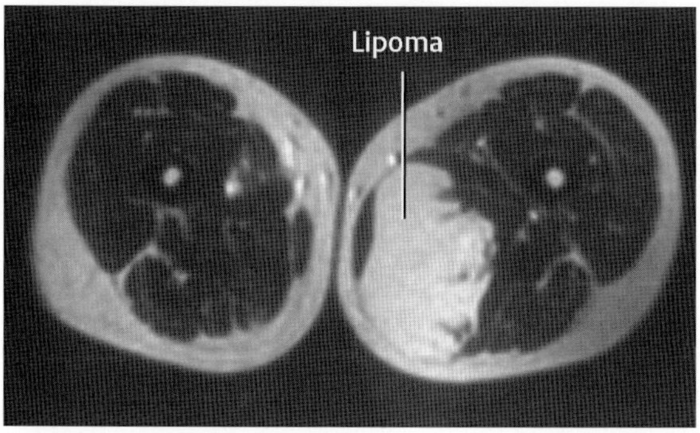

Fig. 3.**111** Lipoma of the thigh (42-year-old woman). T1-weighted SE sequence.

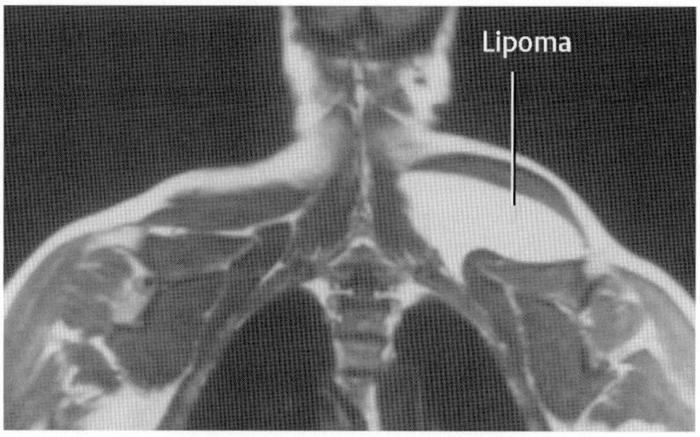

Fig. 3.**112** Lipoma of the shoulder (75-year-old man). T1-weighted SE sequence.

Glossary

The following soft-tissue tumors display an image pattern, especially on MRI, that enables a definitive or, at least, presumptive tissue diagnosis.

Lipoma: Sharply demarcated lesion on MRI with a homogeneous signal of high intensity on T1 **and** T2-weighted SE images. Some lesions may exhibit a delicate capsule of low signal intensity (Figs. 3.**111**, 3.**112**).

Liposarcoma: Detection of fatty components within the tumor. Myxoid components display a very high signal intensity on the T2-weighted image (Fig. 3.**113**).
Caution: Many liposarcomas do not have a characteristic pattern and only display one solid component.

Lymphangioma: The diagnosis generally is made early in life (within the first 3 years). Sonography reveals a hypoechoic lesion with multiple septations. MRI shows a lesion of water signal characteristics, which is low signal intensity on the T1-weighted image and high signal intensity on the T2-weighted image. The lesion may be traversed by delicate septa (Fig. 3.**114**). Absence of, or only faint, enhancement distinguishes this tumor from the hemangioma.

Hemangioma, AV malformation: Hemangiomas are frequent tumors in children and adolescents. Superficial subcutaneous hemangiomas appear as areas of low signal intensity on the T1-weighted image. The T2-weighted image shows numerous confluent punctate areas of high signal intensity, which are partially traversed by septa and undulated structures of low signal intensity. The marked heterogeneous signal pattern reflects the composition of blood-filled vascular channels, fatty deposits, fibrous tissue, and hemosiderin accumulation.

Hemangiomas that are located deep in the musculature are grape-like and cover a relatively large area. They have a very high signal intensity on the T2-weighted image, partially resembling cysts, but are traversed by low signal septa and foci (Fig. 3.**115**).

Color duplex sonography displays vessels, especially in genuine AV malformations. Otherwise, the lesion is very irregular with a mixture of low and high echoes.
Caution: The size of low-flow hemangiomas is frequently underestimated angiographically, and MRI is currently the method of choice in determining the true size of these lesions.

Fibromatoses: These form a group of fibrous tumors that differ in **age** of onset and **location.**

A locally infiltrative growth is characteristic of all these tumors. A capsule is rarely displayed by sonography or MRI, and spreading is not contained by fascial planes. MRI displays these tumors as lesions of very low signal intensity on the T1-weighted images and of variable signal intensity on the T2-weighted image (Fig. 3.**116**). Most of the lesions enhance.

- Fibromas of the aponeurosis and hand are frequent in childhood and adolescence. Involvement of other sites, such as the facial bones, is also possible (Fig. 3.**116**).
- **Aggressive fibromatosis (desmoid):** location: abdominal wall, extremities. All age groups (Fig. 3.**117**).

! Fibromatosis is an aggressive infiltrative tumor, which recurs in up to 70% of cases, even after wide margin resection.

Cysts, ganglions: Cysts and other fluid-filled structures are well demarcated and surrounded by a fibrous capsule of low signal intensity. The signal intensity depends on the type of contained fluid. While the signal intensity of cysts is always high on the T2-weighted SE image, it varies between low and intermediate on the T1-weighted image because of potential blood components. Some ganglion cysts show a connection to the joint. Cysts only have capsular enhancement, and this feature distinguishes them from the diffusely enhancing hemangiomas.

Synovial sarcoma: This is a tumor of the synovial lining. The tumor arises more frequently from the tendon sheath than from the joint capsule. On the T2-weighted image, the tumor shows a relatively high signal intensity, often heterogeneous because of internal calcifications, which can be expected in about 30% of the cases (conventional radiography or CT). The tumor border is mostly sharp, and peritumorous edema absent. A tissue diagnosis is not possible.

Follow-up and Search for Recurrent Soft-tissue Tumors

Sonography and MRI are also the methods of choice for diagnosing recurrent soft-tissue tumors, and MRI assumes a special and dominating role in this setting.

Follow-up and search for recurrent peripheral soft-tissue tumors often proves to be no more difficult than the primary diagnostic evaluation. Remember that surgery or even percutaneous biopsy of a soft-tissue tumor limits the information that can be derived from imaging for about the next 3 months. Edema, hematomas, fibrous bands, and altered anatomy also interfere with the detection of residual tumor. As a general rule, the assessment is severely conditioned for 6 to 9 months after surgical therapy, and only a newly emerging tumor can be considered a reliable finding, as edema alone is a nonspecific finding.

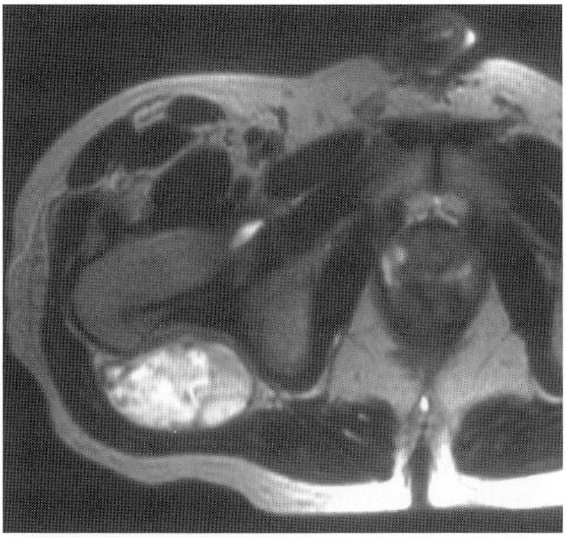

Fig. 3.**113** Myxoid liposarcoma in the gluteal region. T2-weighted SE sequence.

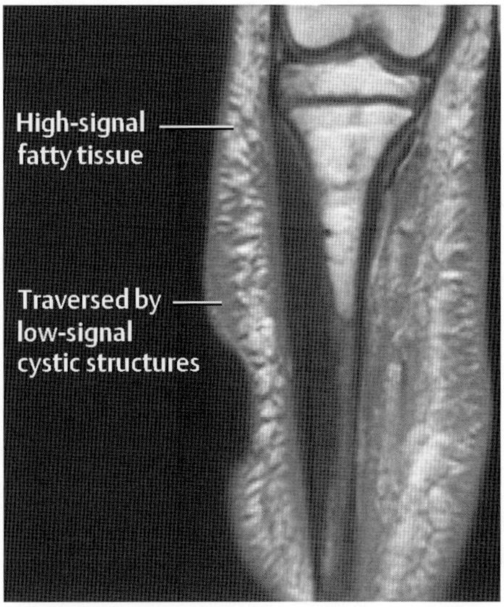

Fig. 3.**114** Lymphangioma in the lower thigh of a 7-year-old girl. T1-weighted SE image.

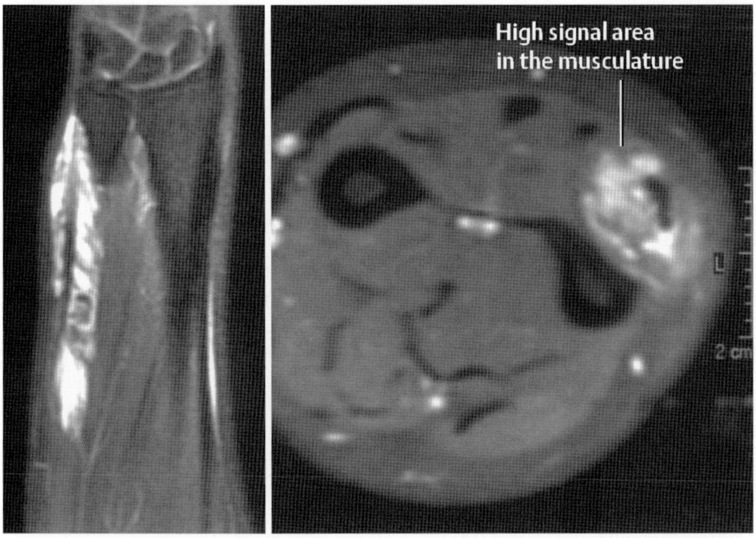

Fig. 3.**115** Hemangioma of the forearm. T1-weighted FSE sequence with fat suppression after enhancement.

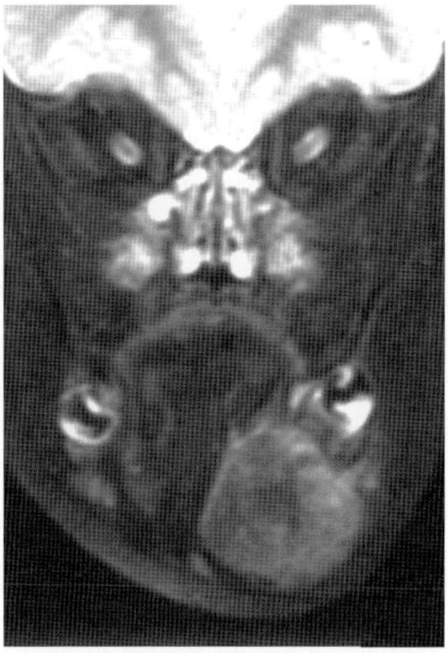

Fig. 3.**116** Fibromatosis of the mandible. Coronal T2-weighted TSE sequence with fat suppression.

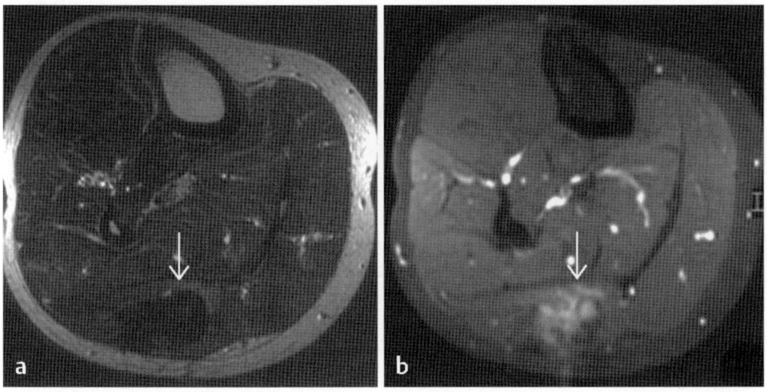

Fig. 3.**117** Desmoid of the thigh. T2-weighted TSE (**a**) and T1-weighted, fat-suppressed sequence after enhancement (**b**).

4 Hematologic Disorders

Plasmocytoma

Synonyms: multiple myeloma, Kahler disease.

■ Plasmocytoma is a monoclonal B cell lymphocytoma characterized by:
- red marrow proliferation,
- bone destruction,
- paraprotein synthesis (immunoglobulin).

The prevailing skeletal manifestations are diffuse osteoporosis and solitary or multiple osteolytic lesions. ■

PATH Neoplastic proliferation of the plasma cells primarily affecting the red marrow which can lead to granulocytopenia, thrombopenia, and anemia. Extraosseous manifestations most frequently occur in the spleen, liver, and lymph nodes. Secondary manifestations include renal failure from tubular damage caused by monoclonal immunoglobulins and amyloidosis.

CLINIC The clinical findings, reflecting the excessive production of abnormal plasma cells, consist of bone pain, weakness, fatigue, fever, weight loss, hemorrhage, and neurologic symptoms. About 6% of the patients develop hepatosplenomegaly in the course of the disease.
Age prevalence: Ages 40 to 80, with men more frequently affected than women.
Location: Multiple lesions are frequently found in the skull, spine, ribs, pelvis, and femur. Diffuse lesions of the peripheral skeleton are usually associated with extensive involvement of the axial skeleton. Lesions of the mandible are frequently present.
Prognosis: Determined by the type of immunoglobulin. The mean survival time after the first symptoms is 3–4 years. Death is caused by renal insufficiency in 60% of patients.
Laboratory values: Detection of paraproteins by means of electrophoresis and of Bence Jones proteins in the urine. Other findings include anemia, elevated sedimentation rate, positive Coombs test, positive rheumatoid factor, hypercalcemia, hyperuricemia, and elevated serum protein from globulin factors. Exception: nonsecretory myeloma (1–3% of myelomas).

X-RAY There are several manifestations, which **coexist:**
- diffuse osteoporosis, especially of the axial skeleton (see 'codfish vertebra' deformity),
- multiple 'punched-out' osteolytic foci, rarely larger than 5 mm,
- confluent moth-eaten pattern of destruction (Fig. 4.**4**),
- permeative destruction pattern,
- large expansile radiolucencies with or without cortical destruction (Fig. 4.**3**),
- reactive osseous changes (sclerotic rim, periosteal reaction) are rare and usually seen following chemotherapy (Fig. 4.**8**),
- rarely 'sclerotic myeloma (plasmocytoma)' may occur (Fig. 4.**6**).

Some locations show typical features:
- skull: multiple lytic lesions of uniform size (Fig. 4.**1**),
- sternum: frequent pathologic fractures,
- spine: predominantly destruction of the vertebral bodies. Paraspinal and extradural tumor extension (Fig. 4.**2**).

NUC Bone scintigraphy does not usually show increased uptake in multiple myeloma. However, the sensitivity of bone scans is not as low as stated in all major textbooks. Bone marrow scintigraphy is considerably more sensitive (detection of 'cold spots') but is less specific since benign lesions likewise show decreased uptake in bone marrow. Furthermore, since they no longer contain hematopoietic bone marrow in adults, the extremities are not imaged with confidence. In conclusion, scintigraphy is not recommended for routinely determining the extent of plasmocytoma (see MRI).

CT MRI has diminished the role of CT, but this modality remains valuable for assessing osseous destruction of the spine and facial bones (Fig. 4.**2**).

MRI Lesions have low signal intensity on T1-weighted and variable signal intensity on T2-weighted images, ranging from high signal intensity to low signal intensity relative to fat.

In general, the bone marrow (especially of the axial skeleton) is homogeneously affected (Fig. 4.**7**), but multiple round foci can occur (Fig. 4.**9**).

By combining conventional and fat-suppressed sequences, high sensitivity can be achieved (though at the cost of low specificity). The major indications

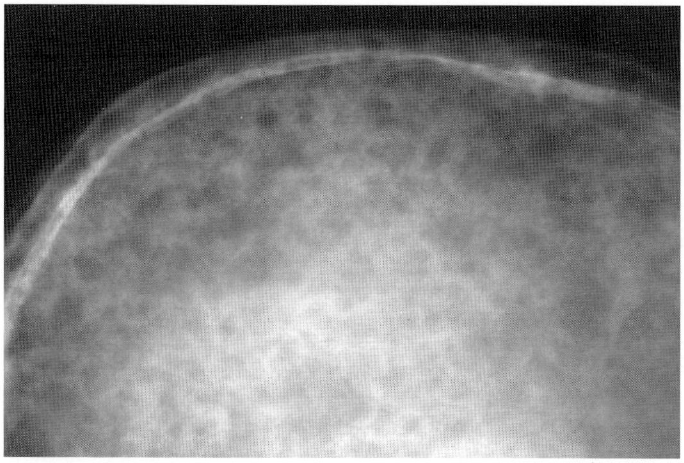

Fig. 4.1 Plasmocytoma of the skull with typical osteolytic lesions.

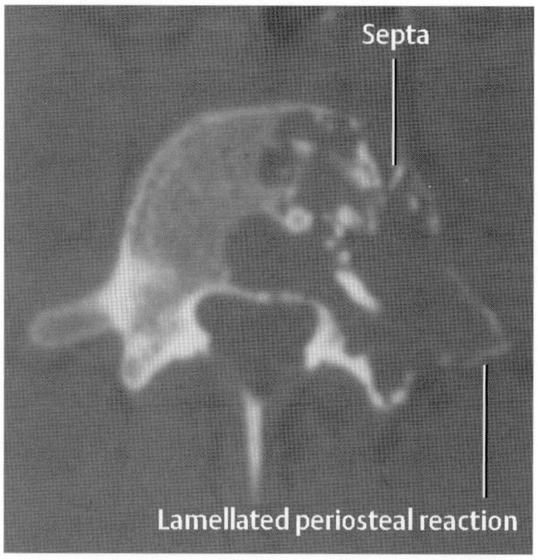

Fig. 4.2 Plasmocytoma. Solitary finding in a 25-year-old man. Septated vertebral destruction with lamellated periosteal reaction.

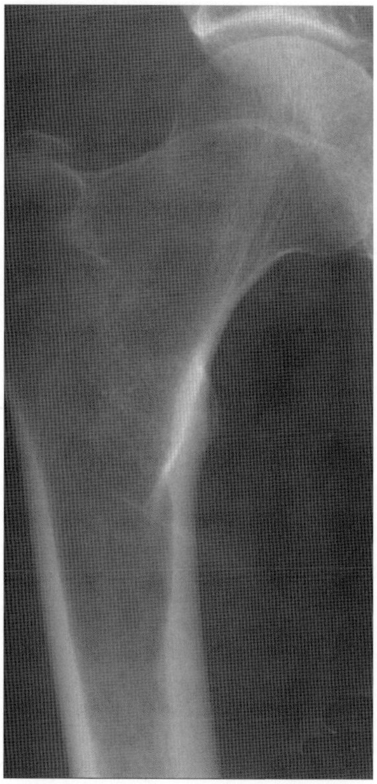

Fig. 4.3 Plasmocytoma. Large osteolytic destruction in the proximal femur. This is a nonspecific radiographic finding.

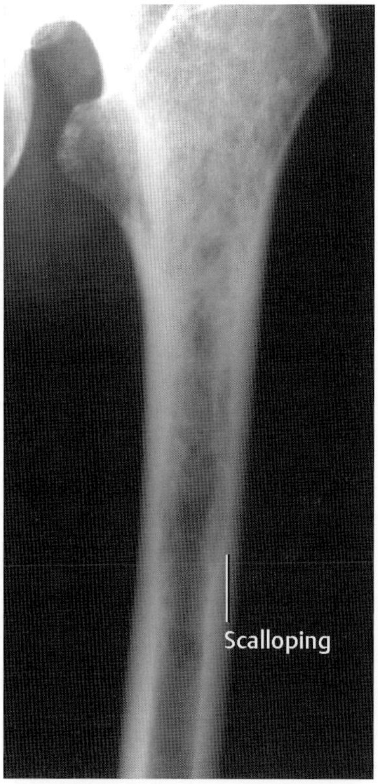

Fig. 4.4 Plasmocytoma of the femur. Extensive osteolytic lesions with medullary and subcortical radiolucencies. Note the endosteal scalloping of the cortex, a finding frequently seen in the proximal femur and humerus.

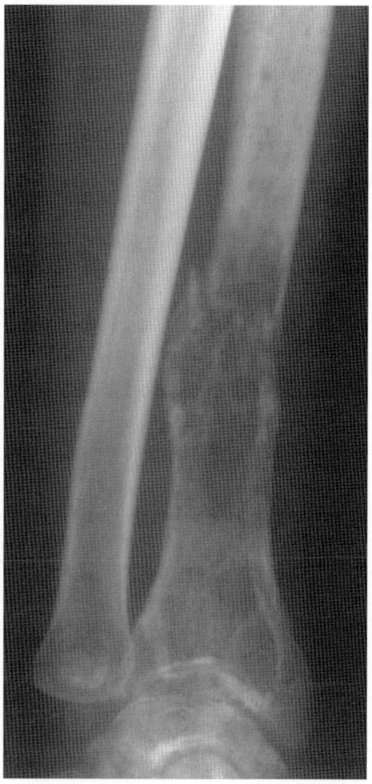

Fig. 4.5 Plasmocytoma of the distal radius. There is osteolysis, medullary expansion with cortical thinning and a pathologic fracture. Note the lack of sclerosis which is typical.

for MRI are assessing the extent of the lesions and their relationship to surrounding anatomic structures. MRI also serves to monitor therapy by following extent, enhancement, and possible fatty conversion during chemotherapy or radiotherapy.

DD A **solitary** lesion or a small number of lytic lesions are indistinguishable from primary osseous lesions, metastases, or infection. **Multiple** small osteolytic foci (less than 5 mm) can be found with

- metastases (often from thyroid or bronchial carcinoma),
- malignant lymphoma,
- leukemia,
- histiocytosis X.

Osteolysis with **expansion** (solitary or multiple) also occurs with:

- metastases (especially from thyroid carcinoma or renal cell carcinoma),
- brown tumors of hyperparathyroidism,
- fibrous dysplasia,
- hemophilic pseudotumors,
- primary bone tumors (e.g., giant cell tumor).

! In 10% of cases plasmocytoma is associated with amyloidoses.

! The literature is incorrect in stating that plasmacytoma spares the vertebral pedicles in contradistinction to metastases. Both of these processes can involve the pedicles.

Table 4.**1** Differential diagnostic criteria of myeloma and metastases

Myeloma	Metastases
Relatively well-demarcated, round to ovoid lesion	Indistinct outlines of different sizes
Cortical scalloping (cortical destruction less frequent)	Cortical destruction frequent
Diffuse involvement of the axial skeleton (see MRI)	Asymmetric involvement of the axial skeleton
Diffuse osteosclerosis rare	Diffuse osteosclerosis possible (osteoblastic metastases)
Diffuse osteoporosis frequent	Diffuse osteoporosis less frequent

Glossary

Solitary plasmacytomas are quite rare and can occur in young patients. They often present with neurologic findings. Skeletal manifestations are more frequent in the spine and pelvis, but can be observed in other skeletal regions and even outside the skeletal system. Many patients found to have a solitary lesion at the time of diagnosis develop multiple lesions during the course of the disease.

The lesions can be lobulated, expansile, or purely osteolytic without expansion. Sclerotic lesions are extremely rare.

Waldenström macroglobulinemia consists of a neoplastic proliferation of B lymphocytes and is characterized by the pathologic production of monoclonal IgM.

Skeletal manifestations are nonspecific and resemble those of plasmacytoma. These include osteoporosis, bone marrow expansion with endosteal erosions, osteolytic destruction, and secondary vertebral compression. Compared to plasmocytoma, osseous destruction is less frequent, but bone marrow expansion is more pronounced. The disease can also be complicated by avascular necrosis of the femoral head caused by 'sludging' from the hyperviscosity of the blood.

POEMS syndrome (**p**olyneuropathy, **o**rganomegaly, **e**ndocrinopathy, **M**-protein, **s**kin changes): Osteosclerotic lesions with osseous proliferations at the entheses (tendon and ligament insertions) are generally found. Irregular bone apposition along the dorsal vertebral elements as well as around the SI and costovertebral joints can help to confirm the diagnosis (Fig. 4.**10**).

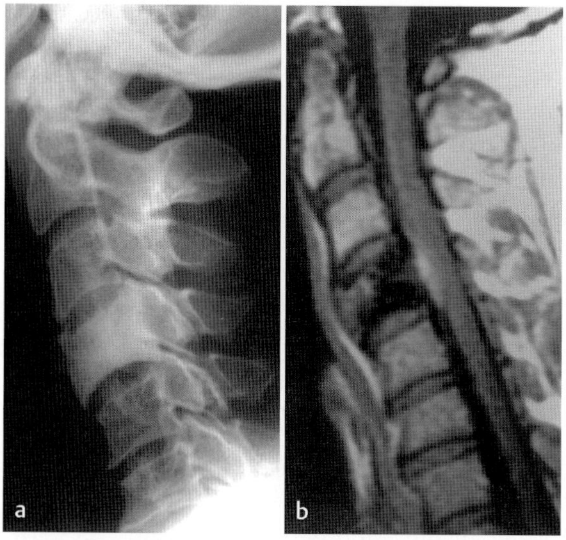

Fig. 4.6 Sclerotic plasmocytoma in a vertebral body, **a** conventional radiograph, **b** MRI, T1-weighted sequence. The low intensity signal reflects the sclerosis.

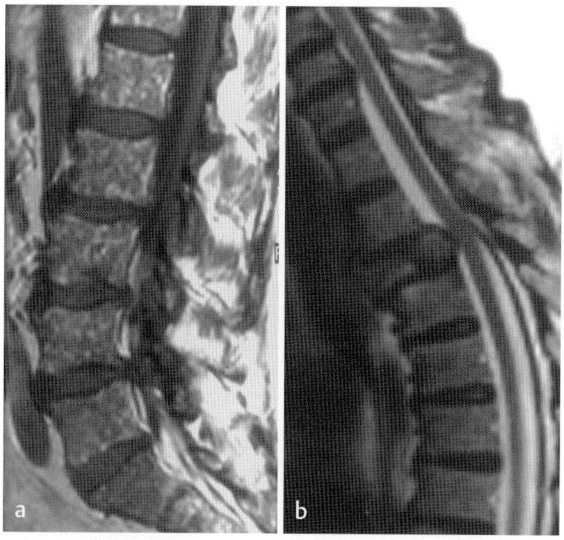

Fig. 4.7 Plasmocytoma of the spine. **a** T1-weighted, **b** T2-weighted SE sequence. Diffuse low signal intensity involving the vertebral bodies. Collapse of the third thoracic vertebral body with compression of the spinal cord.

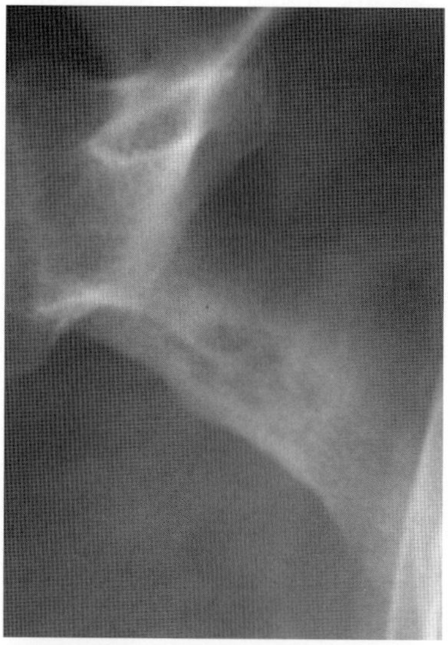

Fig. 4.**8** Plasmocytoma of the scapula with sclerotic rim following chemotherapy. A rare finding.

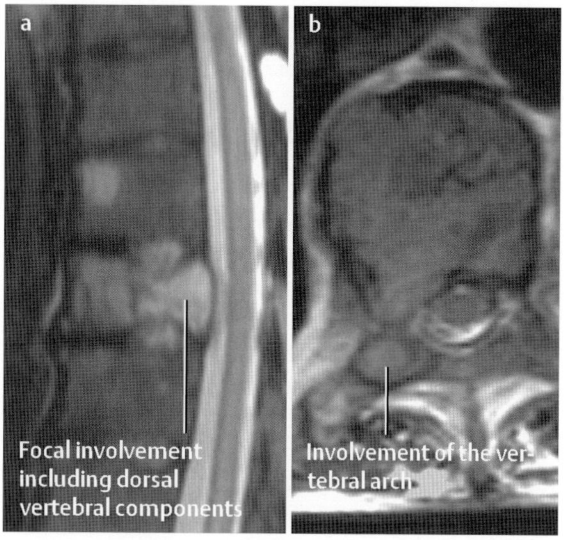

Fig. 4.**9** Atypical plasmocytoma, MRI. **a** STIR sequence: high signal focal involvement including dorsal vertebral components. **b** T2-weighted TSE sequence indicating involvement of the vertebral arch.

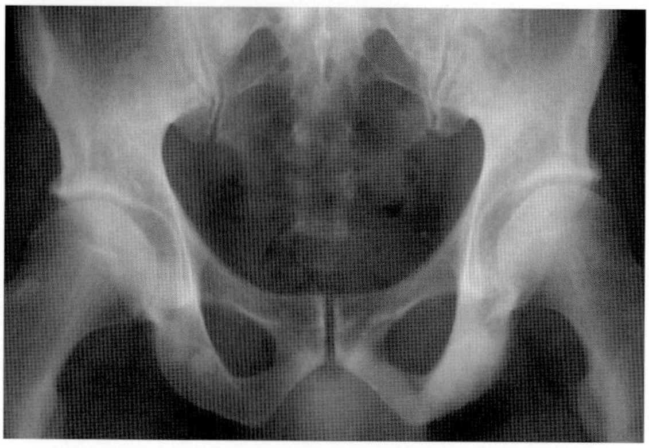

Fig. 4.**10** POEMS syndrome with osteosclerosis.

Leukemias

■ Leukemias consist of autonomous proliferations of hematopoietic cells together with a blocked differentiation caused by neoplastic transformation of the pluripotent hematopoietic stem cells with variable involvement of different cell types. Based on the lineage of the proliferating cell types, lymphatic and myelocytic leukemias are differentiated, each following either an acute or chronic course. ■

CLINIC The clinical signs of **acute** leukemia are manifestations of ineffective hematopoiesis: anemia, hemorrhage, infection, fever. The **chronic** leukemias are clinically dominated by organ infiltration: hepatosplenomegaly, lymphadenopathy (with chronic lymphocytic leukemia), and bone marrow infiltration with anemia. The late stages are characterized by increased susceptibility to infections.

Age distribution: The majority of patients are older than 60 years, and chronic leukemias are rare in children. Acute leukemias can occur at any age, but are most prevalent in patients under 20 (acute lymphocytic leukemia) and over 60 (acute myelocytic leukemia) years of age.

Acute Leukemia in Children

X-RAY Radiologic findings include diffuse osteoporosis, radiolucent metaphyseal bands, osteolytic lesions, periosteal reaction, and osteoporosis (Figs. 4.**11**, 4.**12**). Sutural diastasis of the skull is another, though rarely observed, finding.

Diffuse osteoporosis: Generalized diffuse osteoporosis is always a suspicious finding in children. This process can lead to vertebral compression fractures (Fig. 4.**13**).

Radiolucent metaphyseal bands: These are probably caused by an altered circulation that interferes with regular osteogenesis. If seen after the second year of life, radiolucent metaphyseal bands are fairly characteristic of leukemia. In addition, bands of increased density can be observed adjacent to the radiolucent bands (Fig. 4.**11**).

Osteolytic lesions: These can be observed as permeative or moth-eaten destruction in both tubular and flat bones. Metaphyseal radiolucencies can extend into the diaphysis. Furthermore, osseous destruction can affect the skull, pelvis, ribs, and shoulder girdle (Fig. 4.**12**).

Periosteal reaction: These can accompany lytic lesions and are induced by subperiosteal infiltration by leukemic cells and hemorrhage. Periosteal reaction appears most frequently along the long tubular bones (Fig. 4.**11**).

DD **Radiolucent metaphyseal bands** can also develop with other pediatric systemic disorders such as toxoplasmosis, rubella, cytomegaly, juvenile chronic polyarthritis, rickets, and neuroblastomas. They can also rarely be seen after methotrexate therapy as a result of arrested osteoblastic activity.

In addition, osteolytic lesions and periosteal reactions can be observed in children with sickle cell anemia, metastases (retinoblastoma, embryonal rhabdomyosarcoma) and infections.

Chronic Leukemia in Adulthood

X-RAY The chronic types of leukemia induce less severe and less extensive osseous and articular manifestations than the acute types. The dominating feature is bone marrow hyperplasia with diffuse osteoporosis. Discrete osteolytic lesions (skull and long tubular bones) develop in only 3% of cases (Fig. 4.**14**).

Articular changes are found only in the late stages and include secondary gout, septic arthritis, osteomyelitis, and avascular necrosis (Fig. 4.**16**).

Rare manifestations are large destructive changes, periosteal reactions, acro-osteolysis, discrete subperiosteal erosions, and focal or diffuse osteosclerosis.

CT This is useful primarily for detecting subtle osseous lesions.

MRI The MRI findings are the same as found with other infiltrative disorders such as plasmocytoma, lymphoma, or metastases. These are decreased signal intensity on T1-weighted and increased signal intensity on T2-weighted sequences relative to the normal bone marrow (Fig. 4.**15**).

Above all, MRI can assess the extent of the leukemic process, including any possible soft-tissue involvement, and detect complications such as pathologic fractures, ischemic necrosis (after therapy), or cord compression in cases with vertebral involvement (Fig. 4.**16**). Thus far, MRI has not been used in the clinical setting to monitor the course of the disease and the effectiveness of therapy.

Glossary

Chloroma (granulocytic sarcoma): Local tumor of immature myeloblasts or lymphoblasts with a predilection for bone, periosteum, soft tissues, lymph nodes, and skin.

The radiographic findings of intraosseous infiltration include lytic lesions, especially in the skull, spine, ribs, long tubular bones, and sternum.

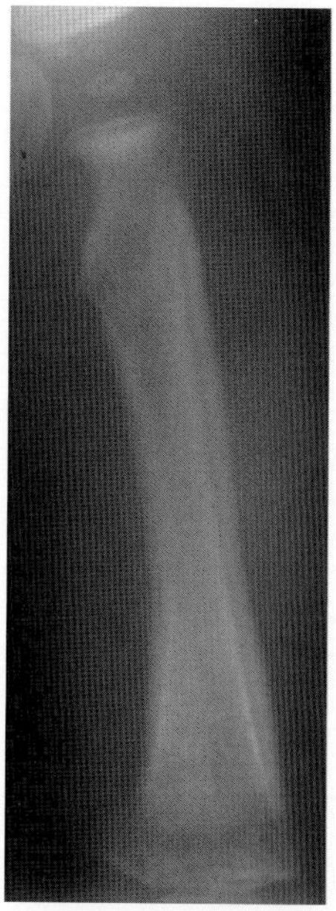

Fig. 4.**11** Acute leukemia in childhood with characteristic radiographic findings: marrow expansion, radiolucent metaphyseal bands, marked periosteal reaction, and lack of normal trabeculae.

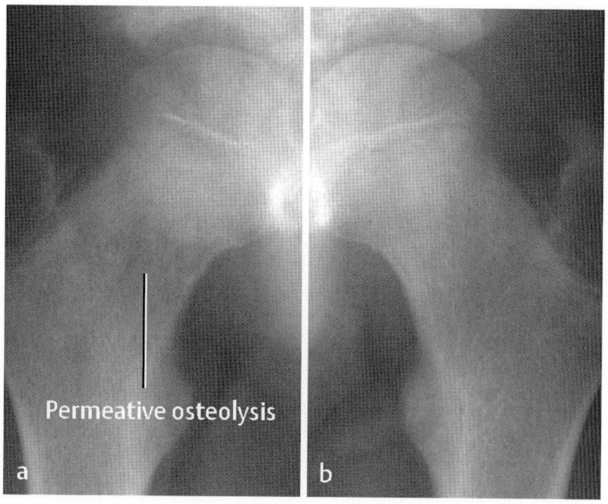

Fig. 4.**12** Acute lymphatic leukemia. **a** Small permeative osteolytic foci in the right femur (MRI showed diffuse bone marrow involvement). **b** Normal contralateral femur for comparison.

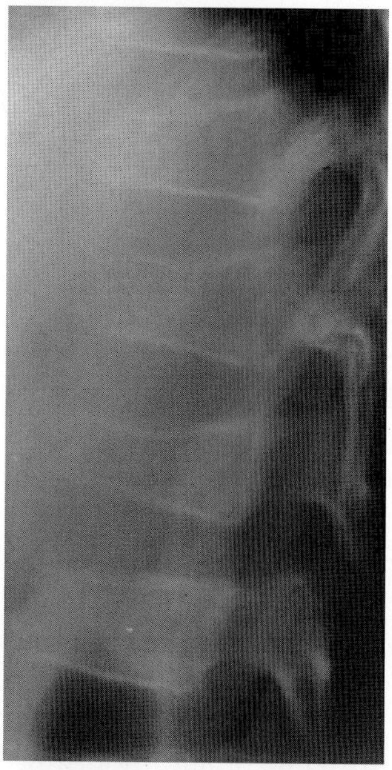

Fig. 4.**13** Acute leukemia in childhood with involvement of the spine: extensive osteoporosis with vertebral compression fracture.

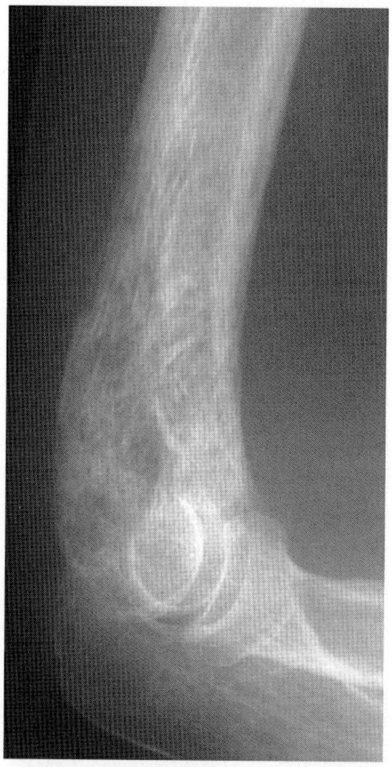

Fig. 4.**14** Chronic myelogenous leukemia with blast crisis. Moth-eaten osteolytic destruction of the marrow space and cortex.

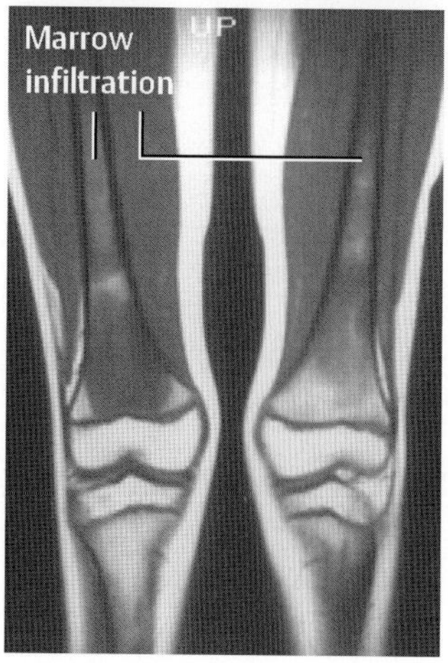

Fig. 4.**15** Marrow infiltration in acute lymphocytic leukemia. T1-weighted SE sequence: clinical suspicion of osteomyelitis with pain in the left thigh and normal radiographs. The lack of soft-tissue reaction does not favor osteomyelitis.

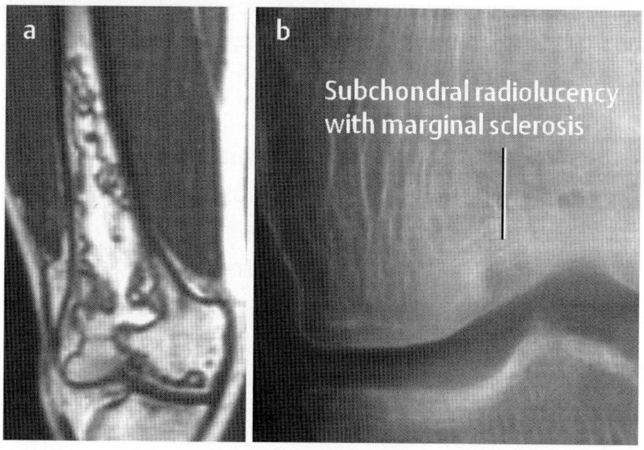

Fig. 4.**16** Acute lymphocytic leukemia following methotrexate therapy.
a T1-weighted SE sequence: typical geographic bone infarct.
b Conventional tomography of the knee: osteonecrosis.

Malignant Lymphoma

■ This is a frequent tumorous lesion, most commonly occurring within lymph nodes, and spread lymphogenously and hematogenously. Malignant lymphomas are subdivided into two main groups: Hodgkin disease and the somewhat more frequent non-Hodgkin lymphoma. ■

PATH The classification of Hodgkin disease and non-Hodgkin lymphoma (NHL) and any subclassification of either type is done histologically and is of the utmost clinical importance because of the different growth patterns. Skeletal manifestations occur in about 20% of patients overall (up to 40% in NHL) and usually reflect the systemic spread of the process.

CLINIC Lymphadenopathy and hepatosplenomegaly are the dominating findings. Frequent symptoms include fever, night sweats, and weight loss ('B symptoms'), which are often associated with a less favorable prognosis.

Age distribution: Hodgkin disease has two characteristic age peaks, one in early adulthood and the other late in life. The age distribution of non-Hodgkin lymphomas depends on the subtype. Men are affected slightly more frequently than women are.

Location: The lesions are most frequently encountered in the spine, pelvis, ribs, and proximal femur and somewhat less frequently in the sternum, clavicle, and scapula. Multiple lesions are slightly more common than solitary lesions.

Prognosis: Determined by subtype and stage at the time of diagnosis. Hodgkin disease has a cure rate of about 70% after combination radiotherapy and chemotherapy.

X-RAY Osteoblastic or osteolytic lesions or a combination of these two are seen (Table 4.**2**). Osteolytic lesions are frequently indistinct in outline and occur preferentially along the long tubular bones with concomitant periosteal reaction. Pathologic fractures and parosseous soft-tissue components are frequent (Figs. 4.**17** – 4.**19**).

Therapy-induced findings: Chemotherapy combined with corticosteroids can cause avascular necrosis within 1 to 3 years after initiation of the therapy and this complication is most commonly seen in the femoral and humeral heads. Methotrexate in particular can cause 'methotrexate osteopathy' consisting of pain, osteoporosis, increased fracture risk, growth lines, and metaphyseal bands of increased and decreased radiolucencies. The pathogenesis is undetermined, but at present, altered circulation is considered the most likely cause.

Table 4.**2** Radiologic manifestations of malignant lymphomas in relation to anatomic location

Location	Manifestation
Pelvis	Multiple well-demarcated osteolytic lesions, with or without sclerosis
Ribs, sternum	Osseous destruction with expansion and periosteal reaction (lamellated or spiculated)
Spine	Predominantly lytic lesions, with possible vertebral compressions. Rarely, mixed or mottled sclerotic lesions or diffuse sclerosis (ivory vertebra of Hodgkin disease)

! The radiographic features of Hodgkin disease and NHL are variable but essentially the same in both conditions except that osteoblastic changes develop more frequently in Hodgkin disease (occurring in up to 40% of all bone lesions).

NUC Bone scintigraphy is better in determining bone destruction in the malignant lymphomas than in plasmocytoma. However, the bone scan is inferior to MRI and has a very low sensitivity for lesions in the axial skeleton.

MRI MRI is the method of choice for evaluating the extent of bone marrow infiltration and for detecting complications, especially in cases with bone marrow involvement without associated bone destruction. The T1-weighted images usually show uniform or slightly heterogeneous decrease in signal intensity. The T2-weighted images exhibit increased signal intensity, especially on the fat-suppressed sequences (Fig. 4.**20**, 4.**21**).

DD **Metastases:** No radiographically distinctive criteria.

Primary bone tumors (osteogenic sarcoma, Ewing sarcoma): These tumors are singular, monostotic tumors.

! If the underlying primary disease is already known, differential diagnostic problems rarely arise. Radiography plays an important role in the detection of osteolytic lesions requiring therapy (stability).

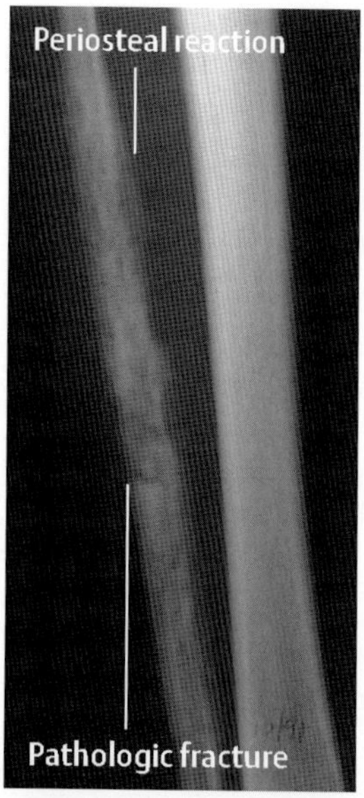

Fig. 4.**17** Malignant lymphoma. Extensive periosteal reaction, expansion, and thoroughly irregular trabecular structure and cortical destruction.

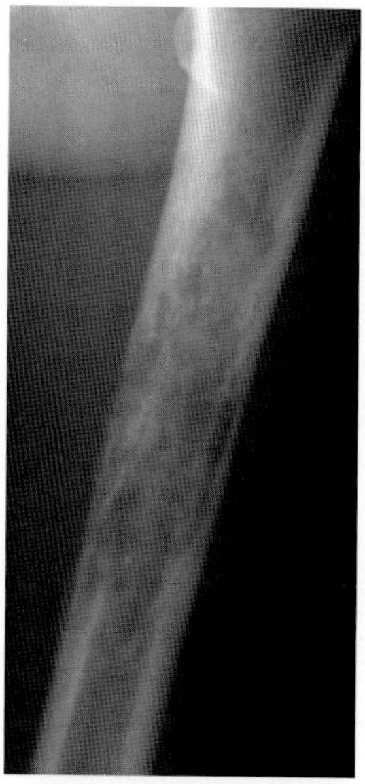

Fig. 4.**18** Non-Hodgkin lymphoma. Moth-eaten osteolytic foci with cortical destruction.

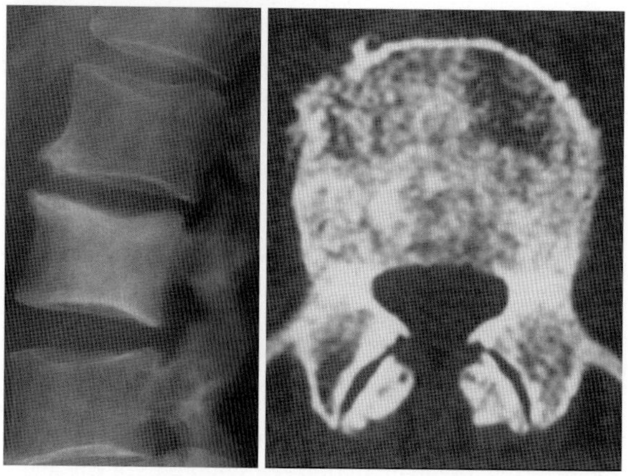

Fig. 4.**19** Non-Hodgkin lymphoma. **a** Homogeneous density on conventional radiograph. **b** CT reveals patchy densities intermixed with radiolucencies.

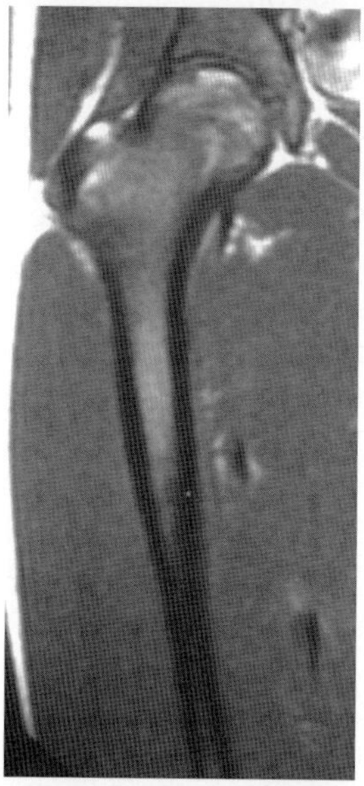

Fig. 4.**20** Hodgkin disease with diffuse bone marrow involvement in a 21-year-old male patient. T1-weighted SE sequence. A diffuse decrease in signal intensity is seen in the femur. Hematopoietic marrow can be seen in the proximal femur at the age of 21 years, but the lack of fatty marrow in the epiphysis is definitely abnormal at this age.

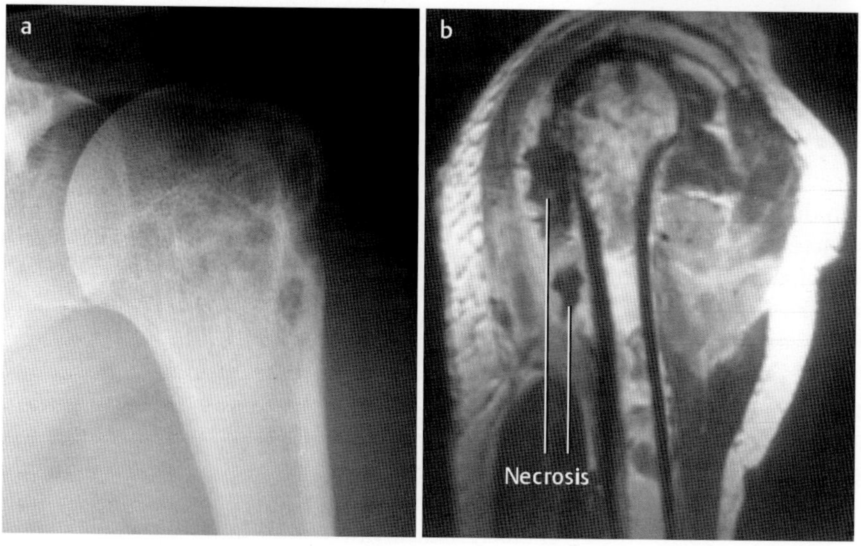

Fig. 4.**21** Non-Hodgkin lymphoma, Stage IV.
a Destruction of the proximal humerus.
b The extent of the soft-tissue component can be appreciated only on MRI (T1-weighted SE sequence after enhancement). The signal voids correspond to areas of tissue necrosis.

Anemias

■ Anemias are caused by impaired production of hemoglobin or erythrocytes, or increased destruction or loss of erythrocytes. The classification of the anemias is based on the underlying pathophysiologic mechanism. The most characteristic osseous manifestations are found in sickle cell anemia and thalassemia. Less prominent and specific changes of the bone and bone marrow develop with iron-deficiency anemia, hereditary spherocytosis, aplastic anemia, and Fanconi anemia. ■

Normal bone marrow development and corresponding MRI findings: The bone marrow of the newborn contains little fat and consists almost exclusively of red marrow. **Conversion** of red to yellow marrow begins in early childhood and progresses from the peripheral skeleton (beginning in the phalanges of the hands and feet) to the central (axial) skeleton. This conversion is completed around the age of 20 years with red marrow then confined to the spine, pelvis, skull, proximal humerus, and proximal femur. Apophyses and epiphyses of the adult skeleton **always** contain yellow bone marrow.

MRI Yellow bone marrow (fat): short T1 and long T2 relaxation times produce a high signal intensity on T1-weighted and T2-weighted SE sequences.

Red bone marrow (higher content of protein and water): The signal intensity may be increased or decreased on T1-weighted and T2-weighted SE-sequences in comparison to muscle tissue, but always shows decreased signal intensity relative to fat. Variable combinations of yellow and red marrow can be encountered, especially in the vertebrae of adults.

Reconversion:

In adults with chronic oxygen deficiency, the proportion of red bone marrow increases. This **reconversion** begins in the spine and flat bones, and follows a patchy or homogeneous pattern.

Bone marrow reconversion accompanies all types of anemias, but can also be present in smokers and patients with pulmonary dysfunction or cardiac insufficiency. Even marathon runners occasionally show evidence of reconversion.

MRI It is difficult to differentiate the MRI findings of reconverted bone marrow from those of pathologic bone marrow processes such as polycythemia vera, hemochromatosis, Gaucher disease, diffuse leukemia and lymphomatous infiltration, myelofibrosis, plasmocytoma, and disseminated metastases.

Sickle Cell Anemia

PATH Sickle cell anemia is an autosomal dominant hereditary hemoglobinopathy. The pathologic hemoglobin S (HbS) induces erythrocytes to acquire a sickle shape in the presence of a fall in pH or oxygen tension. This 'sickling' effect increases blood viscosity and leads to intravascular stasis, which increases the acidosis and hypoxia. Finally, this vicious circle leads to thrombosis and infarction.

The radiologic findings reflect:

1. Marrow hyperplasia: the hypercellularity of the bone marrow is a reaction to the chronic hemolysis. The marrow cavities enlarge, causing trabecular rarefaction.
2. Vascular occlusion: epiphyseal osteonecroses and diaphyseal infarcts of the tubular bones are common complications of sickle cell anemia. The peripheral soft tissues can also show vascular occlusion with secondary hemorrhage and infarcts.
3. Osteomyelitis frequently accompanies sickle cell anemia (common organisms are *Staphylococcus aureus* or *Salmonella typhi*).

CLINIC The clinical course is variable, but homozygous patients only reach middle age even with excellent medical care. The gradual or rapid course of the disease is determined by the destruction of erythrocytes and recurrent organ infarction, the symptoms of which include fever, jaundice, nausea, vomiting, and abdominal pain. Symptomatic crises affecting joints and bones usually occur in the second or third decades.

X-RAY Bone marrow hyperplasia causes diffuse increased radiolucency (= osteoporosis), thickened trabeculae, and marrow expansion of the tubular bones, mandible, and diploë of the skull (Figs. 4.**22**, 4.**23**). Vascular occlusions cause bone infarcts, epiphyseal osteonecroses, and depression of the end plates of the vertebral bodies.

! The 'H-shaped vertebra' is fairly characteristic of sickle cell anemia. In contrast to rounded concavities seen in the osteoporotic 'codfish vertebra', the vertebral end plates exhibit a step-like or squared indentation (Fig. 4.**24**).

Especially in infants, osteonecroses of the small tubular bones lead to dactylitis (so-called 'hand-foot syndrome') in infants and young children. Characteristically there is diffuse marked periosteal

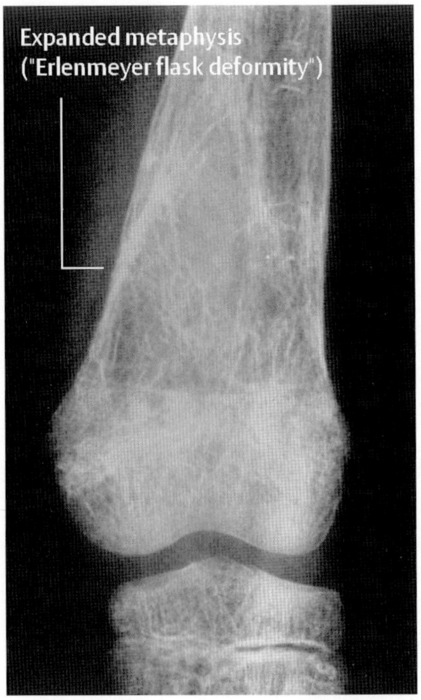

Fig. 4.**22** Sickle cell anemia. Trabecular thickening with 'coarsened' osseous texture, and expansion of the cortex from the hyperplasia of the bone marrow ('Erlenmeyer flask deformity').

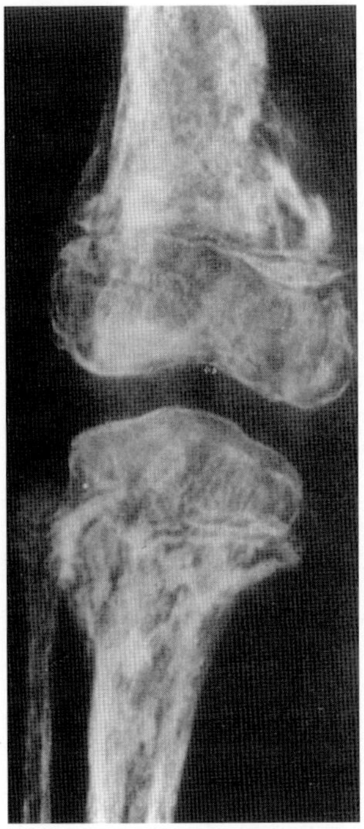

Fig. 4.**23** Sickle cell anemia. Predominantly patchy osteosclerotic lesions attributed to infarcts.

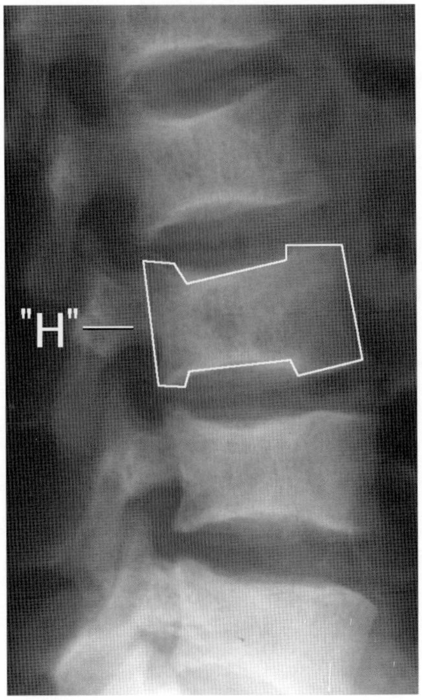

Fig. 4.**24** H-shaped vertebra in sickle cell anemia.

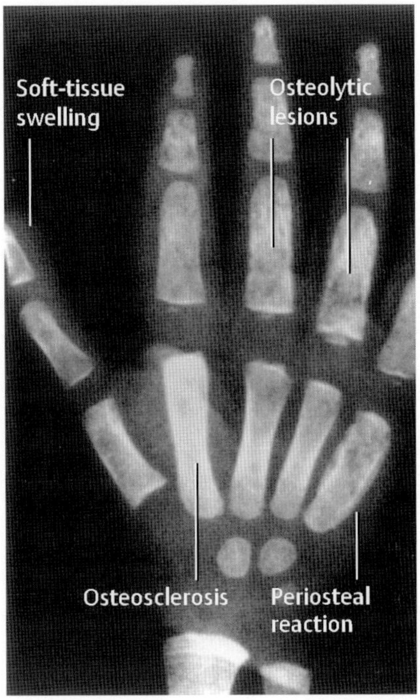

Fig. 4.**25** Dactylitis in a child with sickle cell anemia.

reaction and a mixed pattern of osteoblastic (osteosclerotic) and osteolytic changes, and soft-tissue swelling. The main differential diagnosis is infection, which can often be excluded only by clinical and laboratory findings (Fig. 4.**25**).

NUC Bone scintigraphy plays only a minor role in the diagnostic evaluation. Together with bone marrow scintigraphy, the erythrocyte and iron kinetics measured with radioactive chromium and iron can provide information about the effectiveness of the erythropoiesis and site of hemolytic destruction. This information can also be used to decide whether splenectomy is indicated.

MRI MRI shows diffuse bone marrow reconversion and can detect changes such as infarcts, epiphyseal osteonecroses and, above all, osteomyelitis induced by sickle cell anemia (Fig. 4.**28**).

Thalassemias

Thalassemias are characterized by deficient or lack of synthesis of fetal globulin or, less frequently, the alpha-globulin chain of the hemoglobin molecule. Since fetal HbF contains alpha chains, alpha thalassemia also affects the newborn. In contrast, beta thalassemia only becomes manifest later in life after HbF has been replaced.

PATH Marrow hyperplasia and extramedullary hematopoiesis are the dominating findings. Impaired growth, fractures, infarcts, and epiphyseal osteonecrosis may occur but are less frequent than in sickle cell anemia.

CLINIC The homozygous type is characterized by severe anemia, massive hepatosplenomegaly, and often death in early childhood. The most severe type (lack of alpha chain synthesis) causes 'hydrops fetalis'. The heterozygotic type often leads only to mild clinical symptoms of anemia.

X-RAY The marrow hyperplasia can cause the characteristic and nearly pathognomonic **'hair on end'** appearance of the cranial vault (Fig. 4.**26**). It is characterized by radially thickened trabeculae that traverse the widened diploic space and external table. The facial bones may also be hyperplastic. The phalanges are 'squared' and the long tubular bones are expanded, causing the **'Erlenmeyer flask deformity'** (Fig. 4.**22**).

MRI Indications and signal pattern are like those of sickle cell anemia. Extramedullary hematopoiesis can present as a 'space-occupying' lesion (Fig. 4.**29**).

NUC What has been stated for sickle cell anemia (page 214) also applies to the thalassemias.

Rare Types

Rare types of anemia include hereditary spherocytosis and hereditary elliptocytosis. Their manifestations are essentially the same as those found in sickle cell anemia or thalassemia.

Aplastic Anemia

The bone marrow is acellular or hypocellular. A stem cell defect and possibly an additional stromal defect can lead to marrow hyperplasia or aplasia. Aplastic anemias can have many causes: radiation, paroxysmal nocturnal hemoglobinuria, Fanconi anemia (congenital), hepatitis, pregnancy, thymoma, and medications. Therapy with erythropoietin can lead to a marrow regeneration.

MRI is valuable for diagnosing and following the disease and shows increased signal intensity on T1-weighted sequences caused by heightened fat deposition (Fig. 4.**30**). Hypointense foci can develop during therapy as a manifestation of active marrow. The major differential diagnostic criteria of the anemias are shown in Table 4.**3**.

Table 4.**3** Differential diagnosis of anemias by radiologic signs

Radiologic findings	Differential diagnosis
Extramedullary hematopoiesis	Fibrous dysplasia Tumors
Diffuse osteoporosis	Gaucher disease
Thickened calvaria	Fibrous dysplasia Hyperostosis frontalis interna Paget disease Hyperparathyroidism
Epi- and diaphyseal infarcts	Corticosteroid therapy Collagenosis Idiopathic
'Squared phalanges' (with or without periosteal reaction)	Tuberculosis

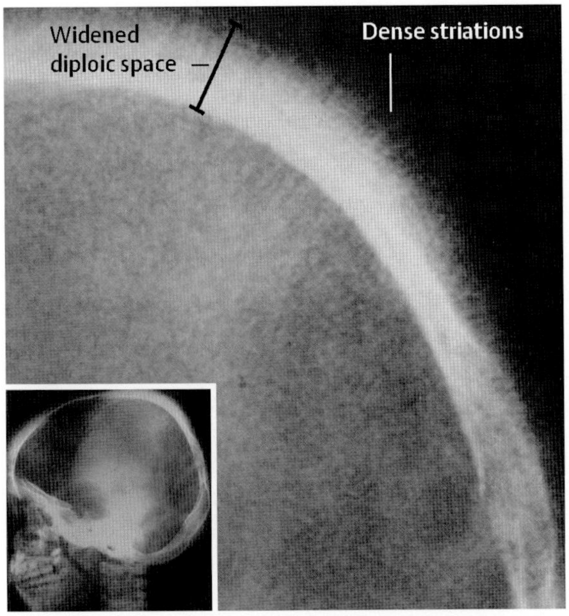

Fig. 4.26 Thalassemia. Typical 'hair-on-end' skull.

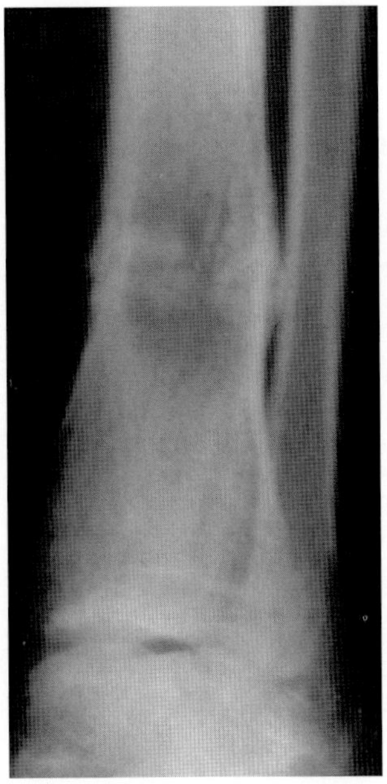

Fig. 4.27 Sickle cell anemia with infarct.

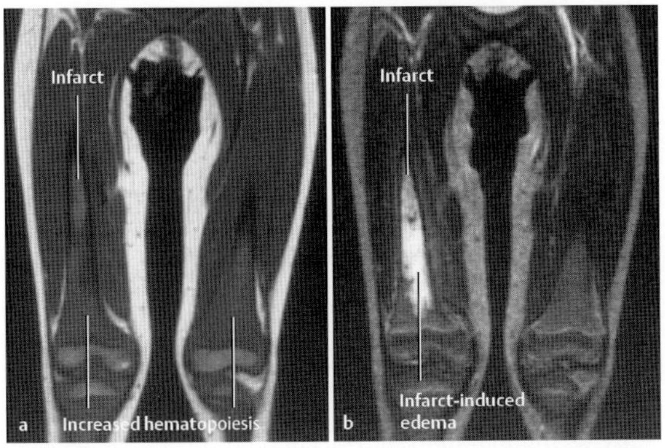

Fig. 4.28 Acute infarct in sickle cell anemia in an 8-year-old boy.

a T1-weighted image: the femoral metaphyses show low signal intensity. (They should be bright because of medullary fat at this age.)

b T2-weighted SE image: infarct-induced edema. The differential diagnosis of osteomyelitis is difficult to exclude in many instances. Hint: infarcts generally lack soft-tissue edema.

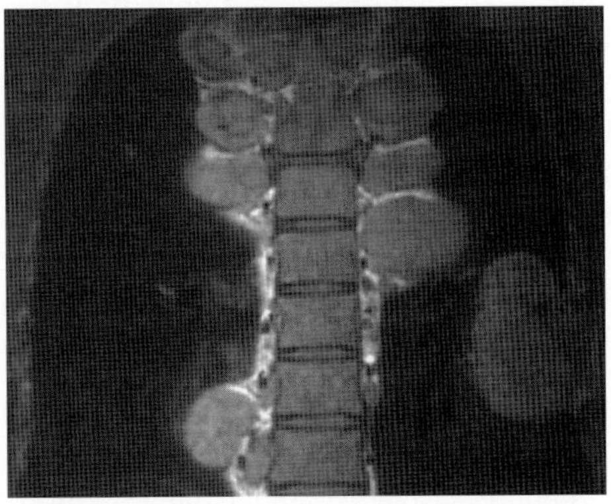

Fig. 4.29 Extramedullary hematopoiesis in thalassemia. Note the multiple paravertebral soft-tissue masses.

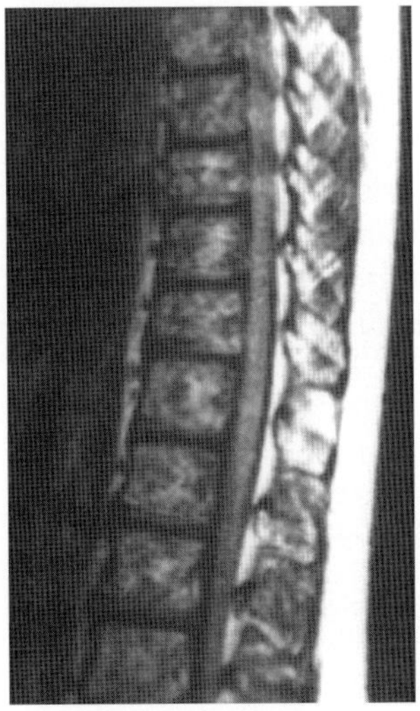

Fig. 4.30 Aplastic anemia in a 16-year-old patient. Fat islands (bright signal) in the vertebral bone marrow (which should be homogeneously dark).

Myelofibrosis

Myelofibrosis is a rare disorder occurring in middle-aged to elderly patients and is characterized by fibrosis and subsequent sclerosis of the bone marrow. The disorder has a predilection for the spine, pelvis, skull, ribs, and proximal femora and humeri.

PATH There are two major groups: primary types (idiopathic) and secondary types (e.g., associated with leukemias, malignant lymphomas). Compensatory extramedullary hematopoiesis can develop, mainly in the liver and spleen.

CLINIC Weakness, weight loss, abdominal pain, vomiting, vertigo, hepatosplenomegaly, and purpura. The diagnosis is established by bone marrow biopsy.

X-RAY Diffuse or focal osteoblastic lesions are dominant, and osteoporosis, osteolytic lesions, and cortical thickening are less frequent. Vertebral bodies often show increased density at the end plates (Figs. 4.**31**, 4.**32**).

! Osteosclerosis of the axial skeleton together with hepatosplenomegaly in patients of middle or later age should suggest the diagnosis of myelofibrosis.

MRI Bone marrow fibrosis causes decreased signal intensity on T1-weighted and T2-weighted SE-sequences (Fig. 4.**32**).

DD Lymphoma and leukemia lead to a less-pronounced sclerosis and usually are monostotic or oligostotic. Mastocytosis has the closest resemblance to myelofibrosis, although there are no distinguishing radiologic features. It is impossible to determine radiographically whether osteosclerosis seen with malignant lymphoma or leukemia is a primary or secondary condition.

Osteosclerosis without splenomegaly should suggest one of the following disorders: metastases, fluorosis, Paget disease, renal osteodystrophy, or osteopetrosis. Osteoblastic metastases are less symmetric, more diffuse, and frequently associated with osteolytic lesions. Carcinoid metastases most frequently produce a purely diffuse osteosclerosis.

Glossary

Mastocytosis (Figs. 4.**33, 34**): This is a disorder characterized by proliferation of mast cells and resultant skeletal changes. The clinical presentation includes urticaria pigmentosa, nausea, and vomiting induced by intermittent release of histamines. The skeletal manifestation of mastocytosis consists of diffuse (rarely focal) osteopenia (possibly the effect of histamine release) or focal or diffuse osteosclerosis (= osseous reaction to mast cells infiltrating the bone marrow).

Polycythemia vera: This is a neoplastic transformation of a hematopoietic stem cell with proliferation of erythropoiesis and involvement of granulogenesis and megakaryogenesis. It is characterized by hepatosplenomegaly, thrombosis, and a hemorrhagic diathesis. The marrow shows generalized hyperplasia and diffuse osteoporosis, and secondary myelofibrosis can lead to diffuse and localized osteosclerosis. Complications are osteonecrosis (usually of the femoral head) caused by intravascular thrombosis. It can be accompanied by hyperuricemia and secondary gout (5%–8%).

Lipidoses

Lipidoses or lysosomal storage diseases are caused by genetically determined defects in the lysosomal enzymes with deposits of incompletely degraded insoluble metabolites within the lysosomes. The clinical manifestations are dominated by storage in the CNS, liver, and spleen.

Glossary

Gaucher disease (Synonym: glucocerebrosidosis, Fig. 4.**35**): This is a rare autosomal recessive disorder with accumulation of glucocerebrosides in the reticuloendothelial cells. The proliferation of so-called 'Gaucher cells' in the liver and spleen leads to hepatosplenomegaly. Accumulated Gaucher cells in the bone marrow produce osseous destruction, hematologic dysfunction, and articular changes. The typical radiologic findings include:

Osseous deformities: Expansion of the contour of the long tubular bones, most frequently affecting the distal femoral shaft, 'H-shaped' vertebrae (as seen with sickle cell anemia), **osteonecrosis** primarily affecting the femoral head, but also the humeral heads and tibial plateaus, **marrow involvement** with accumulation of Gaucher cells in the bone marrow, inducing cellular necrosis, fibrous proliferation, and trabecular resorption. Conventional radiographs show increased radiolucency of all tubular bones. Focal lesions appear as confined osteolytic foci or moth-eaten destruction. Reactive osteosclerosis can also be observed infrequently.

MRI: Its most important role is the detection of complications such as ischemia, necrosis, osteomyelitis, and vertebral fractures. On T1-weighted and T2-weighted SE sequences, there is decreased signal intensity relative to the normal bone marrow. Fat-suppressing sequences (STIR) show increased signal intensity, but the signal pattern and any possible enhancement following administration of contrast medium are determined by the activity of the disease and the degree of marrow infiltration by fibrosis and glucocerebroside-containing cells. MRI and scintigraphy have a high sensitivity, but only a low specificity in this disorder.

Niemann-Pick disease (Fig. 4.**36**): This is a rare hereditary disorder with extensive accumulation of lipids, especially sphingomyelin, in reticuloendothelial parenchymal cells. *Radiography:* Coarsened trabeculae, marrow expansion, and cortical thinning. Its radiographic appearance is similar to that of Gaucher disease, but there is no associated epiphyseal necrosis.

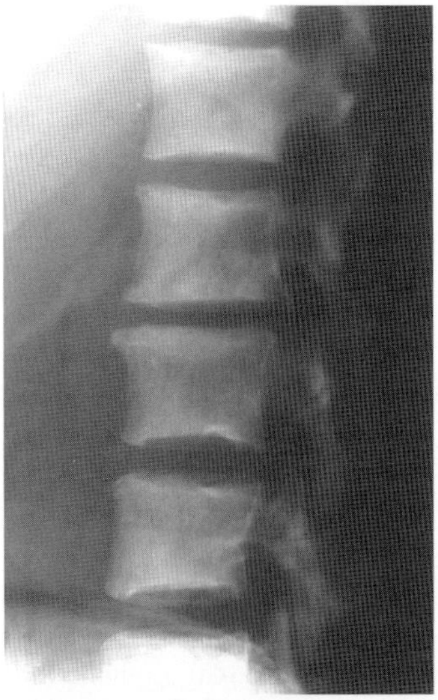

Fig. 4.**31** Diffuse sclerosis due to myelosclerosis. **Caution:** Diffuse processes are often difficult to recognize since normal bone for comparison is absent.

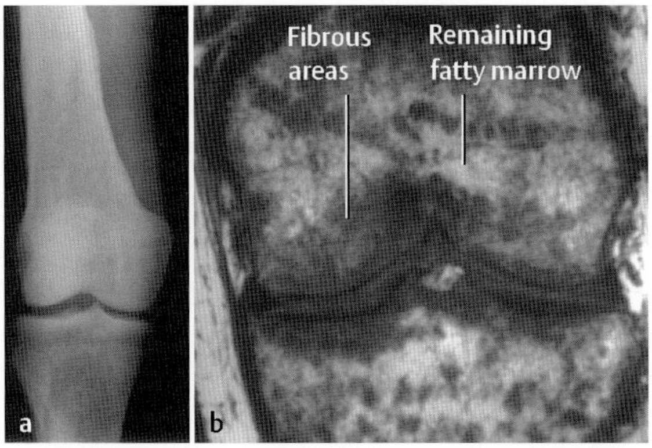

Fig. 4.**32** Myelofibrosis, osteosclerotic type. **a** Diffuse increased density and marked cortical thickening. **b** MRI (T1-SE sequence) shows fibrous areas as hypointensity within the normal hyperintense marrow fat.

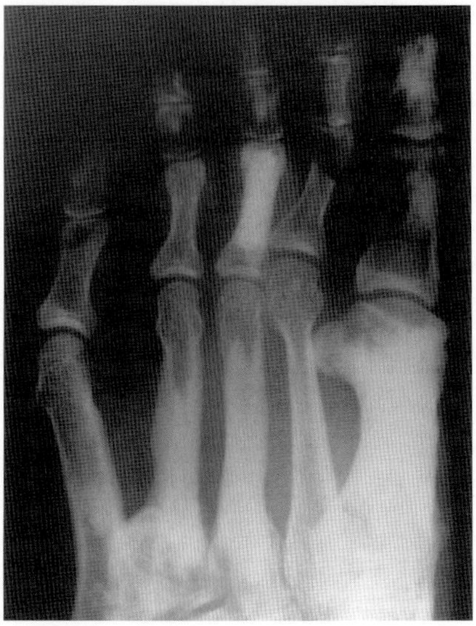

Fig. 4.**33** Mastocytosis with peripheral focal osteosclerosis. The finding is not specific, but the appearance and location are typical.

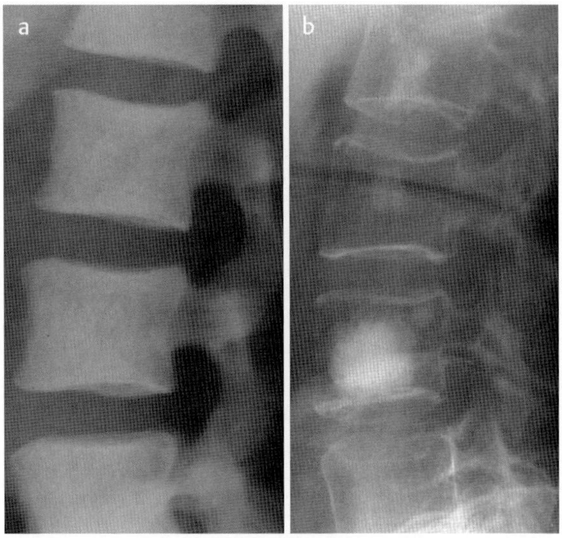

Fig. 4.**34** Different forms of sclerosis in mastocytosis. **a** Diffuse osteosclerosis, **b** Focal osteosclerosis.

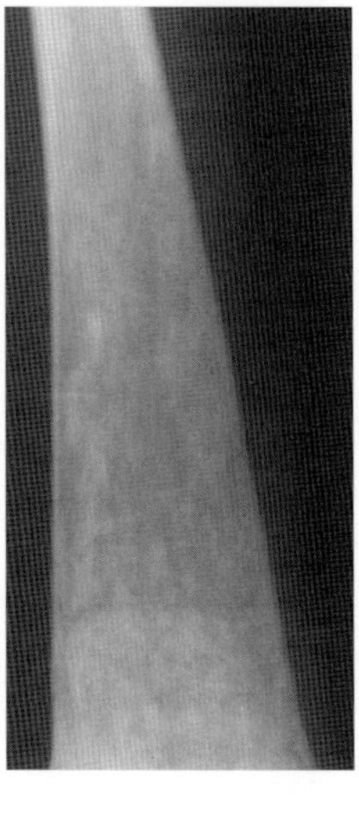

Fig. 4.**35** Gaucher disease. Expansion of the bone with cortical thinning and delicate osteosclerotic areas.

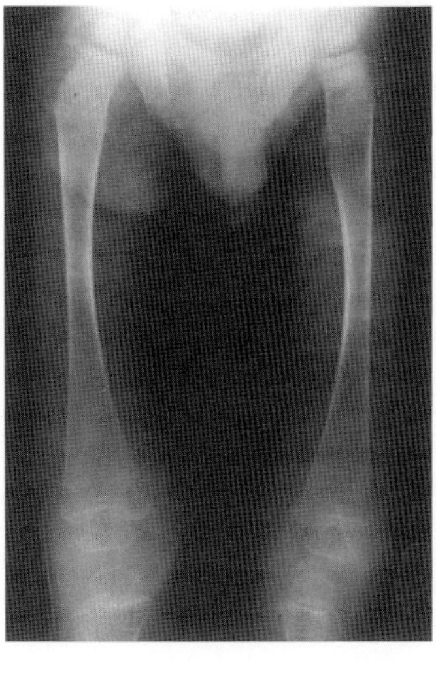

Fig. 4.**36** Niemann-Pick disease. Diffuse marrow expansion, marked osteoporosis and cortical thinning. No epiphyseal osteonecrosis (differential diagnosis: Gaucher disease).

5 Ischemic Bone Disease

Osteonecrosis

Synonyms: avascular osteonecrosis, aseptic osteonecrosis, necrotic bone disease.

Definition: Since in the area of ischemic bone disease there are many terms for the same condition, the term osteonecrosis is best defined as follows:

> ■ Bone is an organ composed of mineralized and nonmineralized tissue. Osteonecrosis is a disease that causes bone death. ■

It has become customary to apply the term osteonecrosis to ischemic injury to the epiphysis and the term bone infarct to ischemic injury to the diaphysis and metaphysis of the tubular bones.

A special manifestation of ischemic bone disease primarily involves the articular cartilage:
- Osteochondritis dissecans, the most common type in adolescents, and
- Legg-Calvé-Perthes disease, the commonest type in infancy.

The basic aspects of ischemic bone disease, such as etiology, pathophysiology, morphology, role of the different imaging methods, and staging, will be presented by using osteonecrosis of the hip, the most common form of osteonecrosis, as an example.

Osteonecrosis of the Hip

Synonym: avascular necrosis of the femoral head.

PATH **Epidemiology:** The peak incidence is at 40 years of age, and bilateral involvement occurs in 30%–70% of cases.

Etiology: The conditions that cause osseous ischemia are listed in Table 5.**1**. Most examples of avascular necrosis of the femoral head are believed to be caused by a variety of factors, and the exact relationship between the risk factors and vascular occlusion is still controversial.

Post-traumatic avascular necrosis of the femoral head (e.g., following a subcapital fracture of the femur or a hip dislocation) causes vascular disruption and acutely deficient perfusion of the femoral head.

The pathophysiologic model explaining the development of necrosis of the femoral head is well described. Recurrent ischemic attacks on bone are followed by an increase in intraosseous pressure. This increased pressure is probably due to edema, since bone marrow functionally represents a closed compartment. The intraosseous capillaries and venules are compromised by this increased pressure, resulting in the vicious circle found in the 'compartment syndrome' of the extremities.

Osseous necrosis can develop from four sources: arterial supply, venous drainage, intraluminal capillary obstruction, and compression of the capillaries and sinusoids in the marrow space (Table 5.**1**). **Course:** The ischemic necrosis passes through stages that can be quite variable in length and can last days to years (Table 5.**2**).

The **initial stage** is reversible, and the necrotic area is not demarcated. Vascular insufficiency is followed by ischemia-induced bone marrow edema, which increases intraosseous pressure. An ischemic period of 12–48 hours damages the bone marrow and, subsequently, the trabecular bone. Restoration of normal blood flow can prevent progression to frank necrosis, whereas persistent vascular insufficiency leads to a demarcation of the necrosis, either through confluence of several small necrotic areas or as an innately large necrotic region.

When this occurs, the **irreversible stage** has been reached. The subsequent course is primarily determined by the mechanical property of the necrosis, which in turn depends on the size of the necrotic area. If the necrosis is small and surrounded by buttressing reactive bone, the bone will not collapse, preventing a fracture of the subchondral plate and any intra-articular extension. A large necrotic area results in mechanical insufficiency of the osseous structure.

This **mechanical insufficiency** begins with a subchondral fracture above the necrosis, initially with the configuration of the femoral head being maintained.

The **late stage** is characterized by collapse of subchondral bone and articular cartilage, with subsequent degeneration that progresses to severe deformity and destruction of the joint.

CLINIC The clinical findings range from no complaints (silent hip) to slight pain on weight bearing to persistent pain with inability to walk. The complaints are usually seen with ischemic attacks, osseous fragmentation, and delayed degenerative changes.

A special manifestation of the initial stage of necrosis of the femoral head is the bone marrow edema syndrome.

Therapy: Untreated, 50% of cases develop fragmentation and destruction of the femoral head within 3 years. Early detection (with MRI) is of utmost importance since the reversible initial stage may heal with conservative therapy such as decompression. Furthermore, necrosis without fragmentation can be treated surgically with preservation of the head.

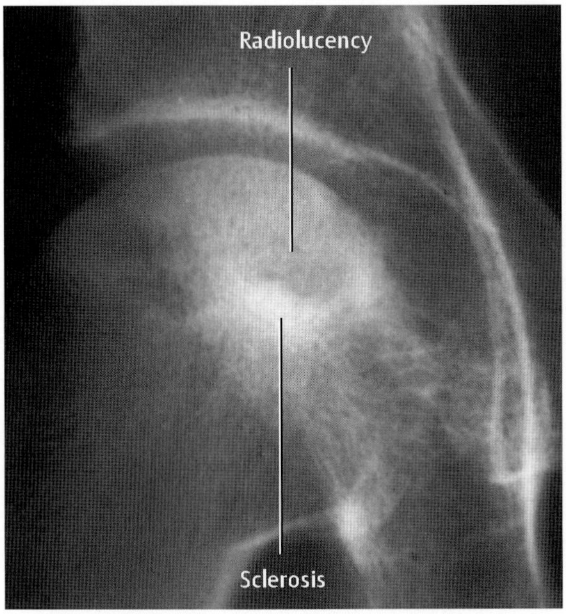

Fig. 5.**1** Typical and diagnostic radiographic features of an avascular necrosis of the femoral head with a localized subchondral radiolucency surrounded by a sclerotic rim (Stage: ARCO II).

Table 5.**1** Etiology of avascular necrosis of the femoral head

Affected vascular component	Etiology risk factors
Arterial	Fracture Hip dislocation Massive arterial embolism, recurrent fat embolism Vasculitis
Venous	Legg-Calvé-Perthes disease Massive venous thrombosis Idiopathic (?)
Intraosseous capillaries	Fat embolism Diabetes mellitus Vasculitis in systemic lupus erythematosus Sickle cell anemia Caisson disease (nitrogen bubbles)
Intraosseous vessels	Abnormal fat metabolism Hypertrophy of fatty tissue (corticosteroids, alcohol) Hyperemia Gaucher disease (glycosylceramide lipidosis)

Table 5.**2** Stages of avascular necrosis of the hip and corresponding radiographic findings according to ARCO. The crescent sign is radiolucent on the radiograph and shows increased signal intensity on the T2-weighted MR image (Mitchell et al., 1986)

Stage	Pathology	Radiography	MRI
0 (initial stage)	Ischemia, small necrotic area	Normal	Normal
I	Large necrotic area, edema	Normal	Bone marrow edema
Early II (irreversible stage)	Large demarcated necrotic area	Possible osteoporosis	Double line sign
Late II	Large demarcated necrotic area	Osteoporosis, osteolysis, demarcated sclerosis	Double line sign
III (mechanical insufficiency)	Fracture	Crescent sign, fracture	Crescent sign (subchondral fracture line)
IV (late stage)	Subchondral collapse, osteoarthritis	Subchondral collapse, secondary degeneration	Subchondral collapse, secondary degeneration

Prognosis: The best prognostic criterion is the percentage of the affected surface circumference of the femoral head. This measurement is best determined by CT or MRI. If the area is calculated to be

- < 30%, the avascular necrosis is stable,
- > 40%, the avascular necrosis has a poor prognosis, i.e., progression should be expected,
- 30%–40%, the avascular necrosis falls in the transitional range with an unpredictable outcome.

X-RAY Technical considerations: Radiographs should be obtained in the AP and lateral projections.

In early necrosis, a subtle **osteopenia** can be observed in the affected region of the femoral head (early Stage II). With progression, the necrosis appears as localized **osteolysis** or diffuse **osteoporosis, subchondral pseudocyst**, and **sclerosis** (Figs. 5.**1** – 5.**3**). The demarcated **band-like sclerosis** may be variable (Stage II). Diagnostic signs of avascular necrosis of the femoral head are the **subchondral location** and demarcation of these changes without signs of mass effect. The radiographic signs of an advanced necrosis are **subchondral fracture** (Stage III), **articular extension** (Fig. 5.**4**), and **secondary degenerative changes** with joint space narrowing and marginal osteophyte formation (Stage IV, Table 5.**2**).

In Stages 0 and I (ARCO), the radiographs are normal. In Stage II, radiographic findings are present, but are often too subtle to diagnose avascular necrosis. Since a negative radiographic finding is unreliable, conventional radiography is not suitable for the detection or exclusion of early avascular necrosis of the femoral head. However, it remains the first step in the diagnostic investigation since it can establish or exclude a variety of other diagnoses.

NUC The three-phase bone scan with Tc 99 m diphosphonate is used. Specific signs of avascular necrosis of the femoral head are decreased accumulation in the initial stage **('cold spot')** and at a later stage increased accumulation in the reactive border zone **('cold in hot spot')**. A frequent nonspecific sign is the **diffuse accumulation** of activity in the femoral head as a manifestation of bone repair (Fig. 5.**6**). The discrete but specific ('cold in hot spot') scintigraphic finding of bilateral avascular necrosis of the femoral head can easily be interpreted as a false-negative finding (Fig. 5.**7**).

A diffuse accumulation of activity in the femoral head with extension into the femoral neck and intertrochanteric region most likely represents bone marrow edema syndrome.

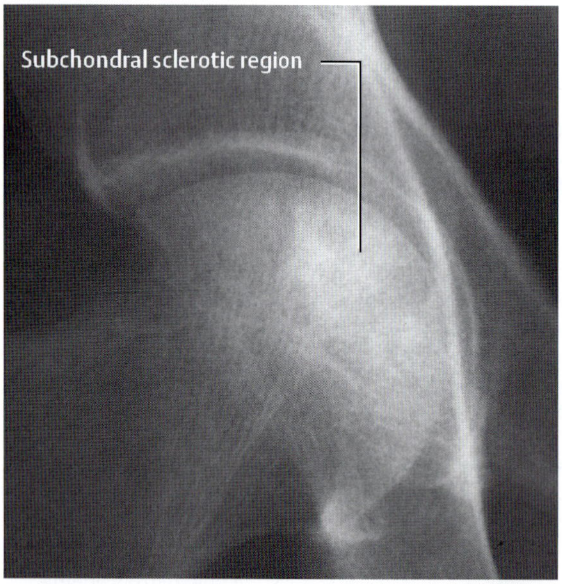

Fig. 5.**2** Small avascular necrotic area of the femoral head with a region of subchondral sclerosis.

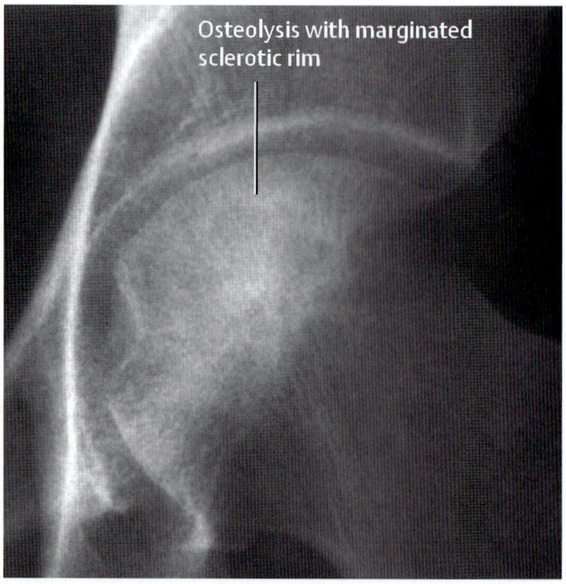

Fig. 5.**3** Avascular necrosis of the femoral head, recognized as osteolysis with a marginated sclerotic rim.

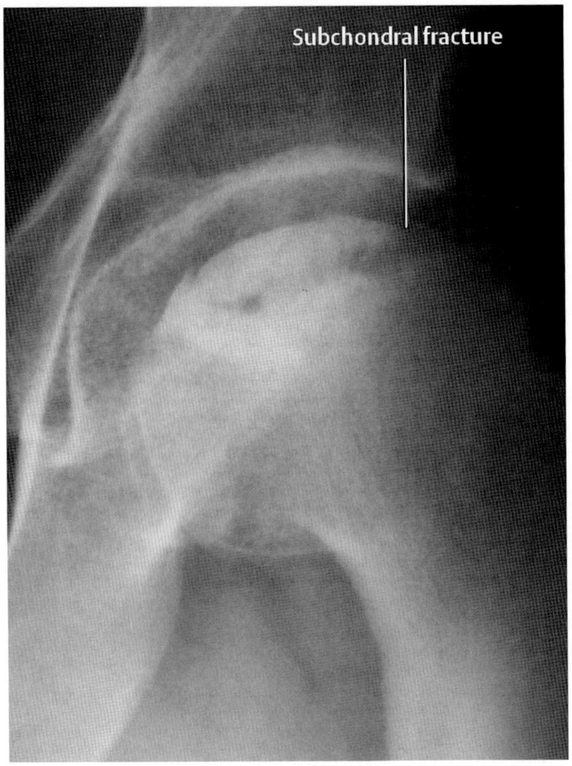

Fig. 5.**4** Avascular necrosis of the femoral head with subchondral fracture (ARCO III).

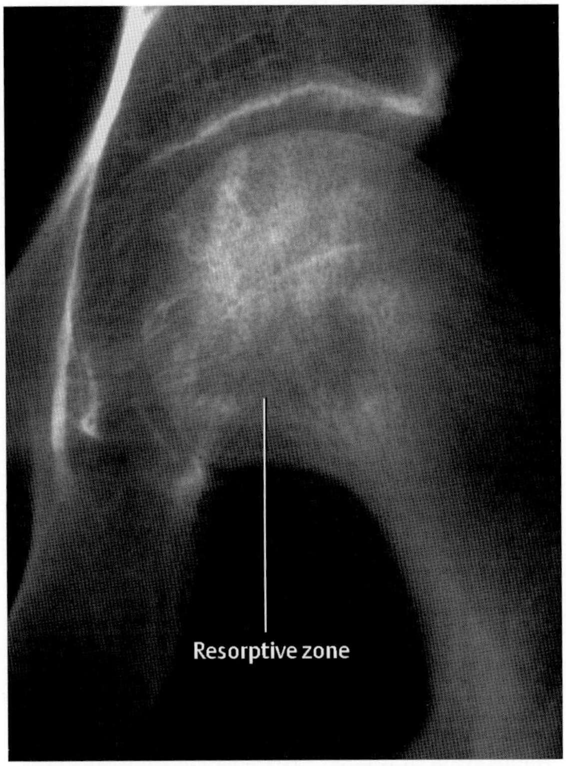

Fig. 5.**5** Avascular necrosis of the femoral head with mixed sclerosis and an especially pronounced region of resorption.

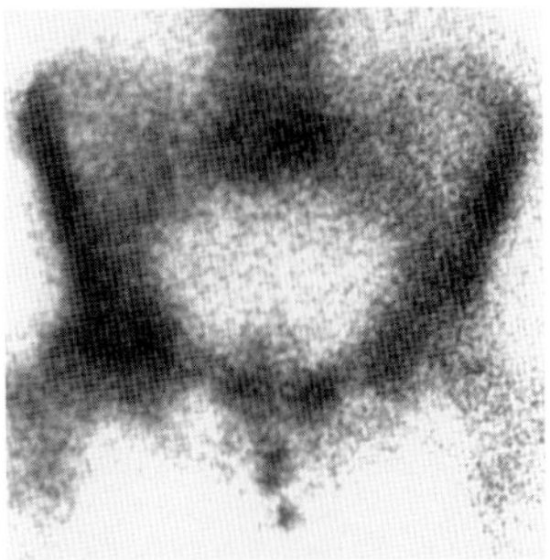

Fig. 5.**6** Bone scan of an avascular necrosis with diffuse uptake on the right (nonspecific).

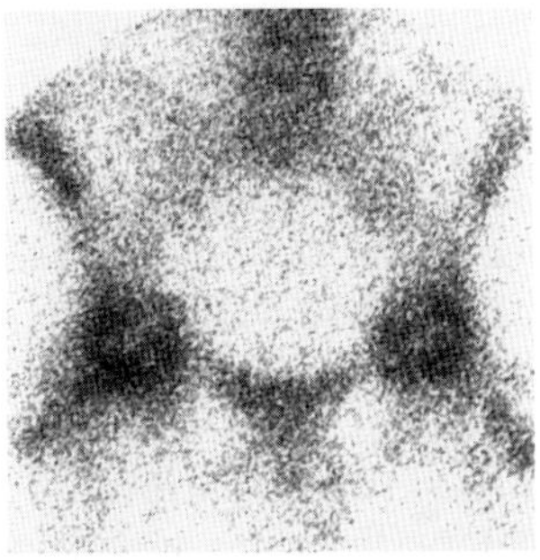

Fig. 5.**7** Bone scan with the specific sign of a bilateral avascular necrosis of the femoral head referred to as 'cold in hot spot'.

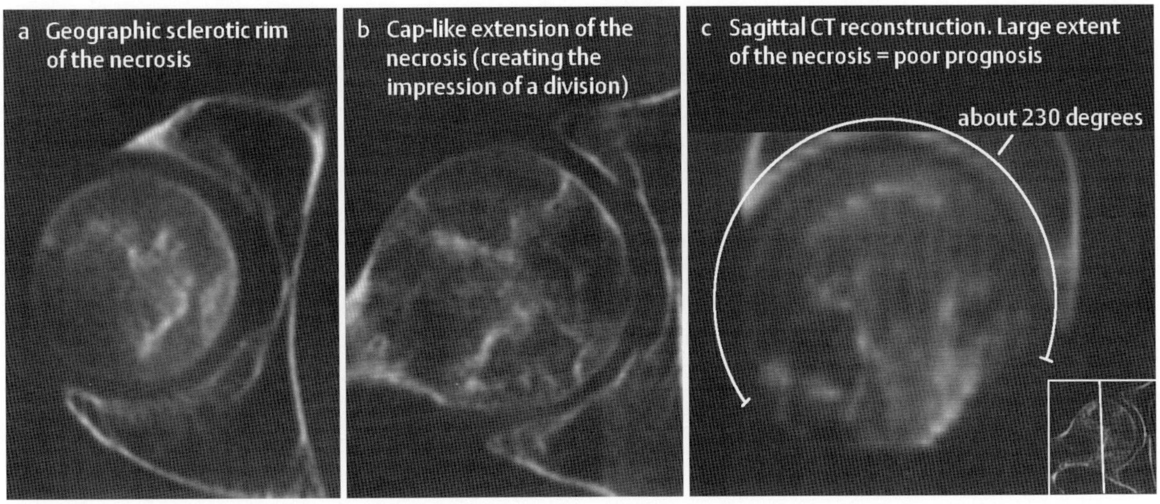

Fig. 5.**8** CT of an extensive avascular necrosis of the femoral head. The reformatted image shows a large area of necrosis and implies a poor prognosis. Moreover, it precludes a displacement osteotomy.

CT CT is performed with thin axial (1–2 mm) and coronal sections, as well as with sagittal reformations (Figs. 5.**8**–5.**10**).

CT enables early detection of a **subchondral fracture** or a **collapse of the articular surface** – both signs of mechanical insufficiency – free of superimposed structures. With the help of 2-D reconstructions, the prognostically relevant **extent of the necrosis** can be accurately determined. The percentage of the affected femoral head surface can be estimated as follows:

$$\text{Size of the necrosis (\%)} = \frac{\sphericalangle \text{sag.}}{180} \cdot \frac{\sphericalangle \text{cor.}}{180} \cdot 100$$

$\sphericalangle$ sag. = angle of the affected femoral head surface in the sagittal plane

$\sphericalangle$ cor. = angle of the affected femoral head surface in the coronal plane

CT is the method of choice for the early detection of a subchondral fracture (Stage III). Both CT and MRI are methods of choice for surgical planning, since both enable an accurate assessment of the extent and location of the necrosis.

MRI For the exclusion of an avascular necrosis of the femoral head, a T2-weighted sequence with fat suppression (e.g., STIR), supplemented by a T1-weighted echo sequence, is used. MRI units designed for the simultaneous application of a body coil and a surface coil are best suited for this examination, since this allows exclusion of bilateral involvement of the femoral heads. A positive finding should be followed with a T1-weighted sequence in the sagittal plane to calculate the quantitative parameters (see CT). Contrast enhancement is not mandatory, but does permit a semi-quantitative assessment of the ongoing reparative processes.

The characteristic findings of avascular necrosis of the femoral head on MRI are the necrosis itself and its surrounding reparative granulation tissue (Figs. 5.**11**, 5.**12**). In (ARCO) Stage I, the necrosis exhibits a pattern of edema with low signal intensity on the T1-weighted image and high signal intensity on the T2-weighted image. In Stage II, a signal pattern of fat or a mixed type is encountered. The fat-equivalent signal pattern consists of high signal intensity on the T1-weighted and T2-weighted images and mimics the signal intensity of healthy fatty bone marrow.

The margin of the necrotic area exhibits a typical pattern on MRI and is critical, since it allows a confident diagnosis. This is a well demarcated line of low signal intensity on the T1-weighted image, accompanied by an inner line of high signal intensity (granulation tissue) along the side of the necrosis and an outer line of low signal intensity (sclerosis, fibrosis) along the healthy bone on the T2-weighted image (= **'double line sign'**). After intravenous injection of contrast medium, the inner line shows strong enhancement (Fig. 5.**11**).

! MRI is indicated in all patients with clinical suspicion of an avascular necrosis of the femoral head and in patients with persistent hip pain of undetermined etiology.
MRI is the best method to distinguish avascular necrosis of the femoral head from other disorders.

MRI is the method of choice to diagnose, stage, and determine the extent of an avascular necrosis of the femoral head. The disadvantage of MRI is its limited differentiation between Stages II and III avascular necrosis of the femoral head.

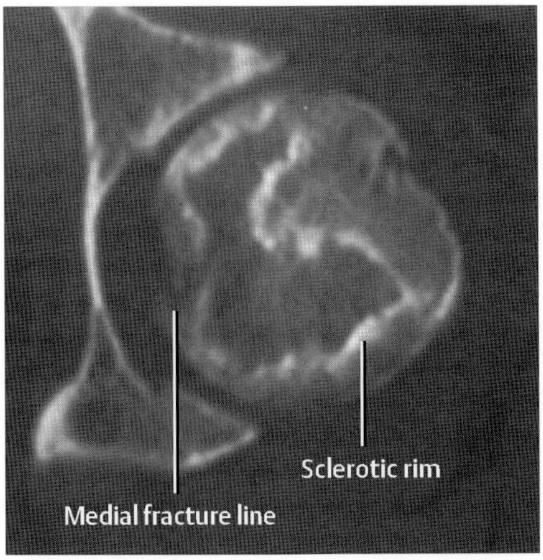

Fig. 5.**9** CT of a typical avascular necrosis of the femoral head with sclerosed border and medial fracture line (ARCO III).

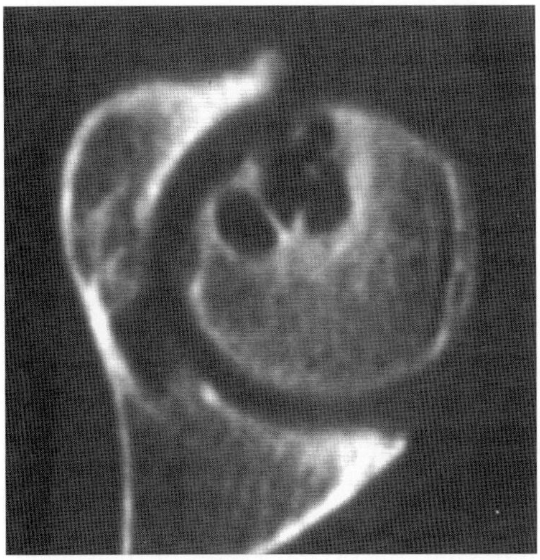

Fig. 5.**10** CT of avascular necrosis of the femoral head with a multicystic or septated pseudocystic appearance and a defect in the anterior subchondral cortex.

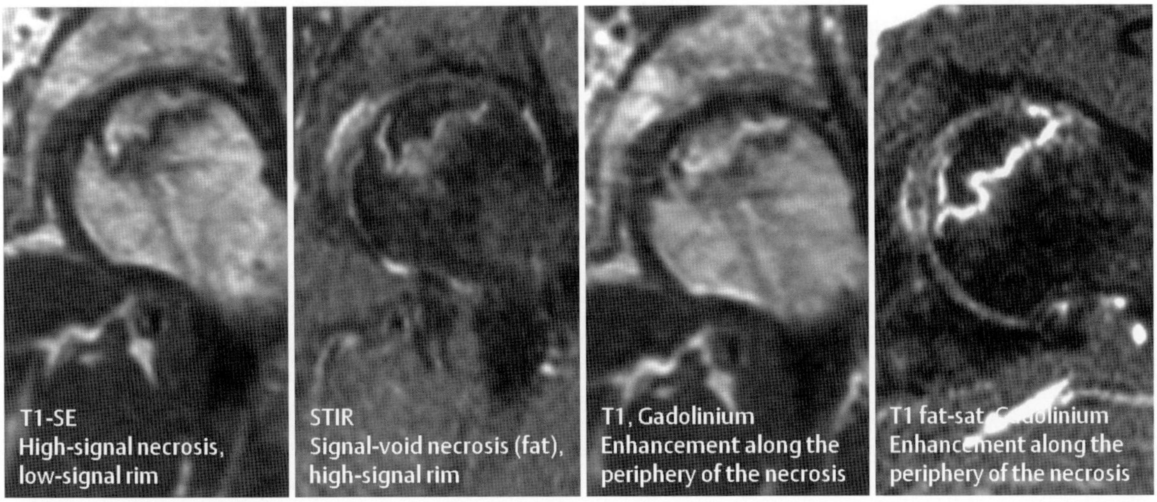

Fig. 5.**11** Several MRI sequences of avascular necrosis of the femoral head. Reparative granulation tissue, which strongly enhances, is seen around the periphery of the necrosis.

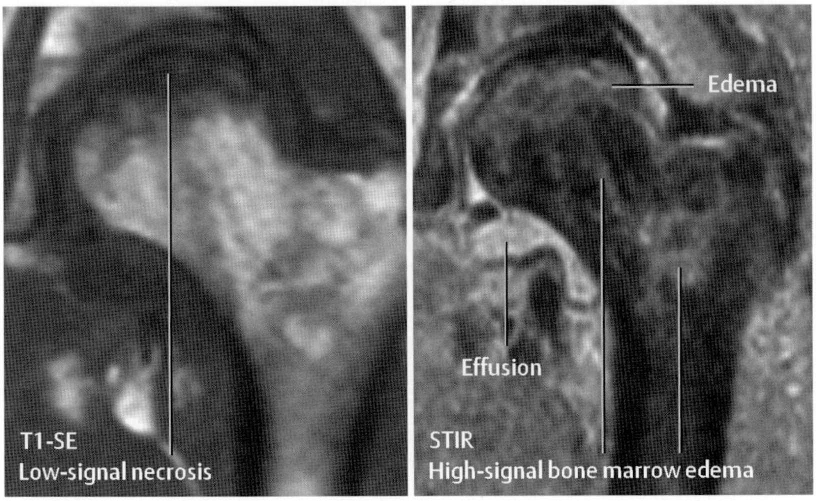

Fig. 5.**12** MRI of an avascular necrosis of the femoral head with flattening of the femoral head. The STIR sequence shows the heterogeneous necrotic area and an area of increased signal intensity in the femoral neck and peritrochanteric region representing bone marrow edema.

Osteonecrosis in other Locations

Osteonecroses in other areas are less common than in the femoral head, but involvement of these locations should be considered in the presence of risk factors or a history of trauma.

The commonest other locations for osteonecrosis are the carpal bones (especially the lunate and scaphoid), the distal femur, and distal metatarsal heads. The humeral head, proximal tibia, patella, talus, and navicula of the foot are less commonly involved (Table 5.**3**) (Fig. 5.**15**). Rarely the sesamoids may also be involved (Fig. 5.**18**).

Osteonecroses of the major joints (knee and shoulder) show an image pattern similar to that found in the hip. The osteonecroses of the smaller bones of the hand and foot are somewhat different in imaging, therapy, and prognosis and will be described in more detail.

Osteonecrosis of the Lunate

Synonyms: Kienböck disease, lunatomalacia.

This condition occurs most often in young men involved in manual labor (e.g., pneumatic hammer operators). Another predisposing factor is the increased pressure on the lunate caused by an ulnar minus variance.

The typical signs of lunate osteonecrosis on conventional radiography and MRI are summarized in Table 5.**4**. In the early stage, MRI is more sensitive and specific than conventional radiography or scintigraphy (Fig. 5.**13**). Intravenous administration of contrast medium adds prognostic information to the MRI.

Table 5.**4** Radiographic and MRI findings of lunate osteonecrosis

Stage	Radiography	MRI
I	Usually normal, but possible linear radiolucency or sclerosis	Altered signal intensities (T1 ↓, T2 ↓↑) in > 50 % of the lunate
II	Normal contour, increased density	Altered signal intensity in up to 100 % of the lunate, crescent sign
III A	Collapse of the lunate	Same as II, additional fragmentation
III B	As III A, additional scapholunate and triquetrolunate subluxation	Same as III A, additional scapholunate and triquetrolunate subluxation
IV	As III B, additional carpal osteoarthritis	Same as III B, additional synovitis

Table 5.**3** Summary of the different osteonecroses

Disorder	Location of Lesion	Age (years)	Probable mechanism	Incidence
Kienböck disease	Lunate	20 – 40	Recurrent trauma?	++++
Scaphoid fracture necrosis	Scaphoid, proximal portion	15 – 40	Proximal fracture	+++
Preiser disease	Scaphoid	Any age	Idiopathic	+
Thiemann disease	Phalangeal bases of the hand	11 – 19	Idiopathic	+
Panner disease	Capitellum	5 – 10	Trauma	+
Humeral head necrosis	Humeral head	Any age	Idiopathic	+
Femoral head necrosis	Femoral head	30 – 50	Idiopathic, corticosteroids, alcoholism, trauma	++++
Legg-Calvé-Perthes disease	Femoral head	4 – 8	Idiopathic	+++
Ahlbäck disease	Medial femoral condyle	> 60	Idiopathic	++
Blount disease	Proximal tibial epiphysis	< 15	Trauma	+
Talar necrosis	Talus	20 – 40	Idiopathic, trauma	++
Köhler I disease	Tarsal scaphoid	3 – 7	Idiopathic	+
Köhler II disease	Metatarsal head	13 – 18	Idiopathic	+++

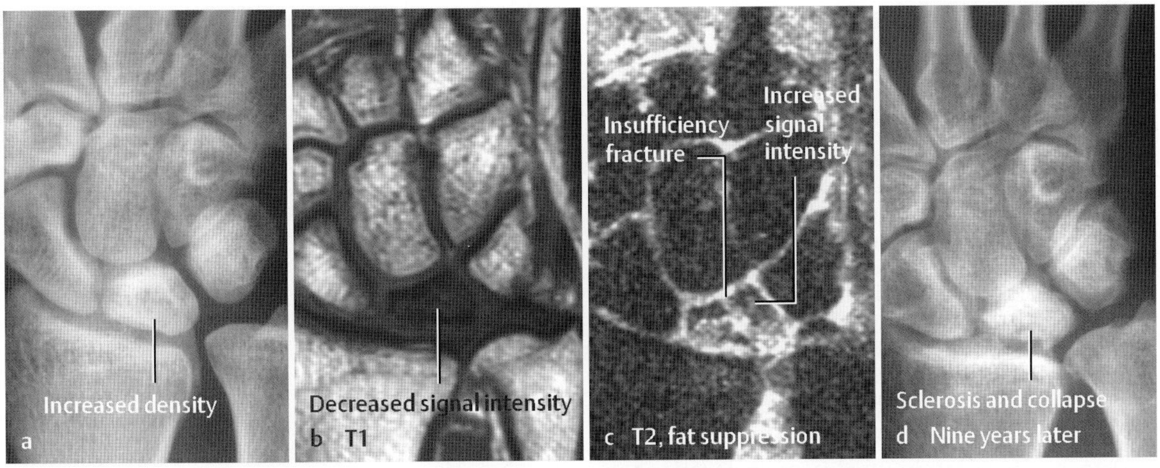

Fig. 5.**13** Osteonecrosis of the lunate. The radiograph (**a**) shows a sclerosis, and MRI (**b, c**) shows decreased signal intensity on the T1-weighted image and increased signal intensity on the fat suppressed T2-weighted image (edema pattern) (Stage II). **d** Nine years later, the lunate is collapsed and sclerotic.

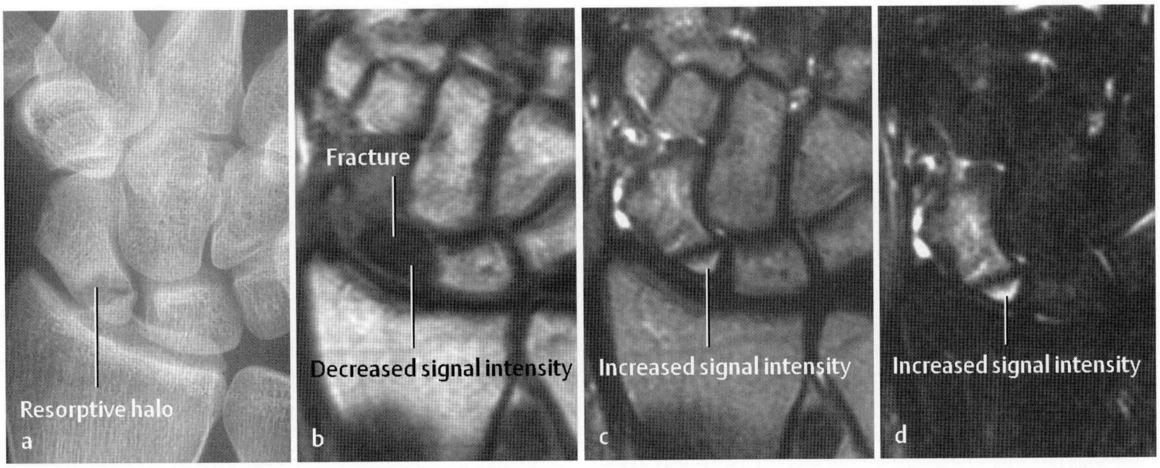

Fig. 5.**14** Avascular necrosis of the scaphoid following a fracture. **a** Delayed healing of the fracture with absent callus formation and resorption along the fracture line. On MRI, the proximal fragment and the areas adjacent to this fragment show a low signal intensity on the T1-weighted sequence (**b**) and high signal intensity on the T2-weighted sequence (**c, d**).

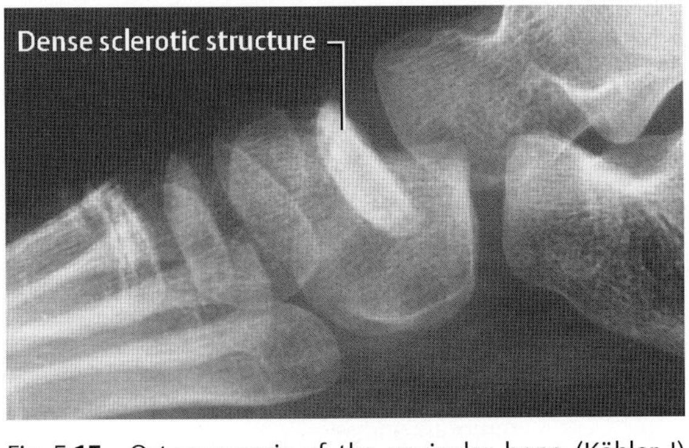

Fig. 5.**15** Osteonecrosis of the navicular bone (Köhler I) with pronounced sclerotic changes.

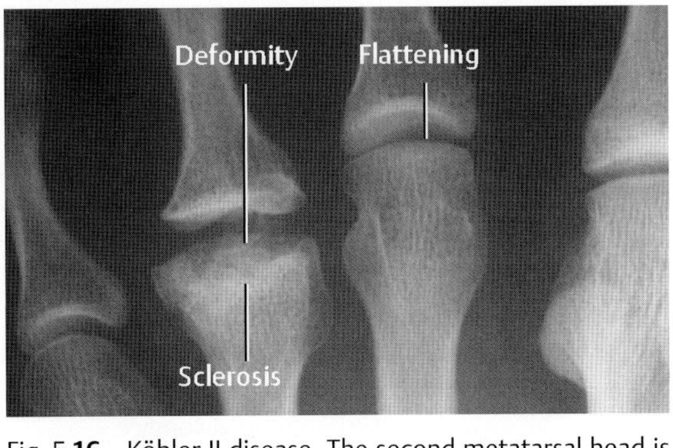

Fig. 5.**16** Köhler II disease. The second metatarsal head is flattened (Stage II), and the third metatarsal head is already deformed and sclerotic (Stage III).

Osteonecrosis of the Scaphoid

Synonym: Idiopathic type: Preiser disease.

PATH The proximal pole of the scaphoid receives its blood supply from vessels entering the distal pole. Therefore, osteonecrosis generally occurs in the proximal fragment following a proximal scaphoid fracture, since the fracture interrupts the distal blood supply. In addition to this fracture-induced osteonecrosis, an idiopathic scaphoid necrosis (Preiser disease) is described, but is quite rare.

The signs and the role of the different imaging methods correspond to those of the lunate (Stage I–IV, Table 5.**4**, Fig. 5.**14**).

Osteonecroses rarely involve other locations in the wrist.

Osteonecrosis of the Metatarsal Heads

Synonyms: Köhler II disease, Köhler-Freiberg disease, Freiberg disease, Freiberg infraction, juvenile metatarsal arthritis, metatarsal osteochondropathy, epiphysitis of the second metatarsal, Panner disease of the second metatarsal.

PATH The cause of idiopathic necrosis of the metatarsal heads (90%) is unknown. Contributing factors reported in the literature include stress, possibly with vascular damage and ischemia. Symptomatic avascular necrosis of the metatarsal head (10%) may be caused by diabetes mellitus, radiotherapy, corticosteroid therapy, trauma, electrical injuries, frostbite, and burns.
Age: Usually seen in adolescents, with a female predominance.
Location: The second metatarsal is most frequently involved, rarely the third metatarsal, and only exceptionally the fourth, fifth, and first metatarsals. In rare instances, osteonecrosis can simultaneously involve two or more metatarsal heads.

X-RAY Staging according to Bragard:
Stage I: The initial radiograph is normal and is followed by subchondral radiolucent lines and flattening of the metatarsal head.
Stage II: Sclerotic and radiolucent areas, fragmentation, progressive flattening, irregular border, and enlargement of the metatarsal head. The epiphyseal line can prematurely fuse, and cortical thickening appears along the adjacent metaphysis and the diaphysis.
Stage III: Deformity, degenerative osteoarthritis (Fig. 5.**16**).

Osteonecrosis of the Distal Femur

Synonym: Ahlbäck disease.

PATH This is an idiopathic osteonecrosis.
Epidemiology: The disease affects middle-aged and elderly patients and mainly involves the weight-bearing portion of the medial femoral condyle.

X-RAY Only weeks after the onset of symptoms (pain), discrete irregularities appear in the subchondral bone of the **medial** femoral condyle. Later, a well-demarcated radiolucency appears and is followed by depression of the subchondral bone (= flattening of the condylar articular surface). This is usually associated with reactive sclerosis, especially along the border zones (Fig. 5.**17 a**). The affected area can measure up to 5 cm in diameter. Bone fragmentation develops in the final stages of this disorder.

MRI Subchondral area of low signal intensity on the T1-weighted and T2-weighted image. The osteonecrotic area is surrounded by a zone of high signal intensity on the T2-weighted image (edema) and is demarcated from the adjacent bone marrow. Later course of the disease enhancement can be seen (Fig. 5.**17 b**).

DD The most important differential diagnosis is osteochondritis dissecans. The distinguishing findings are summarized in Table 5.**5**.

Table 5.**5** Differentiation between Ahlbäck disease and osteochondritis dissecans

Criterion	Ahlbäck disease	Osteochondritis dissecans
Age	After 40 years of age	Adolescents and young adults
Symptoms	Pain, swelling, restricted motion	Variable, may be absent
Typical location	Weight-bearing surface of the medial femoral condyle	Non-weight-bearing surface of the lateral femoral condyle
Probable pathogenesis	Vascular insult	Recurrent microtrauma, impaired ossification?

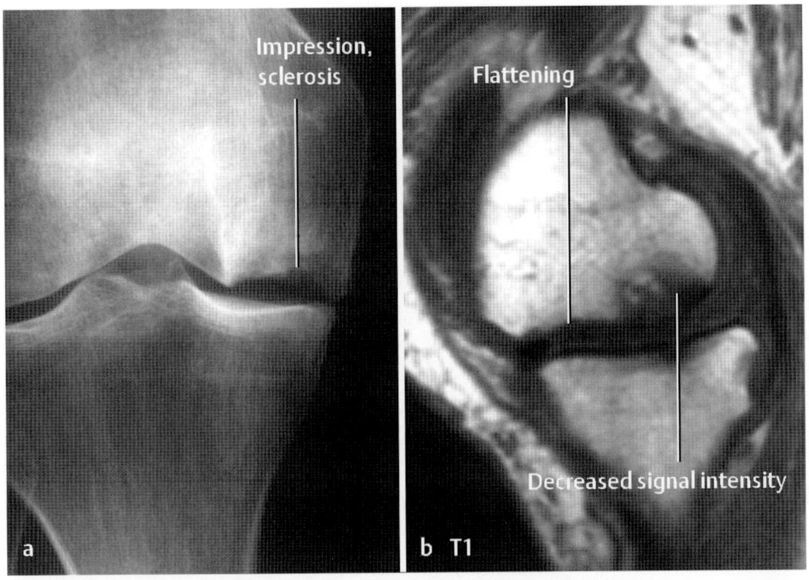

Fig. 5.**17** Ahlbäck disease. Osteonecrosis of the medial femoral condyle has led to subchondral collapse and adjacent reactive sclerosis on the radiograph. Low signal intensity is seen in the subchondral bone and the crater on the T1-weighted MR image.

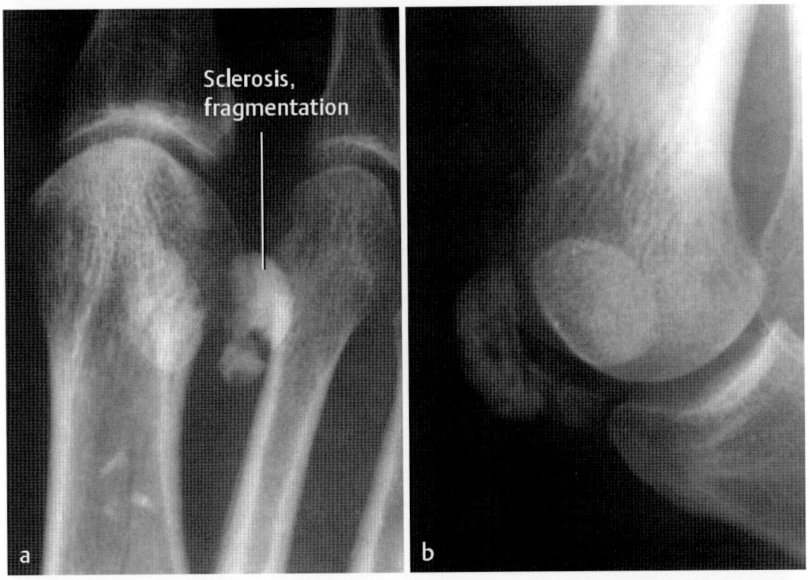

Fig. 5.**18** Rare site of osteonecrosis in a metatarsal sesamoid. The structural sclerosis and fragmentation are well visualized.

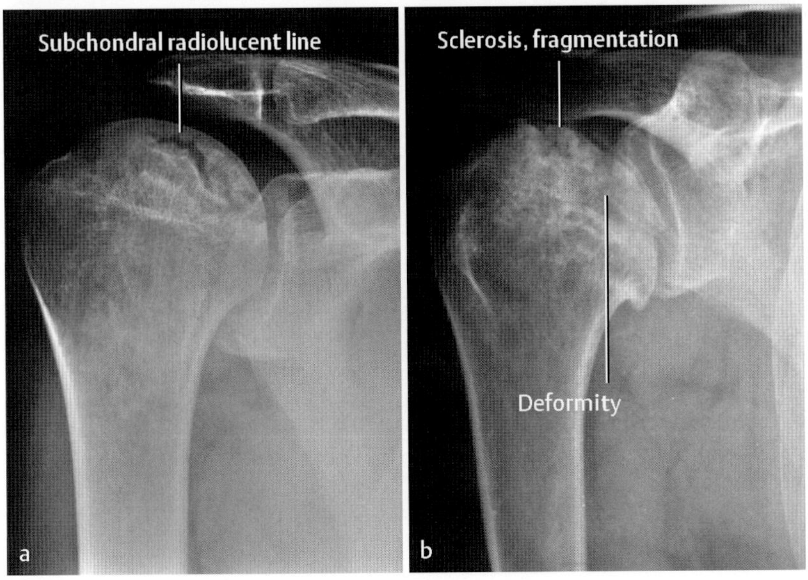

Fig. 5.**19** Osteonecrosis of the epiphyseal region of the humeral head. The typical radiographic findings of sclerosis, fragmentation and deformity are present.

Bone Infarct

■ Bone infarcts result from an interrupted blood supply. Most bone infarcts are asymptomatic, clinically irrelevant, and usually discovered as an incidental finding. ■

The predisposing factors for bone infarcts are the same as those for avascular necrosis and are summarized in Table 5.**1**.

X-RAY Bone infarcts occur centrally in the metadiaphysis or diaphysis. The early stage can be radiographically **unremarkable,** with subtle structural rarefactions (osteopenia, osteolysis) occurring later. Hydroxyapatite is deposited both centrally and peripherally and ultimately causes the typical radiographic findings: serpiginous regions of band-like geographic sclerosis ('resembling a map') (Figs. 5.**20**, 5.**23**, 5.**24**, see also Figs. 4.**15**, 4.**16**).

NUC In the initial phases of vascular compromise decreased uptake is seen in the necrotic area, the so-called **'cold spot,'** followed later in the course of the disease by increased uptake along the periphery, producing the **'cold in hot spot'.**

MRI The rarely observed early stages show decreased signal intensity on the T1-weighted image, and increased signal intensity on the T2-weighted image, representing edema. Later in the disease, MRI shows the typical picture of peripheral zones and the necrosis itself, which 'resembles a map'. As seen in avascular necrosis of the hip, the border of the lesion is important: T1-weighted images show only a low signal intensity line, T2-weighted images an inner high-signal-intensity line (granulation tissue) paralleled by an outer low-signal-intensity line representing fibrosis and sclerosis. Depending on the MRI technique (directional phase encoding, sequence selection), this double line sign can be distorted by superimposed 'chemical shift' artifact. Strong contrast enhancement is generally seen along the entire border zone (Figs. 5.**22**, 5.**23**).

The necrotic area itself shows a largely fat-equivalent signal pattern (high signal intensity on T1-weighted and intermediate signal on T2-weighted images). Cystic degenerations (high signal intensity on the T2-weighted image) are occasionally delineated within the fat.

DD The diagnosis of bone infarct is firmly established by the detection of fat within the lesion on MRI. Infarcts can also contain cystic areas. In rare instances of the homogeneous lesion of low signal intensity (i.e., without fat signal), the differentiation from enchondroma can be extremely difficult (Fig. 5.**24**). If this differentiation is required, the enhancement pattern **within** the lesion can be helpful, as the enchondroma shows many delicate septations reflecting its lobular composition. The bone infarct shows a more patchy and peripheral enhancement.

Caution! Bone infarcts can expand the bone and lead to pronounced periosteal reaction, especially in the sacrum, the ilium and, rarely, also in tubular

Table 5.**6** Differential diagnosis of the bone infarct

Disease	Calcification Morphology	Location	Adjacent structures	MRI findings	Location
Bone infarct	Band-like, geographic sclerotic rim	Eccentric (but also central, geographic	Unremarkable	Fat (high signal), walled-off	Meta-diaphyseal, central
Enchondroma	Popcorn-like (arcs and Cs)	In all areas	Endosteal cortical resorption (occasionally)	Mixed features with bright cartilage and dark calcification on T2-weighted images	Metaphyseal
Fibrous cortical defect	Lobulated, grape-like	Initially marginal	Cortex involved	Signal void on T2 weighting (a few fat components possible)	Metaphyseal, eccentric
Fibrous dysplasia	Sclerotic rim, lysis, ground glass density	In all areas	Cortex thinned	Heterogenous, cystic on T2-weighting	Meta-diaphyseal, central

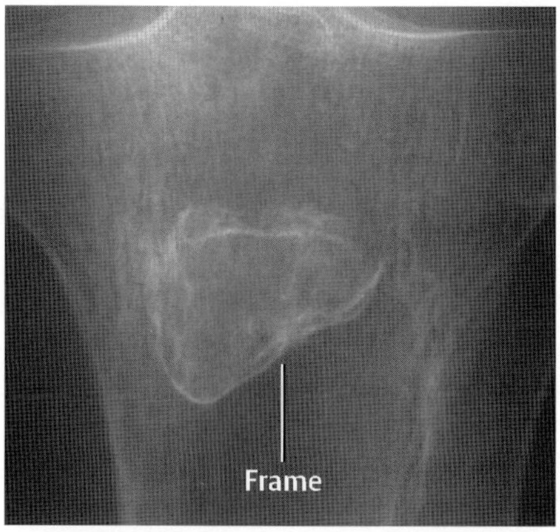

Fig. 5.**20** Bone infarct in the proximal tibia. The sclerosis encloses the infarct like a frame, producing the impression of a 'bone in bone.'

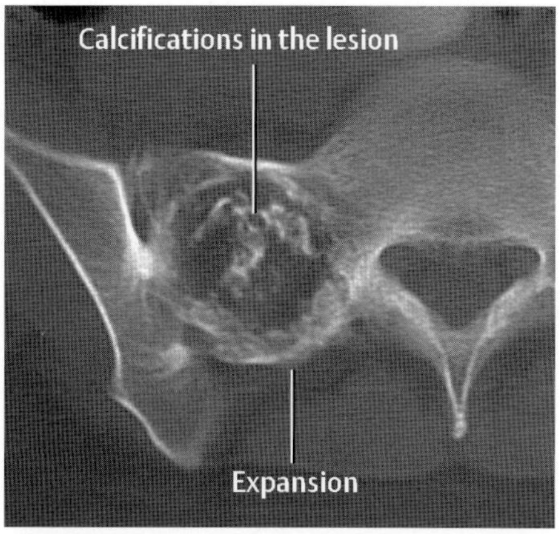

Fig. 5.**21** Bone expansion caused by a bone infarct in the sacrum. Notice the flocculent nature of the calcifications (differential diagnosis: enchondroma).

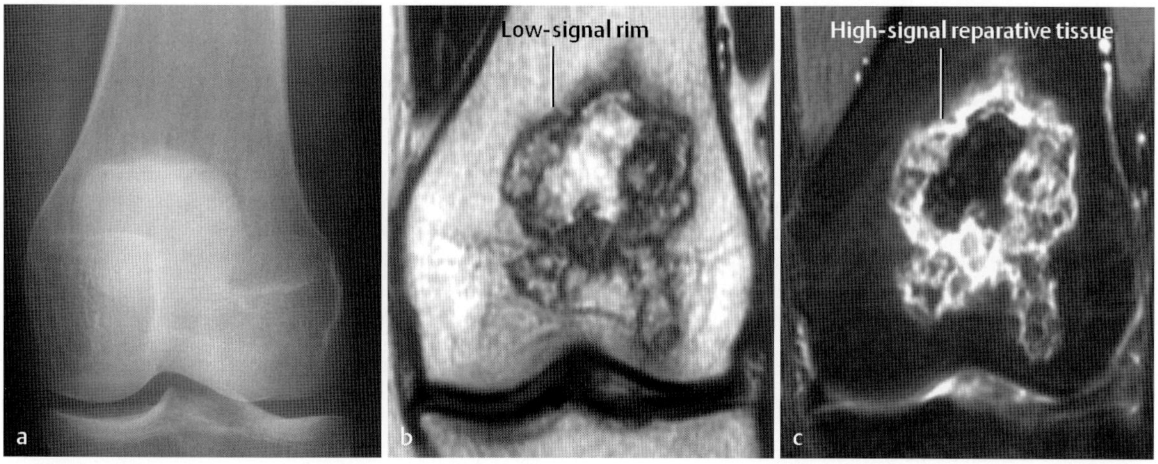

Fig. 5.**22** Bone infarct in an 37-year-old woman. Radiograph is normal. The diagnosis of bone infarct rests on the T1-weighted SE sequence (**b**), since it reveals fat within the lesion. The STIR sequence shows extensively vascularized tissue within the infarct.

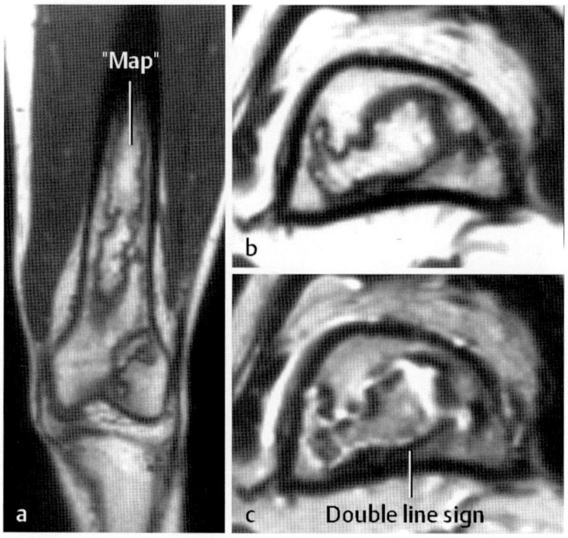

Fig. 5.**23** Typical bone infarct in the femur 'resembling a map'. **a, b** T1-weighted images. The T2-weighted image (**c**) clearly displays the double line sign.

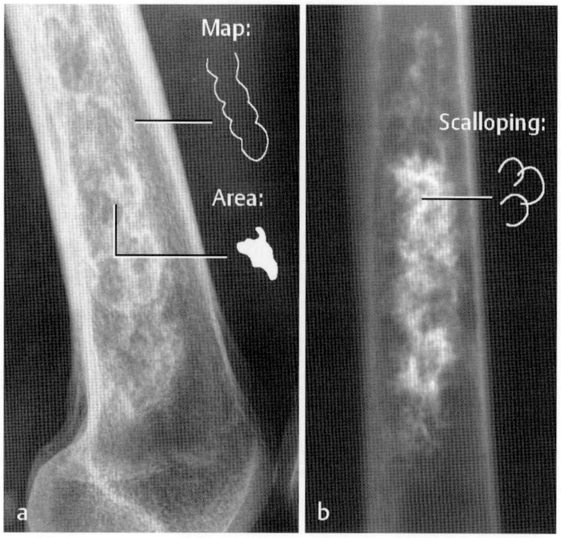

Fig. 5.**24** Comparison between bone infarct (**a**) and enchondroma (**b**), with their respective classic calcification patterns.

bones. The detection of fat **within** the lesion is important for the diagnosis of the bone infarct, and the diagnosis can be established by MRI.

Additional differential diagnoses can be found in Table 5.**6**.

Bone Marrow Edema Syndrome

Synonyms: Transient osteoporosis, transient osteonecrosis, algodystrophy.

■ The bone marrow edema syndrome is usually transient and self-limiting. Since it can rarely progress to osteonecrosis, it should be considered an early stage of osteonecrosis in many instances. ■

PATH The etiology of this disorder, like that of osteonecrosis, is unknown. Histologically, necrotic fat cells, fibrovascular regenerative tissue, and increased osteoid can be found. Histologic proof of the edema itself is difficult.

The mineral content is reduced ('hydroxylapatite shift') and causes increased radiolucency. Since loss of bone substance does not occur, the term 'osteopenia' is more appropriate than 'osteoporosis' in this setting.

Caution! Detection of cell death should not be equated with irreversible necrosis. Bone marrow edema syndrome is a testament to the reparative capability of the bone marrow.

CLINIC Bone marrow edema syndrome predominately involves young and middle-aged men, as well as pregnant women in the third trimester.

The classic chief complaint is pain. Bone marrow edema syndrome mainly involves the hip but can also occur in the femoral condyle, talus, humeral head, and elbow.
Therapy: Conservative and, if extensive, also surgical by means of core decompression, which generally can produce a rapid improvement.

X-RAY The radiographs are normal during the first few days of bone marrow edema syndrome. Later, osteopenia with diffusely increased radiolucency and indistinct and washed-out trabeculae and cortex develop. The pattern of involvement is diffusely patchy and partially band-like. It can be confined to a segment of the femoral head or can involve the entire femoral head, including portions of the femoral neck and trochanteric region. The joint space is preserved, but the subchondral plate does become demineralized. After 4 – 10 months remineralization to a normal appearance is the usual course for this disorder (Figs. 5.**25**, 5.**26**).

MRI MRI is indicated in all patients with clinical suspicion of bone marrow edema syndrome.

The protocol is the same as that for evaluation of avascular necrosis of the femoral head. The bone marrow edema induces changes affecting large areas of the femoral head with variable extension to the femoral neck and intertrochanteric region. Compared to healthy bone marrow, the edema is of low signal intensity on T1-weighted images and high signal intensity on T2-weighted images. Contrast enhancement is moderate to strong and usually heterogeneous. Initially, bone marrow edema syndrome shows a diffuse pattern, with diffuse to patchy, partially confluent to homogeneous changes (Figs. 5.**25** – 5.**27**). With progression, a more focal form develops and is seen as more circumscribed bone marrow edema and a less-pronounced difference in signal intensity. In the final stages of the disease, delicate web-like or linear remnants of low signal intensity remain, or complete restitution occurs.

NUC Scintigraphy is the most sensitive method for detecting bone marrow edema syndrome (diffuse increase involving femoral head, femoral neck, and intertrochanteric region). The finding might be interpreted as falsely negative in cases with bilateral or only moderately severe involvement. However, because of the low specificity of scintigraphy, MRI has become the mainstay for the early diagnosis of bone marrow edema syndrome.

DD The MRI findings must be differentiated from:

- Stress fractures (these bone marrow changes are usually along the inner cortex of the femoral neck, sparing the femoral head and may have a signal-void fracture line),
- Post-traumatic bone marrow edema (clinical history),
- Osteomyelitis (soft-tissue and joint involvement),
- Tumors (evidence of a space-occupying process).

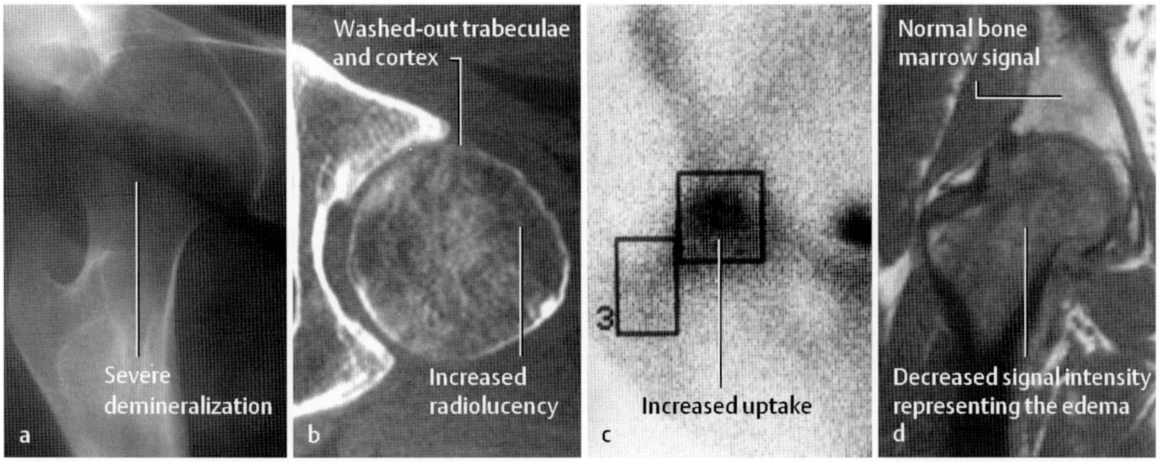

Fig. 5.**25** Bone marrow edema syndrome in the hip with different imaging modalities (different patients). Radiograph (**a**) and CT (**b**) show a diffusely increased radiolucency with indistinct and washed-out appearance of spongiosa and cortex. The bone scan (**c**) shows intense tracer uptake in the femoral head with some extension into the femoral neck region. MRI (**d**) (T1-weighted SE sequence) confirms the bone marrow edema.

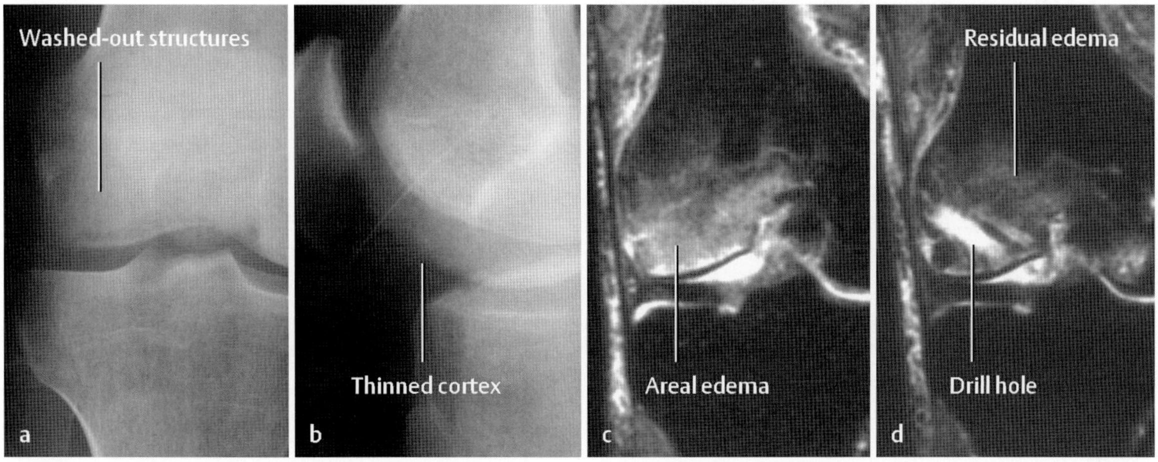

Fig. 5.**26** A 50-year-old patient with spontaneous pain. The radiographs (**a, b**) show a washed-out trabecular pattern with cortical thinning and increased radiolucency. The STIR sequence (**c**) displays the bone marrow edema best. **d** After drilling there is partial resolution of the edema at 2 months. Three years later, the patient developed bone marrow edema syndrome in the contralateral knee, initially involving the medial and later the lateral femoral condyle.

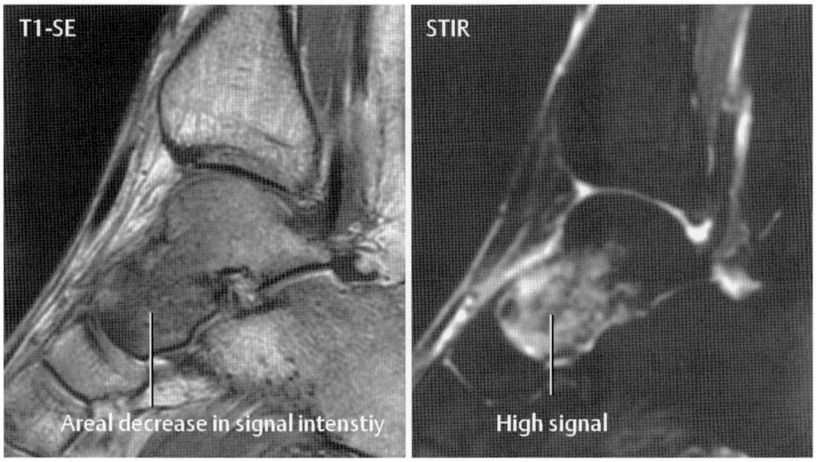

Fig. 5.**27** Altered signal in the talar neck due to bone marrow edema. The edema shows decreased intensity on the T1-weighted SE sequence and marked heterogeneously increased intensity on the STIR sequence.

Legg-Calvé-Perthes Disease

Synonym: Idiopathic osteoporosis of the femoral head.

Legg-Calvé-Perthes disease is an avascular necrosis of the femoral head and is classified under the osteochondroses. It is considered a distinct entity that must be distinguished from avascular necrosis of the femoral head that occurs together with hip dysplasia and epiphysiolysis, and after femoral neck fracture.

PATH At the typical age of involvement (4–7 years), the femoral head is almost exclusively supplied by lateral epiphyseal vessels creating a critical condition of the blood supply ('latent ischemia'). It is, however, unclear why only some cases progress to a manifest avascular necrosis of the femoral head.

Course: In the **initial stage** of the condition, ischemia leads to arrest of the enchondral ossification of the epiphysis, while the articular cartilage, which is mostly nourished by the joint fluid, continues to grow. This insult is accompanied by synovitis and followed by sclerosis of the ossification center, referred to as the **stage of condensation.** In the subsequent **stage of fragmentation,** granulation tissue interposes between the necrotic areas of impaired enchondral ossification, resulting in shrinkage of the epiphysis and fragmentation of the ossification centers.

Regeneration stage: After revascularization of the affected areas new bone is formed, leading to healing with deformity. Only rarely is there complete restoration to normal.

CLINIC The chief complaint is limping. In 4%–18% of cases both hips are involved, but rarely at the same time.

X-RAY Radiographs cannot detect early stages of the disease. For advanced stages, an AP film of the pelvis and a lateral view of the hip are adequate for the diagnosis, gradation, and assessment of the prognosis.

Initial Stage (Fig. 5.**28**):
- Joint space widening,
- Slight difference in density and configuration of the growth plate in comparison to the contralateral hip.

Caution: The radiographic findings at this stage are nonspecific and frequently subtle!

Condensation Stage (Fig. 5.**29**):
- Increased density of the ossification center.

Fragmentation Stage (Fig. 5.**30**):
- Decreased size and rarefaction of the epiphysis,
- Flattening of the femoral head,
- Fragmentation or lysis of the ossification center.

Regeneration Stage (Fig. 5.**31**):
- Appearance of new ossification centers, which gradually fuse to an ossification center of normal density,
- Atypical spatial orientation and widening of the growth plate, with irregular contours. Later, decreased width of the growth plate and possible premature epiphyseal closure,
- Metaphyseal radiolucent bands, densities and cysts.

End Stage (Fig. 5.32):
- Rarely, complete restoration **or**
- widening, flattening, and subluxation of the femoral head ('mushroom configuration', 'Coxa plana') with secondary acetabular dysplasia (predisposition for degenerative osteoarthritis).

Prognostic Criteria:
The risk of healing with deformity and the necessity of surgical intervention can be assessed on the basis of the following radiographic findings:
- congruence of the femoral head and acetabulum ('concentric appearance'): lateral displacement due to a deformed femoral head is unfavorable,
- preserved lateral half of the epiphysis of the femoral head ('lateral column').

Other so-called 'head-at-risk' signs imply a poor prognosis:
- small osteoporotic segment at the outer epiphyseal side in the shape of a recumbent 'V' ('gauge sign'),
- calcification lateral to the epiphyseal plate,
- metaphyseal involvement with cysts and sclerotic areas.

SONO Best for the detection of a joint effusion.

MRI As long as the radiographic findings are normal, MRI is the only modality that can detect early disease by showing edema in the epiphysis (Fig. 5.**28**). MRI can also show the position of the epiphysis within the acetabulum on follow-up examinations.

DD **Coxitis:** (Coxitis fugax or coxitis of other nature): MRI is necessary if the radiographs are normal. In contrast to Legg-Calvé-Perthes disease, coxitis fugax (= transient synovitis) has an acute clinical onset, and MRI shows an unremarkable epiphysis. The differentiation from septic arthritis is best achieved by hip aspiration.

Avascular necrosis of the femoral head of other nature: Simultaneous, bilateral avascular necrosis favors a systemic disease (sickle cell anemia, hypothyroidism, Gaucher disease).

Meyer dysplasia: This constitutes a delayed and irregular ossification, possibly with several ossification centers. The density of the epiphysis is **not** increased, and the metaphysis is unaltered.

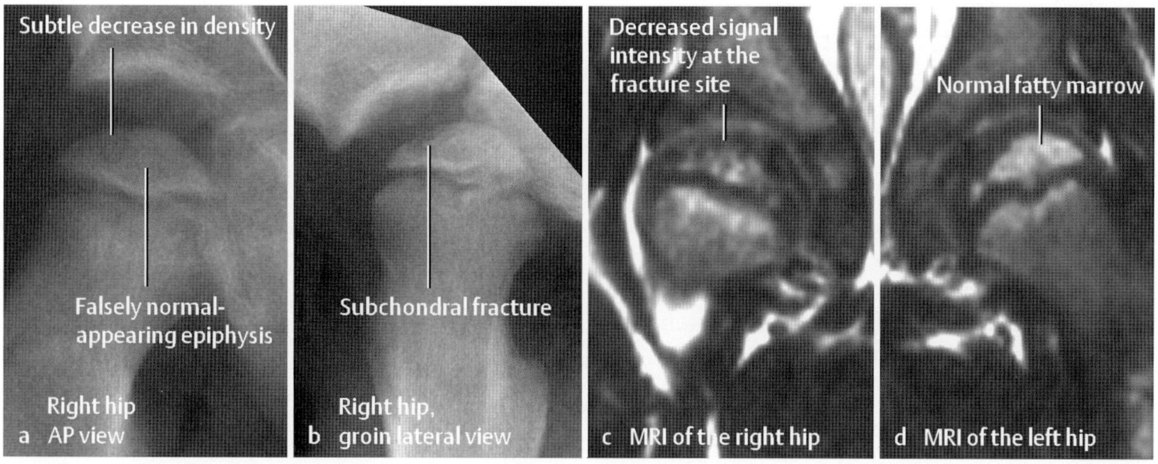

Fig. 5.**28** Initial stage of Legg-Calvé-Perthes disease. Although the AP view shows only subtle changes, the groin lateral view reveals a typical subchondral fracture. On MRI, the signal void on the T2-weighted TSE sequence indicates fatty marrow necrosis.

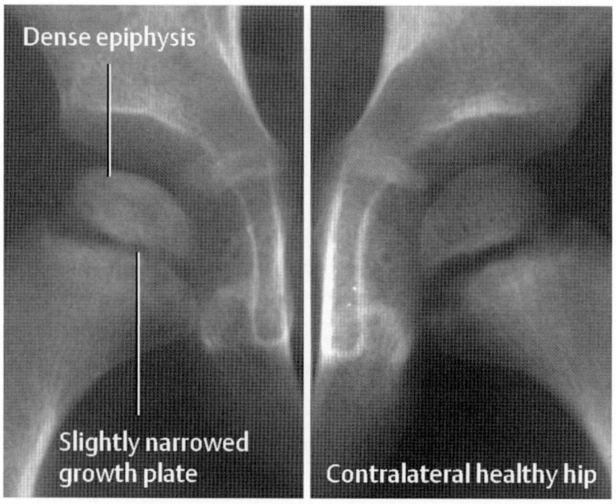

Fig. 5.**29** Condensation stage. Comparison with the contralateral healthy hip reveals the increased epiphyseal density.

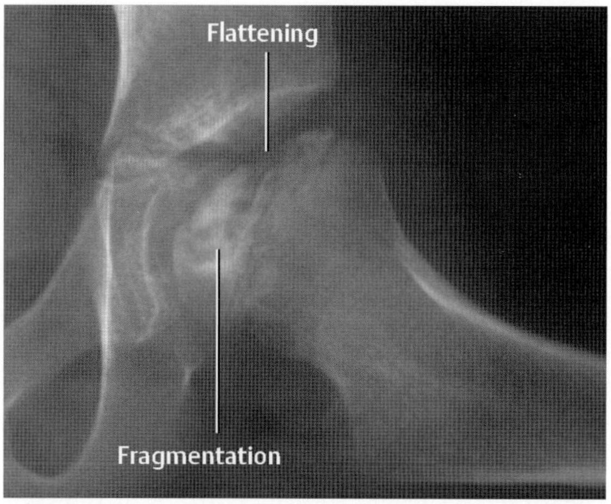

Fig. 5.**30** Fragmentation stage. This stage is characterized by flattening of the epiphysis together with fragmentation.

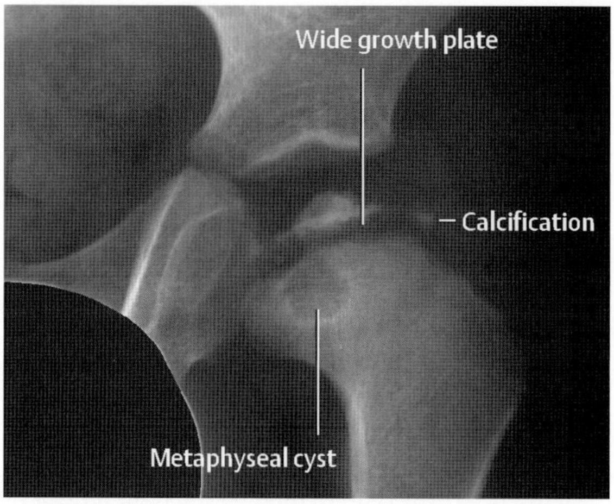

Fig. 5.**31** Regeneration stage. The calcification lateral to the epiphyseal line and the metaphyseal cyst are regarded as the 'head-at-risk' sign and imply a poor prognosis.

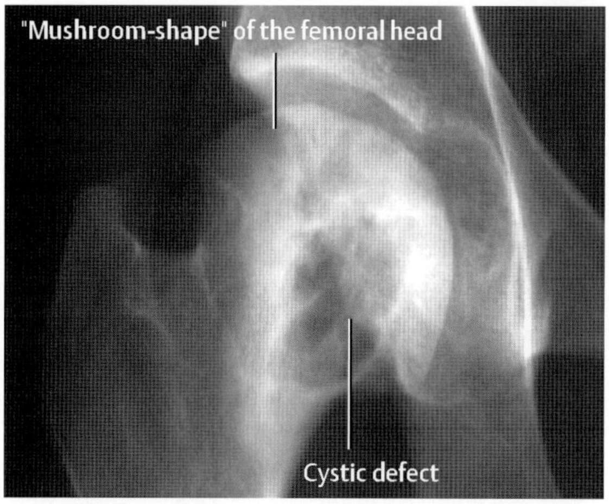

Fig. 5.**32** Late stage. This case exhibits a large defect in the femoral head in addition to the mushroom deformity (predisposition for degenerative osteoarthritis).

Osteochondritis Dissecans (OCD)

Synonym: Osteochondrosis dissecans, ischemic osteochondral infarction.

■ Osteochondritis dissecans is a circumscribed area of subchondral cartilage-bone fragmentation. It is induced by **osseous** ischemia with possible secondary involvement of the cartilage and is distinguished from osteonecrosis by extent, location, patient age, and prognosis. ■

PATH Chronic repetitive overuse or acute mechanical or traumatic factors are important predispositions, but familial clustering of the disease and bilateral involvement in up to 23% of cases suggest other, so far unknown, contributing factors. The natural history follows the stages shown in Fig. 5.**33**.

! In patients under the age of 18 years, the cartilage is frequently still intact at the time of diagnosis, in contrast to young adults.

CLINIC Pain activated by movement and recurrent effusions are the clinical findings. A loose intra-articular body ('joint mouse') can cause typical intermittent pain and locking.

! Clinically, osteochondritis dissecans may be entirely asymptomatic, and it frequently is an incidental radiologic finding (in particular at the talus).

Location: The weight-bearing portions of all major joints tend to be involved (especially the knee and ankle). The classic locations are the inner aspect of the medial **femoral condyle** and the medial facet of the talus.
Age: Osteochondritis dissecans occurs in the second to fourth decades of life.
Therapy: Evaluation of osteochondritis dissecans in stages (see MRI) determines whether conservative therapy (non-weight-bearing, MRI Stage I) or surgical therapy (drilling, fixation of the fragment, MRI Stage II) is appropriate. The integrity of the cartilage is crucial. Before closure of the epiphysis, surgery is rarely indicated.
Prognosis: As long as the cartilage is intact (MRI Stage I), the long-term prognosis is good.

X-RAY
- Diffuse, crescentic subchondral radiolucency (early sign, Fig. 5.**34 a**),
- Subchondral fragments of normal or decreased bone density. The fragments are surrounded by a radiolucent rim (Fig. 5.**34 b**),
- Band-like sclerosis along the radiolucent zone,
- Indistinctly outlined subchondral sclerosis with irregularity of the joint contour (late sign, Fig. 5.**34 c**),
- Cyst formation (late sign),
- Loose intra-articular body and 'mouse bed' (late sign) (Fig. 5.**33**).

! Radiography can establish the diagnosis of osteochondritis dissecans at the time of clinical presentation, but the therapy is determined by MRI or arthroscopy or both.

MRI MRI distinguishes two stages.
Stage I (arthroscopic Stage I):
- The cartilage is intact (visualized with T2-weighted gradient echo and TSE sequences, Fig. 5.**35 a**).
- The ischemic area appears as a crescent of low signal intensity on the T1-weighted SE image.
- The transitional zone separating the low-signal osteochondritis dissecans from the low-signal normal bone has a high signal intensity (T2 TSE image) and enhances.

Stage II (arthroscopic Stage II–IV):
- The cartilage shows tears and defects of variable extent (Figs. 5.**35 b, c**).
- Fluid between fragment and fragment bed (high signal intensity on T2-weighted TSE image, Fig. 5.**35 b**).
- Cystic areas (high signal intensity on T2-weighted TSE image).
- The transitional zone does not enhance after intravenous injection of contrast medium.

DD In adults, the differentiation from osteonecrosis often is clinically inconsequential, since the therapy is identical in view of the extensive involvement generally present in these patients. Classic osteochondritis dissecans occurs in young patients, is small, and has a crescentic manifestation.

In the talus, differentiation from a fresh osteochondral fracture can be problematic.
- An osteochondral fracture is invariably associated with bone marrow edema (MRI!), and edema is rarely seen with osteochondritis dissecans. Associated edema at other osseous sites (tibia) supports the diagnosis of an acute injury.
- Osteochondritis dissecans is usually medial, but acute fractures tend to involve the lateral facet of the talus. The traumatic fragments are elongated, whereas OCD of the talus produces more round, crater-like fragments.

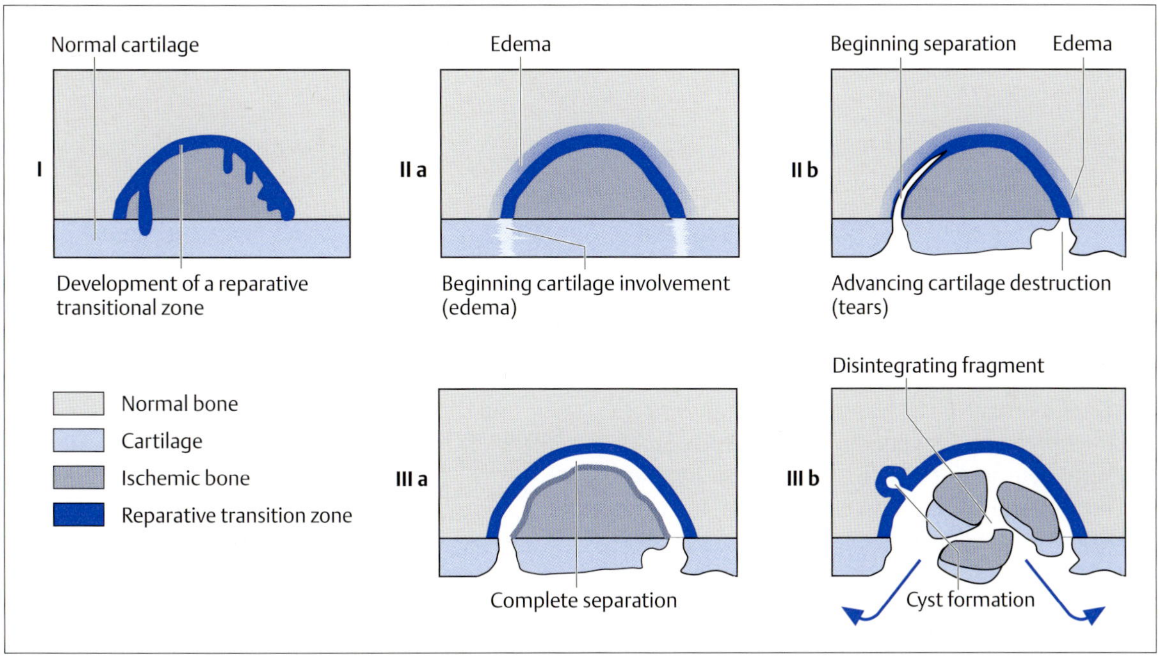

Fig. 5.**33** Stages of the pathologic-anatomic evolution of osteochondritis dissecans.

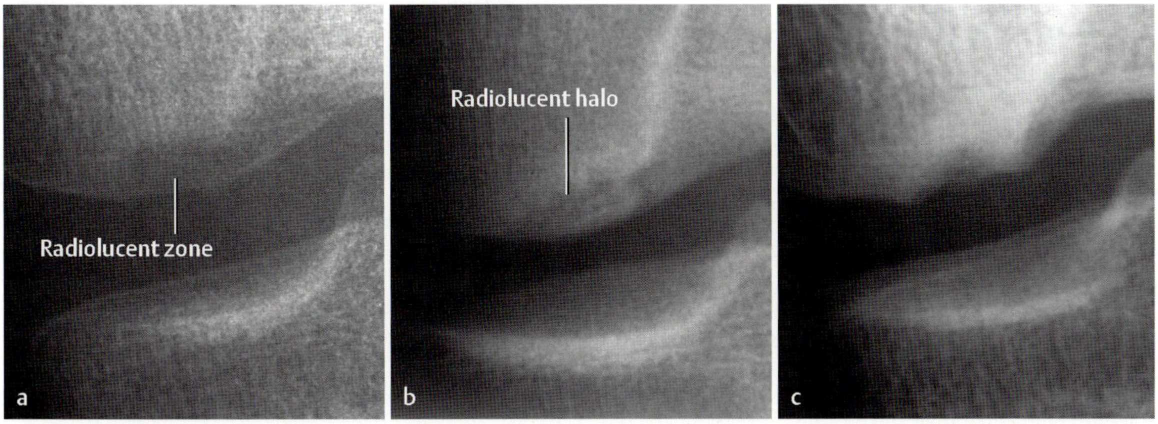

Fig. 5.**34** Radiologic signs of osteochondritis dissecans. **a** Early sign, **b** classic sign with radiolucent halo around the osteochondral fragment, **c** late changes indicating healing with a residual defect ('mouse bed').

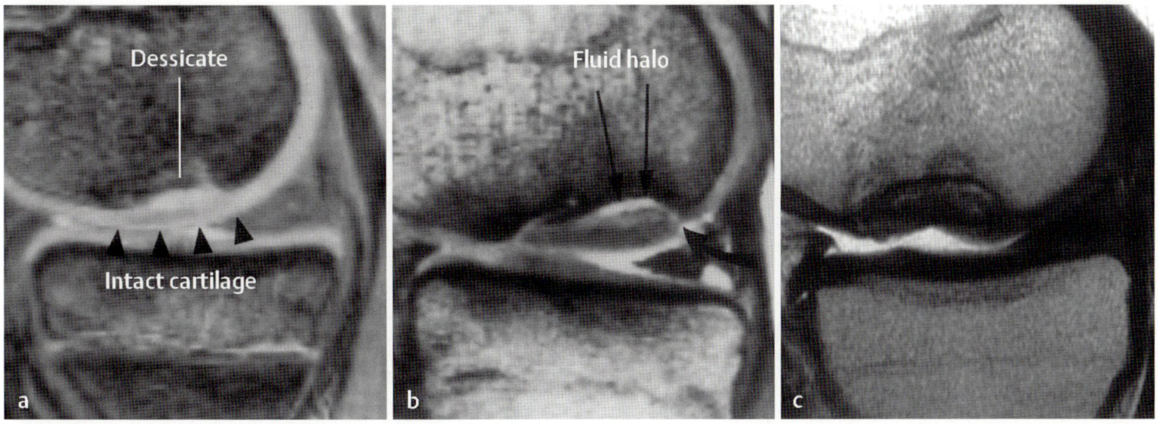

Fig. 5.**35** MRI of osteochondritis dissecans. **a** Stage I, **b** Stage II with cartilage defect (both GE sequences). **c** Late stage with irregular cartilage contour (T2-TSE image).

6 Metabolic, Hormonal, and Toxic Osteopathies

Osteoporosis

■ Osteoporosis is a systemic skeletal disease characterized by low bone mass and microarchitectural deterioration with a consequent increase in bone fragility and susceptibility to fractures (Consensus Development Conference, 1996, Amsterdam). The fractures occur spontaneously or after minor injury. The decreasing bone mass keeps the ratio of mineral content to collagenous matrix unchanged (in contrast to osteomalacia). ■

PATH The entire bone mass of the human is composed of 80% cortex and 20% spongiosa. The spongiosa has by far the larger surface and consequently reacts faster to metabolic changes. Physiologic remodeling takes place in small functional units in which osteoclasts and osteoblasts interact.

The microstructure of normal spongiosa primarily consists of trabecular plates that are broadly connected (Fig. 6.**1**). In osteoporosis, the trabecular plates show deep resorptive lacunae that disconnect the trabeculae, and osteoblasts lack the morphologic substrate for the deposition of new bone. The trabecular plates are gradually reduced to thin rods, which in turn perforate and eventually disappear (Fig. 6.**2**). At this stage, more and more microfractures and reparative microcallus formation are observed. This process is followed by progressive loss of intertrabecular connections and a corresponding increase in brittleness.

Classification of Osteoporosis

Primary Osteoporosis (Idiopathic):

1. Postmenopausal osteoporosis (Type I osteoporosis):
   - Between age 50 and 65 years. Estrogen deficiency induces high bone turnover and leads to accelerated trabecular resorption and perforation, especially within the first five postmenopausal years.
   - Fractures predominantly of the spongiosa and primarily affecting the vertebral bodies.
   - Peripheral fractures (e.g., femoral neck) are less frequent.
   - Gradual transition to senile osteoporosis is possible.
2. Senile osteoporosis (Type II osteoporosis):
   - Decreased bone turnover, inadequate dietary calcium, and age-related decreased synthesis of calcitriol can cause a high bone turnover by means of hyperparathyroidism, even in old age.
   - General loss of bone mass in the spongiosa and cortex of bone.
   - Fractures tend to involve the peripheral skeleton: femoral neck, distal radius, proximal humerus, tibia, and pelvis.

Secondary Osteoporosis:

- Endocrinal: Cushing disease, hyperthyroidism, hypogonadism, primary hyperparathyroidism.
- Corticosteroid therapy, chemotherapy, anticonvulsant therapy, and others.
- Intestinal: malabsorption, pancreas insufficiency.
- Inactivity, weightlessness (Fig. 6.**7**).
- Other conditions, e.g., lactose intolerance, excessive alcohol abuse, heavy smoking, anorexia nervosa, and others.

Caution! Renal osteodystrophy is a separate clinical entity and, strictly speaking, should not be categorized as a secondary osteoporosis.

CLINIC Osteoporosis is clinically silent until the appearance of macrofractures. Specific biochemical markers do not exist for primary osteoporosis, but laboratory tests are important for the differential diagnosis of secondary osteoporosis and other low-calcium osteopathies.

Clinical screening is important and should include all individuals at risk for osteoporosis. This includes the clinical history (hereditary risk factors, low dietary calcium and vitamin intake, physical inactivity, tobacco abuse, slender constitution, etc.), hormonal status (premature menopause, amenorrhea, masculine hypogonadism, corticosteroid therapy, etc.), and bone densitometry.

Peak bone mass is reached at 30–35 years and measures 160 ± 30 mg of calcium HA/ml. The World Health Organization (WHO) has proposed a gradation of the bone mass loss based on densitometry of the lumbar spine in Caucasian women:

- Normal: bone mineral density (BMD) within – 1 standard deviation (SD) of a young normal adult.
- Low bone mass (osteopenia): BMD between – 1 and – 2.5 SD below that of a young normal adult.
- Osteoporosis: BMD is – 2.5 SD or more below that of a young normal adult.
- Established osteoporosis: BMD is more than – 2.5 SD below that of a young normal adult, and one or more fractures are present.

! Since the peak bone mass is the same for women and men, the term 'osteoporosis' can be defined as a bone mineral content of less than 85 mg CaHA/ml.

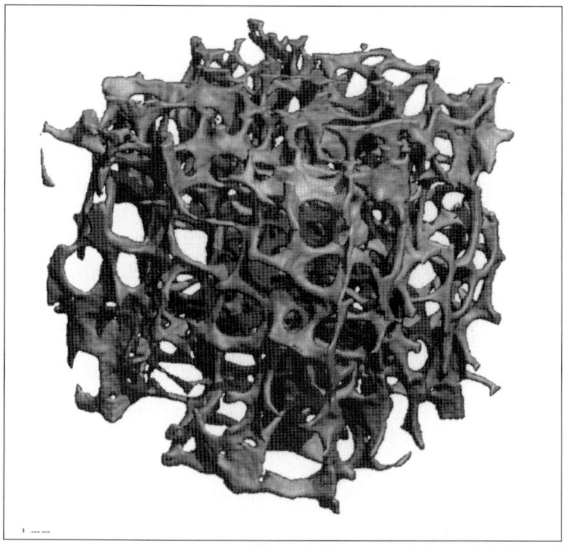

Fig. 6.1 Normal spongiosa of bone with predominately plate-like, broadly connected trabeculae. 3-D CT of a block specimen (4 × 4 mm³) with ultra-high resolution.

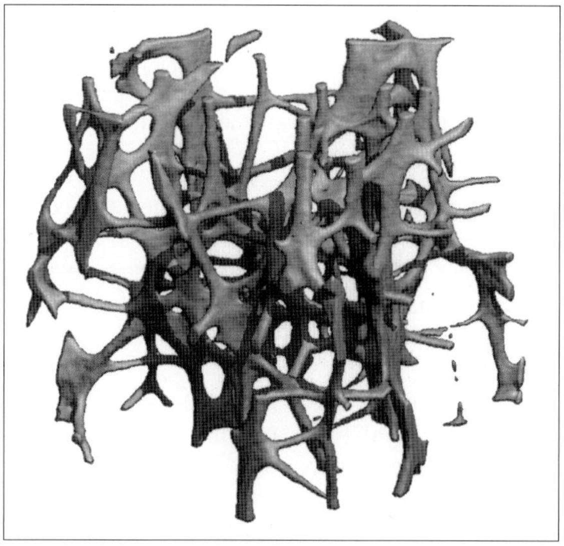

Fig. 6.2 Senile osteoporosis with thin rod-like trabeculae, reduced number of trabeculae, and decreased trabecular connections. 3-D CT of block specimen (4 × 4 mm³) with ultra-high resolution.

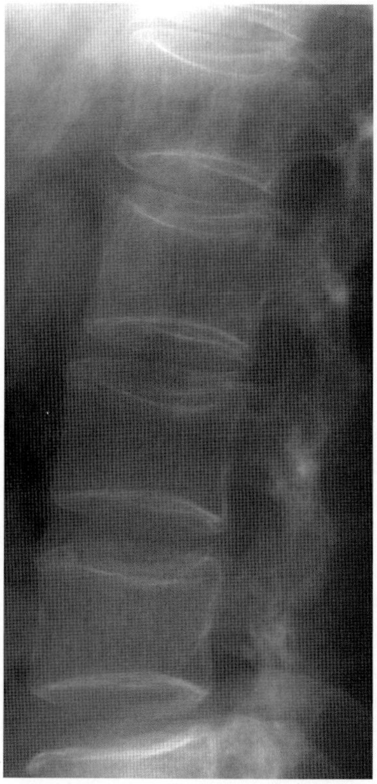

Fig. 6.3 Postmenopausal osteoporosis with marked longitudinal striation caused by accentuated vertical trabeculae. Sharply outlined vertebral bodies ('picture-framing') are also seen.

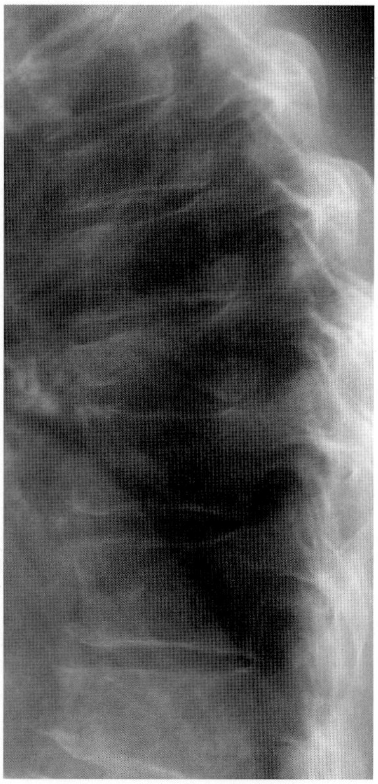

Fig. 6.4 Wedge-shaped thoracic vertebral body in osteoporosis.

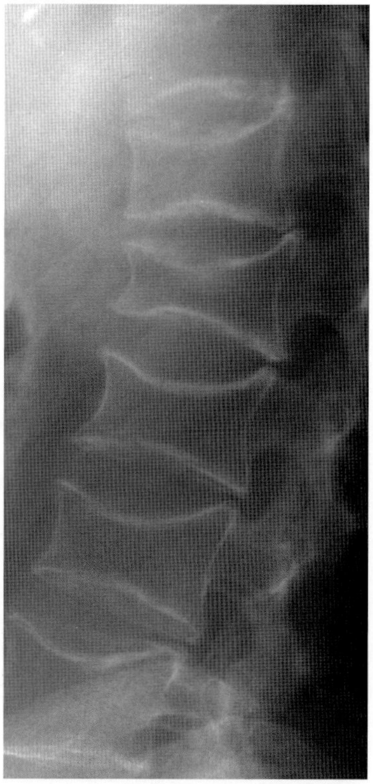

Fig. 6.5 Lumbar 'codfish' vertebral bodies with biconcave indentation. Extreme accentuation of the vertebral outline is seen.

CLINIC Decreased bone mineral density increases the risk of macrofractures. For example, a 1 SD decrease in BMD increases the fracture risk by approximately 1.5 to 2 times normal risk. In the spine, pre-existing vertebral fractures further increase the fracture risk.

X-RAY Osteoporosis is characterized by decreased bone density, rarefied trabecular structure, cortical thinning and fractures.

All types of osteoporosis involve the spine more frequently than other skeletal sites.

Bone Density

Decrease in bone mass corresponds to a decrease in radiographically detected calcium with an increase in the radiolucency of bone.

Radiography does not show decreased bone density until approximately 30% of the bone mass is lost. Consequently, radiography is not appropriate for the early detection of demineralization.

! A decreased bone density is seen not only with osteoporosis, but also with other skeletal diseases. Therefore, it is preferable to use the descriptive term **osteopenia** until the underlying condition has been found.

Caution:
- The radiographic appearance of osteopenia depends on technical factors (kV/mAS, hardening of the X-ray spectrum, etc.), and standardization is necessary to avoid misdiagnoses.
- Interpretation of osteopenia depends on the subjective assessment of the examiner.
- Digital radiography is not suitable for assessing osteopenia since the adjustment of the optical densities by histogram equalization compensates for any increased radiolucency.

Bone Structure

In the vertebral bodies, there is initially attenuation of the horizontal trabeculae and accentuation of the load-bearing vertical trabeculae, resulting in increased longitudinal striation and trabecular thickening on radiography. This so-called 'hypertrophic atrophy,' which is observed mainly in old age, is attributed to microcallus deposition. The trabecular loss results in accentuation of the cortex of the vertebral body, which exhibits a sharply delineated outline in contrast to osteomalacia. These textural changes produce the so-called 'picture-frame' vertebral bodies (Figs. 6.**3**, 6.**5**).

Macrofractures

In **postmenopausal (Type I)** osteoporosis, the fractures tend to involve the vertebral bodies and can even occur without demonstrable decrease in bone density. The vertebral deformities range from subtle indentation of the end plates, wedging, and codfish-vertebra deformity to a complete collapse of the vertebral body (Figs. 6.**4**, 6.**5**). In addition, intravertebral disk protrusion and fractures with intervertebral vacuum phenomenon are observed. The vertebral bodies of the thoracolumbar transition (most frequently T12 and L1) are most commonly involved because of their load bearing. The wedged thoracic vertebral bodies cause an accentuated kyphosis of the thoracic spine. Recent fractures are characterized by increased density along the vertebral end plates (impacted bone substance, reparative callus formation).

The differentiation between osteoporotic, traumatic and metastatic vertebral fractures is discussed on pages 52 – 53.

Fractures due to **senile (Type II) osteoporosis** tend to involve the peripheral skeleton, and typical sites are femoral neck, distal radius, and ribs. In addition, insufficiency fractures can occur in the osteoporotic skeleton, appearing as a band-like sclerosis or radiolucent lines, with or without periosteal reaction. The preferential sites are the spine, sacrum, pelvis (ilium, pubic bone), femoral neck, tibia, and calcaneus (Fig. 6.**6**).

Cortex

Osteoporosis can produce the following findings in the cortex:
- increased endosteal resorption (especially with the increased bone turnover seen in postmenopausal osteoporosis) resulting in cortical thinning due to endosteal scalloping,
- increased intracortical resorption with tunneling (longitudinal striation) and trabecular transformation. Such changes are also seen in the context of primary hyperparathyroidism, renal osteodystrophy, and reflex sympathetic dystrophy (Sudeck atrophy).

DD An osteoporotic appearance that is practically indistinguishable from genuine osteoporosis can be observed in:
- diffuse plasmocytoma (additional osteolytic foci can help in the differentiation; the moth-eaten or permeative pattern is usually not as uniformly distributed throughout the skeleton as in osteoporosis),

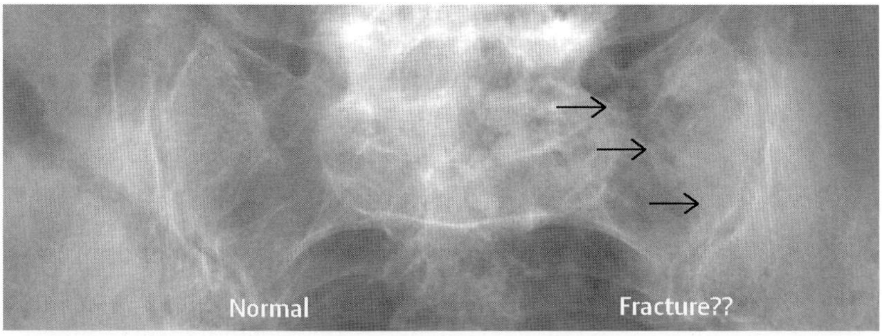

Fig. 6.**6** Insufficiency fracture of the left sacrum. Confirmation by CT or MRI.

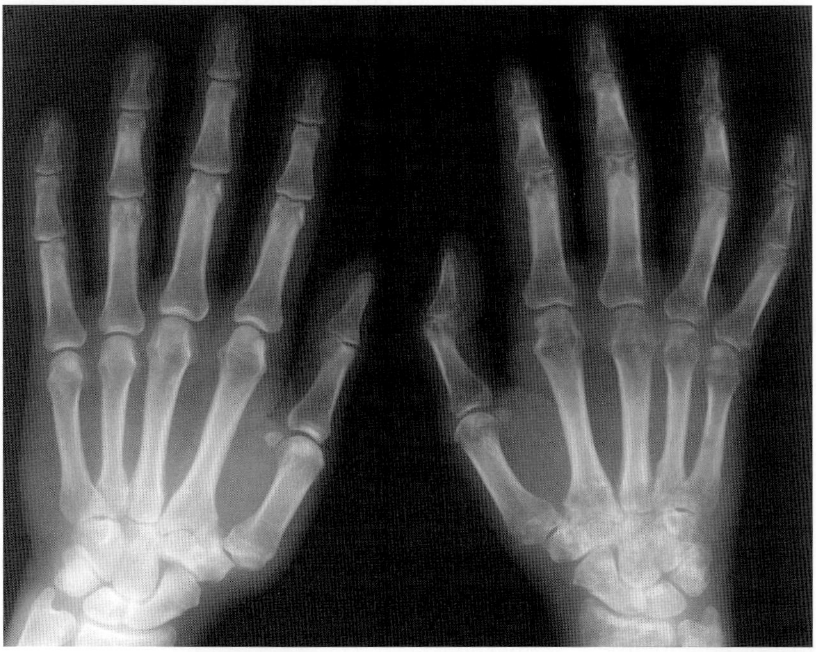

Fig. 6.**7** Severe patchy osteoporosis of the right hand due to longstanding immobilization in hemiplegia.

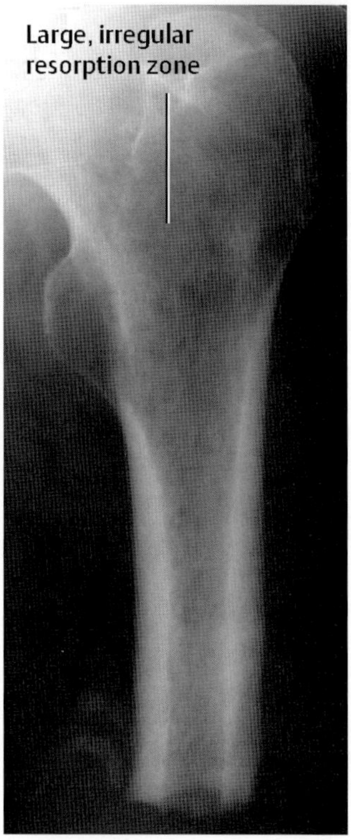

Fig. 6.**8** Moth-eaten osteoporosis in the femoral stump following amputation for osteosarcoma.

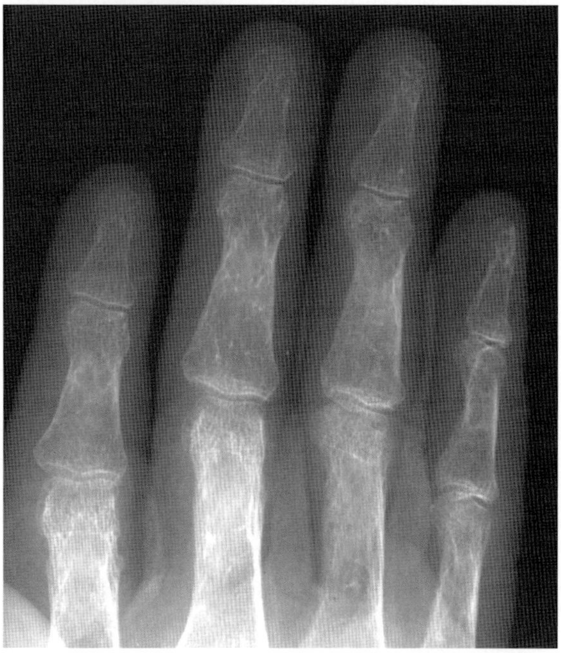

Fig. 6.**9** Senile osteoporosis. Cortical thinning with corresponding enlargement of the marrow space.

- diffuse bony metastases, e.g., small-cell bronchial carcinoma, breast carcinoma (mistaken for osteoporosis only in diffuse bone marrow carcinomatosis since tumors tend to cause larger destructive lesions),
- osteomalacia (with washed-out osseous appearance, Looser zones),
- systemic mastocytosis (types associated with pure osteoporosis cannot be differentiated on the basis of radiographic features).

! Osteoporosis occasionally produces a moth-eaten or permeative pattern and can then appear rather 'malignant', especially in cases of localized disuse osteoporosis (Figs. 6.**8**, 6.**10**). Clinical history and the detection of fat in the bone marrow by CT or MRI usually enables differentiation in radiographically equivocal cases.

X-Ray Absorptiometry and Osteoporosis

Many methods have been proposed for measuring the extent of demineralization with radiography. Indices that consider both severity of vertebral deformity and the number of affected vertebral bodies can be helpful to monitor therapy. However, they are all unsuitable for the early diagnosis of osteoporosis.

Bone Densitometry: It is the goal of bone densitometry to determine the fracture risk **before** fractures have occurred. It is used in subjects at risk of osteoporosis or suspected of having increased bone loss.

Bone densitometry basically measures bone mineral density and content. The two requirements for this measurement are a representative site and a reliable, reproducible method. Preferred sites are the lumbar spine, proximal femur, distal radius, and calcaneus. For the assessment of fracture risk, the lumbar spine should be measured, since measurements of the peripheral skeleton do not always predict the fracture risk in the axial skeleton.

Types of Bone Densitometry

Planar methods (area density in g/cm^2):
- Single x-ray absorptiometry (SXA),
- Dual x-ray absorptiometry (DEXA).

Volumetric methods (quantitative computerized tomography [QCT], true bone density in mg/ml):
- Single energy QCT (SE-QCT),
- Dual energy QCT (DE-QCT),
- Peripheral QCT (pQCT)

Quantitative sonography (QUS)
Quantitative MRI (QMR)
The major criteria for determining the quality of any measurement technique are absolute precision and reproducibility. Which measurement error is more critical depends on the goal of the examination. If an individual measurement is obtained to determine the mineral content of the patient relative to subjects of the same age and sex (early detection, risk analysis), the reliability rests primarily on absolute precision. If the rate of loss is the most important measurement in a specific patient (e.g., for monitoring therapy), reproducibility is the most crucial criterion. To determine a loss rate of 2.5%, the reproducibility error of the method should not exceed 1%.

Absorptiometry and computed tomography are the most common methods in widespread use and play a practical role. Both of these are based on the attenuation of the radiation beam passing through the skeleton.

Technical Principles and Clinical Role of the Various Methods

Single X-ray Absorptiometry (SXA)

This measures the attenuation of an X-ray beam at a peripheral site, most commonly the radius. It is relatively simple and inexpensive but has been abandoned because of suboptimal precision and reproducibility.

Dual X-ray Absorptiometry (DEXA)

This technique measures the attenuation of an X-ray beam from two energy peaks (Fig. 6.**11**). Measuring the attenuation of two different energy peaks compared with a standard reference material enables the calculation and subtraction of the soft-tissue component of the X-ray attenuation. This increases the precision of the measured bone density in comparison to single X-ray absorptiometry. Dual X-ray absorptiometry has become the standard method for diagnosing and following osteoporosis and is used to measure the lumbar spine, hip, or distal forearm. In the lumbar spine, erroneous measurements due to overlying calcific structures (calcified aortic plaques, osteophytes), compression fractures, and scoliosis may be encountered, and comparison with current lumbar spine radiographs are important to avoid misdiagnosis.

Quantitative CT (QCT)

With the gantry appropriately angled, the mid-level of three lumbar vertebrae (usually L1 – L3) is scanned, provided they are not fractured. A region of interest is automatically and, consequently, reproducibly placed in the spongiosa of each vertebral body. The bone density is determined by comparing the average of the measured Hounsfield units with the measured Hounsfield units of the known densities of a reference phantom. Single X-ray QCT measures the attenuation at one energy level, and dual X-ray QCT adds a second measurement at another energy level by changing the X-ray tube voltage. Analogous to DEXA, the dual X-ray QCT can eliminate the error introduced by the marrow fat, but places more demand on the software needed for analysis.

The advantage of quantitative CT is the selective measurement of a small volume of spongiosa of bone and the simultaneous display of its structure (microcallus, microcalcifications). Extraneous calcifications, such as aortic calcifications, do not present a problem in measuring the bone density. The disadvantage is that the radiation dose delivered is higher than that of DEXA.

Practical remark: The report of a QCT should read as follows:

'The bone mineral density was calculated from representative axial sections of three lumbar vertebral bodies.... The absolute bone mineral density averaged over the three vertebral bodies is... mg/ml. This value is... standard deviations below the average in a population of the patient's age and sex (Z score) and... standard deviations below the peak bone mass of a young adult (T score).

Conclusion: No osteoporosis/osteopenia/osteoporosis/manifest osteoporosis.'

(Note: One standard deviation corresponds to 30 mg/ml; consequently, a calcium content of less than 85 mg of CaHA corresponds to osteoporosis.)

Peripheral Quantitative CT

A small, specially designed unit measures the bone density of the distal radius using the principle of quantitative CT. This method enables clinical follow-up and requires an experienced technologist. Moreover, this method can provide information about the biomechanical property of the bone but alone is unsuitable for establishing the initial diagnosis of osteoporosis.

Quantitative Sonography and Quantitative MRI

Both of these methods are currently being investigated and are not yet used in clinical practice.

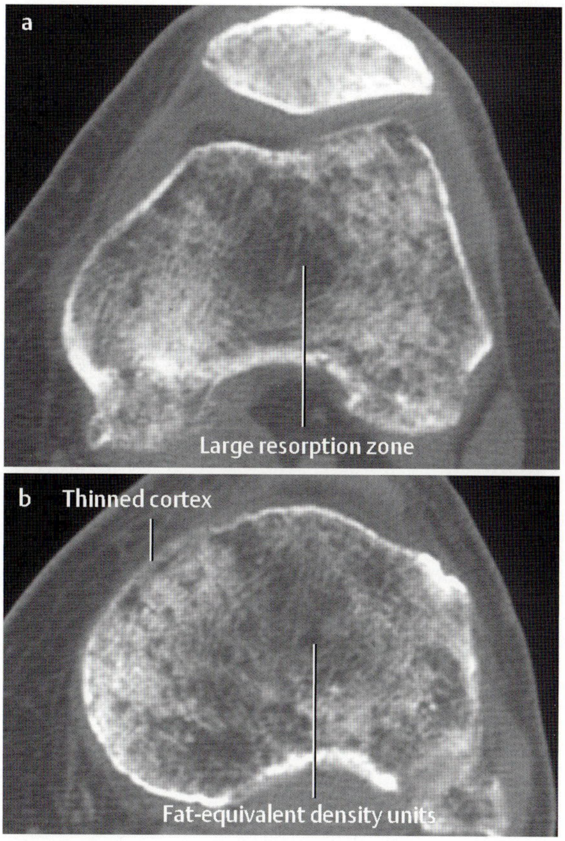

Fig. 6.**10** Disuse osteoporosis of the knee after trauma. **a** Femoral condyles, **b** tibial plateau. The fat-equivalent density in the region of the trabecular resorption is indicative of osteoporosis.

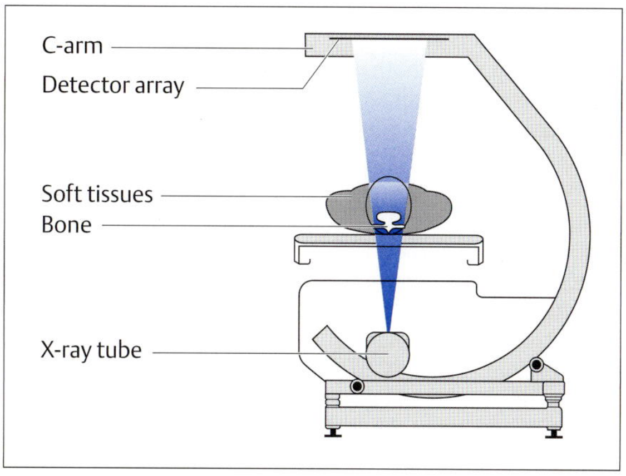

Fig. 6.**11** Schematic drawing of a DEXA unit.

Rickets and Osteomalacia

■ This is a group of conditions with inadequate mineralization of the osteoid due to vitamin D deficiency or hereditary disorders of vitamin D metabolism. In the growing skeleton, this interferes with the normal development of the growth plates, causing rickets, and in the mature skeleton leads to a delayed mineralization of the spongiosa and cortical bones, causing osteomalacia. ■

PATH **Calcium metabolism** is regulated by parathyroid hormone, calcitonin, and vitamin D.

Parathyroid hormone is synthesized in the parathyroid glands, and its secretion increases with **hypocalcemia.** Parathyroid hormone

- stimulates the osteoclasts to release calcium and phosphate from bone,
- stimulates vitamin D synthesis in the kidney, resulting in increased intestinal resorption of calcium,
- increases resorption of calcium in the kidney and decreases resorption of phosphate.

Calcitonin is synthesized in the C cells of the thyroid gland and secreted as a response to **hypercalcemia.** Calcitonin

- activates the osteoblasts to deposit more calcium in bone,
- increases renal calcium secretion.

Vitamin D is synthesized in three steps:

1. Formation of the precursor 7-dehydrocholesterol in the liver,
2. Formation of cholecalciferol through ultraviolet light in the skin, and
3. Double hydroxylation to 1,25-$(OH)_2$-cholecalciferol in the liver and kidney, respectively.

The synthesis is stimulated by parathyroid hormone and calcium and phosphate deficiency. Vitamin D

- increases mineralization of bone,
- increases intestinal resorption of calcium.

Rickets or osteomalacia develops if the amount of either vitamin D or calcium is inadequate. In the past, insufficient supply of vitamin D due to **inadequate sunlight (UV light) exposure** ('rickets') was most prevalent. The important predispositions today are:

- inadequate resorption of calcium in conditions with gastrointestinal malabsorption (e.g., after gastric and intestinal surgeries, in pancreas insufficiency),
- loss of phosphate due to renal tubular defects (e.g., congenital, hemodialysis, transplant),
- premature neonates requiring about 3 to 6 times more vitamin D than normal neonates,
- liver diseases,
- anticonvulsant therapy (Phenytoin).

In **normal bone growth** (Fig. 6.**12**) the chondrocytes proliferate along the diaphyseal side of the growth plate, and a large amount of intercellular cartilage substance accumulates. The chondrocytes align in longitudinal columns (columnar cartilage), and fluid accumulates from the intervening cartilage matrix. This leads to swelling of the chondrocytes (lacunar cartilage) and precipitation of calcium in the cartilage matrix. This is the signal for the osteoclasts to become active and to remove the intercellular substance ('tidemark'). Osteoblasts appear in the remnants of the calcified cartilage matrix, where they first form osteoid. This osteoid mineralizes later and is transformed into woven bone. Finally, lamellar bone is formed.

In **rickets,** the zone of chondrocytes becomes disorganized, increases its number of cells, and undergoes hypertrophy. This increases the length and width of the growth plate. In addition, the osteoid produced is inadequately mineralized, and there is a decrease in the normal formation of osteons.

CLINIC In children, the most striking findings are disproportionate growth retardation of the peripheral skeleton in relation to the axial skeleton and bone deformities:

- Widening of the growth zones (e.g., 'rosary of rickets'),
- Basal invagination of the skull (= the dens projects more than 1 cm above the bimastoid line),
- Tibial bowing,
- Scoliosis,
- Deformed pelvis.

Furthermore, these children are susceptible to infections and tetany during the healing phase.

The leading biochemical markers are hypocalcemia and hypophosphatemia.

X-RAY **Rickets:** The changes are most pronounced at the zones of increased bone transformation. Primarily affected are:

- costocartilage junction of the mid-ribs (Fig. 6.**13**),
- proximal humerus,
- distal femur and tibia,
- distal forearm.

The growth plates are widened, cup-shaped, and frayed (Figs. 6.**14**, 6.**15**).

Various bone deformities are variably present, and skeletal growth is delayed.

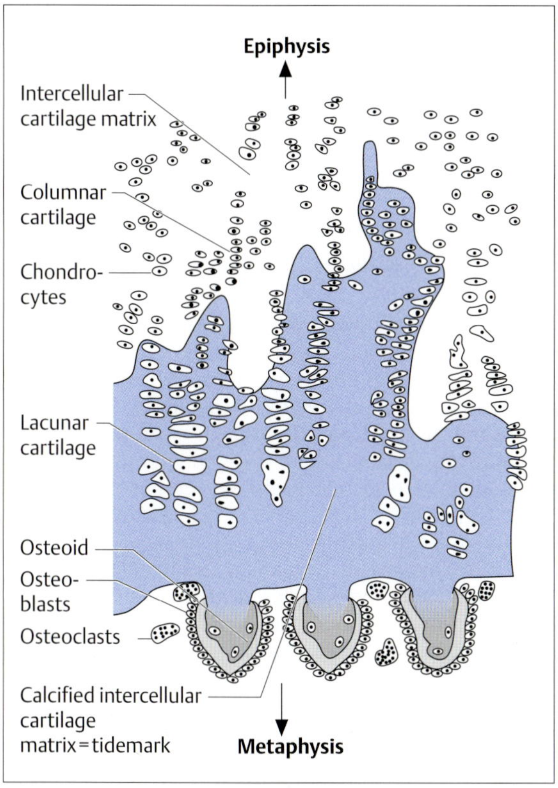

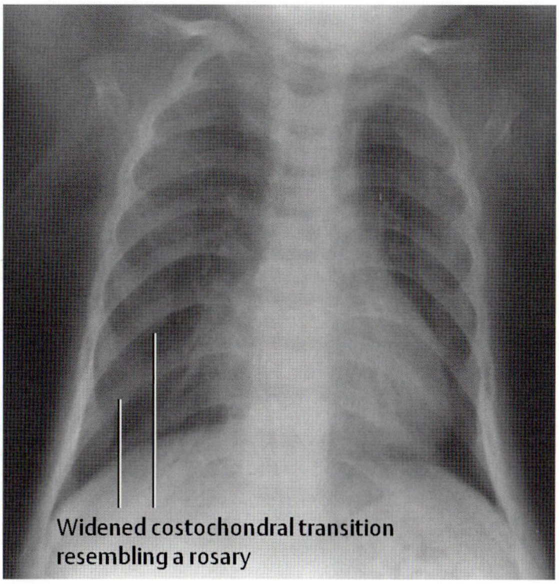

Fig. 6.**13** Bony thorax of a 10-year-old boy with rickets.

Left:
Fig. 6.**12** Normal structure of the epiphyseal plate.

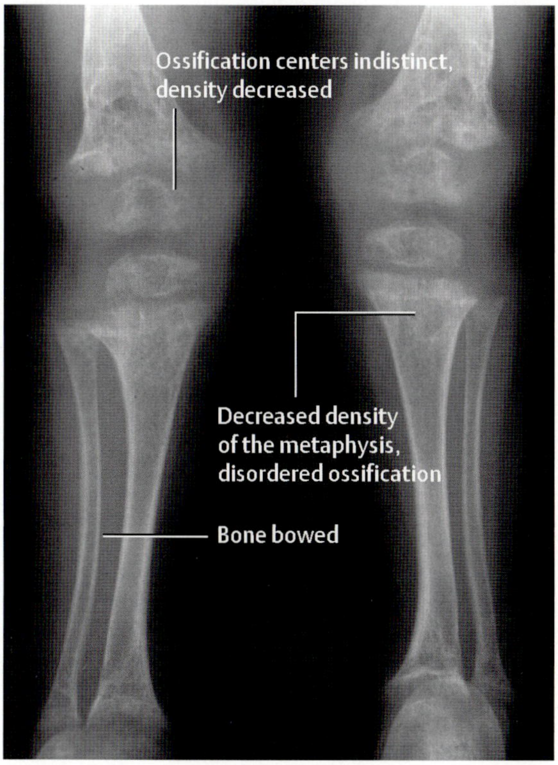

Fig. 6.**14** Knee and lower leg of a 10-year-old boy with rickets. Notice the cup-like deformities and widening of the epiphyseal plates.

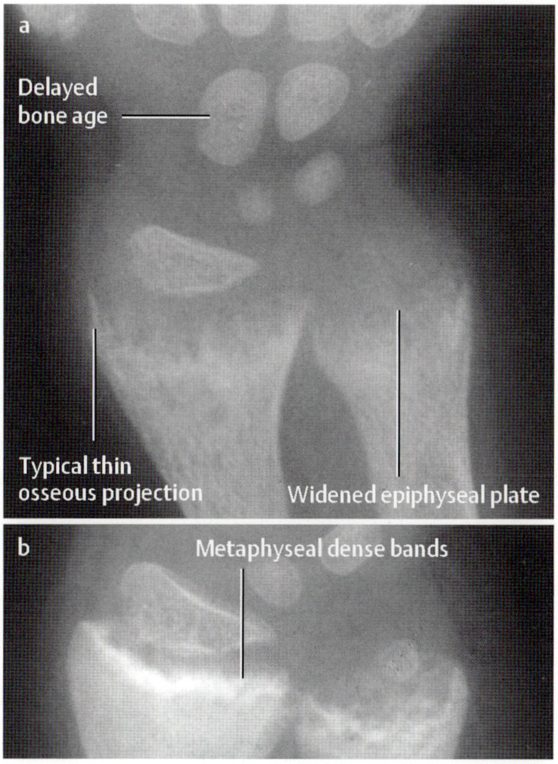

Fig. 6.**15** **a** Hand of a 10-year-old boy with rickets. Since the periosteal reaction is more apparent than the endosteal reaction, typical marginal osseous projections are seen. **b** After vitamin D therapy for 1 year, metaphyseal bands of increased density due to massive ossification of the osseous matrix have appeared.

Osteomalacia: A decreased number of trabeculae and an oversupply of nonmineralized osteoid produce nonspecific osteopenia with a 'washed-out' appearance (Fig. 6.**16**). Localized radiolucencies can correspond to osteoid accumulations or dilated Haversian canals. Moreover, subperiosteal deposition of osteoid takes place along the tubular bones, characteristically leading to widening and fissuring of the dorsal contour of the femur. Finally, bowing of the bone can be seen because of insufficiency (Fig. 6.**17**).

Looser zones are a characteristic feature of osteomalacia. They represent incomplete insufficiency fractures, which appear radiographically as radiolucent lines. They often are symmetric and perpendicular to the cortex and characteristically only affect a portion of the bone circumference. They differ from stress fractures because of their frequent bilateral occurrence and retarded healing and persistent incomplete osseous bridging over time. Characteristic sites are the scapula, ribs, pubic bone, femur, and proximal ulna (Fig. 6.**18**).

NUC The bone scan shows the distribution of systemic involvement in osteomalacia and is a suitable screening examination for the detection of Looser zones.

Glossary

Vitamin D-resistant rickets (= 'phosphate diabetes', 'hypophosphatemic rickets') is a hereditary condition. Dwarfism, calcifications of parenchymal organs, and osteosclerosis are the manifestations of this condition.

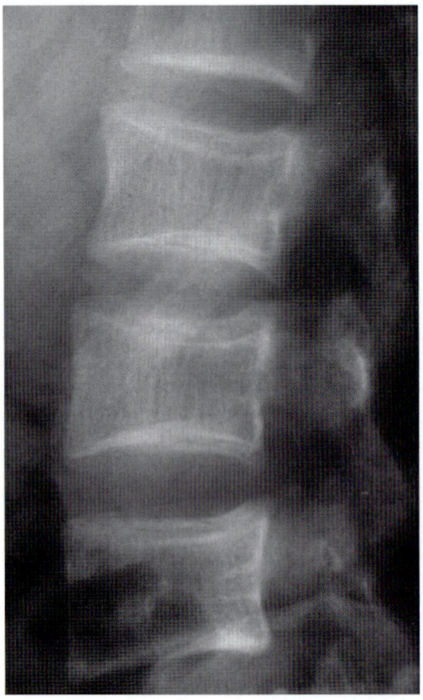

Fig. 6.**16** Lumbar spine of a 22-year-old woman with osteomalacia. The 'washed-out' appearance of the vertebral bodies is characteristic.

Hyperparathyroidism

Synonyms: secretory fibro-osteoplasia, osteitis fibrosa cystica generalisata Recklinghausen.

■ Hyperparathyroidism is characterized by increased parathyroid hormone levels in the blood and produces a typical pattern of bone resorption and transformation. ■

PATH **Primary hyperparathyroidism** is caused by autonomous hypersecretion of the parathyroid gland (solitary or multiple adenomas, hyperplasia, carcinoma) and is characterized by hypercalcemia.

Secondary hyperparathyroidism is caused by longstanding hypocalcemia. Underlying conditions are chronic renal insufficiency, malabsorption, or abnormal phosphate metabolism. Hyperplasia of the parathyroid glands is found in the majority of cases.

Tertiary hyperparathyroidism represents the autonomous function of the parathyroid gland induced by longstanding secondary hyperparathyroidism. In this condition, the hyperplastic parathyroid glands have become adenomatous.

CLINIC Hyperparathyroidism is usually discovered by its complications of renal stones, peptic gastrointestinal ulcers, and pancreatitis. Pain and swelling of the joints are infrequent complaints. Today's more advanced diagnostic approach has made clinically severe forms a rare occurrence.

X-RAY Early diagnosis and follow-up examinations can be produced by conventional or digital magnification radiography of the hands, often best accomplished by using mammography technique (Fig. 6.**19**). Other imaging methods do not play a major role in hyperparathyroidism.

The radiographic features are:

- increased bone resorption (Table 6.**1**),
- deposition of calcium pyrophosphate and urate,
- osteosclerosis.

The cardinal radiographic features in the fingers are subperiosteal resorption, tunneling, and trabecular resorption.

In **subchondral resorption,** subchondral bone is replaced with inferior and less resilient fibrous tissue, leading to fractures of the joint-bearing bone and, in advanced stages, osteolytic destructions.

A **sclerotic component** can be dominant, especially in the axial skeleton. Characteristic bands of increased densities are seen along the vertebral end plates, causing the so-called 'rugger-jersey spine' (Fig. 6.**28**). In addition, periosteal bone appositions can develop.

Primary hyperparathyroidism is characterized by high incidence of **chondrocalcinosis** and **brown tumors** (Fig. 6.**22**).

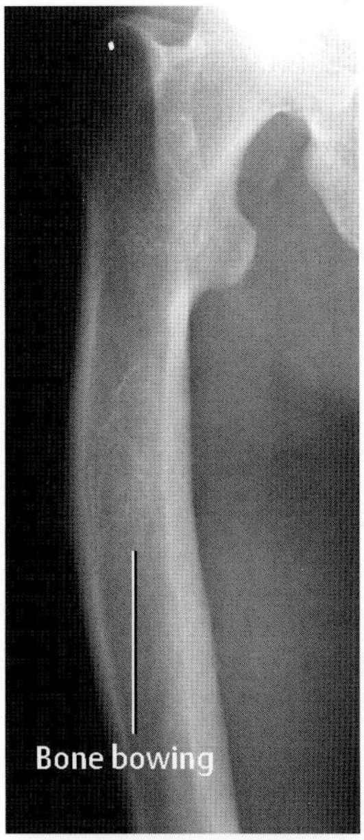

Fig. 6.**17** Femur of a 48-year-old woman with osteomalacia. Notice the periosteal osseous apposition along the inner aspect of the femoral shaft.

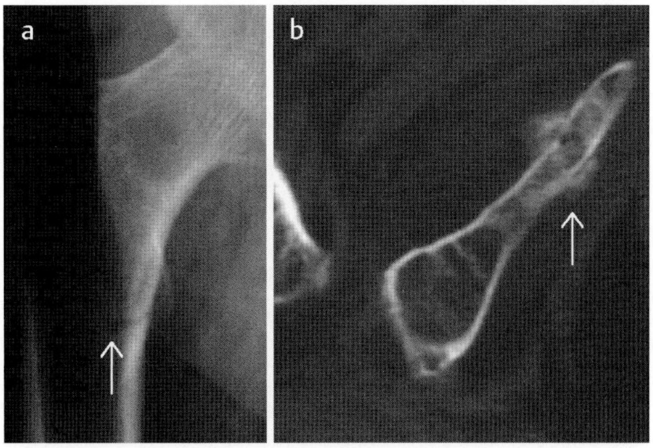

Fig. 6.**18** Looser zones. **a** Femur of a 43-year-old woman. This patient had osteomalacia due to renal osteodystrophy. The findings are bilateral and **symmetric**. **b** Unilateral Looser zone seen on CT of the pelvis (pubic ramus) in a female patient with osteomalacia.

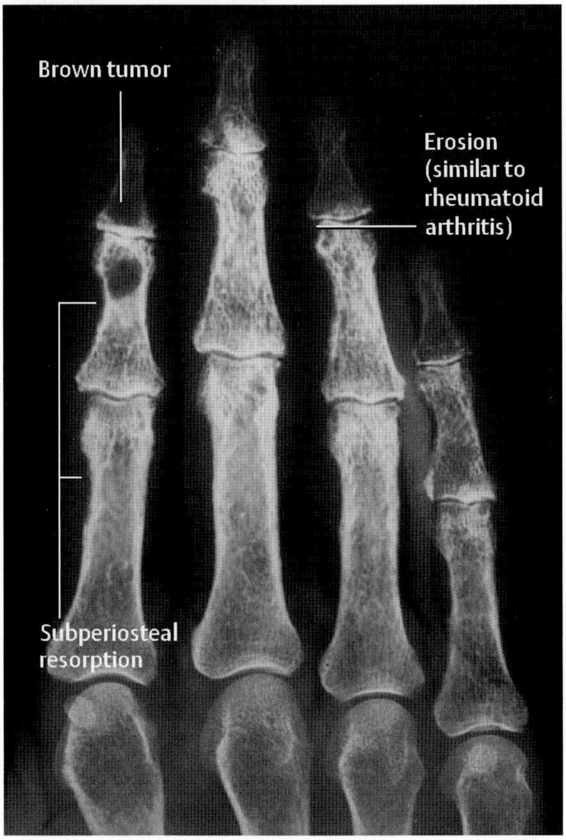

Fig. 6.**19** Finger of a 21-year-old woman with secondary hyperparathyroidism.

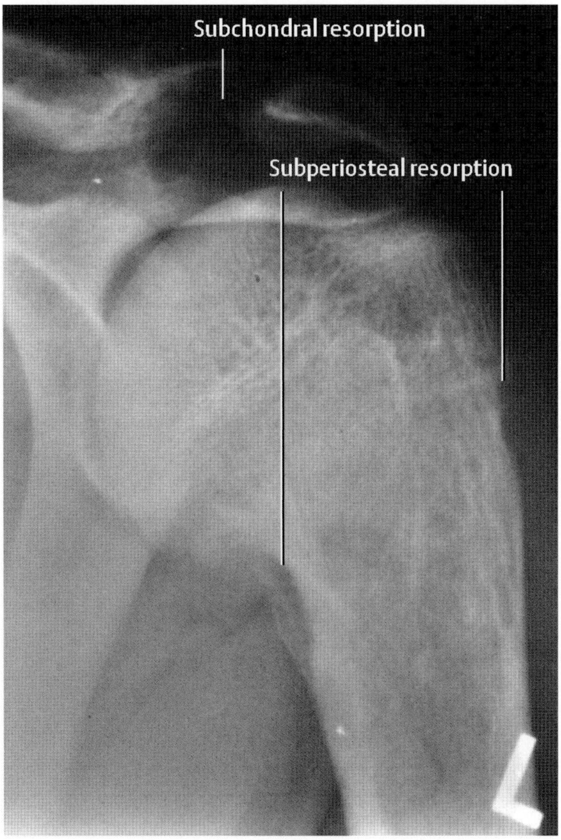

Fig. 6.**20** Subperiosteal resorption around the shoulder in a 61-year-old man with primary hyperparathyroidism.

After therapy (e.g., resection of the parathyroid glands or renal transplantation), the periosteal resorptions reverse, and there is ossification at the insertion sites. As part of the healing process, the pseudowidening of the symphysis and SI joints might become a synostosis. The brown tumors develop calcifications, which only years later are replaced by lamellar bone (Fig. 6.**24**).

DD Differentiation from other articular diseases, especially rheumatoid arthritis, is guided by the typical distribution pattern of involvement observed with each entity (Table 6.**2**).

Calcium pyrophosphate deposition disease (CPPD) can be associated with hyperparathyroidism, but can also occur as an isolated entity (idiopathic, see page 368).

Table 6.**1** Manifestations of **increased bone loss** in hyperparathyroidism

Pathomechanics	Radiography	Location
Subperiosteal resorption (Figs. 6.**19**, 6.**20**)	Irregular superficial cortical defects	Radial aspect of the middle phalanx of fingers 2 and 3, ungual process, femoral neck, proximal tibia, proximal humerus, ribs; submarginal at the joints: acromioclavicular, sternoclavicular, and sacroiliac joints, symphysis
Intracortical resorption	Tunneling of the cortex Widening of the Haversian canals	Radial aspect of the middle phalanx of fingers 2 and 3, metacarpal 2
Subchondral resorption (Fig. 6.**23**)	Thinned or absent lamella	Sacroiliac, sternoclavicular, and acromioclavicular joints, symphysis, vertebral end plates, major and minor joints of the extremities
Subtendinous resorption (Fig. 6.**21**)	Insertional defects with stippled soft-tissue calcifications	Heavy mechanical load at the insertions of tendons and ligaments
Trabecular resorption (Fig. 6.**25**)	Loss of spongiosa, fibrous replacement	Skull, pelvis, tubular bones, fingers
Brown tumors (rarely observed today) (Figs. 6.**19**, 6.**20**, 6.**24**)	Focal, solitary or multiple, eccentric or cortical resorption	Facial bones, pelvis, ribs, femur

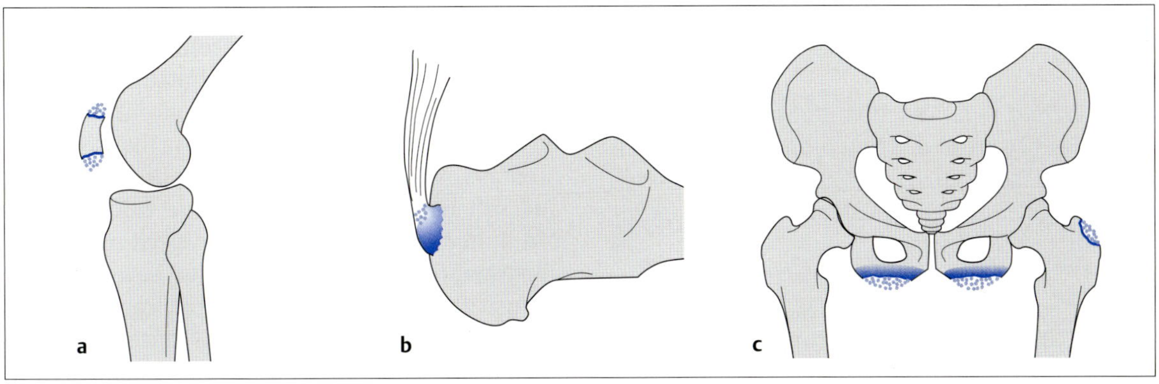

Fig. 6.**21** Subtendinous resorption in hyperparathyroidism.

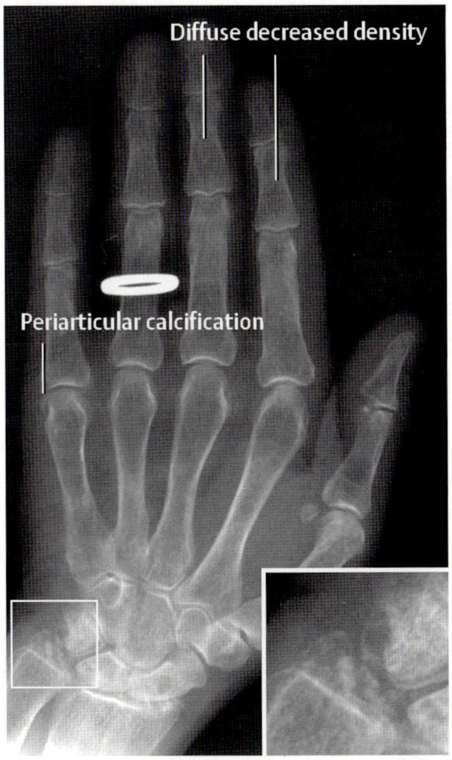

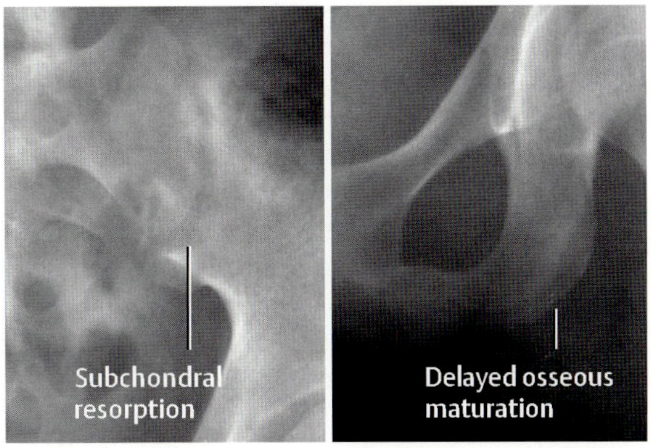

Fig. 6.**23** Pelvis of a 23-year-old woman with secondary hyperparathyroidism.

Left:

Fig. 6.**22** Hand of a 72-year-old woman with primary hyperparathyroidism. The insert shows calcifications in the triangular fibrocartilage complex.

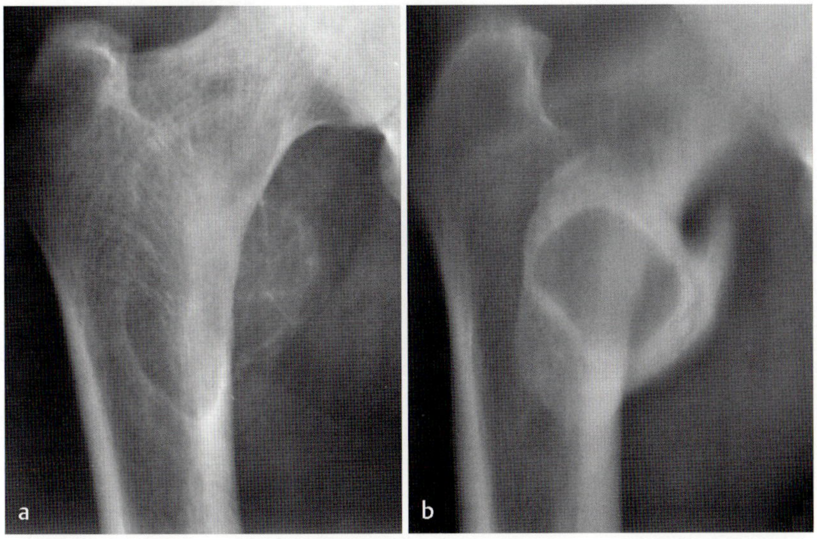

Fig. 6.**24**

a Femur of a 30-year-old woman with a brown tumor due to primary hyperparathyroidism.

b Conventional tomography of the femur. The brown tumor is surrounded by a sclerosis 6 years after resection of the parathyroid glands.

Renal Osteodystrophy

Impaired renal function and end-stage renal insufficiency treated with chronic hemodialysis induce osseous changes that are characterized by expanded osteoid, osteoclastic resorption, and altered bone mass.

PATH Renal osteodystrophy is caused by a variety of illnesses and is characterized by:
- secondary hyperparathyroidism (in the presence of unchanged phosphate intake, reduced glomerular filtration leads to an increase in serum phosphate, resulting in decrease in serum calcium, which leads to increased parathyroid hormonal secretion),
- decreased vitamin D formation (osteomalacia component of renal osteodystrophy),
- parathyroid hormone resistance of the skeleton.

X-RAY The radiographic features of primary hyperparathyroidism are also seen in renal osteodystrophy. Periosteal resorption in the hands and subchondral bone loss at the acromioclavicular joints predominate (Figs. 6.**26**, 6.**27**). Osteosclerotic changes (Fig. 6.**28**), periosteal osseous proliferations, and vascular calcifications are more pronounced in primary hyperparathyroidism. Chondrocalcinosis is rare.

The changes caused by the osteomalacic component of renal osteodystrophy lead to:
- Osteopenia,
- Looser zones,
- Bowing deformities of the bones.

In children with renal insufficiency, widening of the epiphysis (rickets) is invariably seen. In addition, epiphysiolysis is frequent (Fig. 6.**29**).

In addition to osteopenia and subperiosteal resorption, the cortical bone becomes osteoporotic, and there is an increased risk of fracture.

When the product of calcium concentration and phosphate concentration exceeds the solubility products, calcium phosphate deposits in bones and soft tissues. These **soft-tissue calcifications** can mimic articular symptoms caused by osseous abnormalities. They often involve several joints, are usually bilateral, and may rarely cause osseous erosions. Liquid calcifications can cause fluid levels (visible primarily on CT), and these findings can be rather extensive ('pseudotumorous calcinosis,' Fig. 6.**30**).

Other changes that are associated with dialysis and renal transplants are **avascular necrosis** and **amyloidosis.**

! Amyloidosis in patients with end-stage, dialysis-dependent renal insufficiency is caused by a decrease in β_2-microglobulin elimination and is not directly related to renal osteodystrophy (see page 254).

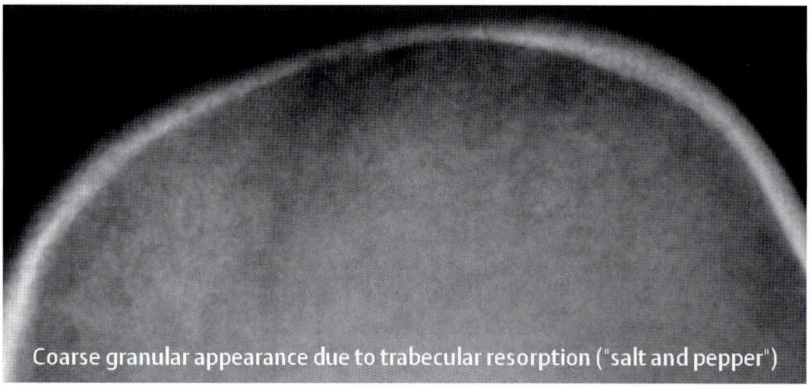

Fig. 6.**25** Skull of a 30-year-old woman with renal osteodystrophy.

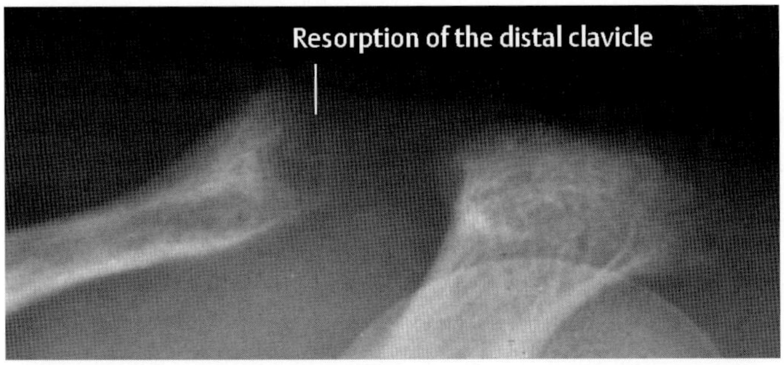

Fig. 6.26 Acromioclavicular joints in a 17-year-old male patient with renal osteodystrophy.

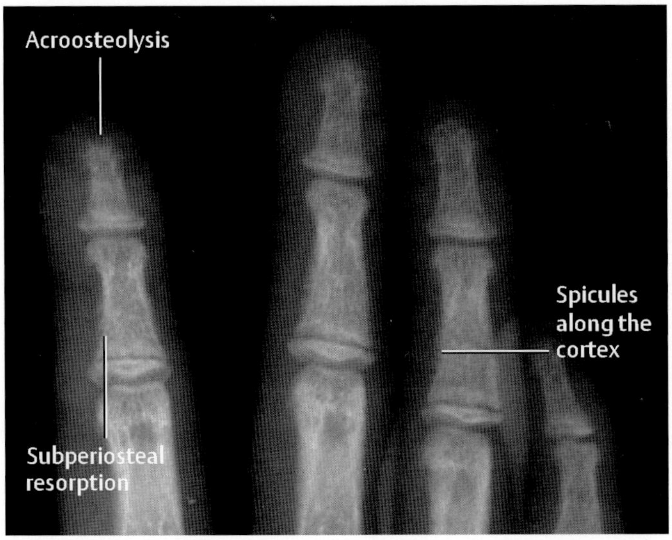

Fig. 6.27 Hand of a 17-year-old male patient with renal osteodystrophy.

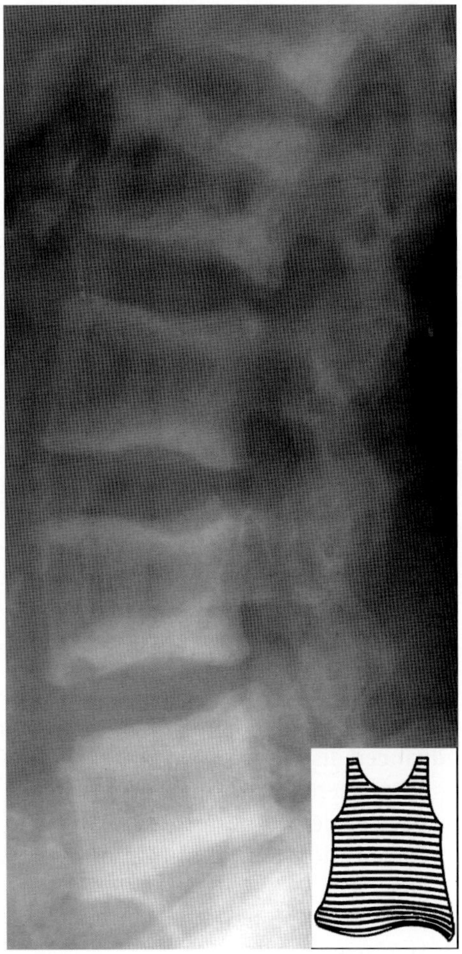

Fig. 6.28 'Rugger jersey spine' in renal osteodystrophy, 30-year-old woman. (Rugger jersey = typically striped jersey of a rugby football team.)

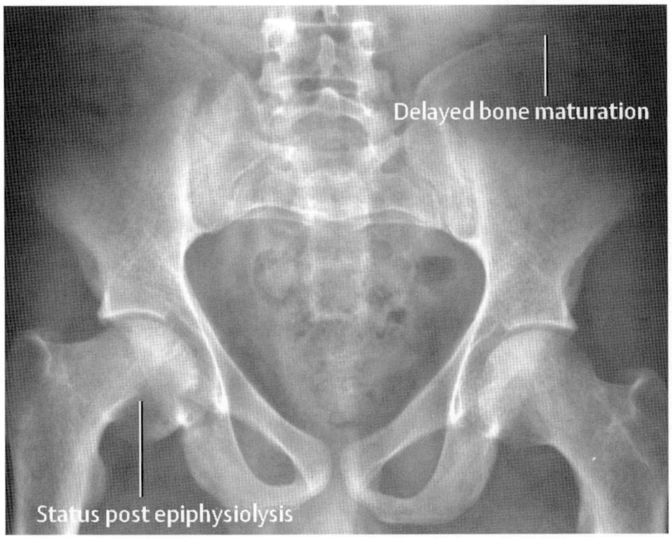

Fig. 6.29 Pelvis of a 22-year-old man with renal osteodystrophy. Status post-epiphysiolysis.

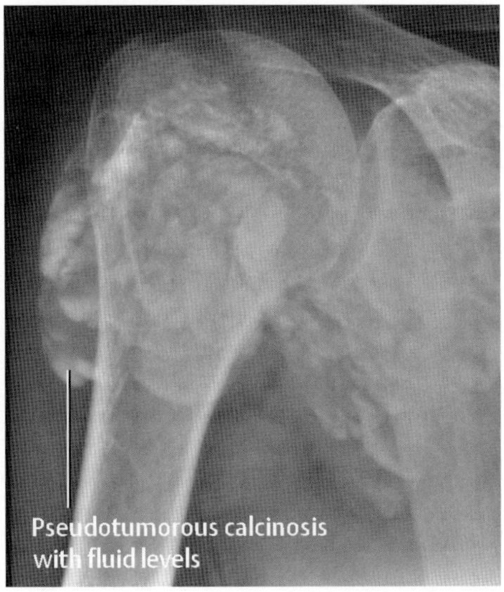

Fig. 6.30 53-year-old man with renal osteodystrophy and shoulder pain.

Hypoparathyroidism

■ In hypoparathyroidism, the serum parathyroid hormone levels are decreased, resulting in hypocalcemia and hyperphosphatemia. ■

PATH The deficiency of parathyroid hormone may be iatrogenic (e.g., thyroidectomy with injury to the parathyroid glands or their vascular supply) or secondary to aplasia or atrophy associated with autoimmune disease.

Pseudohypoparathyroidism is a genetically determined end organ resistance with characteristic phenotype (Albright osteodystrophy).

CLINIC Hypocalcemia leads to increased neuromuscular irritability and often to tetany (carpopedal spasm). Basal ganglia calcifications also occur (Fahr disease). The hereditary types are associated with stunted growth, a strikingly round face, mental retardation, obesity, brachydactyly, and epiphyseal disturbances.

X-RAY Radiographs do not contribute to the **early** diagnosis. The radiographic findings of **advanced** disease are:

- Osteosclerosis,
- Dentine defects of the teeth,
- Calcifications in the soft tissues and basal ganglia,
- Premature epiphyseal fusion,
- Thickened calvaria.

In pseudohypoparathyroidism, metacarpal and metatarsal shortening, exostoses projecting at right angles from the longitudinal bone axis, and bone bowing may also be seen (Fig. 6.**31**).

Toxic Osteopathies

Metal Poisoning (Lead, Bismuth, Phosphorus)

■ Acute and chronic metal poisoning has become extremely rare due to heightened safety rules today. It occurs after prolonged exposure to toxic substances at increased doses. ■

X-RAY Characteristic features are symmetric metaphyseal bands of increased density or patchy areas of sclerosis (Fig. 6.**32**). Metal poisoning might also cause metaphyseal widening. Since lead passes the placenta after the 13th gestational week, the newborn of mothers exposed to high lead levels during pregnancy also develop metaphyseal bands of increased density, delayed dental and skeletal development, and often generalized osteoporosis.

Bismuth can also cause avascular necrosis in addition to the above-mentioned metaphyseal bands of increased density.

DD The sclerotic lines of metal poisoning are considerably broader and more conspicuous than the physiologic lines of increased density in the tubular bones and vertebral bodies (growth lines, Park or Harris lines) and can persist throughout life.

Aluminum Bone Disease

The major causes are aluminum hydroxide antacid therapy or administration of aluminum-containing phosphate binders in uremic patients. Aluminum inhibits bone mineralization. Thus, the radiographic features are osteopenia, Looser zones, and periosteal appositions. Children also show rickets-like changes at the metaphyses.

Fluorosis

■ Fluorosis represents a metabolic bone disease induced by long-term exposure to fluorides. Today, this primarily is an after effect of osteoporosis therapy with sodium fluoride. Rarely, it may be a manifestation of an abnormally high fluoride levels in the drinking water. ■

PATH Fluoride leads to increased new-bone formation by hyperstimulation of osteoblastic activity. Osseous resorption is suppressed by the incorporation of the relatively stable compound, fluoroapatite.

CLINIC Joint pain and ankle swelling occur.

X-RAY About one year after commencement of the therapy with sodium fluoride, there is an increased bone density associated with thickening of the cortex, coarsened trabecular texture (Fig. 6.**33**), and ligamentous calcifications. The features of fluoride intoxication are:

- Osteosclerosis,
- Osteophytes and spondylophytes,
- Ligamentous calcifications,
- Periostitis.

The findings are reversible and disappear 10–15 years after cessation of fluoride exposure. Long-term fluoride therapy over several years can also increase bone fragility.

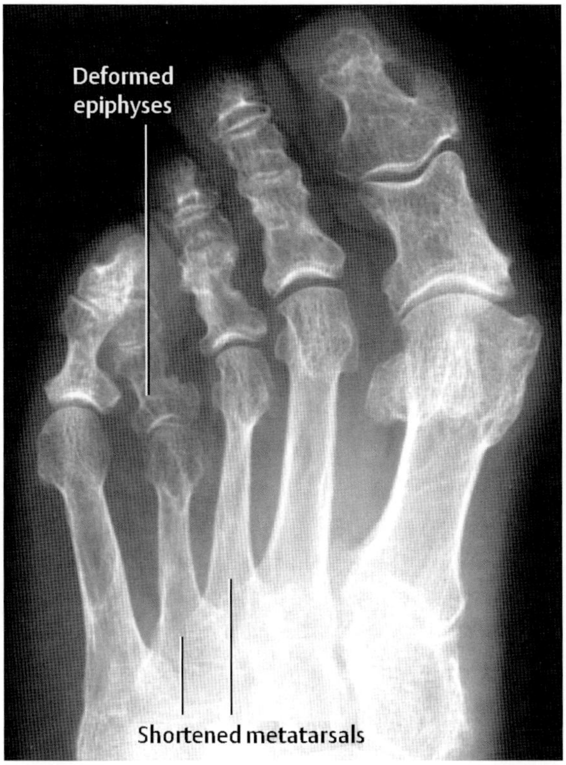

Fig. 6.**31** Forefoot of a 45-year-old woman with pseudohypoparathyroidism.

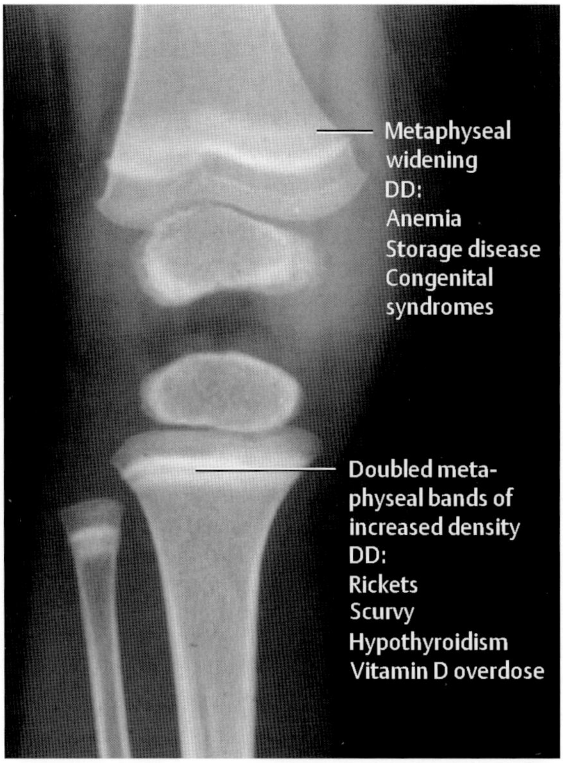

Fig. 6.**32** Knee of a boy with two episodes of lead intoxication. Other less-frequent differential diagnoses of dense metaphyseal bands are leukemia in remission and transplacental infections.

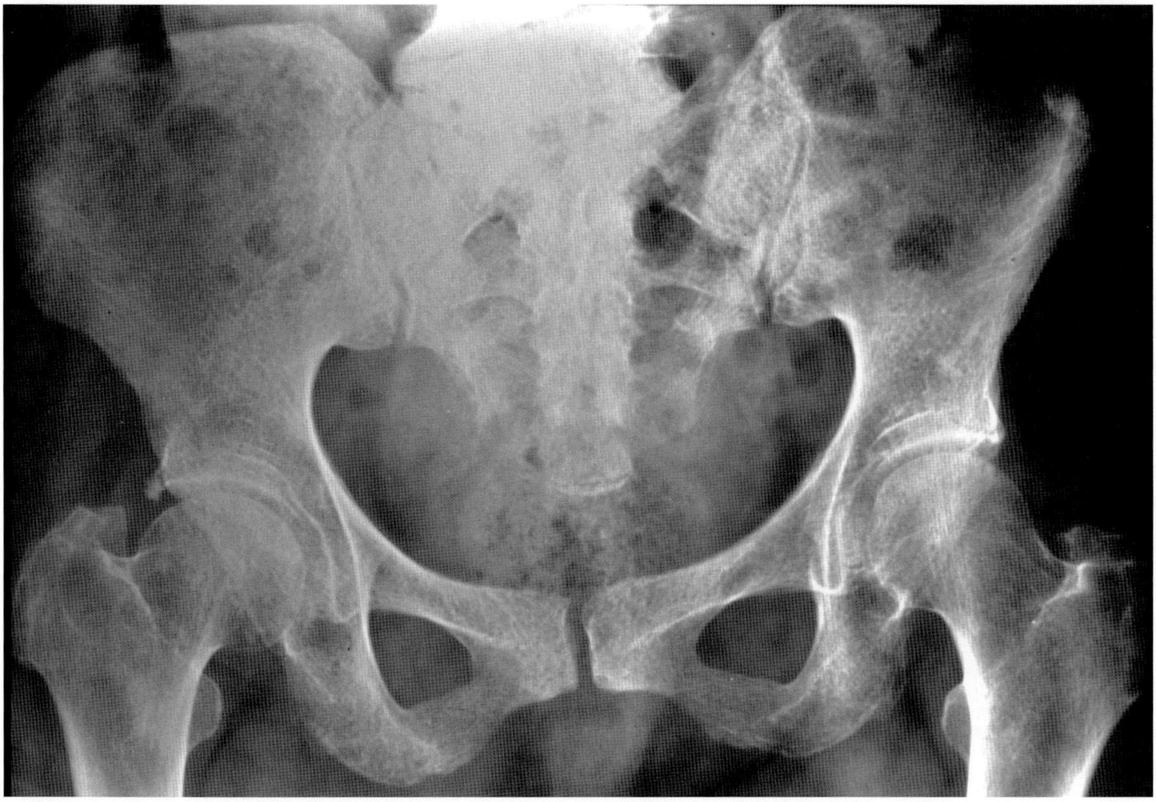

Fig. 6.**33** Pelvis of a 76-year-old woman after sodium fluoride therapy for osteoporosis for 4 years. Note the coarsened trabecular texture.

Corticosteroids

Therapy with corticosteroids can induce numerous side effects in the musculoskeletal system (Table 6.**3**). To a great degree, they are independent of dose and duration of application.

PATH Not all aspects of the pathogenesis of corticosteroid-induced changes are known. Therapeutic side effects cannot always be clearly distinguished from the outcome of the natural history of the underlying disease. Corticosteroids probably induce secondary hyperparathyroidism due to reduced calcium reabsorption and tubular hypercalciuria. Numerous data also indicate that steroids have a direct effect on the number and activity of osteoblasts.

CLINIC There are many clinical findings associated with corticosteroid administration. These include fractures, which can remain asymptomatic over a long period, noninfectious joint effusions containing low-protein fluid, tendon tears, intra-articular and periarticular calcifications, and mediastinal and epidural lipomatosis. Some of the changes are reversible after cessation of the therapy.

X-RAY **Insufficiency fractures** caused by corticosteroid-induced **osteoporosis** characteristically heal with exuberant callus formation (Fig. 6.**34**). Vertebral compression fractures are solitary or multiple and show sclerosis along the end plates (Fig. 6.**35**). Due to reduced pain perception, fractures of the ribs and calcaneus are characteristically asymptomatic for an extended period of time.

Avascular necrosis which appears 2 to 3 years after initiation of therapy is especially common in renal transplant patients.

Osteomyelitis and septic arthritis have a predilection for the knee joints, but can affect several bones. *Staphylococcus aureus* is the commonest infecting organism.

Repeated intra-articular corticosteroid injections over several years can induce calcifications in the periarticular fatty tissue, bordering ligaments, synovial lining, and articular cartilage and can cause chronic joint irritation.

SONO High-resolution sonography can distinguish between degeneration and rupture of the tendon when the clinical findings are equivocal.

CT CT can make a valuable contribution by detecting changes in areas difficult to evaluate by radiographs. This is especially true in insufficiency fractures of the sacrum, in the evaluation of neurologic complications, and in the search for epidural lipomatosis.

MRI This is the method of choice to evaluate avascular necrosis and infections.

Other Medications

Bone changes caused by other medications are rare (Fig. 6.**36**). The imaging findings are summarized in Table 6.**4**.

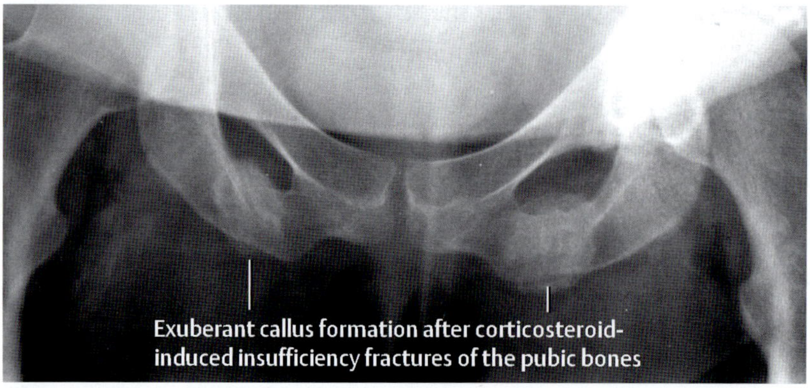

Fig. 6.**34** Pelvis of a 34-year-old woman with corticosteroid-induced Cushing syndrome. Exuberant callus formation after bilateral corticosteroid-induced pubic insufficiency fractures. The overlying abdominal soft tissues indicate massive obesity.

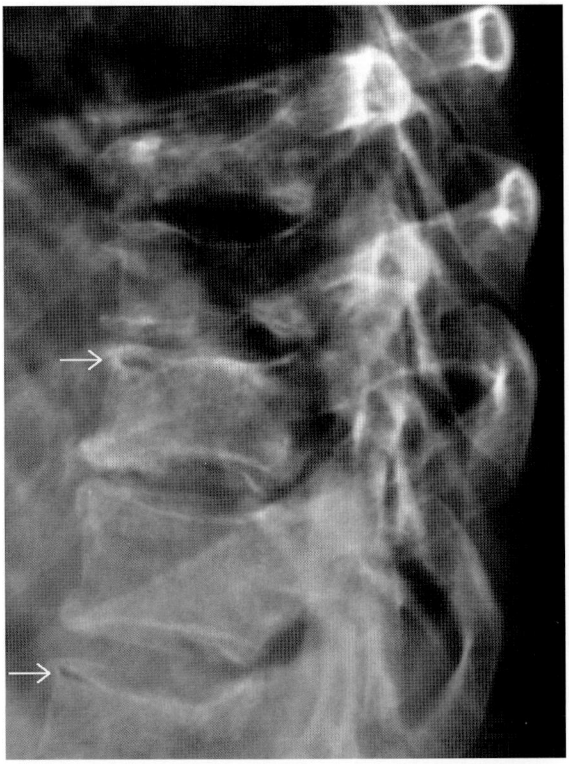

Fig. 6.**35** Thoracic spine of a 66-year-old woman after corticosteroid therapy. Multiple corticosteroid-induced vertebral compressions with subdiskal vacuum phenomenon (→). The vacuum phenomenon enables the differentiation from osteoporotic, neoplastic and traumatic vertebral compressions to be differentiated.

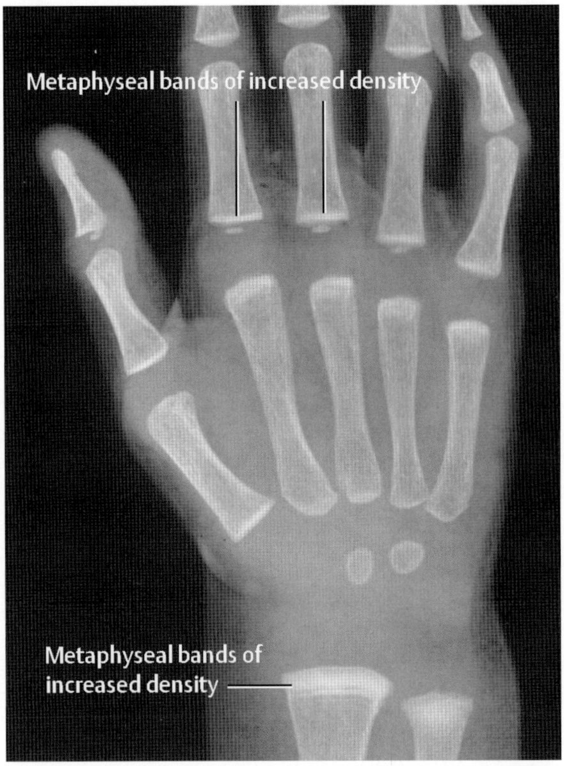

Fig. 6.**36** Hand of a 4-year-old boy with vitamin D overdose.

Table 6.**3** Effects of corticosteroids on the musculoskeletal system

Pathomechanics	Effect
Increased bone resorption	Osteoporosis
Vasculitis, fat embolism, microfractures	Avascular necrosis
Pain loss	Neuroarthropathy (see page 360)
Immune deficiency	Septic arthritis, osteomyelitis
Biochemical alteration	Tendinopathy, soft-tissue atrophy, Peri- and intra-articular hydroxyapatite deposition, Mediastinal and epidural fat accumulation

Table 6.**4** Medication-induced changes of the musculoskeletal system

Agent	Effect
Dopamine	Gangrene, avascular necrosis
Calcium gluconate	Soft-tissue calcifications
Heparin	Osteoporosis, stress/insufficiency fractures
Phenytoin (Dilantin)	Rickets and osteomalacia, thickening of the calvaria, and enlargement of the heel pad
Vitamin A, isoretinoids	Periostitis of the ulna and metatarsals, hyperostosis
Vitamin D (Fig. 6.**36**)	Osteoporosis, metaphyseal thickening, periarticular calcifications
Prostaglandins	Periostitis
Methotrexate	Osteopenia, rickets
Aluminum	Osteopenia, Looser zones, metaphyseal fraying

Amyloidosis

■ Amyloidosis is the generalized or local deposition of amyloid in various organ systems. ■

PATH Amyloid consists of heterogeneous glycoproteins with a β-pleated sheet structure that are deposited in interstitial tissue.

Amyloid osteoarthropathy is caused by amyloid deposits in the joint capsule, articular cartilage, periarticular soft tissues, and juxta-articular bones. Among other factors, amyloidosis is caused by or associated with:
- malignant monoclonal gammopathy (plasmocytoma, Waldenström disease),
- chronic inflammatory diseases (rheumatoid arthritis group),
- chronic hemodialysis (β_2 microglobulin depositions).

CLINIC Amyloid osteoarthropathy is characterized by joint pain, especially at night. The joints show restricted motion. Soft-tissue swelling and effusions occur. Amyloid deposits can also cause carpal tunnel syndrome.

X-RAY **Carpal bones, femoral head, acetabulum, humeral head:**
- 'cyst-like', smoothly marginated radiolucencies with thin sclerotic rims. In some instances, a connection to the articular cavity can be seen on radiographs (see erosion, Fig. 6.**37**),
- the joint space is frequently normal in width but rarely can be widened due to amyloid deposition or narrowed due to a destructive arthropathy (amyloid-induced synovitis).

Cervical and lumbar spine:
- narrowing of the intervertebral disk spaces,
- erosions, destructions of adjacent end plates (Fig. 6.**38**),
- minimal osseous reaction,
- barely widened paravertebral soft tissues.

CT The erosive character of the radiographically visualized 'cyst' is well delineated.

MRI MRI shows low signal intensity, on both T1-weighted and T2-weighted images, that is nonspecific.

DD **Interosseous ganglion cyst:** MRI displays fluid (high signal intensity) rather than amyloid (low signal intensity) in the osteolytic lesion.

Plasmacytoma: The osteolytic foci in plasmocytoma are multiple and lack a sclerotic rim.

Rheumatoid arthritis: Clinically and radiographically, the destructive type of amyloidosis is difficult to distinguish from rheumatoid arthritis, especially if it is a reactive amyloidosis complicating rheumatoid arthritis. Dense sclerosis around the lesions favors amyloidosis.

Pigmented villonodular synovitis (PVNS): PVNS involves one joint, and amyloidosis, especially of the hand, involves several joints. The radiographic features, however, are identical to a large extent.

Brown tumors: The radiographic features are almost identical. CT or MRI generally reveals connections to the joint in amyloidosis.

Spondylodiscitis: Differentiated mainly by MRI. The soft tissues have a low signal intensity in amyloidosis in contrast to spondylodiskitis.

Acromegaly

■ Acromegaly is caused by excess somatotropin secretion by the pituitary gland. Osseous and articular changes represent only a few of many manifestations. ■

CLINIC Complaints usually begin in the third and fourth decades and consist of extremity and lumbar spine pain. Joint swelling occurs, and articular crepitation is frequent. Joint pain and restricted articular motion appear only later with the development of secondary osteoarthritic changes.

X-RAY The major radiographic features of acromegaly are summarized in Table 6.**5**. In clinical practice, acromegalic arthropathy is most important and characteristically presents with osseous overgrowth similar to that seen in degenerative joint disease. However, in acromegaly the joint space is preserved or may even be widened. The shoulder, elbow, hip, and knee are the most severely involved joints. Premature degeneration with corresponding joint space narrowing makes the differentiation of acromegaly from 'ordinary' degenerative osteoarthritis difficult.

! Unusually advanced degenerative changes in non-weight-bearing major joints (shoulder, elbow) should suggest the diagnosis of acromegaly. This diagnosis can also be a consideration if the joint space is remarkably well preserved (Fig. 6.**39**).

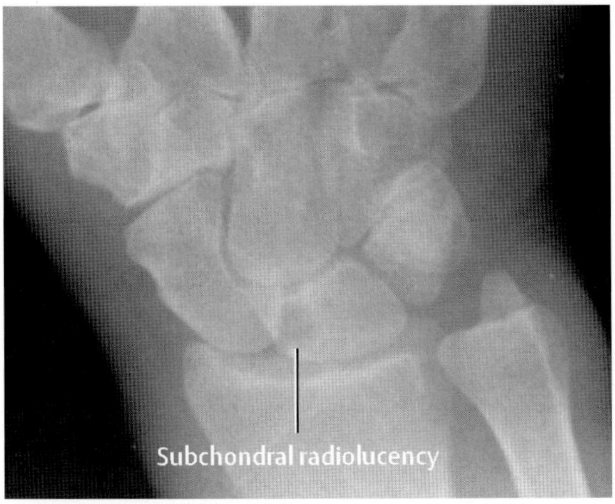

Fig. 6.37 Hand of a 58-year-old woman with amyloidosis. The differential diagnosis of the radiolucency in the lunate includes interosseous ganglion cyst, post-traumatic cyst, osteonecrosis, gout, and brown tumor.

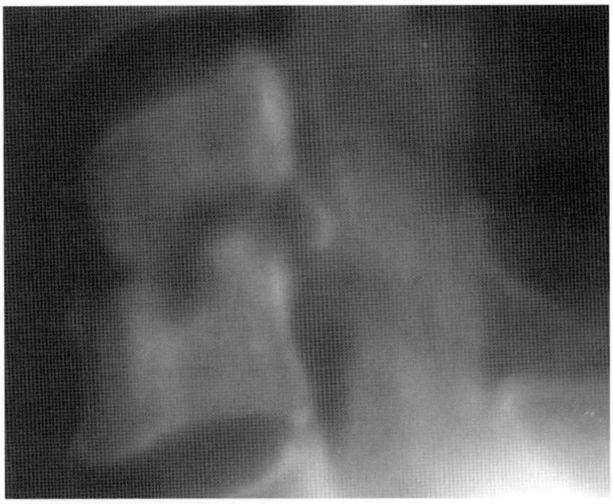

Fig. 6.38 Erosive spondyloarthropathy in a patient with renal insufficiency on long-term dialysis. The cause of the erosive changes is not entirely determined. Amyloidosis is the most likely cause, but secondary hyperparathyroidism can also induce such destructions in the end plates.

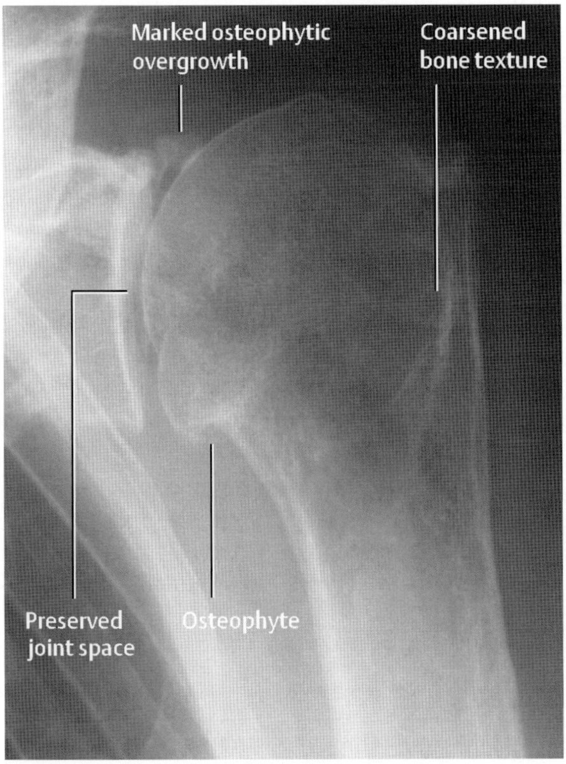

Fig. 6.39 Acromegaly. Aside from the structural changes of the humerus, the discrepancy between extensive osteophytic overgrowth and preserved width of the joint space is noticeable.

Table 6.5 Major radiographic findings of acromegaly

Bone
- Cortical thickening, most marked at the metacarpals and metatarsals
- Coarsened trabecular pattern
- Enlarged sesamoids
- Enlarged, anchor-shaped ungual processes
- Increased anteroposterior and transverse diameter of the vertebral body with preservation of vertebral height
- Osseous resorption at the tendinous, ligamentous, and capsular insertions
- Osteophytes and periarticular soft-tissue calcifications of the metacarpophalangeal joints
- Enlarged sella turcica

Soft tissues
- Soft-tissue thickening, most pronounced at the heel

Joints
- In the early stage, joint space widening (cartilage proliferation); in the late stage, degeneration with joint space narrowing
- Marked osteophytic osseous apposition, especially at the major joints, including the non-weight-bearing joints

7 Constitutional Disorders of Bone Growth

The constitutional disorders of bone growth encompass a vast number of congenital conditions associated with disturbed bone growth and development in all or parts of the skeleton. This category of disorders includes more than 100 well-defined entities and more than 1000 not-yet-categorized symptom complexes. The original summary and categorization of constitutional disorders of bone were described in the Paris Nomenclature of 1986, and the latest revision was reported in 1992. According to this nomenclature, the category of constitutional disorders of bone growth includes skeletal or osteochondrodysplastic dysplasias, primary metabolic disorders, chromosomal aberrations, dysostoses, and idiopathic osteolyses.

■ **Skeletal dysplasia (synonym: osteochondrodysplasia)** is a **generalized** abnormality of cartilage and bone development.
Dysostosis is an abnormal development of **individual** bones, isolated or combined.
The term 'osteodystrophy' has been abandoned. ■

This chapter describes the most frequent conditions selected from the vast number of congenital skeletal conditions, and outlines the most characteristic features of these diseases for better detection and appropriate categorization. The selection criteria in Table 7.**1** follow the International Nomenclature and Caffey's designation. Overlapping of the proposed classifying features is unavoidable. The literature should be consulted for detailed information related to the various entities.

Skeletal Dysplasias

Synonym: Osteochondrodysplasias

The important **clinical manifestation** of osteochondrodysplasias is inferior bone growth. The height reached in adulthood generally is below 140 cm (approximately 55 inches). The disturbance in bone growth is disproportional and, depending on the relative involvement of the spine or trunk, the trunk or the limbs are shortened. Disproportionate limb growth can lead to **rhizomelic** (proximal), **mesomelic** (medial) or **acromelic** (distal) types of micromelia. Kyphoscoliosis, deformities of the extremities, and misalignment of the joints are prominent features.

Diagnosing skeletal dysplasias is often difficult and relies on clinical, genetic, histologic, and histochemical methods. Radiographs are very important and often essential for the diagnosis. Discriminating radiographic features are deviation in size, shape, and bone density of particular skeletal segments. A singular anomaly generally excludes a skeletal dysplasia, but two or more identified deviations might suffice for diagnostic assignment to a skeletal dysplasia. The prerequisite is the systematic analysis of the radiographic features to address the following questions:

- **How many skeletal segments** are involved: single or multiple alterations?
- **Where is the alteration:** long bones, short tubular bones, axial skeleton?
- **Which growth zones** are involved: epiphysis, metaphysis, diaphysis?
- **How is the bone density:** normal or changed locally or diffusely; increased or decreased?

The radiographic examination of patients with suspected skeletal dysplasia consists of three or four views of the most frequently involved skeletal sites. Supplementary views should be added if needed.

Survey radiographic views:
- AP film of the hand,
- AP film of the pelvis,
- AP and lateral films of the lumbar spine and pelvis,
- Lateral film of the skull in certain instances,
- AP film of the entire skeleton, the so-called 'babygram', in neonates and infants.

Table 7.**1** Constitutional diseases of bone (based on Caffey and the International Paris Nomenclature)

I. Skeletal dysplasias

A. Identifiable at birth
1. Thanatophoric dysplasia
2. Achondroplasia
3. Chondrodysplasia punctata
   3.1 Rhizomelic form
   3.2 Conradi-Hünermann form
4. Asphyxiating thoracic dysplasia
5. Dyschondrosteosis (Léri-Weill disease)
6. Cleidocranial dysplasia

B. Identifiable later in life
Predominantly epiphyseal dysplasias:
1. Multiple epiphyseal dysplasia

Predominantly metaphyseal dysplasias
2. Hypochondroplasia
3. Metaphyseal chondrodysplasias:
   3.1 Schmid type
   3.2 McKusick type
   3.3 Schwachman type

Predominantly spondyloepiphyseal or metaphyseal dysplasias:
4. Spondyloepimetaphyseal dysplasia congenita
5. Spondyloepimetaphyseal dysplasia tarda

C. Skeletal dysplasia with disorganized development of cartilage and fibrous components
1. Multiple cartilaginous exostoses (Diaphyseal aclasis)
2. Enchondromatosis (Ollier)
3. Polyostotic fibrous dysplasia
4. Congenital generalized fibromatosis

D. Abnormal density of osseous structures
Decreased bone density:
1. Osteogenesis imperfecta
2. Hypophosphatasia
3. Hereditary rickets
   3.1 Phosphate diabetes
   3.2 Pseudodeficiency rickets

Increased bone density:
4. Osteopetrosis
5. Pyknodysostosis
6. Osteopoikilosis
7. Osteopathia striata
8. Melorheostosis

II. Dysostosis multiplex group

1. Mucopolysaccharidoses
2. Mucolipidoses, gangliosidoses

III. Dysostoses

1. With predominant craniofacial involvement
2. With predominant axial involvement
3. With predominant limb involvement

IV. Idiopathic osteolyses (very rare)

Early Onset Types

Many skeletal dysplasias can be diagnosed *in utero* or in the neonatal period. These are characterized by a disproportion between the head, trunk, and limbs. Identifying fetal disproportions by obstetrical sonography can suggest a skeletal dysplasia. Stillbirths or death in the neonatal period due to associated anomalies with impaired vital functions is common. Postnatally, the **radiographic evaluation** is crucial for establishing the diagnosis. A definitive diagnosis is mandatory for the **genetic counseling** of parents who wish to have more children.

Thanatophoric Dysplasia

CLINIC **Mode of inheritance:** Autosomal dominant with spontaneous mutation.
Prevalence: Occurring in 1:26000 to 1:58000 births, this is the most common lethal skeletal dysplasia. Its name means 'death bearing,' referring to the incompatibility with life due to the severe narrowing of the thorax.
Manifestation: Growth disturbance is disproportionate, as the trunk is of normal length and the extremities shortened. The thorax is extremely narrow, and the head is large with a depressed nasal root. Affected neonates that are not stillborn die within a few days after birth.

X-RAY Attention should be directed to the characteristic changes of the bony thorax, axial skeleton, and extremities (Figs. 7.**1**, 7.**2**):
- Extremely small bony thorax with very short ribs,
- Markedly flattened vertebral bodies with ossification defects in the end plates. Ratio of disk spaces to vertebral bodies is 3 : 1 (normally 1 : 1),
- Height of the ilium decreased, giving squared iliac wings,
- Extreme micromelia with concomitant broadening of the shaft. Widened metaphyses with flaring and cupping. So-called 'French telephone' deformity of the curved and shortened femur,
- Prominent cranial vault, possibly combined with a severely disturbed ossification of the sutures, producing the so-called 'cloverleaf skull'.

DD Similar but less-extensive skeletal changes are observed in **achondroplasia,** which has less-pronounced vertebral flattening and less shortening and bowing of the long tubular bones. **Achondrogenesis** has even more poorly developed and often absent ossification centers.

Achondroplasia

CLINIC **Mode of inheritance:** Autosomal dominant with a spontaneous mutation rate of 80%.
Prevalence: Occurring in 1 : 13500 live births, it is the most common skeletal dysplasia. The synonym 'fetal chondrodysplasia' has been abandoned, but the now-accepted term achondroplasia is strictly not appropriate either, since cartilage is formed.
Manifestation: Affected individuals show disproportionate, micromelic, and rhizomelic dwarfism with a final body height not exceeding 122 cm (approximately 48 inches). The head is enlarged and shows a prominent forehead and a flattened nasal bridge. Characteristic features are a thoracolumbar kyphosis and protruding buttocks due to an increased pelvic tilt. The fingers are shortened and have a three-pronged or trident appearance.

X-RAY Attention should be directed to the characteristic deformities of the pelvis and posterior vertebral arches, to the disproportionately short extremities, and to the severely disturbed ossification in the epiphyseal growth zone:
- Squared pelvis ('elephant ears') already present in early childhood; an extremely small sacroiliac notch and an almost horizontally oriented acetabular roof (Fig. 7.**3**),
- Short and broad tubular bones with rhizomelic exaggeration; characteristic oval radiolucency of the upper ends of the femur in neonates; widened and medially enlarged distal femoral metaphyses (Fig. 7.**4**); partial metaphyseal invagination of the epiphyses, so-called 'ball-in-socket epiphyseal-metaphyseal junction,'
- Short and flattened vertebral bodies with posterior scalloping; progressive decrease in the interpediculate distance of the lumbar spine from cranial to caudal (Fig. 7.**5**),
- Large cranial vault resting on a small cranial base, constricted foramen magnum and dilated CSF space by CT,
- 'Overlapping fibula' due to overgrowth of the fibula relative to the tibia.

DD The common **heterozygotic** type has easily recognized features, whereas the less common homozygotic type resembles thanatophoric dysplasia; the changes of hypochondroplasia are variable and less severe.

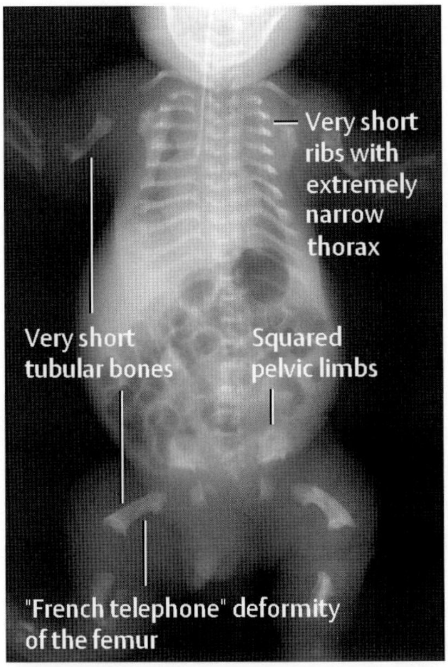

Fig. 7.1 'Babygram' of thanatophoric dysplasia.

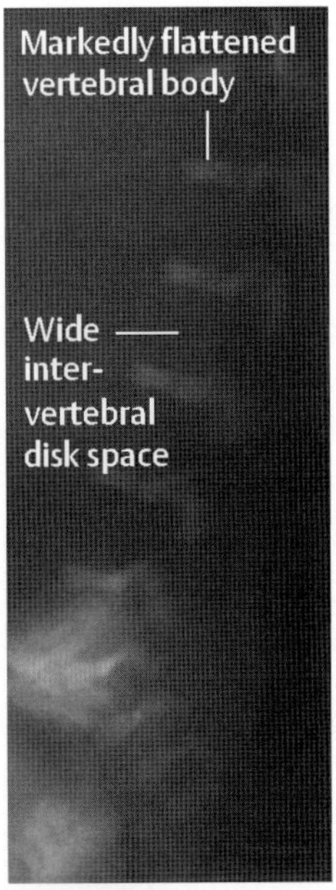

Fig. 7.2 Lateral spine of thanatophoric dysplasia in the same child as in Fig. 7.1.

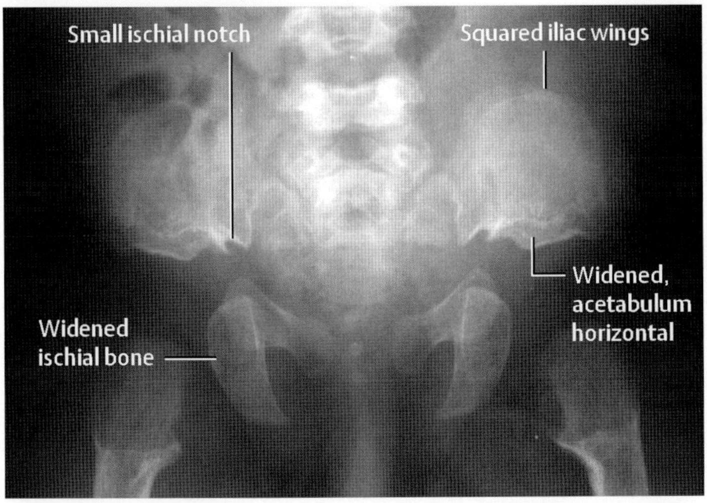

Fig. 7.3 Pelvis of a 5-month-old child with achondroplasia.

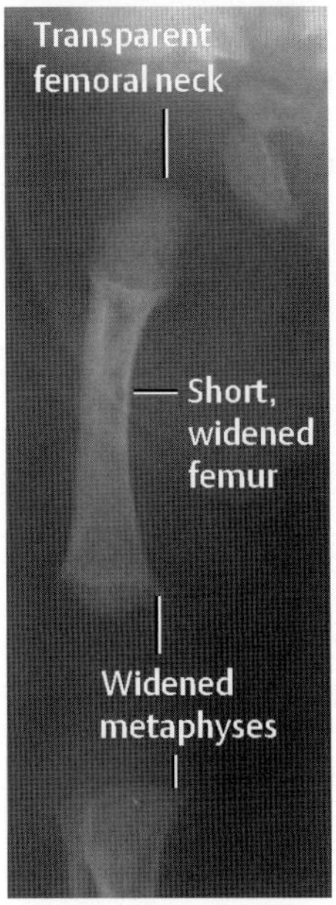

Fig. 7.4 Achondroplasia, same child as in Fig. 7.3.

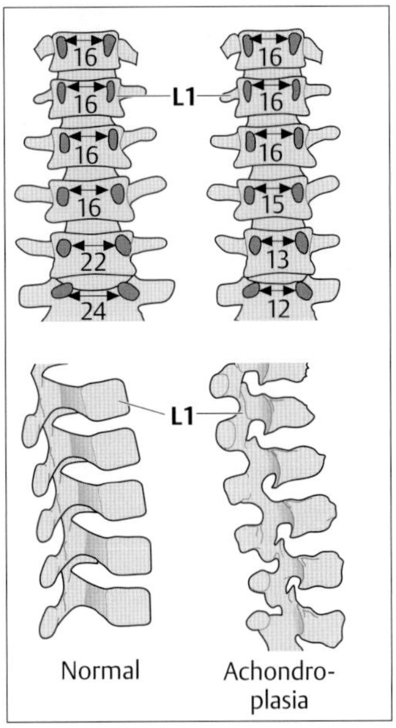

Fig. 7.5 Differences in interpediculate distances and the configuration of the vertebral bodies in a normal child and in a child with achondroplasia (after Caffey).

Chondrodysplasia Punctata

Stippled calcifications seen in the growth zones of the long tubular bones, in the axial skeleton and in the tracheal cartilage give this condition its name. Fifteen different types of dysplasia with these radiographic features have been differentiated so far. The most frequent types are the rhizomelic type and the Conradi-Hünermann type.

CLINIC **Mode of inheritance:** The rhizomelic type is autosomal recessive, and the Conradi-Hünermann type is X-linked dominant.
Manifestation: Whereas the rhizomelic type has symmetric rhizomelic limb shortening, the Conradi-Hünermann type has asymmetric limb shortening. Both types are associated with craniofacial dysmorphism and cataracts.
Prognosis: The rhizomelic type follows a more severe clinical course, and death usually occurs within the first year of life due to severe infections and cerebral damage.

X-RAY Attention should be directed to the characteristic stippled calcifications in the skeletal cartilage of the newborn and, later in life, to the various manifestations of limb shortening:
- stippled calcifications in the cartilage of the extremities and, in the Conradi-Hünermann type, also in the axial skeleton, larynx, trachea, and joint capsule; disappearance of the stippled calcifications within the first year of life (Fig. 7.**6**),
- symmetric shortening of the long tubular bones, especially of the humeri and femora in the rhizomelic type, and asymmetric limb shortening in the Conradi-Hünermann type,
- division of the vertebral bodies in the lateral projection by a so-called 'coronal cleft,' which slowly regresses later in life.

MRI Severely abnormal myelinization with cortical atrophy in the rhizomelic type.

SONO This technique can directly display the relationship between the stippled calcifications and the epimetaphyseal growth zone (Fig. 7.**7**).

DD Other types of chondrodysplasia punctata should be included in the differential diagnosis, including fetal warfarin syndrome in infants born to mothers who took coumarin derivatives during pregnancy, fetal alcohol syndrome, and Zellweger syndrome.

Asphyxiating Thoracic Dysplasia

Synonyms: Jeune syndrome, thoraco-pelvic-phalangeal dysplasia.

CLINIC **Mode of inheritance:** Autosomal recessive.
Prevalence: 1 : 100 000 live births.
This condition has a broad clinical spectrum ranging from the lethal type in neonates with a narrow thorax to the mild type without respiratory difficulties. The outstanding findings are short-limbed dwarfism and polydactyly (in some instances). Progressive nephropathy develops later in life.

X-RAY Attention should be directed to the characteristic changes of the bony thorax and pelvis (Fig. 7.**8**):
- narrow, bell-shaped thorax with very short ribs that show parasternal flaring,
- squared pelvis with shortened sacroiliac notch and an inferior spur,
- micromelia of the long and short tubular bones with irregular metaphyses.

DD In the newborn period, all skeletal dysplasias associated with a narrow thorax enter the differential diagnosis and include Ellis-van Creveld syndrome, thanatophoric dysplasia, and achondroplasia, and, in later infancy, all of the skeletal dysplasias with predominantly metaphyseal growth disturbances.

Dyschondrosteosis

Synonym: Léri-Weill disease

CLINIC **Mode of inheritance:** Autosomal dominant.
Manifestation: Mesomelic dwarfism with shortened forearms combined with Madelung deformity.

X-RAY Attention should be directed to the characteristic shortening and bowing of the forearm with Madelung deformity:
- shortened radius (Fig. 7.**9**),
- ulnar and radial epiphyses are slanted toward each other with posterior dislocation of the ulna (Madelung deformity, Fig. 7.**10**),
- Tibial shortening may be present in some instances.

DD Other mesomelic growth disturbances with shortened bones of forearm and lower leg should be taken into consideration. Turner syndrome can also show similar changes.

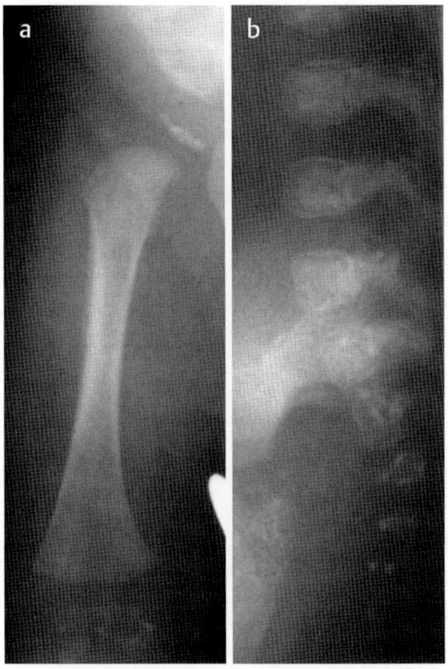

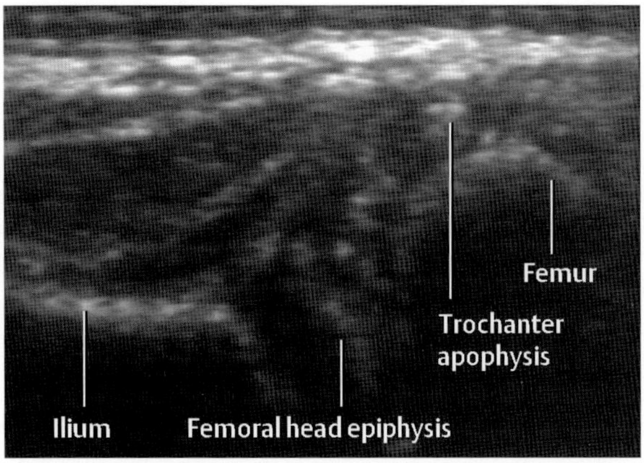

Fig. 7.**7** Lateral section of sonogram in same child as in Fig. 7.**6**. Note the small coarse calcifications in the cartilaginous epiphysis of the femoral head and in the apophysis of the trochanter.

Left:
Fig. 7.**6** Chondrodysplasia punctata, Conradi-Hünermann type, 2-month-old child. Typical 'stippled' calcifications.

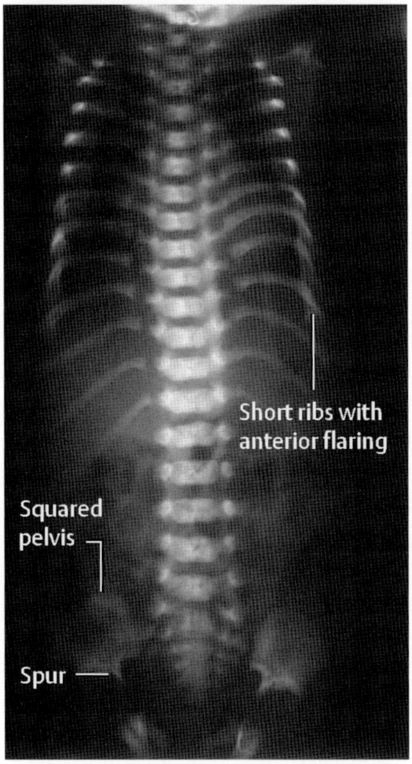

Fig. 7.**8** Asphyxiating thoracic dysplasia in a newborn: AP radiograph of the trunk (babygram) shows short ribs with resultant very narrow thorax.

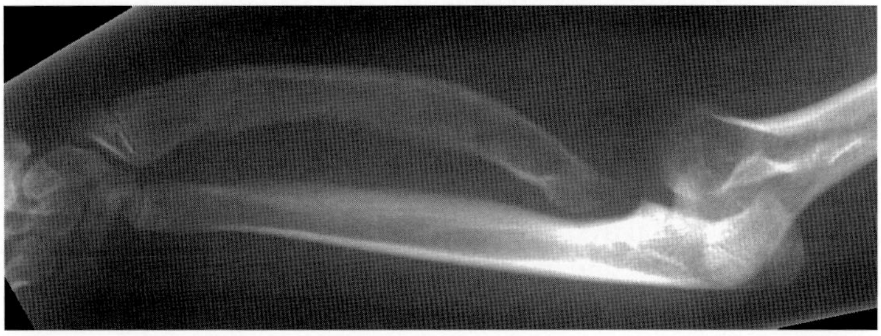

Fig. 7.**9** Dyschondrosteosis in an 11-year-old girl. The forearm is shortened and the radius bowed.

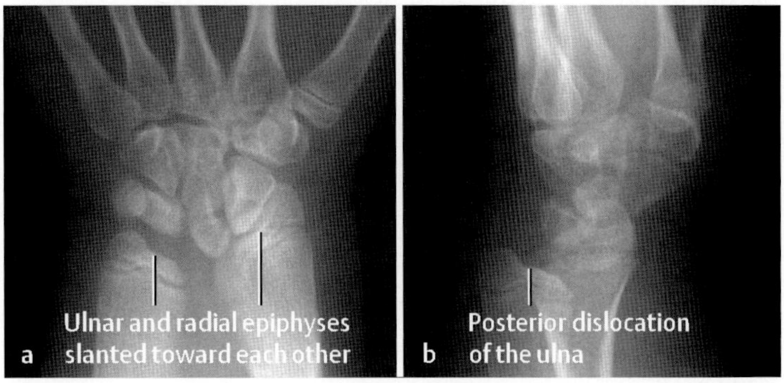

Fig. 7.**10** Dyschondrosteosis in the same child as in Fig. 7.**9**. The distal articular surfaces of the radius and ulna are slanted toward each other. The ulna is posteriorly dislocated.

Cleidocranial Dysplasia

Synonym: Pelvico-cleidocranial dysostosis.

CLINIC **Mode of inheritance:** Autosomal dominant.
Manifestation: The outstanding findings are the large head with an open or late-fusing anterior fontanelle, disturbance of teeth development, and anterior approximation of the shoulders in cases with aplastic or hypoplastic clavicles.

X-RAY Attention should be directed to the characteristically delayed ossification of the cranial vault and to the clavicular aplasia or hypoplasia:
- widely patent anterior fontanelle and sutures with multiple intercalary bones (Fig. 7.**11**),
- aplasia or hypoplasia of both clavicles or pseudarthrosis of hypoplastic clavicles (Fig. 7.**12**),
- narrow thorax with descending ribs (Fig. 7.**12**),
- steep, high iliac wings with marked coxa vara.

DD Congenital clavicular hypoplasia and pseudarthrosis in neurofibromatosis and pyknodysostosis.

Late-Onset Types

Late-onset skeletal dysplasias often are only identified after infancy and during early school years when disproportionate growth becomes apparent. They are differentiated by the variable involvement of the osteochondral growth zones and the involvement of different skeletal regions. This was considered in the selection of the differentiating criteria for the following classification of skeletal dysplasias.

Predominantly Epiphyseal Dysplasias

Multiple Epiphyseal Dysplasia

Synonym: Fairbank disease, Ribbing disease.

CLINIC **Mode of inheritance:** Autosomal dominant.
Prevalence: Occurring in 1 : 11 000 births, this is the most common nonlethal skeletal dysplasia.
Manifestation: Affected patients show stunted growth and slightly disproportionate limb shortening. Later manifestations are increasing stiffness and pain in the hip, knee, and ankle due to premature degenerative osteoarthritis. The diagnosis is often not made until late in childhood.
Prognosis: Some authors distinguish between patients with a mild clinical course, the Ribbing type, and patients with a severe clinical course, the Fairbank type.

X-RAY Attention should be directed to the characteristic changes in shape and size of the epiphyses, especially in the lower extremities:
- delayed ossification of all epiphyses (precluding the determination of skeletal bone age),
- small, flat, and irregularly fragmented epiphyses, especially around the hip, knee, and ankle (Figs. 7.**13**, 7.**14**),
- slight irregularities of the vertebral end plates and mild anterior vertebral flattening.

MRI Normal signal intensity of the small and irregularly outlined epiphyses.

DD All conditions with regional or generalized epiphyseal growth disturbances, including Meyer dysplasia, Legg-Calvé-Perthes disease, spondyloepiphyseal dysplasia, chondrodysplasia punctata, hypothyroidism, and growth hormone deficiency.

Predominantly Metaphyseal Dysplasias

Hypochondroplasia

Synonym: Mild or incomplete achondroplasia, chondrohypoplasia.

CLINIC **Mode of inheritance:** Autosomal dominant.
Prevalence: Because of its variable clinical manifestations, it is often incorrectly diagnosed as 'constitutionally short stature'. It is one of the five commonest skeletal dysplasias.
Manifestation: Affected patients show a mild, disproportionate growth disturbance with limb shortening that is less severe than observed in achondroplasia.

X-RAY Attention should be directed to the characteristic changes of the posterior arches of the lumbar vertebrae and of the metaphyses of the long tubular bones:
- craniocaudal decrease in the interpediculate distances of the lumbar spine, which might be the single radiographic abnormality in some cases. Posterior scalloping and decreased AP diameter of the vertebral body (similar to achondroplasia, but less severe, see Fig. 7.**5**),
- slight shortening of the long tubular bones, with slight metaphyseal widening,
- short, broad femoral necks with relatively large femoral head epiphyses,
- overgrowth of the fibula relative to the tibia (overlapping fibula).

DD Achondroplasia, metaphyseal chondrodysplasias of the Schmid type and McKusick type.

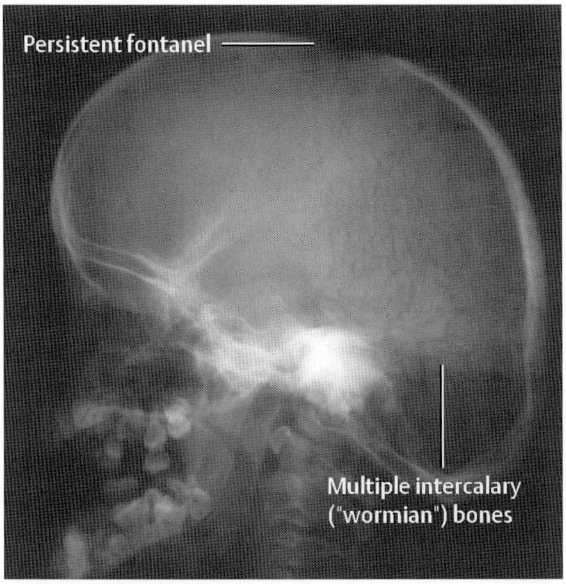

Fig. 7.**11** Cleidocranial dysplasia, 15-year-old patient. Multiple intercalary (wormian) bones and persistent fontanelles are apparent.

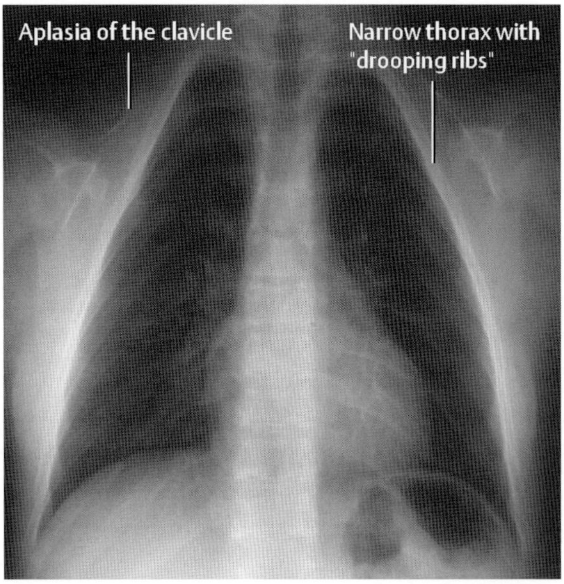

Fig. 7.**12** Cleidocranial dysplasia: narrow thorax with downward inclining ribs, aplasia of the clavicles (same child as in Fig. 7.**11**).

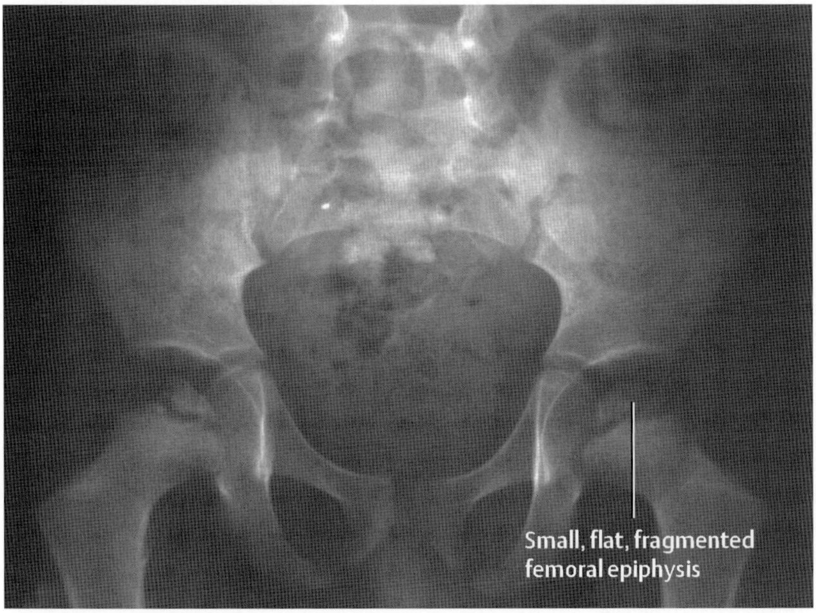

Fig. 7.**13** Multiple epiphyseal dysplasia in a 5-year-old patient. Small, flat, fragmented femoral epiphysis.

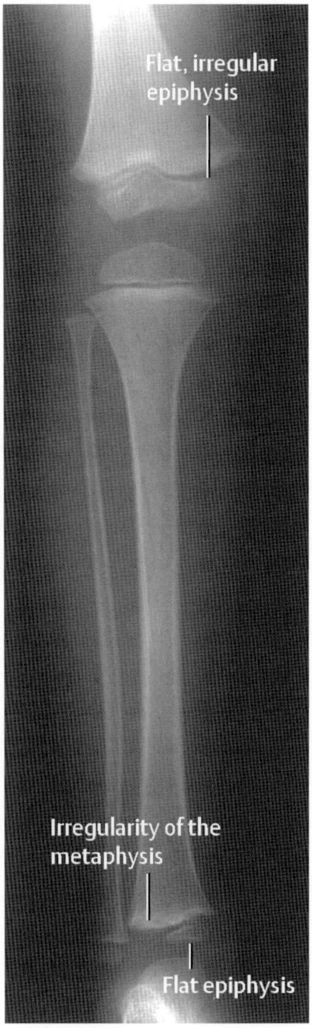

Right:
Fig. 7.**14** Right lower leg of the same child as in Fig. 7.**13**. Femoral and distal tibial epiphyses are flat. Irregular femoral epiphysis and distal tibial metaphysis.

Metaphyseal Chondrodysplasias

This group of skeletal dysplasias includes changes that predominantly involve the metaphyseal growth zones of the long tubular bones. They vary only in extent, clinical manifestation, and mode of inheritance.

Schmid Type

CLINIC **Mode of inheritance:** Autosomal dominant.
Prevalence: According to the literature, this is the most common metaphyseal dysplasia, especially if less severe manifestations are included.
Manifestation: Progressive growth retardation with waddling gait and bowed legs.

X-RAY Attention should be directed to the characteristic metaphyseal changes of the lower extremities:

- shortening and widening of the femoral neck with coxa vara and a large epiphysis of the femoral head (Fig. 7.**15**),
- widening of the distal femoral metaphysis with irregular ossification zone and varus deformity of the femur (Fig. 7.**16**),
- frequent widening and indistinctness of the costochondral junctions of the ribs,
- the pelvis, spine and hands generally not affected.

DD Various types of rickets, especially phosphate diabetes, as well as other types of metaphyseal dysplasias and spondylometaphyseal dysplasia.

Glossary

Two rare metaphyseal chondrodysplasias of autosomal recessive inheritance are the McKusick type and Schwachman type.

The chief features of the **McKusick type** are metaphyseal growth disturbances, especially of the short tubular bones of the hands and feet, together with fine, sparse hair on head and body.

The **Schwachman type,** or MMN chondrodysplasia, has an additional exocrine pancreatic insufficiency and cyclic neutropenia. The metaphyseal changes are seen primarily in the hip and knee.

Predominantly Spondyloepiphyseal or Metaphyseal Dysplasias

These types of skeletal dysplasias are dominated by changes in the spine and in the epiphyses and metaphyses of the long tubular bones.

Spondyloepimetaphyseal Dysplasia (Early Type)

Synonym: Spondyloepimetaphyseal dysplasia congenita

CLINIC **Mode of inheritance:** Autosomal dominant.
Prevalence: Infrequent (exact incidence unknown).
Manifestation: It is recognizable in early childhood, in some cases even at birth. Trunk and neck are short, with progressive kyphoscoliosis and a barrel, keeled chest. Later in life, limb shortening becomes apparent, and muscle hypotonia and retinal detachment are observed.

X-RAY Attention should be directed to the characteristic changes of the vertebral body, epiphyses of the femoral head, and dens.

In the neonatal period:

- ovoid to pear-shaped vertebral bodies in the lateral projection (Fig. 7.**17**), absent ossification of the femoral epiphyses.

In childhood and later:

- platyspondylia with irregular end plates,
- marked coxa vara with delayed ossification of the femoral head, flattened acetabular roof with a small spur along the acetabular rim (Fig. 7.**18**),
- hypoplastic dens.

DD Mucopolysaccharidosis type IV (Morquio), spondyloepimetaphyseal dysplasia tarda.

Spondyloepimetaphyseal Dysplasia (Tarda Type)

Synonym: Spondyloepimetaphyseal dysplasia tarda.

CLINIC **Mode of inheritance:** X-linked recessive.
Prevalence: Infrequently encountered.
Manifestation: It is diagnosed later in life by severe growth failure that becomes apparent at school age or adolescence. Later, pain due to premature degenerative changes develops in the back, hips, and shoulders.

X-RAY The radiographic features consist of generalized platyspondylia with anterior loss of height and 'buckling' of the vertebral body and complete absence of the ring apophyses; the epiphyseal changes resemble those seen in the early type.

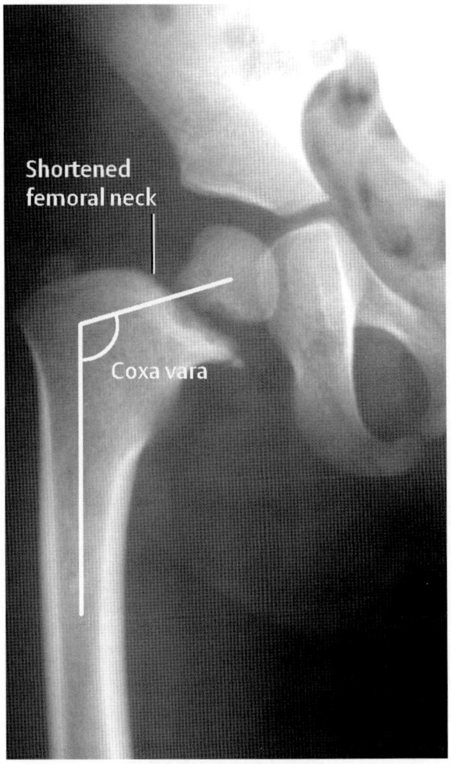

Fig. 7.**15** Metaphyseal dysplasia, Schmid type, 3-year-old child.

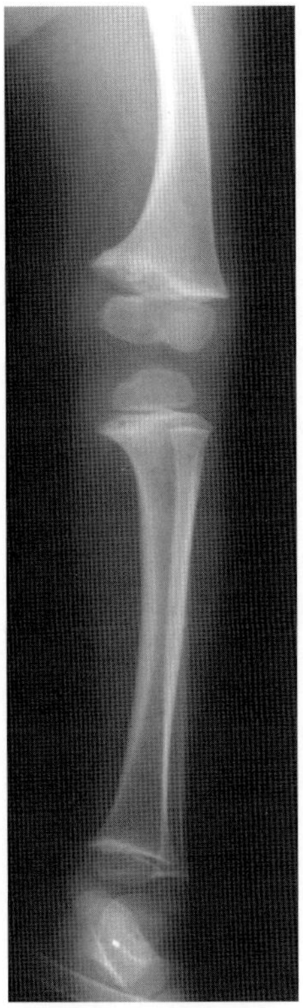

Fig. 7.**16** Same child as in Fig. 7.**15**, left leg: irregular ossification zone, varus deformity of femur and tibia, widening of the metaphysis.

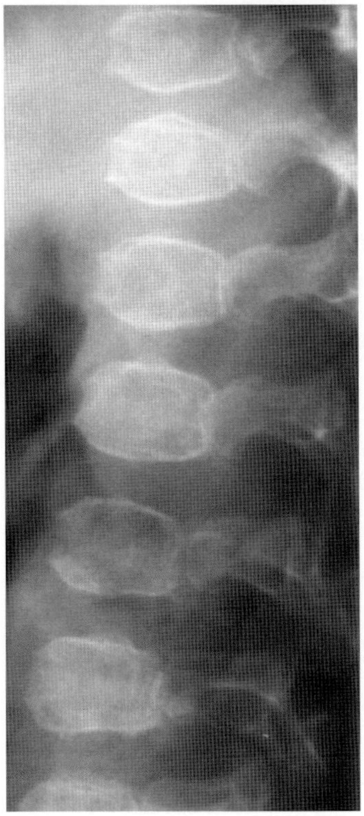

Fig. 7.**17** Spondyloepiphyseal dysplasia (early type) in an 18-month-old child. Typical 'pear-shaped' deformity of the vertebral bodies.

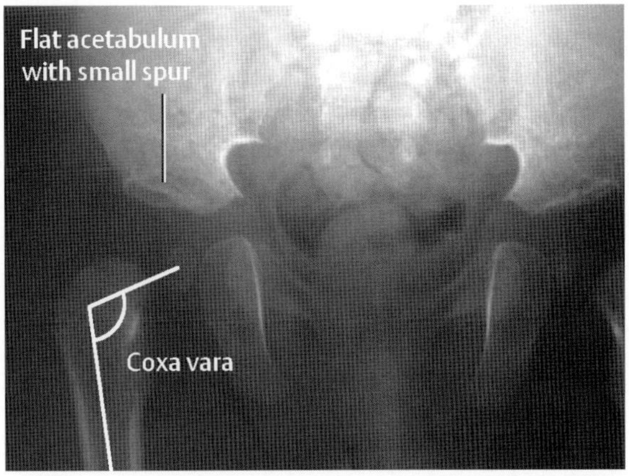

Fig. 7.**18** Same child as in Fig. 7.**17**. There is a coxa vara deformity in the proximal femur, and the acetabular roofs are flat and have a small marginal spur.

Skeletal Dysplasia with Disorganized Development of Cartilage and Fibrous Components

Multiple Cartilaginous Exostoses

Synonym: Osteochondromatosis, diaphyseal aclasia.

CLINIC **Mode of inheritance:** Autosomal dominant.
Prevalence: 1 : 10 000 to 1 : 100 000.
Manifestation: The exostoses are multiple, occasionally cause pain, arise next to the growth plate, and continue to grow until epiphyseal closure. Complications are secondary shortening and deformity of the tubular bones and misaligned joints, most frequently observed as 'Madelung-like' deformity of the forearm. The incidence of malignant transformation (chondrosarcoma, osteosarcoma) has been reported to be as high as 10% in old reports, but is now believed to be less than 1% overall.

X-RAY Attention should be directed to characteristic deformities of the metaphyses of the long tubular bones, as well as to characteristic deformities of anterior rib ends, medial scapula, iliac wings, and vertebral borders:
- broad-based or narrow osseous projections arising from the metaphyses and directed away from the nearest joint (Fig. 7.**19**),
- exostosis with a smooth cortical outline and spongiosa with a homogeneous or partially irregular calcification pattern; cartilage cap seen on CT or MRI during the growth period,
- secondary deformity and shortening of the long tubular bones,
- sudden onset of growth after epiphyseal closure and an indistinct outline of an exostosis is always suspicious for malignant transformation (see CT/MRI).

DD It rarely coexists with enchondromatosis; when this occurs, differentiation is difficult.

Enchondromatosis

Synonym: Ollier disease, multiple enchondromatosis

CLINIC **Mode of inheritance:** Unknown.
Prevalence: Not established but probably underestimated.
Manifestation: It is diagnosed as asymmetric growth disturbance at the age of 2 to 10 years. Hands and feet show localized swelling, and occasionally pathologic fracture can occur. The rate of malignant transformation is about 30%.

X-RAY Attention should be directed to the characteristic largely intraosseous lesions in the metaphyses of the tubular bones and in the scapula and ilium:
- sharply demarcated, oval, linear or pyramidal radiolucencies in the metaphyses of the tubular bone and in flat bones, such as the scapula and pelvis (Figs. 7.**20**, 7.**21**),
- secondary shortening and occasional bizarre deformity of the tubular bones.

DD Multiple cartilaginous exostoses can coexist with enchondromatosis. Fibrous dysplasia and infantile myofibromatosis also enter the differential diagnosis.

Polyostotic Fibrous Dysplasia

Synonyms: Jaffé-Lichtenstein disease, osteitis fibrosa disseminata.

Fibrous dysplasia may be monostotic or polyostotic. Polyostotic fibrous dysplasia together with pigmented skin lesion (*café au lait* spots) and pubertas praecox (precocious puberty) in girls is referred to as McCune-Albright syndrome.

Congenital Generalized Fibromatosis

Synonyms: Infantile myofibromatosis.

The osseous manifestation with or without visceral involvement has multifocal fibrous proliferations that appear as cystic defects with a thin sclerotic rim. The strictly osseous manifestation frequently regresses spontaneously, and the visceral manifestation is often lethal.

Skeletal Dysplasias with Abnormal Density of Osseous Structures

Decreased Bone Density

Osteogenesis Imperfecta

Synonyms: About 40 names, including Lobstein type, osteopsathyrosis, Vrolik type, Bruck syndrome.

The term 'osteogenesis imperfecta' includes a heterogeneous group of conditions with defective bone formation of varying severity; four major types are recognized today (Table 7.**2**).

CLINIC **Mode of inheritance:** Depending on the type, autosomal dominant or autosomal recessive.
Prevalence: 1 : 25 000.
Manifestation: All four types share increased bone fragility. Multiple fractures of the tubular bones can lead to deformity of the extremities. Vertebral fractures often result in shortened stature and kyphoscoliosis. The characteristic clinical findings are a triangular face, blue sclerae, and defective dentinogenesis.

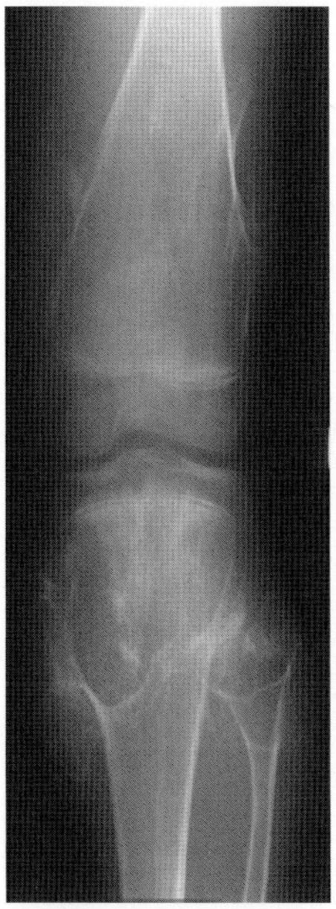

Fig. 7.**19** Multiple cartilaginous exostoses, 12-year-old child. Typical diaphyseal orientation of the exostosis.

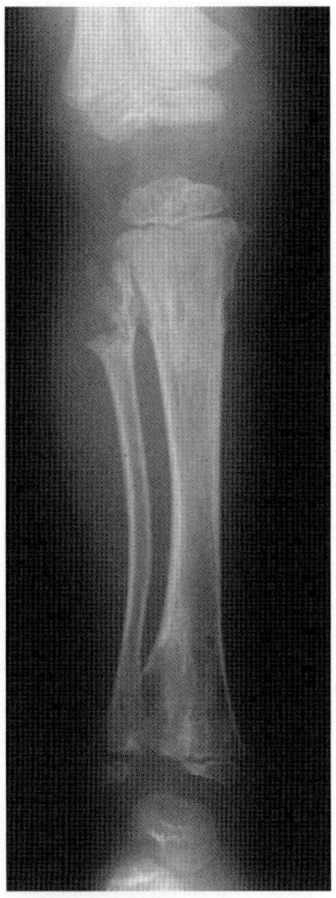

Fig. 7.**20** Enchondromatosis, 2-year-old child. Growth disturbance of the distal femoral epiphysis. The metaphyseal defect zones are smoothly marginated.

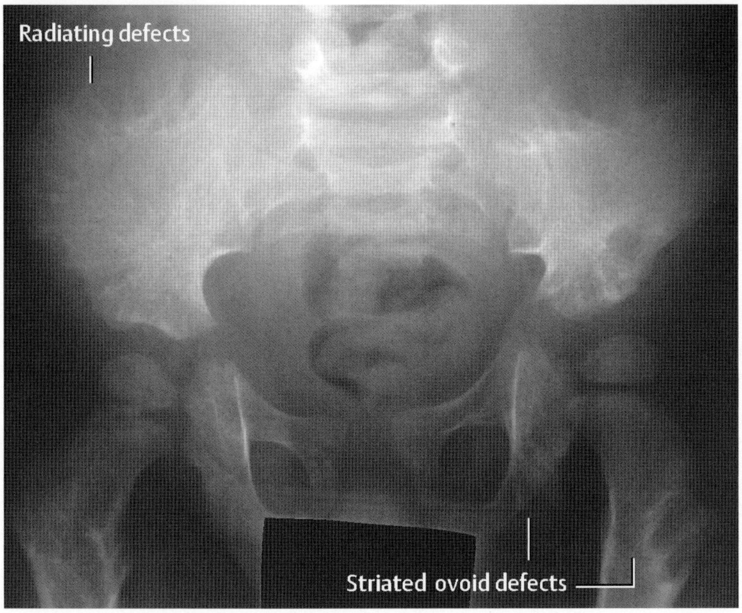

Fig. 7.**21** Same child as in Fig. 7.**20**, typical radiating defect in the ilium, as well as linear to ovoid defects in the femoral neck and ischium.

Table 7.**2** Types of osteogenesis imperfecta in detail (according to Sillence)

Type	Mode of Inheritance	Fractures, deformities	Natural history
I (a, b)	AD	+	Mild
II (a, b, c)	AD/AR	+++	Lethal
III	AR	++	Severe
IV (a, b)	AD	+/–	Variable

X-RAY All types have the following features (Figs. 7.**22**, 7.**23**):

- decreased bone density,
- thin cortex,
- multiple intercalary bones, so-called wormian bones, in the skull,
- fractures with abundant though rapidly resolving callus,
- displaced and deformed bones following fractures,
- vertebral compression fractures with 'codfish' deformity of the vertebral bodies.

Hypophosphatemia

CLINIC **Mode of inheritance:** Autosomal recessive, but autosomal dominant occurs.
Prevalence: 1 : 100 000.
Manifestation: Genetically determined decrease in the activity of alkaline phosphatase in the blood and in the tissues, resulting in incomplete ossification of the cartilage along the osseous growth zones and increased urine excretion of phosphoethanolamine.
Clinical Course: Four types with a different course can be distinguished:

a) Lethal type with stillbirth or death soon after birth due to respiratory insufficiency,
b) Infantile type with failure to thrive, fever of unknown origin, and seizures,
c) Mild, late type in childhood with premature loss of the incisors, pain, and stiffness,
d) Latent adult type.

X-RAY Lethal type with extremely diminished mineralization, barely ossified cranial vault, shortened and deformed tubular bones, with death due to hypoplastic bony thorax,

- infantile type with decreased mineralization of the entire skeleton, especially with 'rickets-like' irregularities at the metaphyses and occasionally severe ossification defects (Figs. 7.**24**, 7.**25**),
- late type with mild rickets-like changes.

DD The lethal type of hypophosphatemia must be distinguished from the lethal type of osteogenesis imperfecta, while the infantile and late types of this disorder should be differentiated from the various types of rickets and metaphyseal osteochondrodysplasias.

Hereditary Rickets

The cause of hereditary rickets can be either a deficient vitamin D metabolism (pseudodeficiency rickets or vitamin-D-dependent rickets) or phosphate loss due to a renal tubular defect (phosphate diabetes or vitamin-D-resistant rickets). The distinguishing criteria of both types of rickets are listed in Table 7.**3**.

Table 7.**3** Criteria for distinguishing between hypophosphatemic rickets and pseudodeficiency rickets

	Pseudodeficiency rickets	Hypophosphatemic rickets
Cause	Enzyme defect	Renal tubular defect
Mode of Inheritance	Autosomal recessive	X-linked dominant
Onset	First year of life	Second year of life
Natural history	Impaired growth and failure to thrive, muscle hypotonia	Bowing of long bones
Laboratory:		
Serum phosphate level	Decreased/normal	Markedly decreased
Serum calcium level	Decreased	Normal
Aminoaciduria	Increased	Normal

X-RAY **Pseudodeficiency rickets:** Often severe rickets-like changes in early childhood with widening of the epiphyseal growth plate, cup-like and irregular metaphyseal zones, and demineralization.
Vitamin D-resistant rickets: Less severe rickets-like changes at the metaphyses, bowing of the long tubular bones, especially of the lower extremities (Figs. 7.**26**, 7.**27**), coarse trabecular texture, Looser zones and fractures.

DD Both types of hereditary rickets should be distinguished clinically, biochemically, and radiographically from the other types of rickets, such as vitamin D-deficiency rickets, renal osteodystrophy, Fanconi syndrome, tubular acidosis, and cystinosis. Metaphyseal osteochondrodysplasias must be differentiated the same way.

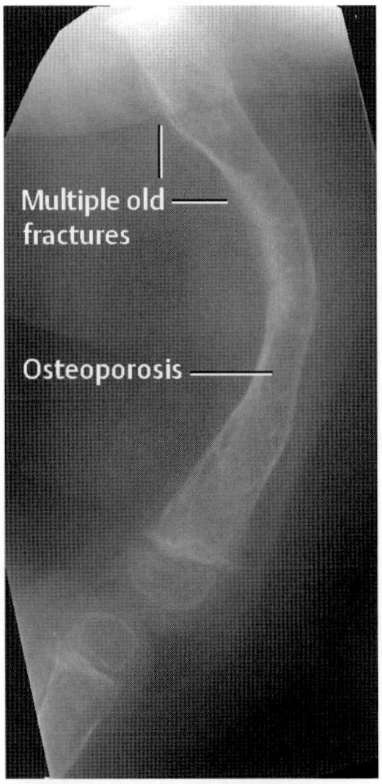

Fig. 7.**22** Osteogenesis imperfecta, Type III, 15-month-old child. Severe anterior bowing of the femur and multiple old fractures.

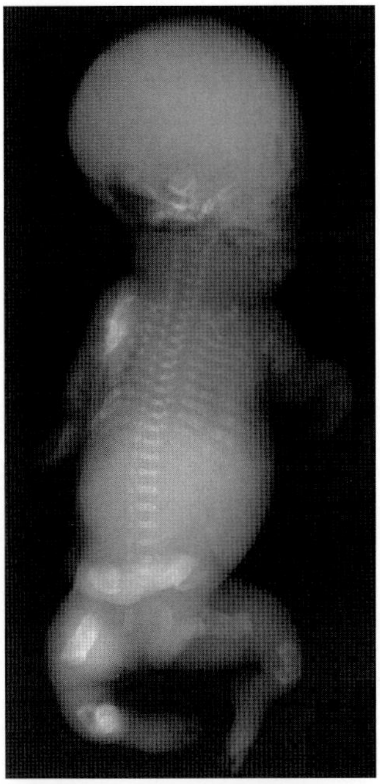

Fig. 7.**23** Osteogenesis imperfecta Type IIa. Lethal type, postnatal death. Postmortem whole-body radiograph (babygram). No ossification of the cranial vault, multiple rib fractures, 'telescoped' tubular bones due to intrauterine fractures.

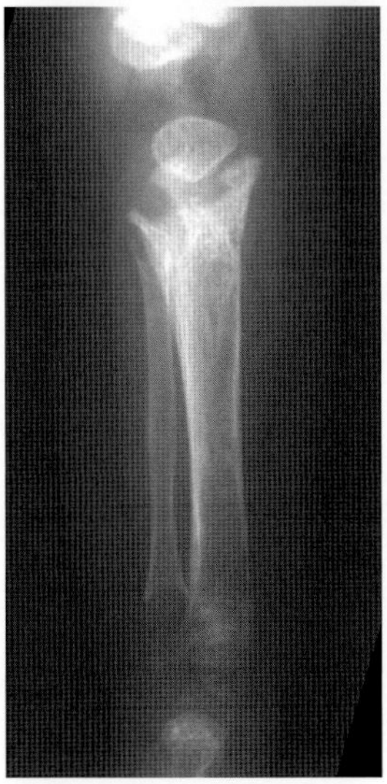

Fig. 7.**24** Hypophosphatemia, infantile form, 9-month-old child. Severe ossification defects are seen in the metaphysis.

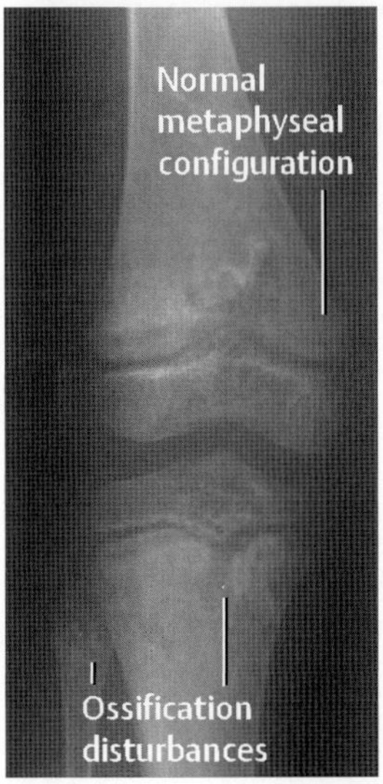

Fig. 7.**25** Same child as in Fig. 7.**24** at 7 years. Solely metaphyseal ossification disturbances in the tibia and femur, without severe metaphyseal deformities.

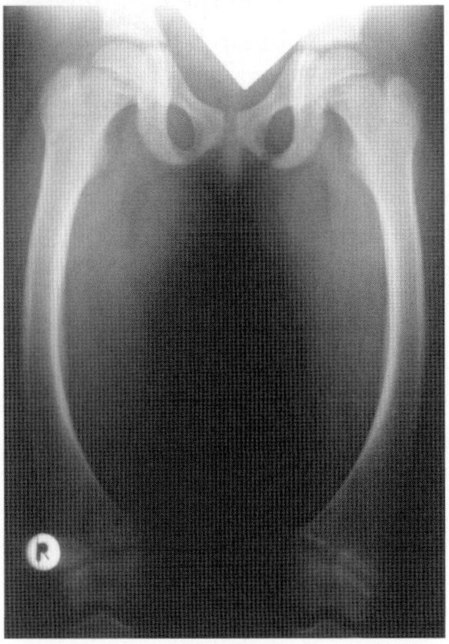

Fig. 7.**26** Phosphate diabetes in a 10-year-old child. Varus deformity of the femur.

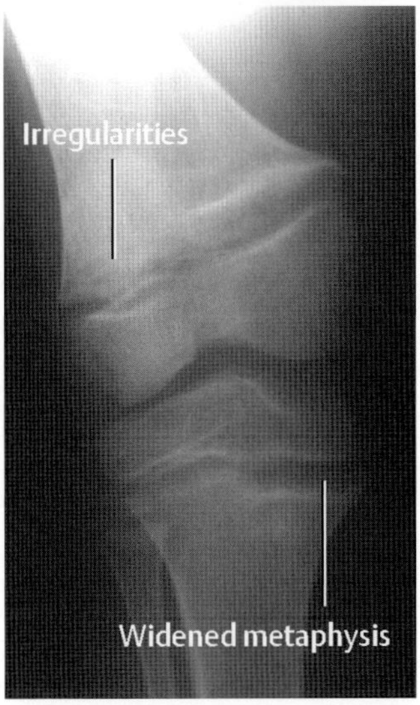

Fig. 7.**27** Same child as in Fig. 7.**26**. Widening and irregularity of the metaphyses.

Increased Bone Density

Osteopetrosis

Prevalence: 1 : 20 000 births

Osteopetrosis is a group of disorders characterized by increased bone density. Four different types with autosomal dominant or recessive inheritance have been described. Based on clinical and radiographic criteria, only two types, the early and the late types, are distinguished.

Precocious Manifestation (= early type)

Synonyms: Marble bone disease, congenital osteosclerosis.

PATH Defective osteoclast function inhibits bone absorption and leads to persistence of the normally resorbed calcified cartilage matrix with resultant narrowing of the marrow space. The bone becomes brittle, and medullary hematopoiesis is severely compromised.

CLINIC **Mode of inheritance:** Autosomal recessive.
Manifestation: The dominating findings are anemia and pancytopenia, hepatosplenomegaly, fractures, cranial nerve palsies, and infections, often with a lethal outcome.

X-RAY Attention should be directed to the increased density of the entire skeleton:

- demarcation between cortex and medullary cavity is lost (Fig. 7.**28**),
- clubbing of the metaphyses,
- transverse metaphyseal radiolucent bands or 'bone within a bone' pattern of the tubular bones and 'Oreo cookie' pattern of the vertebral bodies, indicative of a course with intermittent exacerbation and remission,
- thickened and markedly sclerotic cranial vault and base, and hypoplastic paranasal sinuses, but normal mandible.

Delayed Manifestation (= late type)

Synonyms: Albers-Schönberg disease, osteosclerosis of late onset, benign type.

CLINIC **Mode of inheritance:** Autosomal dominant, rarely recessive.
Clinical Course: Depends on the age of initial manifestation: onset in childhood leads to cranial nerve symptoms due to nerve compression, anemia, fractures, and osteomyelitis. In the adult, the condition often remains asymptomatic; bone pain, periapical dental abscesses, and carpal tunnel syndrome can occur.

X-RAY The increased sclerosis of the skeleton is similar to but less severe than that seen in the precocious manifestation, and the cortex is usually distinguishable from the medullary space (Fig. 7.**29**).

DD Conditions included in the differential diagnosis are sclerotic dysostoses with similar radiographic features without anemia, such as pyknodysostosis, Paget disease, osteoblastic metastases, and physiologically increased bone density in neonates.

The following skeletal dysplasias with increased bone density are rarely encountered:

Pyknodysostosis

The disease of Toulouse-Lautrec!

CLINIC **Mode of inheritance:** Autosomal recessive.
Manifestation: Rare condition with short stature and short limbs and fingers.

X-RAY Generalized osteosclerosis, distal hypoplasia of the terminal phalanges and the acromial ends, craniofacial dysplasia with sclerosis of the cranial vault.

Osteopoikilosis

Synonym: Spotted bones.

CLINIC **Mode of inheritance:** Autosomal dominant.
Prevalence: 1: 16 500.
Manifestation: Usually of slightly short stature; cutaneous and subcutaneous nodules can occur, but are rare.

X-RAY Multiple small sclerotic foci of various shapes (round, oval) in the spongiosa of the pelvis, metaphyses, and epiphyses of the tubular bones and in the carpal and tarsal bones (Fig. 7.**30**).

Osteopathia Striata

X-RAY Longitudinal streaking of the metaphyseal zone of the long tubular bones, without clinical symptoms.

Melorheostosis

CLINIC It is asymptomatic in childhood, but in adulthood pain can develop at the sites of osseous involvement, with swelling and atrophy of the overlying soft tissues.

X-RAY Monostotic or polyostotic, longitudinal hyperostotic strips along the cortex of the tubular bones extending across the joints, resembling flowing honey or molten wax (Fig. 7.**31**).

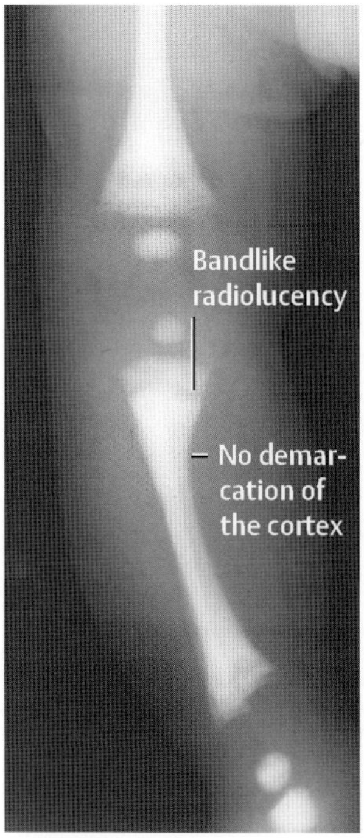

Fig. 7.28 Osteopetrosis, precocious manifestation (early type) in a 3-month-old child. Massively increased bone density, broad metaphyseal bands of decreased density.

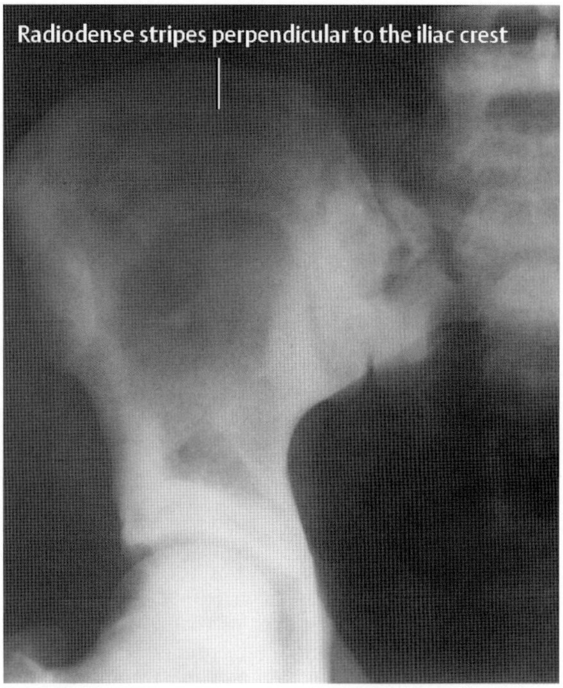

Fig. 7.29 Osteopetrosis, delayed manifestation (late type), adult.

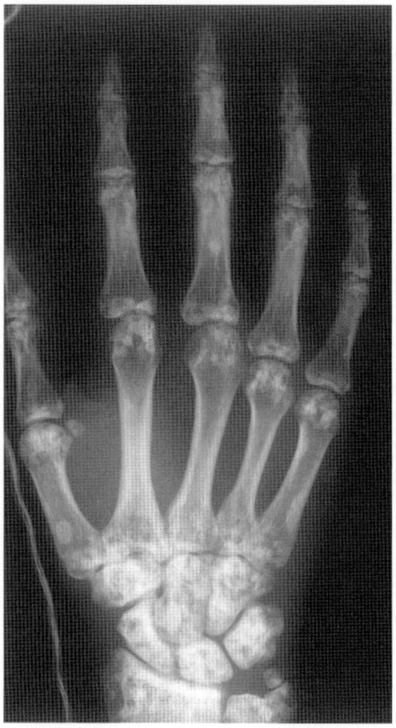

Fig. 7.30 Osteopoikilosis, adult. Multiple punctate sclerotic foci.

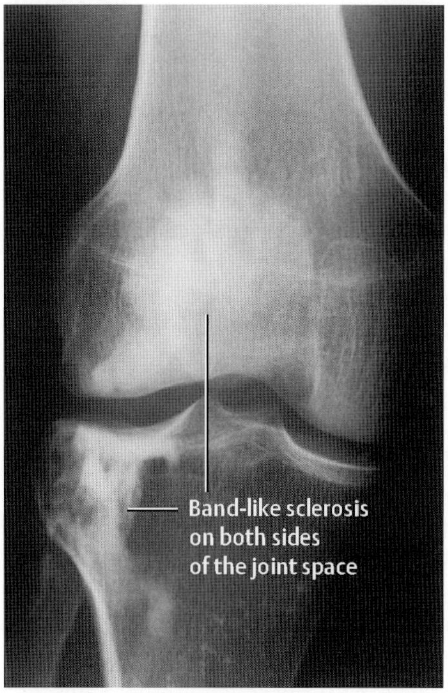

Fig. 7.31 Melorheostosis, adult.

Dysostosis Multiplex

The term 'dysostosis multiplex' applies to the radiographic features of the skeletal manifestation of all hereditary disorders with lysosomal storage of heteroglycans. The heteroglycanoses include mucopolysaccharidoses (MPS), glycoproteinoses, gangliosidoses, and sphingolipidoses. In these disorders, the heteroglycans are deposited in the lysosomes of the cells of the fasciae, tendons, vessels, cardiac valves, muscles, cornea, osteocytes, chondrocytes, meninges, ganglion cells, kidneys, liver, spleen, and lymph nodes. The particular enzyme defect determines the organ involvement.

Mucopolysaccharidoses

CLINIC Twelve types have been defined. The severity of clinical findings, such as coarse facial features (gargoylism), mental retardation, peripheral neuropathy, short stature, joint contractures, hepatomegaly, and clouding of the cornea, vary according to the type of the enzyme defect.

X-RAY The typical skeletal changes are encompassed in the term **dysostosis multiplex.** Attention should be directed to characteristic changes of the pelvis, spine, hand, and skull (Fig. 7.**32**):

- hook-shaped deformity of the upper lumbar vertebra due to an anterosuperior ossification defect, persistent ovoid vertebral configuration, development of wedge vertebrae (Fig. 7.**33**),
- hypoplasia of the ilium at its base with flaring of the iliac wing resembling mouse ears; widened iliac angle when lateral edge of the acetabular roof is absent,
- widened second through fifth metacarpals with characteristic proximal pointing. Proximal and middle phalanges are short and wide, lack normal diaphyseal tubulation, and are wider proximally than distally with distal tapering ('sugar loaf configuration'). Hypoplastic distal phalanges and finger contractures may be present (Fig. 7.**34**).
- macrocephaly with thickened cranial vault, enlarged sella turcica, and sclerosis of the cranial base. Hypoplastic dens with occipitocervical instability,
- thorax: 'oar-shaped ribs' due to posterior widening of the ribs.

CT Hydrocephalus and impaired myelinization of white matter.

DD The diagnosis is established by measuring the excretion of abnormal amounts of mucopolysaccharides in the urine and by detecting the enzyme defect in cultured fibroblasts. Table 7.**4** shows the different forms of mucopolysaccharidoses.

Table 7.**4** Mucopolysaccharidoses (summary based on Spranger)

Designation	Onset (age in years)	Dysostosis multiplex	Mode of Inheritance
MPS I-H	0.5–1	Severe	AR
MPS I-S	6	Mild	AR
MPS I-H/S	2–4	Moderate	AR
MPS II	1	Severe	XR
MPS III-A	2–6	Mild	AR
MPS III-B	2–6	Mild	AR
MPS III–C	2–6	Mild	AR
MPS III–D	2–6	Mild	AR
MPS IV-A	2	Platyspondylia	AR
MPS IV-B	2	Platyspondylia	AR
MPS VI	2–3	Severe–moderate	AR
MPS VII	Variable	Moderate	AR

Mucolipidoses and Gangliosidoses

Mucolipidoses are rare hereditary dysostoses with lysosomal storage of carbohydrates and radiographic features of a dysostosis multiplex. In particular, many features of mucolipidosis II, III, and IV resemble those of a dysostosis multiplex. To a different degree, the same applies to GM1 gangliosidosis and to the oligosaccharidoses (mannosidoses and fucosidosis).

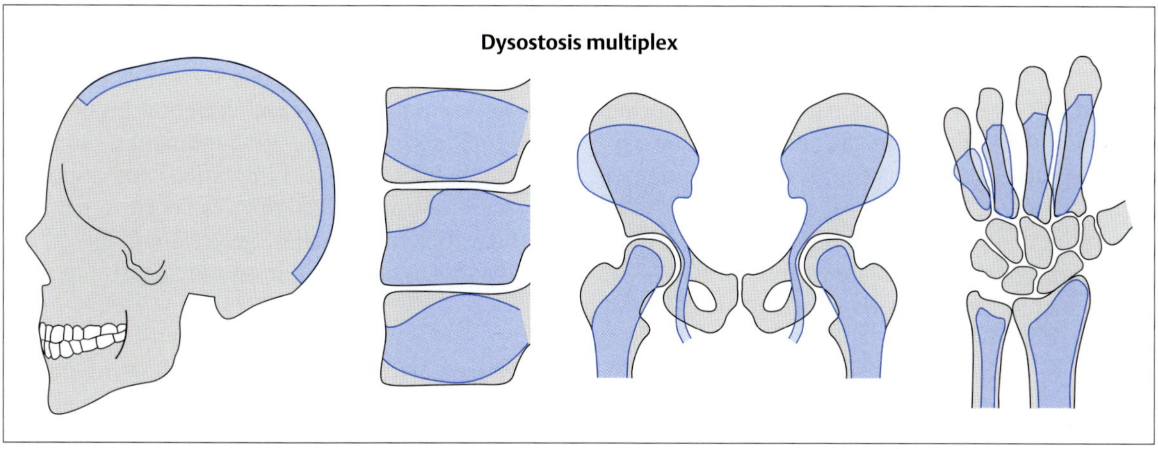

Fig. 7.**32** Characteristic radiographic changes in dysostosis multiplex (according to Spranger).

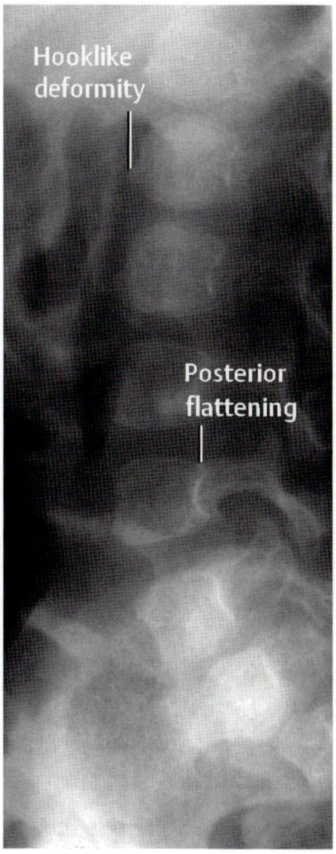

Fig. 7.**33** MPS II, age 3 years, 6 months.

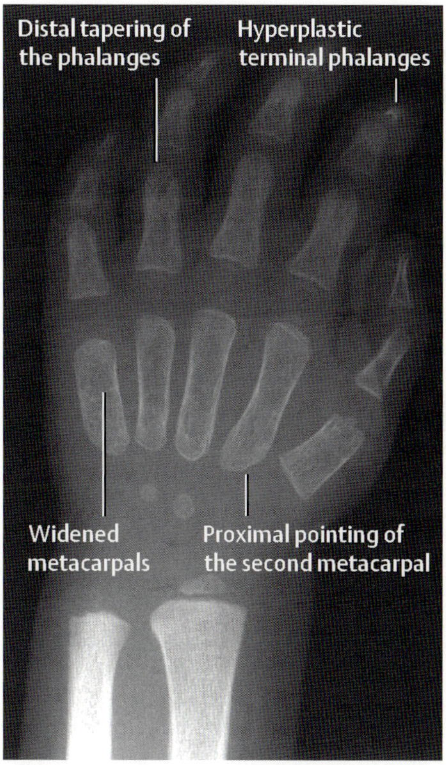

Fig. 7.**34** Same child as in Fig. 7.**33**.

Dysostoses

Dysostoses are congenital failures of normal growth and development of individual bones, either singly or in combination. They are segregated and categorized according to their location (Table 7.**5**). In individual cases, the differentiation from a generalized skeletal dysplasia can be difficult. The causes include both genetic and exogenous factors due to prenatal damage.

Table 7.**5** Classification of dysostosis

Predominant involvement:
A Craniofacial involvement
– Craniosynostoses
– Craniofacial dysostosis (Crouzon)
– Acrocephalosyndactyly (several types)
– Mandibulofacial dysostosis (Franceschetti)
B Axial involvement
– Vertebral segmentation defects (including Klippel-Feil and Sprengel deformity)
– Spondylocostal dysostosis
– Oculovertebral syndrome
C Involvement of limbs
– Underdevelopment anomalies (aplasia and hypoplasia)
– Hyperplasia of limbs (lipomatous macrodystrophy, Klippel-Trenaunay syndrome)
– Segmentation anomalies and synostoses, e.g., radioulnar synostosis, syndactylies
– Connatal camptomelias and pseudarthroses
– Conditions associated with limb anomalies

Dysostoses with predominant craniofacial involvement appear as dyscephalies of the face, isolated or combined with dysplasia of the facial bones. The neurocranium shows craniostenosis due to premature closure (synostosis) of individual or several sutures.

The autosomal dominant craniofacial dysostosis (Crouzon disease) and acrocephalosyndactyly (Apert-syndrome) are dominated by synostosis of the coronal and lamboid sutures with hypoplasia of the anterior and middle cranial fossa, resulting in markedly deformed facies. In acrocephalosyndactyly, this is associated with total syndactyly of the hands and feet (Figs. 7.**35**, 7.**36**).

Dysostoses with predominant axial involvement appear as segmentation abnormalities of the spine, such as hemivertebrae, wedge vertebrae, block vertebrae, sagittal clefts of the vertebral bodies, and vertebral assimilations. Rib anomalies, such as aplasia and hypoplasia, bifurcation, and supernumerary ribs (e.g., cervical ribs), can occur separately or as additional anomalies. Severe anomalies of the spine and ribs are found in spondylocostal dysplasia.

Dysostoses with predominant limb involvement are characterized by a wide range of variations. The all-inclusive term applied to all limb deformities is **dysmelia.**

- **Reduction anomalies** are divided into transverse and longitudinal limb deficiencies (Fig. 7.**38**).
- **Hyperplasias of limbs** can affect an individual skeletal element such as the finger in macrodystrophia lipomatosis, or a part of a limb as in the Klippel-Trenaunay syndrome combined with a vascular malformation.
- **Segmentation anomalies and synostoses** are frequent and often hereditary anomalies. Hypersegmentation duplicates portions of a limb, largely affecting hands and feet **(polydactyly).** Synostoses of the hands and feet appear as **syndactyly** (fusion or incomplete separation of fingers and toes), **symphalangy** (fusion of two adjacent phalanges), or carpal and tarsal **coalition. Radioulnar synostoses** frequently are bilateral and usually affect the proximal forearm (Fig. 7.**37**).
- **Congenital bowing** of the long tubular bones generally is caused by faulty fetal positions, and pseudarthrosis due to local fibrous degeneration of bone.
- **Disorders in combination with limb anomalies** can occur as:

Fanconi anemia (pancytopenia): This is an autosomal recessive hereditary disease with reduction anomaly of the radial ray of the forearm and hand, combined with a severely disturbed hematopoiesis.

Poland syndrome: This is a unilateral aplasia of the sternal portion of the pectoralis major, together with ipsilateral brachyphalangia and hypoplasia of the forearm.

Rubinstein-Taybi syndrome: Wide phalanges of the thumb and first toe occur, together with unusual facial features and mental retardation.

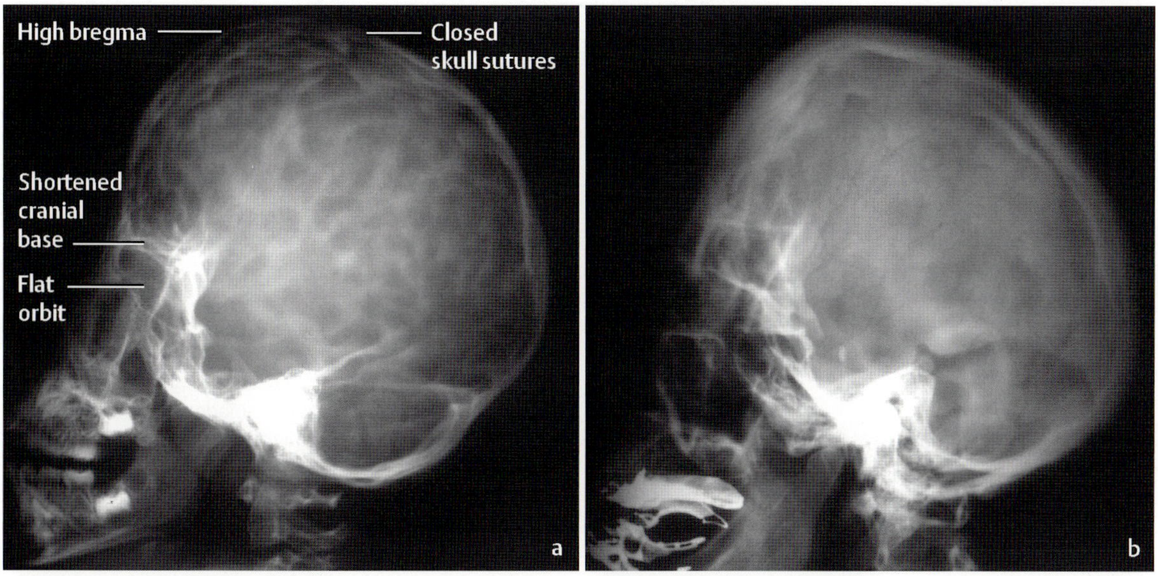

Fig. 7.**35** Crouzon disease. **a** Child, 3 years old, 'cotton-wool skull.' **b** Mother, 30 years old.

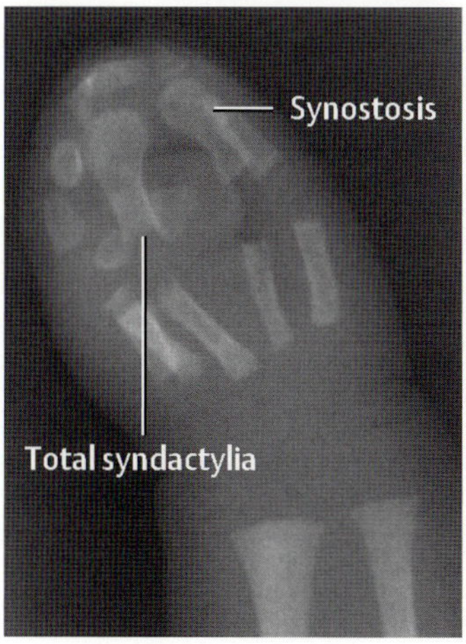

Fig. 7.**36** Acrocephalosyndactyly (Apert syndrome). Newborn with skull changes analogous to Crouzon disease associated with syndactyly of hands and feet.

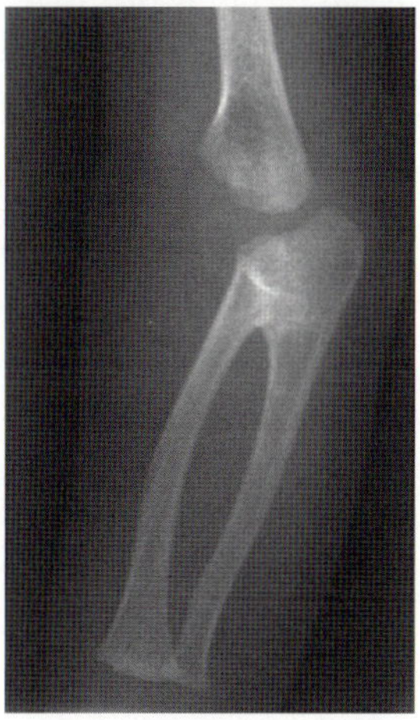

Fig. 7.**37** Radioulnar synostosis, 1-month-old child.

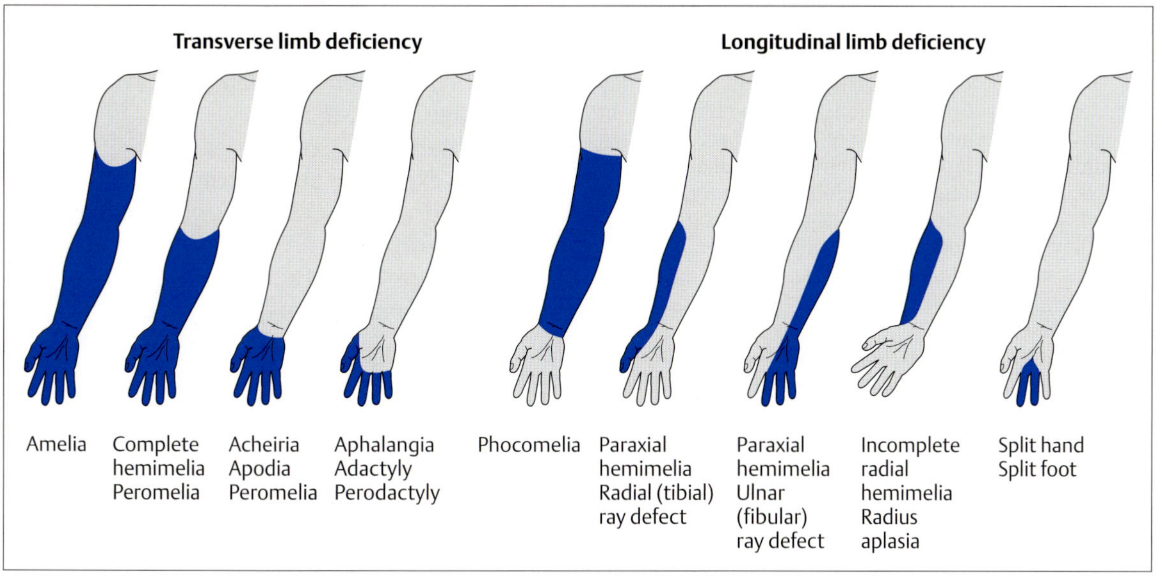

Fig. 7.**38** Reduction anomalies (after Caffey).

8 Various Bone and Soft-Tissue Disorders

Paget Disease

Synonym: Osteitis deformans.

■ Paget disease is a chronic condition, commonest in the elderly and characterized by enlarged, often deformed, coarsely trabeculated bone. The etiology of the condition has not been proven conclusively. ■

PATH The most widely accepted theory is that Paget disease is caused by a virus. According to this theory, the osteoclasts infected with the virus become activated after many years of 'infection' and thus cause rapid bone resorption. Compensatory activation of osteoblasts and fibroblasts induces reactive new bone production with the formation of a more primitive woven bone. Eventually, the bone production predominates, resulting in bone of increased volume and density. Lytic, mixed, and sclerotic stages of the condition are identified.

Paget disease has a prevalence for the axial skeleton (skull, spine, pelvis) and the femur and tibia (Fig. 8.**1**), but any bone can be involved. The involvement can be polyostotic, oligostotic or, less frequently, monostotic.

Osteoporosis circumscripta corresponds to the lytic phase of Paget disease and is an early manifestation.

CLINIC With a prevalence of about 3% in patients older than 40 years of age, Paget disease is a common bone condition. However, in about 90% of cases it is asymptomatic and is discovered as an incidental finding. The condition becomes clinically apparent when bone pain develops, or if complications develop (Table 8.**1**). In the active stage, urine excretion of hydroxyproline (corresponding to osteoclast activity) and serum alkaline phosphatase (corresponding to osteoblast activity) are increased, and these values fall in the osteosclerotic stage.
The radiographic interpretation should address:
- extent and location of the process,
- pathologic fractures,
- joint deformities.

In patients complaining of progressive pain, signs of
- degeneration (especially to sarcoma or giant cell tumor)

have to be looked for diligently.
Therapy: Calcitonin, diphosphonate.

Table 8.**1** Possible complications of Paget disease

Lesion	Cause
Pathologic fractures	Statically inadequate bone Frequently involving the proximal tibia
Paget arthropathy	Premature degenerative changes most frequently in the hip and knee (Fig. 8.**6**)
Neurologic findings	Bony expansion with compression of cranial nerves, spinal canal or root compression
Neoplastic transformation	In less than 1% of cases. Usually osteosarcoma, fibrosarcoma or giant cell tumor

X-RAY Strictly lytic or sclerotic stages of Paget disease are rarely observed. It is this coexistence of lytic and sclerotic changes seen in the mixed stage that enables the diagnosis of Paget disease.

Lytic stage (Figs. 8.**2**, 8.**7**):
- loss of the trabecular texture,
- sharply demarcated, V-shaped or flame-shaped radiolucency (also referred to as 'candle flame' or 'blade of grass'),
- subarticular onset with diaphyseal extension.

Mixed stage (Figs. 8.**3**, 8.**5**):
- coarse trabecular pattern,
- osseous expansion and deformity,
- thickened cortex with striations; 'bubbly' pattern in small bones

Sclerotic stage (Fig. 8.**4**):
- patchy or homogeneous thickening.

Assessment: Radiographs are generally adequate to diagnose and follow Paget disease.

NUC Extensive osseous turnover with increased vascularity corresponds to massive uptake in areas involved with Paget disease. Bone scanning is suitable to determine the extent of pagetic involvement and also, in some cases, to differentiate Paget disease from metastases on the basis of its typical distribution pattern.

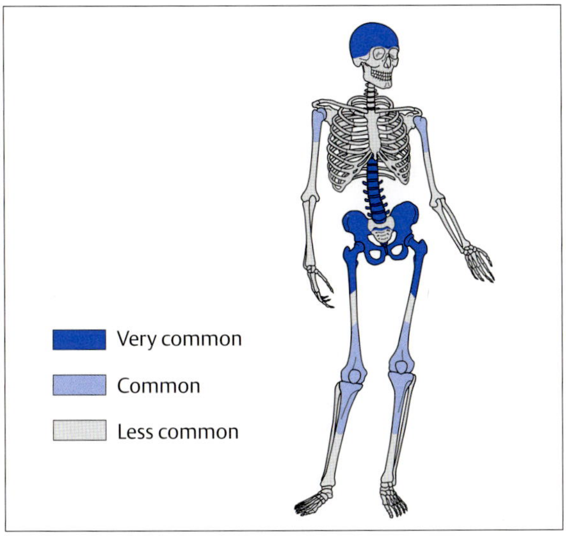

Fig. 8.1 Preferred sites of Paget disease.

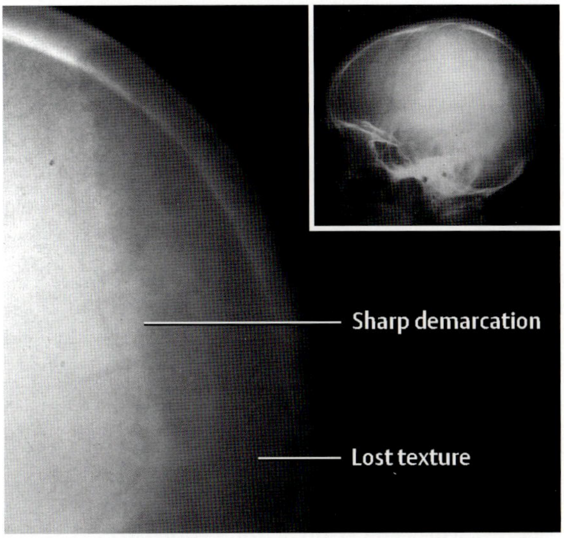

Fig. 8.2 Lytic state of Paget disease in the skull (osteoporosis circumscripta).

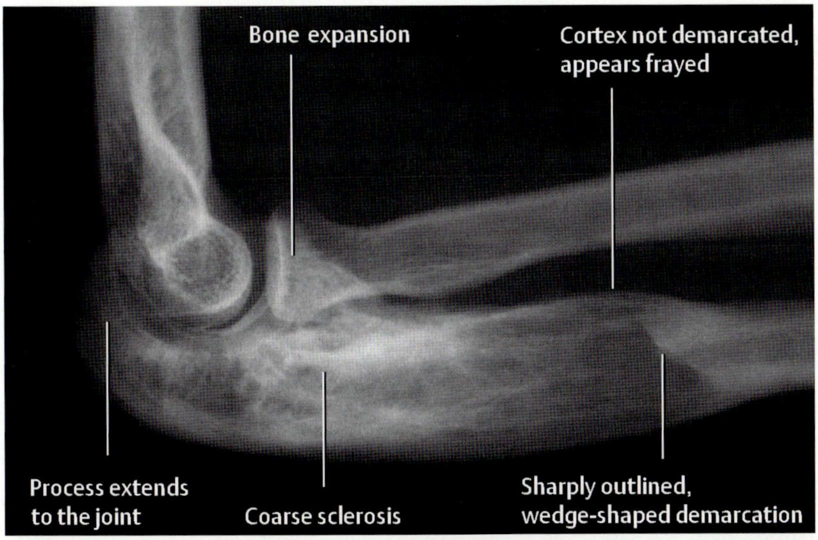

Fig. 8.3 Characteristic radiographic findings of the mixed stage of Paget disease.

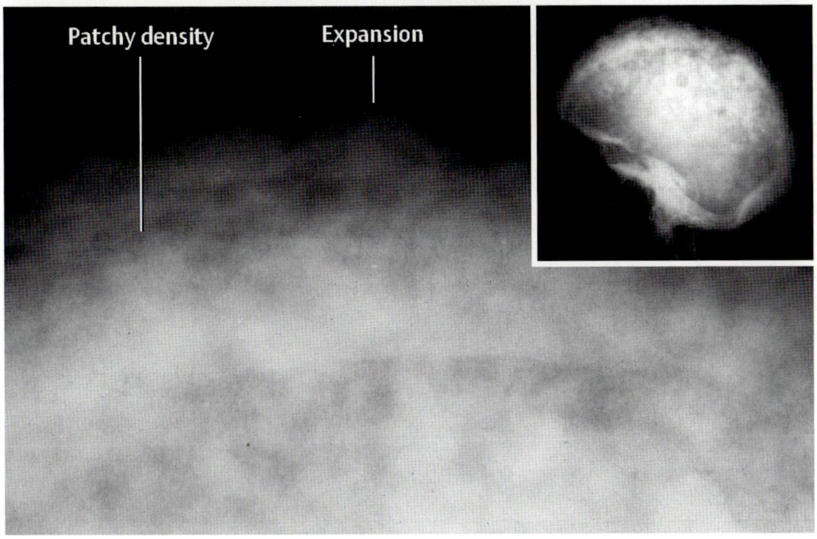

Fig. 8.4 Sclerotic stage of Paget disease in the skull ('cotton-wool' appearance).

CT CT rarely contributes to the diagnosis of Paget disease. However, it can be used to evaluate complications (nerve compression, malignant transformation) and to segregate it from other conditions.

MRI The cortex is thickened but also shows a permeative striated or granular pattern (Fig. 8.**9b**). The striated or granular areas show high signal intensity on T2-weighted images and enhance (Fig. 8.**9c**). The enhancing zones correspond to fibrovascular tissue. Furthermore, the fibrovascular tissue encroaches on the marrow, which is permeated with striated or granular fat marrow remnants.

DD The typical presentation of Paget disease does not pose a diagnostic problem. Atypical presentation or the clinical context can raise differential diagnostic questions.

Differential Diagnosis of Paget Disease

Metastasis
Sarcoma
Hemangioma of vertebra
Fibrous dysplasia
Post-traumatic transformation

The criteria helpful in differentiating Paget disease from metastases are listed in Table 8.**2**.

Sarcomatous transformation must be suspected if new lytic areas develop in areas of sclerotic bone and if parosseous soft-tissue extension develops. Soft-tissue widening or newly formed bone within the surrounding soft tissues is highly suspicious for tumor and must be further evaluated by biopsy. Suspicious clinical findings are pain and soft-tissue swelling. Aside from providing a more exact evaluation of tumorous soft-tissue infiltrations, CT and MRI enable differentiation of the tissues within osteolytic areas; Paget disease contains preserved fatty marrow, and tumorous destruction has to be suspected in cases of its complete absence.

In the spine, increased AP diameter and framing of the affected vertebrae suggest Paget disease (Fig. 8.**8**). Inconclusive cases should be further evaluated by cross-sectional imaging.

Post-traumatic changes generally induce less pronounced enlargement of the bone, but the differentiation can be difficult in individual cases. The bone scan might support the diagnosis by showing additional areas with characteristic pagetic uptake.

Table 8.**2** Differential diagnostic criteria distinguishing Paget disease from metastases

Paget disease	Metastases
Few lesions covering a large area (scintigraphy)	Multiple small lesions (scintigraphy)
Sharp demarcation	Indistinct demarcation
Coarse sclerosis	Often homogeneous, faint sclerosis
Epiphysis invariably involved (most frequent exception: tibia)	
Pelvis: often unilateral involvement	Pelvis: usually diffuse involvement
Enlarged bone	

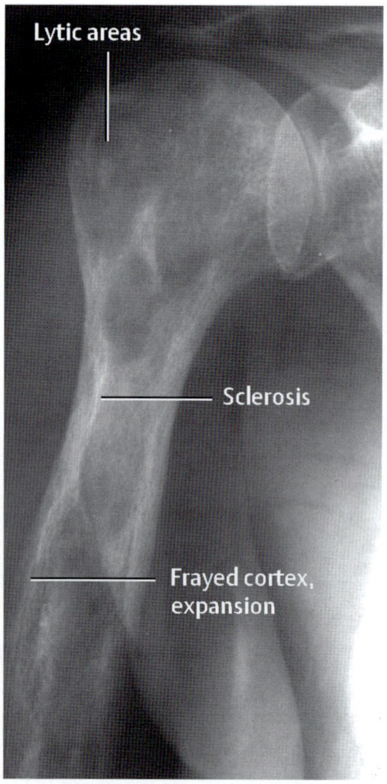

Fig. 8.**5** Mixed stage of Paget disease. Large lytic areas, primarily in the humeral head.

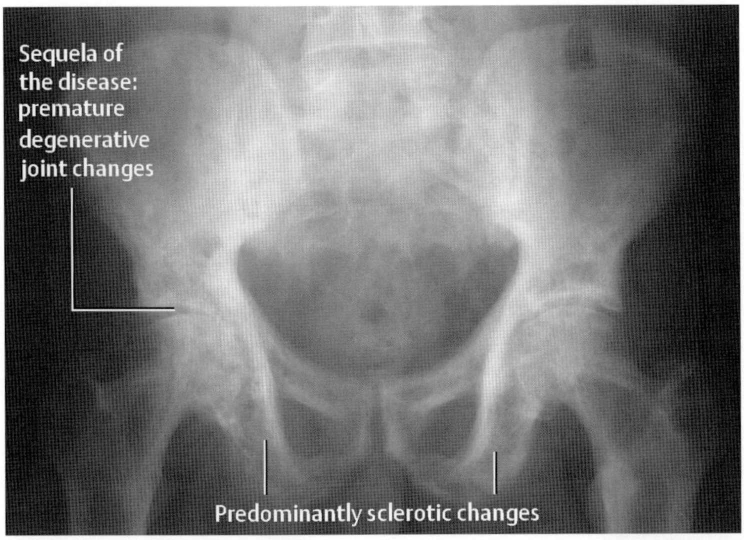

Fig. 8.**6** Sclerotic manifestation of Paget disease in the pelvis with severe Paget arthropathy.

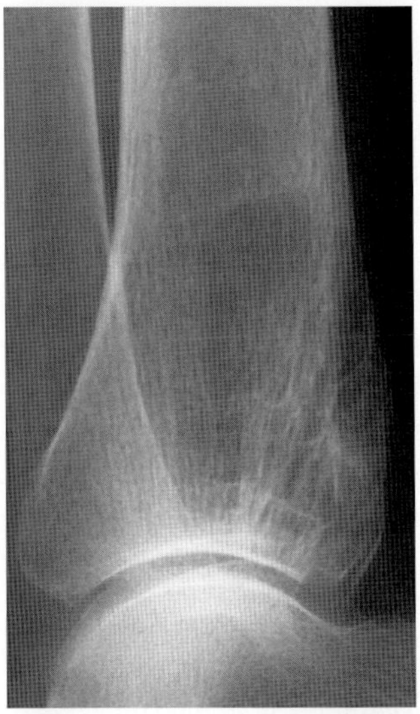

Fig. 8.**7** Rare location of Paget disease in the distal tibia with coarse linear sclerosis (transition from lytic to mixed stage).

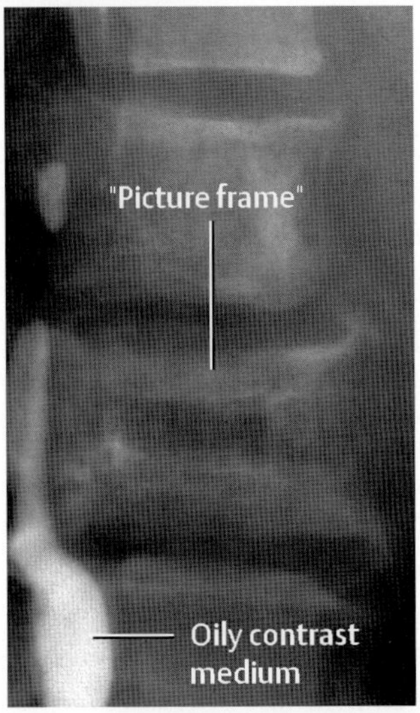

Fig. 8.**8** Characteristic appearance of a pagetic vertebra with picture framing and osseous **expansion** (oily contrast medium is incidentally noted in the spinal canal).

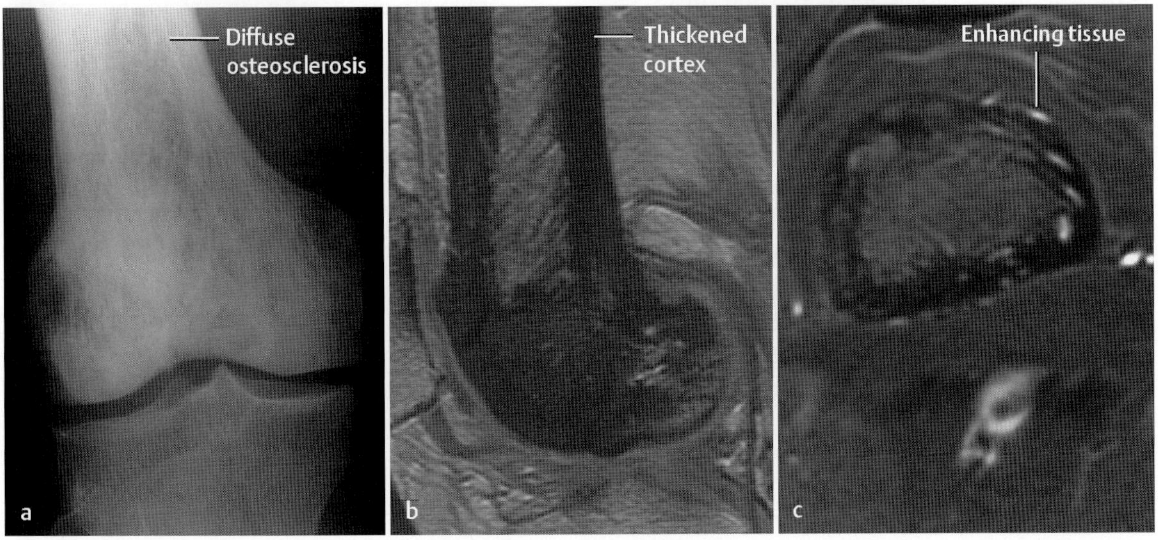

Fig. 8.**9** Paget disease of the distal femur (**a**). The T1-weighted GE sequence (**b**) clearly delineates the thickened and striated cortex. **c** Enhancement of the fibrovascular tissue after administration of contrast medium (T1-weighted SE sequence with fat suppression).

Sarcoidosis

Synonym: Boeck disease.

■ Osteitis cystitis multiplex Jüngling: polycystic type of bone sarcoidosis.
Sarcoidosis is a systemic inflammatory condition of unknown etiology. It can involve any organ and is characterized by noncaseating epithelioid granulomas. Infectious or autoimmune etiologies are the most likely causes.
A distinction is made between:
- sarcoidosis of **bones** with granulomas in the bone marrow and
- the more common sarcoidosis of **joints,** a granulomatous inflammation of the synovial membrane. ■

CLINIC Sarcoidosis can occur at any age, but has a definite predilection for the ages of 15 to 40 years. Osseous involvement is seen in about 5% and joint involvement in up to 10% of patients with sarcoidosis.

Osseous sarcoidosis most commonly involves the hands (metacarpals and phalanges). Its clinical manifestation usually is confined to soft-tissue swelling of the affected areas. Articular sarcoidosis usually involves the wrist, ankle, knee, and elbow, as well as the minor joints of the hand. It causes transient, possibly recurrent bouts of arthralgia. Chronic involvement rarely causes persistent restriction of movements or deformities of the joints.

X-RAY Radiographically detectable changes can be asymptomatic, and clinical findings might not correspond to radiographic changes. The radiographically detectable changes of **osseous sarcoidosis** can be placed into three groups:

1. Diffuse changes of the spongiosa and cortex.
   These changes begin with osteopenia and progress to a lacelike trabecular pattern, as well as to fissuring and thinning of the cortex. The changes may resemble permeative destruction (Fig. 8.**10**).
2. Cystic lesions.
   These can be centrally located, characteristically in the epimetaphyseal region of the phalanges, and are surrounded by thin marginal sclerosis. Eccentrically located lesions cause marginal scalloping with bulging of the overlying cortex (Fig. 8.**11**). Rarely, acro-osteolysis can also occur in sarcoidosis (Fig. 8.**12**).
3. Osteosclerosis.
   In contrast to the aforementioned changes, which are primarily found in the metacarpals and phalanges of the hands, osteosclerosis tends to occur in the central skeleton (spine, pelvis, skull, ribs, and proximal ends of the long tubular bones). This pattern is rare, often occurs long after resolution of the pulmonary sarcoidosis, and is usually in a local or generalized patchy distribution. Acro-osteosclerosis can occur.

For **articular sarcoidosis,** the same criteria as those for acute and chronic synovial arthritis apply.

NUC This is rarely indicated, except for cases requiring differentiation from osteoblastic metastasis (old sarcoidosis lesions show no increased uptake on the bone scan).

DD Sarcoidosis tends to be bilateral but asymmetrical. The important differential diagnoses of sarcoidosis are listed in Table 8.**3**. Especially for differentiating from malignancies (sarcoma, plasmocytoma, metastases, and others), it is important to remember that sarcoidosis almost never induces a periosteal reaction.

The best method for diagnosis of sarcoidosis is bronchoalveolar lavage with determination of the ratio of T4/T8 suppressor cells. The serum concentration of the angiotensin converting enzyme (ACE) is simpler but is less specific.

!
- Osseous sarcoidosis without evidence of pulmonary sarcoidosis is extremely rare.
- Acute articular sarcoidosis is generally associated with erythema nodosum and bilateral hilarnodal adenopathy (Löfgren syndrome).
- Except for typical changes in the phalanges of the hand, the radiographic findings of sarcoidosis are nonspecific, and the diagnosis can only be made in context with a known underlying disease.

Table 8.3 Important differential diagnoses of sarcoidosis

Morphology	Differential diagnoses	Criteria
Permeative bone destruction	Malignancy Osteomyelitis	Frequent periosteal reaction, history, age Frequent periosteal reaction, clinical findings, laboratory
Cystic changes	Bone cyst Brown tumor Enchondroma Metastasis	Solitary, in contrast to sarcoidosis Laboratory Periosteal reaction, cortical destruction (rare in sarcoidosis) Distribution pattern (scintigraphy), age
Osteosclerosis, acro-osteosclerosis	Malignancy Hematologic disease Renal osteodystrophy Myelofibrosis Paget disease Scleroderma Systemic lupus erythematosus	Distribution pattern (scintigraphy), age Laboratory Laboratory Involvement of other organs Involvement of other organs
Acute or chronic arthritic changes	Entire spectrum of arthritic causes	History, clinical course, distribution pattern

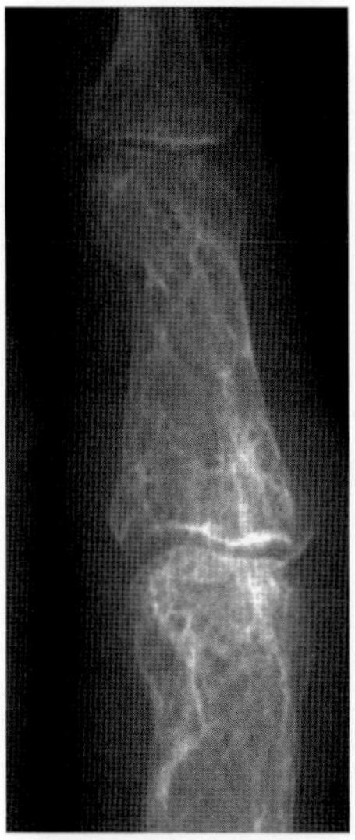

Fig. 8.**10** Lacelike trabecular pattern of sarcoidosis in the finger.

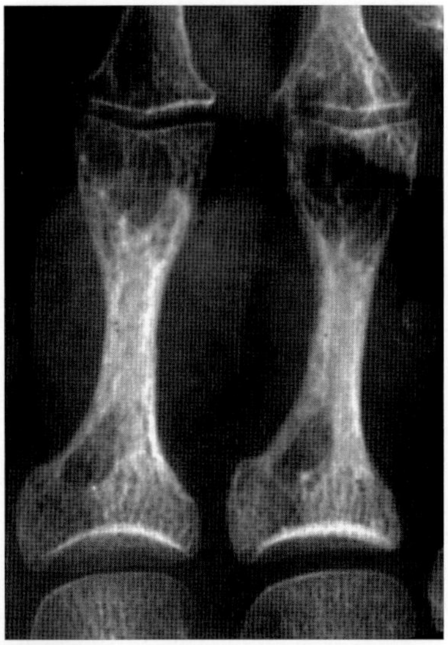

Fig. 8.**11** Lytic, cystic lesions of sarcoidosis in the phalanges of the foot.

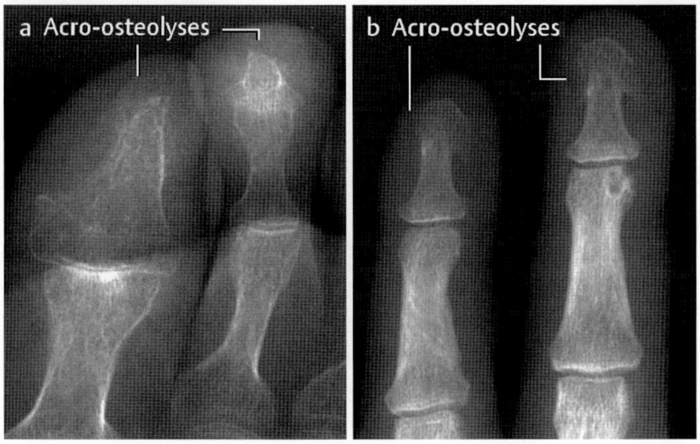

Fig. 8.**12** Typical acro-osteolysis at the toes (**a**) and fingers (**b**). This finding, however, is nonspecific for sarcoidosis.

Hypertrophic Osteoarthropathy

Synonym: Pierre-Marie-Bamberger disease.

■ This is a secondary periostitis and synovitis of unknown etiology with relatively characteristic periosteal proliferations. ■

In the majority of cases, hypertrophic osteoarthropathy is associated with intrathoracic disease, of which bronchial carcinoma and pleural mesothelioma are by far the most frequent. The association with other intrathoracic or extrathoracic conditions (other malignancies, chronic inflammatory intestinal diseases, mucoviscidosis in children, and others) is less common. After therapy for the underlying condition, the osteoarthropathy usually resolves slowly.

! Osseous changes can precede the clinical manifestation of the underlying condition. Thus, hypertrophic osteoarthropathy without known underlying disease should prompt a search for tumor.

CLINIC Some patients are asymptomatic, but arthritic changes that mimic rheumatoid arthritis are common. Clubbing of the fingers can also occur.

Location: The tibia and fibula are almost always involved. The radius, ulna, tubular bones of the hands and feet, and femur are less commonly affected. These changes are **invariably bilateral and symmetric.**

X-RAY Periosteal proliferations may be of the lamellar, undulating, or solid types (Fig. 8.**13**). The periosteal proliferations terminate at the metaphyses.

NUC Increased activity is seen in the regions of periosteal new bone formation. This linear, symmetric tracer uptake along the tubular bones is so distinctive that it can be considered diagnostic (Fig. 8.**14**).

DD The diagnosis of hypertrophic osteoarthropathy generally is unequivocally established in the presence of typical radiographic and scintigraphic findings. The major determining criterion is the bilateral, symmetrical appearance.

In **chronic venous stasis,** the isolated location along the affected extremity is characteristic, and the periosteal proliferation is often nodular.

Glossary: Types of Localized Idiopathic Hyperostosis

Pachydermoperiostosis ('primary hypertrophic osteoarthropathy'): This condition shows periosteal proliferation identical to hypertrophic osteoarthropathy that, however, extends into the epiphysis. Characteristic skin thickening is also present.

Hyperostosis frontalis interna: This condition is more common in women over 40 years old and has no clinical relevance.

Osteitis condensans ilii (hyperostosis triangularis ilii): This is attributed to an osseous reaction to mechanical stress that induces a triangular sclerosis in the ilium along the inferior aspect of the SI joint (Fig. 8.**15**). Women are by far more frequently affected. This condition is frequently associated with degenerative changes of the SI joints, which might explain the associated pain.

Sternocostoclavicular hyperostosis: This process involves the sternal rib ends and usually causes painful swelling. This condition is frequently associated with skin diseases, especially palmoplantar pustulosis.

Diffuse idiopathic skeletal hyperostosis (DISH): As part of DISH (see detailed presentation in Chapter 9), ossifications can occasionally develop at the capsular, ligamentous, and tendinous insertions of the peripheral skeleton.

Infantile cortical hyperostosis (Caffey disease): This is a rare disease of unknown etiology generally seen in children under the age of 5 months. These children usually present with fever, swelling, and tenderness of the affected bones. Periosteal reaction with thickening of the bone up to twice its normal diameter is seen radiographically (Fig. 8.**16**). The mandible, clavicle, and ribs are most commonly involved, but involvement of the pelvis, skull, and the long tubular bones can be seen. These changes can resolve within months to years, but persistent and chronic recurrent episodes can occur and lead to growth disturbances of the affected bones. The major differential diagnoses associated with periosteal reaction in children are listed in Table 8.**4**.

Osteopathia striata, osteopoikilosis: See page 270: Osteochondral dysplasias with abnormal bone density.

Table 8.**4** Differential diagnosis of periosteal reaction in children

- Infantile cortical hyperostosis
- Physiologic periosteal reaction in infants
- Acute osteomyelitis
- Child abuse
- Acute leukemia
- Neuroblastoma metastases
- Prostaglandin therapy

Melorheostosis

This is a rare hyperostosis of unknown etiology characterized by solid and very dense bone formation arising adjacent to the periosteum. Its typical appearance is that of 'dripping candle wax' along the inner or outer cortical surfaces (Fig. 8.**17 a**). It is almost always found in the extremities, is characteristically unilateral, and may cross joints (**regional** disease, Fig. 8.**17 c**).

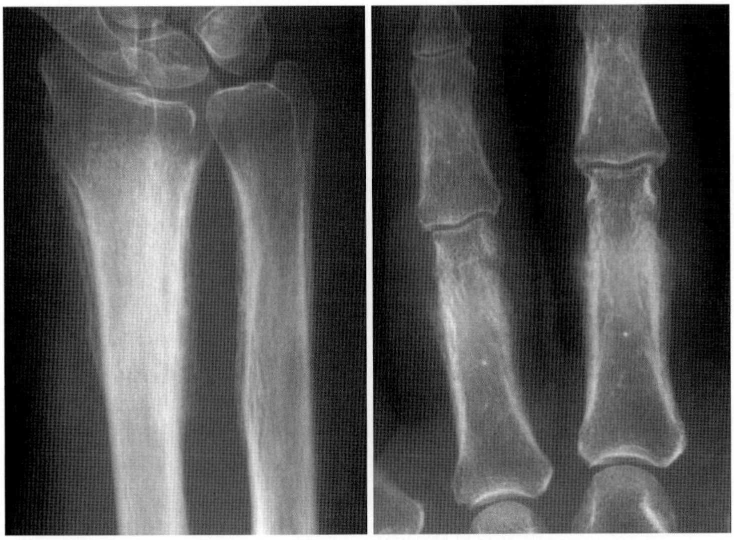

Fig. 8.**13** Classic periosteal reaction of hypertrophic osteoarthropathy (76-year-old female patient with pleural mesothelioma).

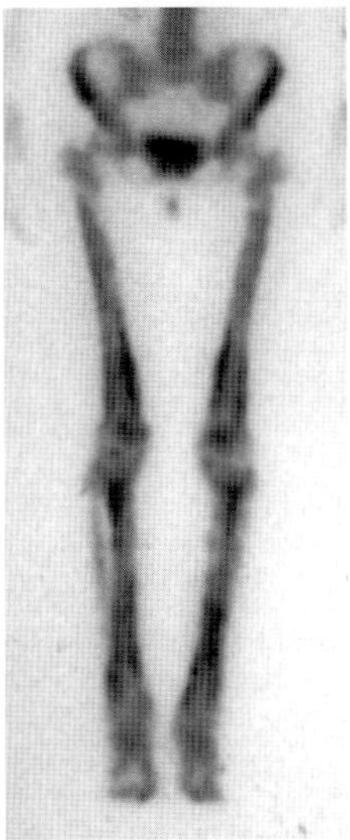

Fig. 8.**14** Bone scan of hypertrophic osteoarthropathy with typical pattern of cortical tracer uptake.

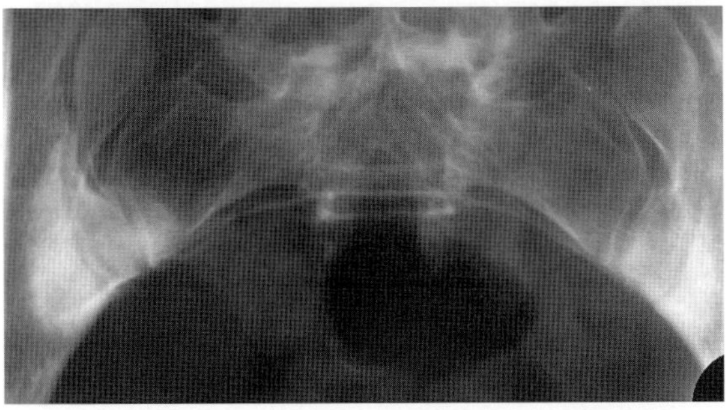

Fig. 8.**15** Typical osteitis condensans ilii in a 36-year-old patient.

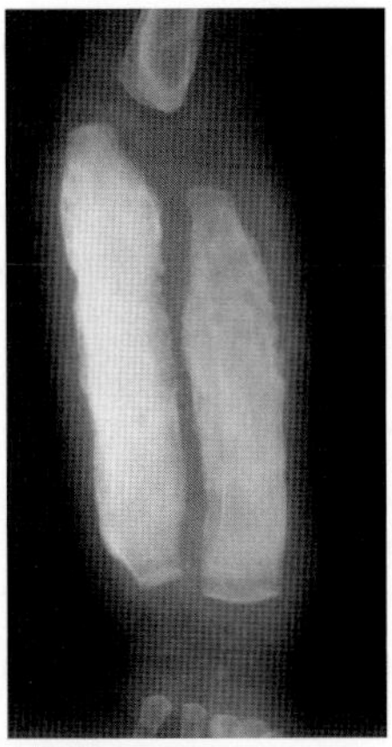

Fig. 8.**16** Infantile cortical hyperostosis with massive periosteal reaction involving the radius and ulna.

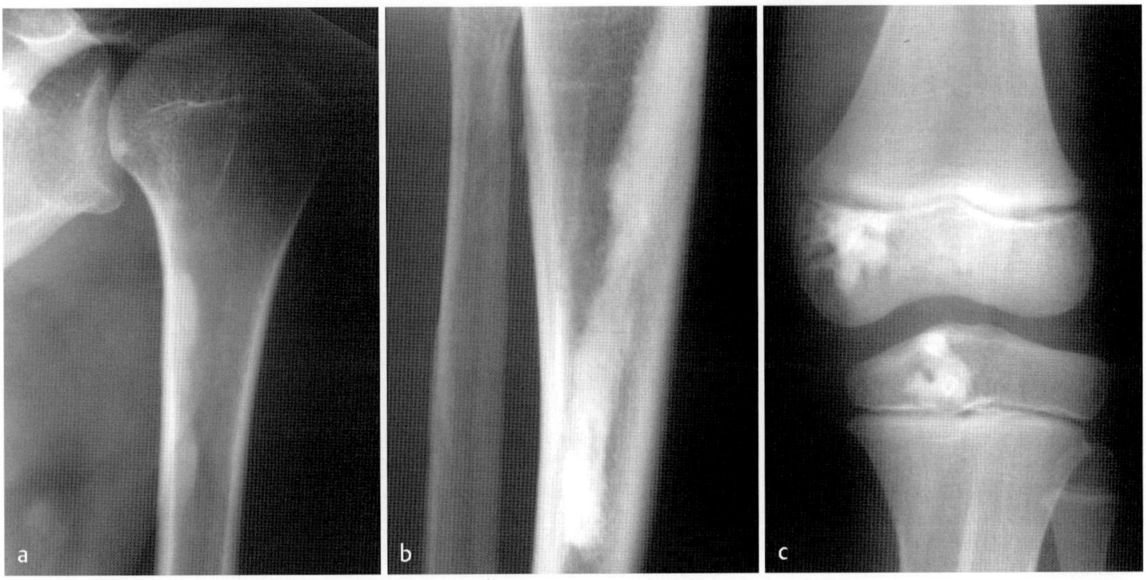

Fig. 8.**17** Melorheostosis in several patients. **a** Shows the typical 'dripping candle wax' configuration and **b** a more rope-like appearance. **c** Demonstrates a localized type that crosses the joint.

Melorheostosis is usually associated with complaints of joint swelling, pain, muscle atrophy and skin changes, and possibly growth disturbances.

Calcifications and Ossifications of the Soft Tissues

Calcifications can be categorized by site (diffuse or local) and by cause:

- soft-tissue calcifications secondary to disturbed calcium-phosphate metabolism,
- soft-tissue calcifications with a normal calcium-phosphate metabolism, and
- soft-tissue calcifications in dystrophic or necrotic tissue

(see Table 8.**5**).

The radiographic features of calcifications are not often diagnostic, and the distribution pattern and laboratory parameters are usually more informative.

Ossifications are genuine new bone formations, which, if advanced enough, show a trabecular pattern. The most common condition is myositis ossificans and less commonly encountered are ossifications due to chronic venous stasis, tendon ossifications in tendonitis, and neoplastic ossifications.

Since discrete trabeculation is often difficult to recognize radiographically, the differentiation between ossification and calcification is not always possible.

Calcifications and ossifications frequently **coexist** in:

- chronic venous stasis,
- paraplegia,
- frostbite,
- trauma,
- compartment syndromes.

! In principle, any calcification can be transformed into an ossification through secondary ossification.

Soft-tissue Calcification Secondary to Imbalanced Calcium-Phosphate Metabolism

Synonym: Metastatic calcifications.

The commonest causes are primary and secondary hyperparathyroidism; less common causes are listed in Table 8.**5**. All types can occur, ranging from delicate stippled to coarse calcifications. Hyperparathyroidism usually causes periarticular calcifications (Fig. 8.**18**).

Soft-tissue Calcifications with Normal Calcium-Phosphate Metabolism

Synonym: Idiopathic calcinosis.

This can be local ('circumscript' calcinosis) or general ('universal' calcinosis). A special form is the so-called pseudotumorous (tumoral) calcinosis that occurs between the ages of 20 and 40 and predominantly in men. The major manifestation is bulky calcifications around major joints. Frequently, swelling is the only clinical finding, but restricted joint motion and pain can develop. Radiographically, the calcifications appear as a cluster of many 1–20 cm calcific nodules demarcated individually by fine radiolucent lines (Fig. 8.**20**).

Dystrophic Calcifications

Dystrophic calcifications can be secondary to any type of tissue necrosis but especially necrosis that is due to burns and frostbites. Additional causes can be found in Table 8.**5** (Fig. 8.**19**).

Table 8.**5** Summary of causes of soft-tissue calcifications

'Metastatic' calcifications (disturbed calcium-phosphate metabolism)	**'Idiopathic' calcifications** (normal calcium-phosphate metabolism)	**'Dystrophic' calcifications** (normal calcium-phosphate metabolism)
– Hyperparathyroidism – Renal osteodystrophy (Fig. 8.**18**) – Excess vitamin D – Hypoparathyroidism – Sarcoidosis – Massive bone loss with plasmocytoma, leukemia, or extensive metastases	– Collagenoses (e.g., systemic lupus erythematosus, dermatomyositis, CREST syndrome, Fig. 8.**20**) – 'Tumorous' calcinosis – Calcinosis universalis (in children)	– Burns – Frostbites – Severe soft-tissue injuries – Compartment syndrome – Tumors (Fig. 8.**19**) – Osteonecroses, infarcts – Tuberculosis

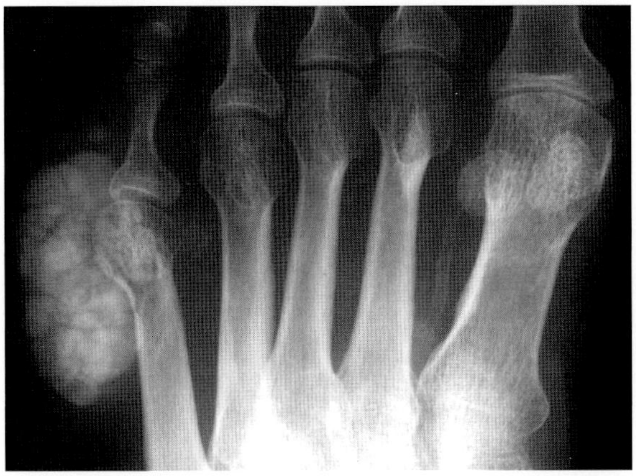

Fig. 8.**18** 'Metastatic' soft-tissue calcifications in secondary hyperparathyroidism due to renal insufficiency. The calcification is very dense and coarse.

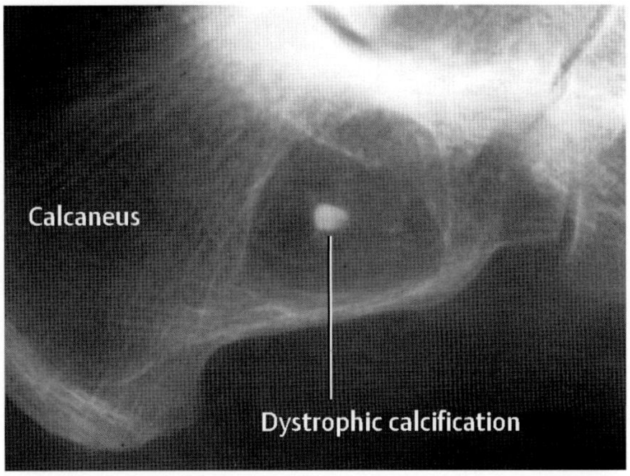

Fig. 8.**19** Dystrophic calcification in a lipoma. The calcification pattern is very variable. In this case, it is dense and relatively homogeneous.

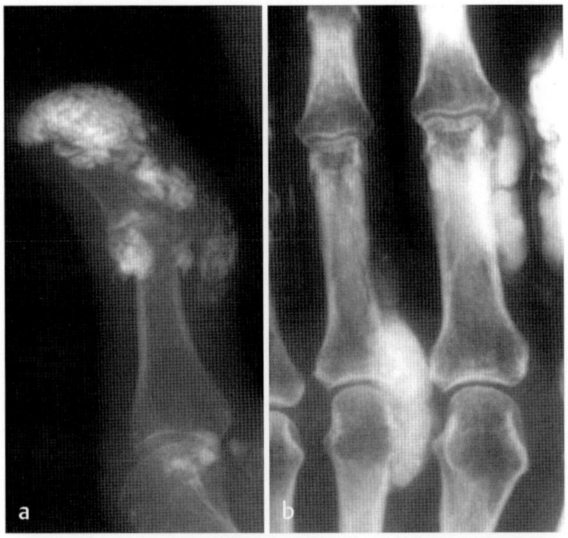

Fig. 8.**20** Idiopathic calcinosis in scleroderma (**a**) and dermatomyositis (**b**).

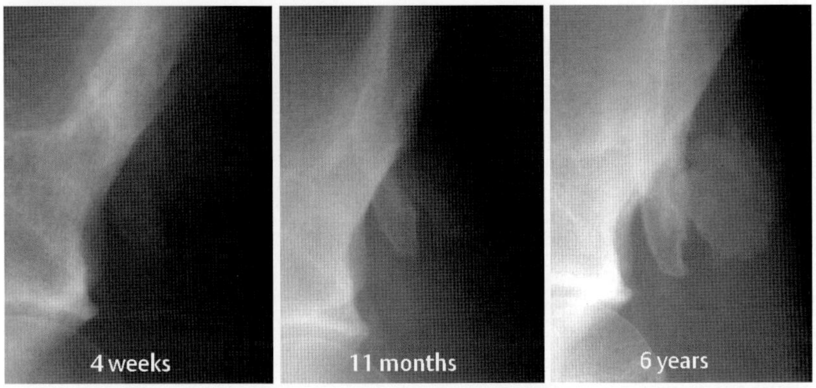

Fig. 8.**21** Myositis ossificans after pelvic injury, pattern of evolution. The ossification can progress long after the trauma, as illustrated in the radiograph obtained 6 years later.

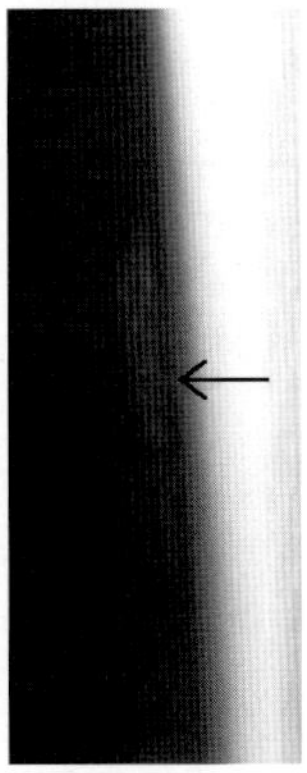

Fig. 8.**22** Discrete finding of myositis ossificans. The ossification is separated by a small stripe from the cortex.

Myositis Ossificans

■ Myositis ossificans is heterotopic, metaplastic formation of bone and cartilage in juxtacortical soft tissues (usually in muscle). ■

PATH The commonest cause is trauma, though often the antecedent trauma is unrecognized. It is formed by undifferentiated mesenchymal cells that produce a matrix of osteoid ground substance that calcifies and ossifies. It is neither an inflammation (as the ending '-itis' might suggest) nor a simple calcification of a hematoma.

CLINIC In the first few weeks, a painful and warm soft-tissue swelling develops. Later the induration increases and the pain becomes less severe.

Location: Myositis ossificans can occur anywhere, but has a predilection for the thigh and elbow.

Therapy: No therapy is required. In fact, the patient should be spared from surgical intervention, especially during the early stages of development, since the condition tends to recur and risks misdiagnosis as a sarcoma.

X-RAY Myositis ossificans and its radiographic features follow an evolutionary process, which can be quite variable.

Early signs: Fluffy, patchy, linear densities adjacent to bone. A fine radiolucent line is generally discernible between the cortex and the lesion (Figs. 8.**22**, 8.**26**).

After 4–6 weeks: The peripheral structures become more radiodense, and the lesion matures centrifugally ('zonal pattern'). A more homogeneous density, however, may also develop. The lesion may then attach to the cortex and no longer be separate from it.

After 4 months: The maturation of the ossification progresses, and the lesion shrinks (Fig. 8.**21**).

! The cortex remains intact or, less frequently, is extrinsically eroded by the process. A lamellar or solid periosteal reaction may also result.

SONO The early stage shows a hypoechoic space-occupying mass. Calcifications may not be sonographically detectable, and the lesion may be indistinguishable from a tumor.

CT CT allows far more effective visualization of the radiographic findings because of the lack of superimposition. The characteristic zonal pattern (dense capsule and less-dense center, Fig. 8.**24**) and the sometimes lamellated composition are much more easily recognized by this technique. Remember that CT, and **not** MRI, is the method of choice for detailed evaluation.

MRI The MRI findings also follow a temporal pattern, as do those of radiography and CT. MRI shows a space-occupying lesion with a progressing decrease in signal intensity (representing calcium) on T1-weighted and T2-weighted TSE images. The lesion shows strong enhancement. The intense edema surrounding this process is characteristic and may by far exceed the size of the lesion (Fig. 8.**25**).

After 6–8 weeks, the lesion becomes increasingly demarcated within the edema. Liquid areas, often with fluid levels, may be seen centrally in some lesions.

DD The differentiation from osteosarcoma and osteochondroma is critical (Fig. 8.**27**).

! Myositis without extensive edema is rare except in the late stage. In this instance, MRI may assist in the distinction between parosteal osteosarcoma, osteochondroma and periosteal chondroma in showing no edema.

Chronic Venous Stasis

The findings in chronic venous stasis can be divided into:

- nodular or undulating periosteal ossification due to periostitis, and
- genuine soft-tissue ossification due to metaplastic new bone formation (Fig. 8.**23**).

In general, the diagnosis is easily made because the disease is known clinically.

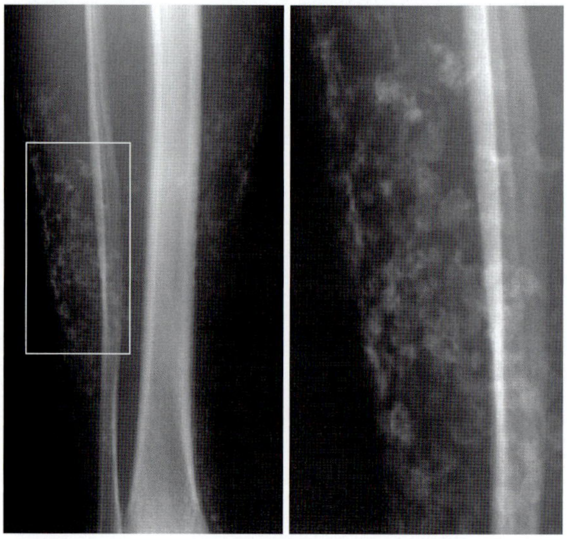

Fig. 8.**23** Soft-tissue ossifications with latticework pattern in chronic venous insufficiency.

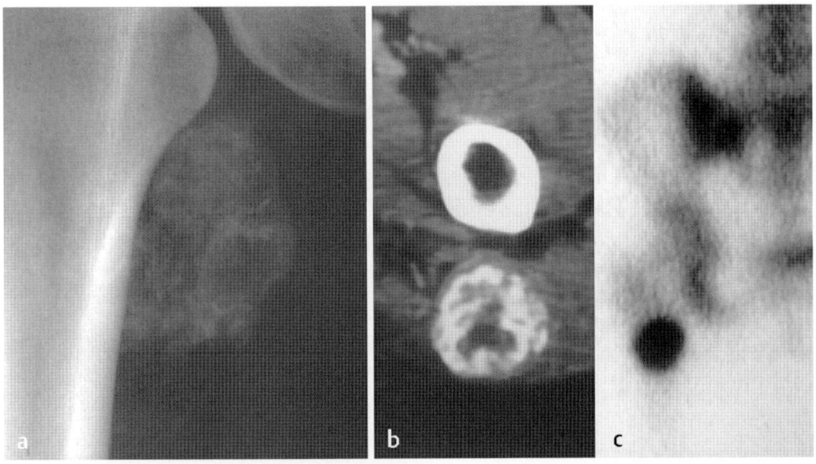

Fig. 8.**24** Myositis ossificans of the proximal femur. Conventional radiography (**a**) suggests a spongiosal pattern. CT (**b**) shows a definite zonal pattern. The lesion also shows intense uptake on the bone scan (**c**).

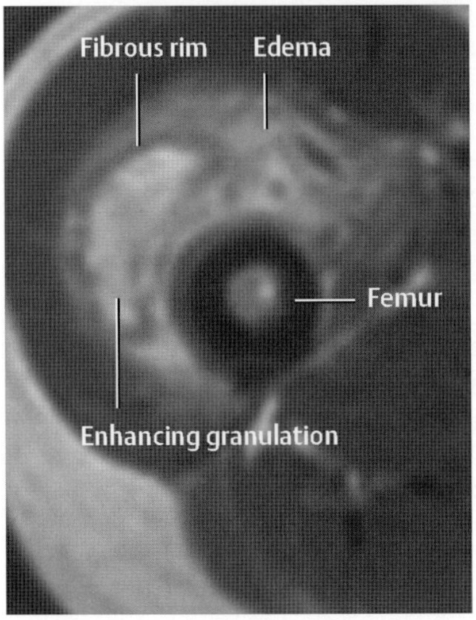

Fig. 8.**25** Extensive enhancement in early myositis ossificans (T1-weighted SE sequence after injection of contrast medium).

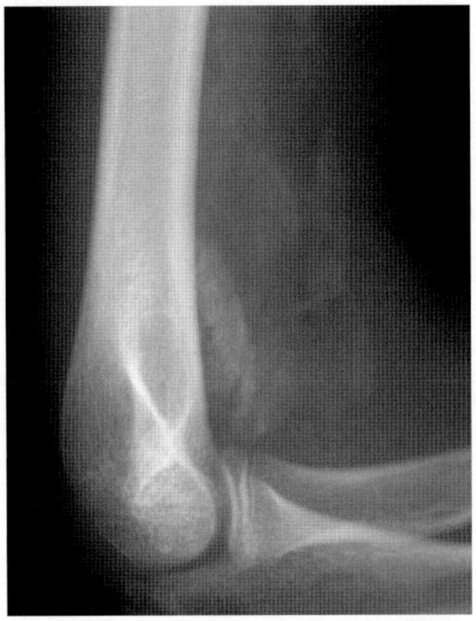

Fig. 8.**26** Typical finding of myositis ossificans in the antecubital fossa. Note that the ossifications are separate from the cortex.

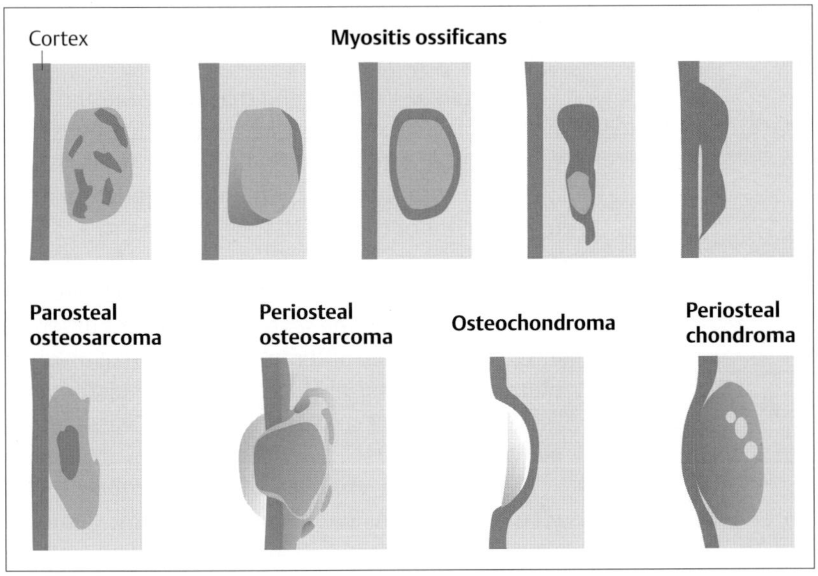

Fig. 8.**27** Radiographic signs of myositis ossificans and its differential diagnoses.

Pustulotic Arthro-osteitis

Synonyms: SAPHO syndrome; spondylarthritis hyperostotica pustula-psoriatica (Schilling), acquired hyperostosis syndrome (Dihlmann, see Glossary).

■ This is found in patients with plantopalmar pustulosis, with additional inflammatory destructive and hyperostotic proliferations of the bones and joints (in about 10% of patients). This osteoarticular involvement is commonest at the sternoclavicular joint (lead or vanguard joint). ■

! Controversy exists as to whether the definition should be more restrictive ('pustulotic arthro-osteitis') or more general ('acquired hyperostosis syndrome', see Glossary). The frequently used term 'SAPHO' (= synovitis, acne, pustulosis, hyperostosis, osteitis) is incorrect, since acne is not part of plantopalmar pustulosis.

PATH The etiology of pustulotic arthro-osteitis is not known. The plantopalmar pustulosis by itself may represent a specific clinical course or a variant of ordinary psoriasis.

Histologically, a subacute or chronic inflammation is detected in the bones, synovial membrane, fibrous joint capsule, and ligamentous and tendinous insertions. The basic reactive changes are:
- Hyperostosis with or without a destructive component,
- Inflammatory enthesopathy,
- Erosive arthropathy, similar to seronegative spondyloarthropathies,
- DISH-like calcifications of the longitudinal ligaments.

CLINIC The condition occurs in adults and has no gender preference.

Symptoms:
- Spontaneous pain and tenderness of the affected joints,
- Local swelling, erythema,
- Painfully restricted movements,
- Skin changes: plantopalmar pustulosis. This is to be differentiated from acne conglobata and fulminans.

Laboratory: Elevated C-reactive protein.

Location:
- Sternoclavicular joints (about 80%),
- Spine, including costovertebral joints,
- Sacroiliac joints,
- Tubular bones, flat bones.

! Skeletal and joint changes can precede the skin changes (as occurs with psoriasis vulgaris).

X-RAY **Sternocostoclavicular joint**
- erosive destruction of the articular cavity,
- irregularity and partial widening of the joint space,
- enlargement and sclerosis of the medial clavicular ends,
- ossification of the costoclavicular ligaments.

Spine, sacroiliac joints
- diffuse vertebral sclerosis
- syndesmophytes and mixed osteophytes, ossification of the longitudinal ligament,
- 'variegated picture' of the sacroiliac joints,
- inflammatory Andersson lesion in the intervertebral space (compare Chapter 9, page 298),
- concomitant erosive arthritis of the costovertebral joints.

Tubular bones, flat bones
- 'mixed' picture of sclerotic and small osteolytic lesions (especially in the scapula),
- massive solid periosteal reactions.

Insertional sites of tendons and ligaments
- bone destructions with erosions,
- later calcifications.

NUC This is the method of choice for known plantopalmar pustulosis associated with 'arthritic complaints'. The diagnosis can be established almost invariably by intense uptake seen in the delayed bone phase of the three-phase bone scan. The sternocostoclavicular joint shows the so-called 'bullhead sign' (Fig. 8.**28**). If intense uptake is also seen in the thoracic and lumbar vertebral bodies, the diagnosis is confirmed by the presence of typical skin changes.

CT The advantages and disadvantages are the same as those of other inflammatory joint disorders (see page 293).

It should be kept in mind that vertebrae and sternocostoclavicular joints can have periosseous and periarticular soft-tissue findings that bear resemblance to accompanying tumorous or inflammatory involvement of the soft tissues.

DD **Infectious arthritis and spondylodiscitis:** The bone scan may indicate a different etiology due to the different distribution of involvement, since bacterial infections are generally confined to one joint and associated skeletal findings are very rare.

Degenerative changes of the sternocostoclavicular joint: Aside from radiographic features (erosive destructive changes versus osteophytic overgrowth), intense uptake on the bone scan suggests pustulotic arthro-osteitis. As a guide, the posterior view of the bone scan displays the uptake in degeneratively altered sternocostoclavicular joints, but clearly shows the hyperostotic uptake as 'shine through.'

Metastases: Radiographically, it may be difficult to differentiate destructive pustulotic arthro-osteitis from metastases. The distribution pattern found in pustulotic arthro-osteitis (sternoclavicular involvement, characteristic bullhead pattern, and involvement of the sacroiliac joints) helps in differentiation.

It should be remembered that pustulotic arthro-osteitis can be accompanied by inflammatory soft-tissue infiltration, making it difficult to segregate it from tumors with conventional radiography and CT.

Diffuse idiopathic skeletal hyperostosis (DISH): Ossifications of the longitudinal ligaments are found in both conditions, but DISH rarely shows decreased height of the disk spaces or ankylosed intervertebral joints. Furthermore, destructive components (erosions, Andersson lesion) do not occur in DISH.

Glossary

Acquired hyperostosis syndrome: The term acquired hyperostosis syndrome coined by Dihlmann restricts the terminology to the basic morphologic finding: hyperostosis. Dihlmann refers to his experience that skin diseases are found in only about two-thirds of the patients with this syndrome. Moreover, he puts stronger emphasis on transitions of this disease to seronegative spondyloarthropathies and also to chronic recurrent multifocal osteomyelitis (see there) in childhood and adolescence.

Acne conglobata, acne fulminans: These are severe dermatologic conditions that cannot be equated with ordinary chronic acne. They can be associated with radiographic features that resemble reactive arthritis: sacroiliitis, spondylitis, erosive enthesopathies, erosive oligoarthritis, and polyarthritis. Furthermore, they can develop hyperostoses, especially at the clavicles. Dihlmann places these radiographic manifestations under the acquired hyperostosis syndrome.

Hyperostosis (osteitis) condensans of the clavicle: This is a stress-induced, noninflammatory, painful hyperostosis of the medial ends of the canicule. Osseous expansion is minimal and the sternoclavicular joint is uninvolved (Fig. 8.**29**).

Tietze syndrome: Etiologically unclear, painful swelling of the sternocostal junctions, primarily of the second to fourth ribs. There are no pathologic radiographic findings. It generally resolves spontaneously.

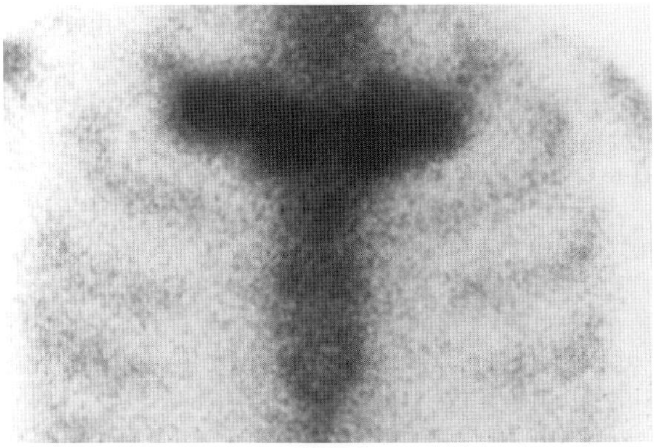

Fig. 8.**28** Scintigraphic 'bullhead sign' of pustulotic arthro-osteitis.

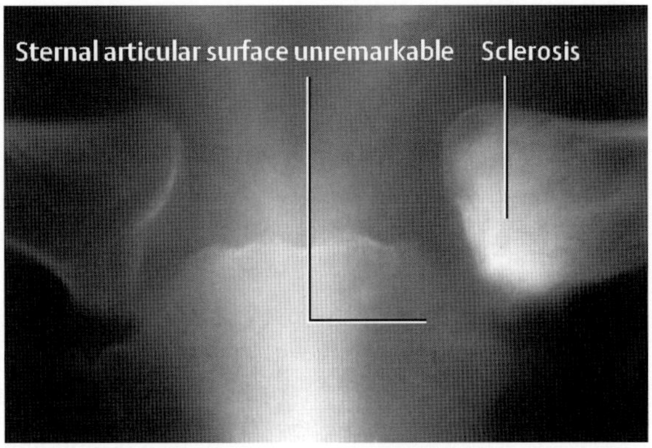

Fig. 8.**29** Hyperostosis (osteitis) condensans of the clavicle. The finding is confined to the medial end of the clavicle. The sternal articular surface is unremarkable.

Congenital Hip Dysplasia

■ Congenital hip dysplasia is a developmental dysplasia of the acetabulum. It causes joint instability that can lead to partial or complete dislocation of the femoral head. ■

PATH With an incidence of 1%, instability of the newborn hip is one of the most common congenital dysplasias, and considerable regional differences and familial clustering are found. Female infants are affected eight times more commonly than male infants, and the dysplasia is bilateral in up to one quarter of the cases.

In congenital hip dysplasia, the acetabulum is too shallow and slanted upward. Subluxation of the femoral head can damage the posterior aspect of the acetabular roof and deform the cartilaginous labrum (Fig. 8.**30**). Complete dislocation with the femoral head out of the acetabular cavity can induce the formation of a false acetabulum, which pushes the cartilaginous acetabular labrum medioinferiorly into the acetabular fossa and stretches the joint capsule. This malposition leads to contractures, especially of the iliopsoas tendon. Moreover, the fibrofatty tissue of the acetabulum becomes hypertrophic (known as 'pulvinar') without the normal pressure provided by the femoral head.

A genetic predisposition and intrauterine factors, such as breech presentation, small uterus (e.g., primipara or oligohydramnios), and increased estrogen levels are considered potential causes. The preferential involvement of the left hip is attributed to breech presentation, in which the fetus tends to lie with the left side against the mother's sacrum.

CLINIC With the hip truly dislocated, the gluteal and inguinal skin folds are asymmetric, and the affected leg is shortened and less active. The **Ortolani** maneuver (reduction of the dislocated hip by abduction of the flexed hip under simultaneous traction) and the **Barlow** maneuver (diagnostic dislocation of the femoral head by adduction of the flexed hip under simultaneous pressure) indicate instability. The clinical signs, however, are often unreliable.

Therapy: If hip dysplasia is diagnosed early, development of a normal and stable hip requires only maintenance of the correct position of the reduced femoral head in the acetabulum for several weeks. Depending on the severity, this can be achieved by triple diapers or by a positioning device (spica cast, abduction splint, or harness). The later the therapy is initiated, the longer it takes and the less satisfactory the results. In children over 6 months of age, a reduction of the hip can often be achieved only with muscle relaxation. Surgical correction is indicated in older children.

Prognosis: If the dysplasia is detected early, normal development of the hip can be expected in about 98% of the affected children. If diagnosed at the age of 3 months, the rate of healing without sequelae declines to about 70%. Healing with residual deformities causes leg shortening with its own consequences, and predisposes to avascular necrosis and early degenerative arthritis.

X-RAY After only 3–6 months, the ossification of the hip has progressed enough to enable reliable detection of hip dysplasia. Consequently, radiographic views are mainly used **after the first year of life**, when sonography no longer adequately demonstrates the acetabulum. The diagnosis rests on measuring the geometry of the hip. Longstanding dislocation or subluxation can produce osseous changes of a false acetabulum at the ilium.

SONO In the newborn and infants, sonography is the method of choice for diagnosing and following hip dysplasia. Its advantages are the visualization of cartilage and the ability to perform a dynamic examination in search of instability. In most cases, the therapeutic abduction can also be monitored sonographically.

The diagnosis and grading according to Graf (relevant for therapeutic decisions) is based on measuring the hip in predefined imaging planes. The auxiliary lines and their diagnostic implications can be found in the literature (Fig. 8.**31**).

When searching for instability, it should be remembered that subtle posterior subluxation is still normal within the first week of life.

Interpretation of sonography requires an experienced examiner, since only slight deviations of the imaging planes (tilting, displacement) yield erroneous measurements that might lead to diagnostic errors.

MRI MRI is indicated if the sonographic findings are inconclusive, in patients with hips resistant to conservative therapy, and preoperative planning with three-dimensional reconstructions. An additional indication is the search for avascular necrosis of the femoral head.

Technique: T1-weighted SE sequences and GE sequences in axial and coronal planes are performed, as they enable adequate differentiation between bone, cartilage, ligaments, and adjacent soft tissues (Fig. 8.**32**).

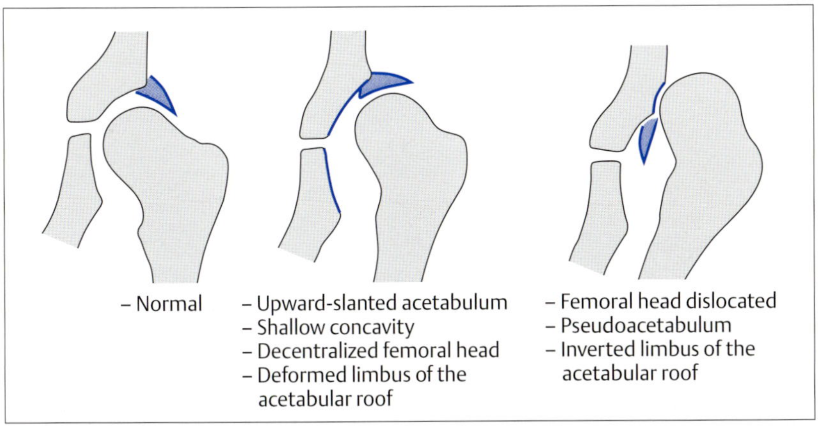

Fig. 8.**30** Different manifestations of hip dysplasia.
a normal finding,
b dysplastic hip,
c dislocation of the femoral head.

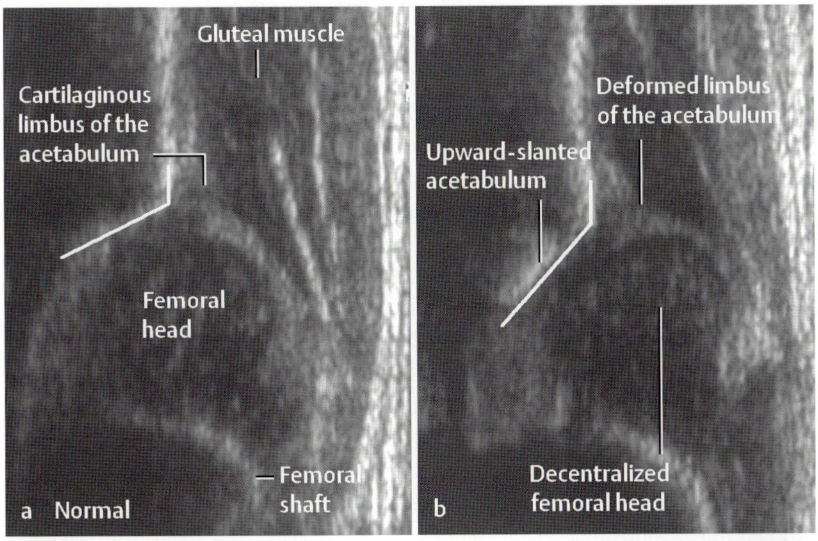

Fig. 8.**31** Comparison of normal neonatal hip (**a**) with a dysplastic hip with slight decentralization (**b**).

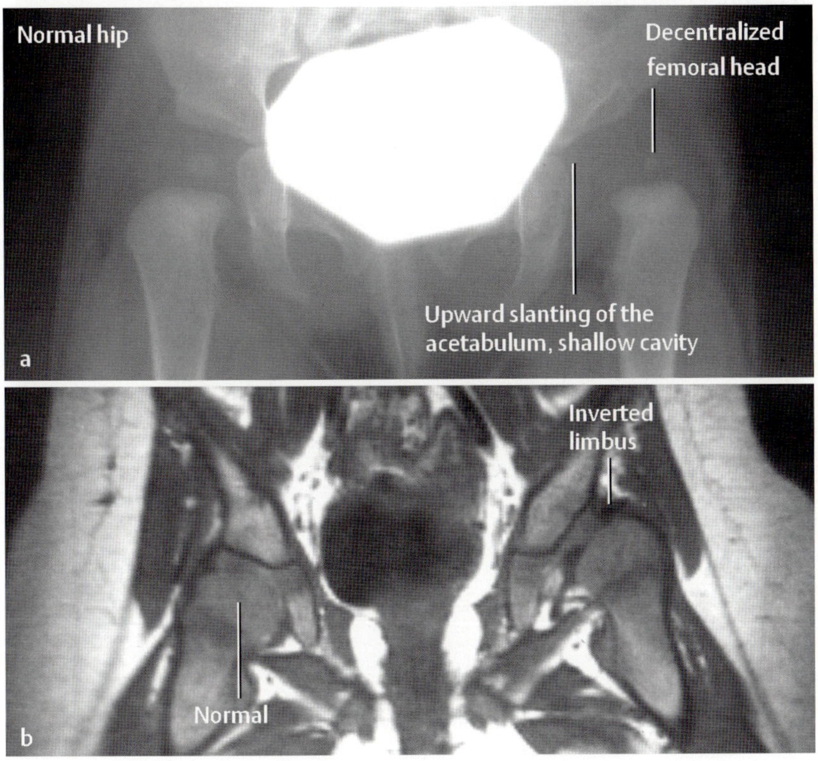

Fig. 8.**32** AP radiograph of the pelvis (**a**) shows the dysplastic configuration of the acetabulum and the decentralization of the femoral head. MRI (**b**) T1-weighted SE sequence) shows the deformity of the cartilaginous acetabular roof, including limbus, covering only 50% of the femoral head.

9 Joints

Introduction and Synopsis

Diseases of the joints comprise a clinically important, heterogeneous group of diseases with numerous overlapping pathologic, radiologic, and, above all, clinical manifestations.

Degenerative and **traumatic** joint lesions are by far the most commonly encountered entities. Articular **inflammations** follow an aggressive course and generally are not infectious. Septic arthritis is relatively uncommon. Neurogenic, metabolic, and hematologic diseases also can lead to joint destruction.

The classifications of joint diseases are not always universally accepted and are the subject of ongoing scientific discussion. Classifications are based on qualitative (presence or absence of radiographic finding) and quantitative (degree of severity) aspects, and are correlated with the pattern of anatomic distribution. The fact that joint diseases affect the soft tissues primarily (above all the synovial lining, articular cartilage, and tendons) and the bones secondarily is common to all joint disorders.

Anatomy of the Synovial Joints

A synovial joint consists of (Fig. 9.**1**):
- epiphysis (articular end of the bone),
- articular cartilage,
- joint capsule,
- joint fluid.

These entities together with muscles, tendons, and ligaments form an anatomic unit.

The epiphyses of the articulating bones: The trabeculae of the epiphyseal and metaphyseal spongiosa commonly follow characteristic courses **(trajectories)** along lines of compression forces.

The cortex of articulating bones gradually decreases in width toward the joint. Where bone is covered by articular cartilage, the cortex is reduced to a very thin osseous layer that appears radiographically as a delicate line, referred to as the **subchondral bone plate.** It can be seen free of any superimposed structures along convex articular surfaces.

Articular cartilage: With few exceptions, this consists of hyaline cartilage, which is nourished by diffusion from the joint fluid. In the calcified zone of the cartilage, small vessels arising from the subchondral bone region have been detected as well. Healthy cartilage is strikingly **elastic** and serves the role of shock absorber. With normal use, a liquid film always remains between the articulating cartilage surfaces.

Joint capsule: By enveloping the joint, the capsule creates an intra-articular and extra-articular space. It inserts at the epiphysis of the articulating bone slightly outside the cartilage cover, creating an intra-articular area not covered by cartilage, referred to as the **bare area.**

The joint capsule consists of an outer, predominately collagenous connective tissue, the **fibrous**

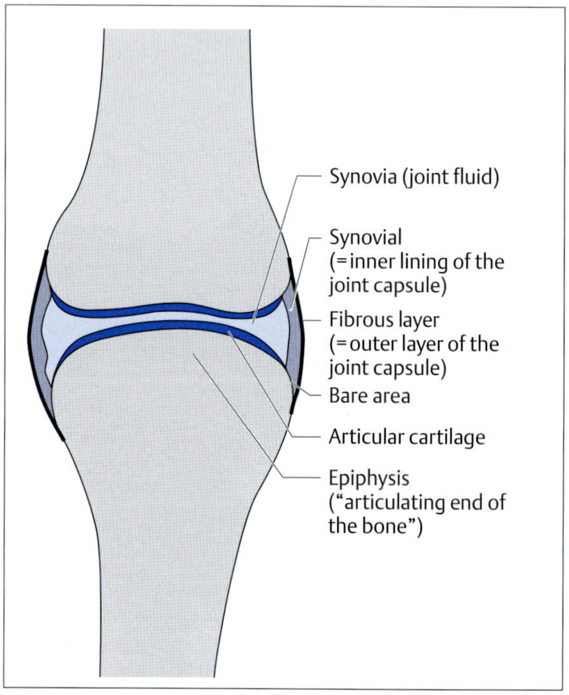

Fig. 9.**1** Anatomy of the synovial joint.

capsule, and an inner **synovial lining,** also referred to as the synovial membrane. The synovial lining also covers all of the intra-articular osseous structures except the articular cartilage. It secretes synovial fluid, determines the fluid's components, and phagocytizes any foreign material, such as organisms or cartilage fragments.

Synovial fluid: The synovial fluid is the 'grease' of the joint and supplies nutrients to the articular cartilage by diffusion.

Signs of Joint Diseases on Radiography and CT

Technical considerations and indications:
Conventional radiography still plays a central role in diagnosing and monitoring joint disorders and in planning therapy. The routine examination consists of at least two views obtained in different projections, frequently with comparison views of the contralateral side. **Digital radiography** has the advantage over conventional film-screen systems of displaying the findings of interest at a brightness that is optimal for interpretation.

> **!** For the interpretation of radiographs, a bright spotlight with circular collimation (to bring out the soft tissues) and a magnifying glass (to analyze delicate osseous structures) should always be available.

Magnification radiography is reserved for special situations and has been largely replaced by sonography and MRI.

Fluoroscopy with spot film is helpful only in selected cases, e.g., visualizing radiolucent halos around implants or displaying soft-tissue calcifications free from superimposed structures.

Conventional tomography has largely been replaced by computed tomography and is performed only to address specific questions, e.g., in the region of the occipitocervical and cervicothoracic transition.

Computed tomography is indicated for evaluating the sacroiliac, sternoclavicular, and temporomandibular joints and the atlanto-occipital transition, and for assessing specific problems related to degenerative changes of the spine. A special application is the combination of CT with myelography ('CT myelography') to achieve a detailed analysis of the nerve roots.

Image analysis should concentrate on four primary features of the joint's anatomic structure:

1. **Alignment of the joint**
   - varus or valgus position; antecurvature or retrocurvature,
   - in the axial skeleton: scoliosis; antetorsion, and retrotorsion.
2. **Soft-tissue density**
   - metallic density: foreign body,
   - calcific density: degenerative, post-traumatic or metabolic calcification
   - fluid equivalent: edema, effusion. Often recognized only by displaced periarticular fat planes,
   - fat equivalent: lipoma,
   - air equivalent: degenerative (intra-articular gas, so-called 'vacuum phenomenon'), or infectious.
3. **Joint space**
   - widening
   - narrowing: generalized or localized
4. **Articular end of the bone (joint socket)**
   Destructive bone changes:
   - juxta-articular demineralization (osteoporosis),
   - loss of the subchondral bone plate,
   - erosions (central, peripheral, juxta-articular),
   - osseous resorptions at the tendon and ligament insertions, osteolysis,
   - joint destruction.

   Proliferative bone changes:
   - subchondral sclerosis,
   - protuberances, osteophytes, and syndesmophytes,
   - calcifications or ossifications at tendon and ligament insertions,
   - calcifications of ligaments (at the spine),
   - ankylosis.

For the large joints, computed tomography can delineate the radiographic features without superimposition of other structures.

Arthrography, performed alone or combined with CT or MRI, is primarily used for the evaluation of the shoulder, wrist, and hip. The indications today center on post-traumatic and degenerative changes.

Radiographic Signs of the Peripheral Joints and Their Role in the Differential Diagnosis

The fundamental radiographic signs are described here to avoid repetition in subsequent chapters. The differential diagnostic implications are merely summarized.

Soft-tissue Swelling (Fig. 9.**2**)

Soft-tissue swelling is recognized by an altered silhouette and by displaced or obliterated fat planes.

- The characteristic sign of **active arthritis** is the voluminous **fusiform** soft-tissue swelling, often with a bulged and indistinctly outlined joint capsule. Under favorable circumstances, it might become visible only several days after the onset of the arthritis and is then the only radiographic 'early sign' (only in the hands).
- In osteoarthritis, soft-tissue swelling is less voluminous and becomes rather nodular at the fingers. If it is accompanied by an inflammatory component (active osteoarthritis), an 'arthritic' soft-tissue swelling develops.
- In periarticular **soft-tissue inflammation** (bursitis, tenosynovitis, infection), soft-tissue swelling is asymmetric but can still be uniform at the fingers and toes (Fig. 9.**2 b**).

Juxta-articular Osteoporosis (Fig. 9.**3**)

This indicates juxta-articular bone loss. It appears as heterogeneous to patchy demineralization, indistinct spongiosa texture, and decreased number of trabeculae. These findings have a gradual transition to the variably wide homogeneous band of demineralization involving the opposing articulating end of the bone.

- As part of an **arthritis,** it is referred to as the 'collateral phenomenon'. The arthritis induces bone resorption by means of neurocirculatory reflexes, increased perfusion, and activated osteoclasts. This process, which is not visible until weeks after the onset of the inflammation, indicates direct bone destruction.
- This is an unusual finding in **osteoarthritis.**
- **Disuse osteoporosis** is not confined to the juxta-articular areas. Since longstanding arthritis leads to pain-induced immobilization of the joints, these types of osteoporosis frequently overlap.
- The osteoporosis of **sympathetic reflex dystrophies** (in particular with Sudeck disease) is, like the soft-tissue swelling in these conditions, a diffuse phenomenon and not confined to the joints. Elevated inflammatory serum parameters are not associated with these diseases.
- **Bone marrow edema syndrome** involves only **one** of the bones on each side of the joint (most commonly the femoral head) and is confined to one joint. The diagnosis can be established by MRI and scintigraphy.

Loss of the Subchondral Bone Plate (Fig. 9.**4**)

Loss of the subchondral bone plate precedes erosions ('pre-erosion' according to Dihlmann). The cause can be either a trophic demineralization (from hyperemia) or a direct effect of pus or pannus ('direct sign').

- Absence of a subchondral bone plate is a specific sign of **arthritis.** In particular, this applies whenever the mineral content of the bones is well preserved in the remaining skeletal regions. Partial loss of the joint silhouette is more indicative of arthritis than complete loss, as the latter can also represent a normal variant.
- This is observed in **osteoarthritis** only with extensive destruction.
- **Systemic demineralization** (e.g., hyperparathyroidism, rickets, osteomalacia) is associated with destruction of the subchondral bone plate.
- Cell death of **osteonecrosis** close to the joint causes fractures of the subchondral bone plate.
- **Bone marrow edema syndrome** ('transient osteoporosis') causes loss of the subchondral bone plate as in arthritis, but the finding is generally monoarticular, and the joint space is not narrowed.

Erosion (Figs. 9.**5**, 9.**6**)

An **erosion** is a confined osseous defect involving the articulating end of the bone ('joint socket'). Seen in profile, it is a defect, and seen end on, it appears as a 'cyst.' Depending on the activity of the disease process, the erosion can have an indistinct, distinct, or even sclerotic border.

- In **arthritis,** the erosions begin at the 'bare areas' and, consequently, are located in the region of the capsular insertions. If a tenosynovitis is present, superficial defects relatively distant from the joint can appear in the region of the inflammatory tendon sheath. Some locations are a relatively specific indication of a synovial origin of the disease.
- In **osteoarthritis,** the erosions occur primarily centrally as pressure erosions. (The abnormal pressure load due to articular destruction can induce osseous resorption.)
- **Gouty** erosions are often located away from the joint (they are not 'erosions' in the true sense of the definition) and can be quite large.

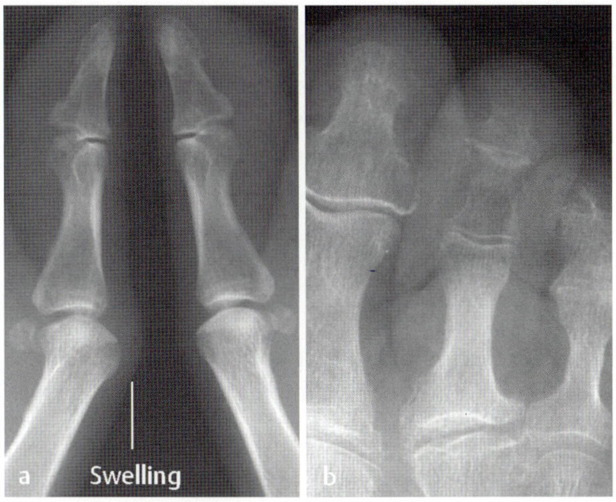

Fig. 9.**2** **a** Arthritis of the metacarpophalangeal joint with localized fusiform soft-tissue swelling. **b** Soft-tissue infection, however, shows diffuse soft-tissue swelling. Notice the demineralization of the phalanges.

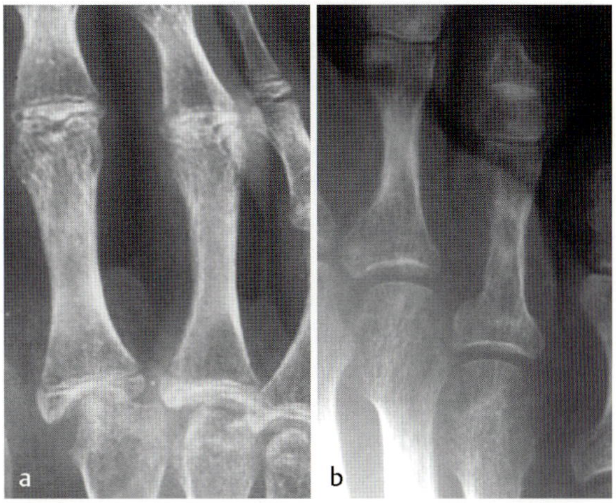

Fig. 9.**3** **a** Juxta-articular osteoporosis in rheumatoid arthritis. For comparison: the osteoporosis in Sudeck disease (**b**) involves all bones.

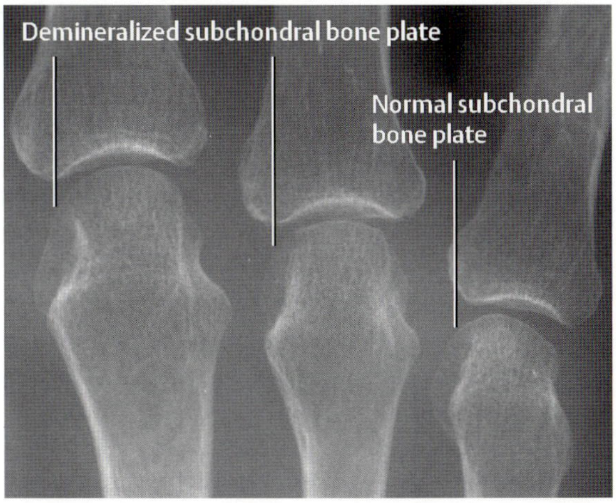

Fig. 9.**4** Loss of subchondral bone plate in rheumatoid arthritis.

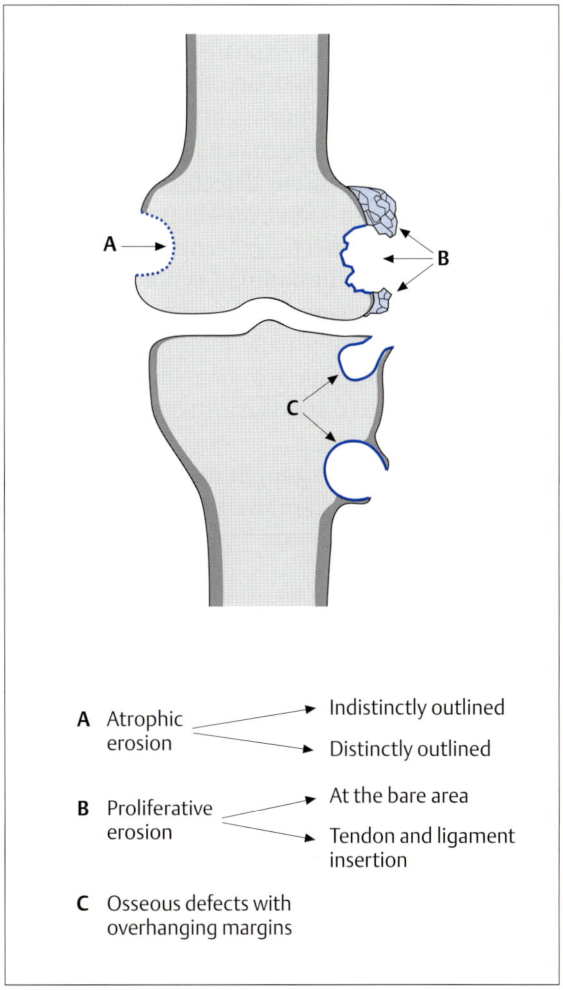

Fig. 9.**6** Erosion and its differential diagnosis.

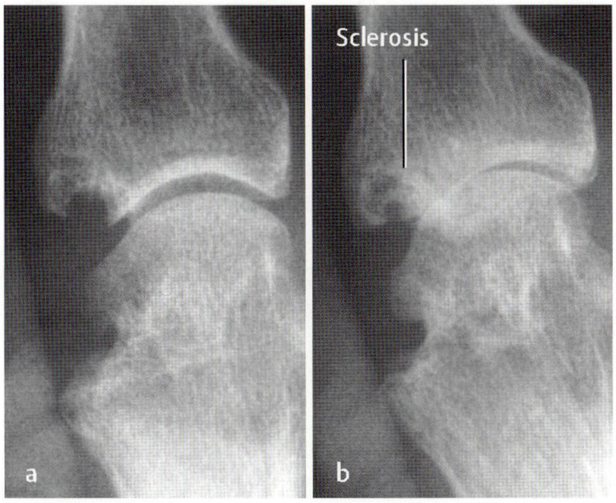

Fig. 9.**5** **a** Acute erosion from rheumatoid disease. **b** Same erosion with marginal sclerosis formed after methotrexate therapy and, as a result, less distinctly demarcated.

- **Destruction caused by an adjacent tumor** presents as a solitary, broad erosion without any additional joint changes.

Circumscribed Osteolytic Foci ('Subchondral Cysts,' 'Geodes') (Fig. 9.7)

These are round, partially confluent defects in the articular ends of the bone. In arthritic conditions, they are also referred to as 'signal cysts'.

- In **rheumatoid arthritis,** they are rarely larger than 1 cm. Marginal sclerosis develops only after therapy. To consider a subchondral cyst as a direct sign of arthritis, the finding must be seen in context with other direct signs.
- Subchondral cysts in **osteoarthritis** ('detritic cyst') usually are multiple, are located in the load-bearing zone, can be larger than 1 cm, and always have marginal sclerosis.
- Sharply demarcated subchondral osteolytic defects are found in **metabolic** diseases such as amyloidosis or pyrophosphate arthropathy. A fusiform soft-tissue swelling is frequently present. The joint space, however, is of normal width. Intraosseous **gouty** tophi may have a variety of appearances. Punched-out defects can occur alone or together with ovoid osteolytic lesions, and they can be septated or trabeculated.
- In **pigmented villonodular synovitis (PVNS),** the osteolytic changes arise from the articular margins. They are usually multiple and almost always have sclerotic margins. Joint-space narrowing and juxta-articular osteoporosis are absent (see page 376).
- In the **intraosseous ganglion,** the connection to the joint space is not always visible (see page 374).

Joint-space Narrowing (Fig. 9.8)

This indicates cartilage destruction.

- In **arthritis,** the narrowing is uniform and involves the entire joint space or large portions of it.
- In **osteoarthritis,** the joint-space narrowing is characteristically confined to a segment of the joint, most severely affecting the weight-bearing zones. This is an early sign of osteoarthritis.
- Joint-space narrowing also occurs in **chondrocalcinosis.** Additional chondral calcifications assist in the differential diagnosis.

Subchondral Sclerosis (Fig. 9.9)

This is a reactive osteosclerosis formed by a coarse, often disorganized framework of lamellar bone.

- It is unusual in **arthritis** and, if present, is usually observed after reparative intervals in chronic arthritic inflammation.
- Subchondral sclerosis is a characteristic sign of **osteoarthritis.**

Lamellar Periosteal Reaction (Fig. 9.10)

Single or multiple metadiaphyseal lamellar reactions are often present and often occur in the vicinity of the affected joints.

- It is observed close to the joint in some types of **arthritis** (particularly in seronegative spondylarthritis and juvenile rheumatoid arthritis), probably as a result of a periosteal edema.
- Other differential diagnoses are osteoarthritis, tumors, hematologic conditions, chronic venous insufficiency, and post-traumatic conditions.

Reactive Bone Apposition (Fig. 9.11)

Reactive bone apposition occurs as osteophytes and protuberances. The shape and distribution of these are often clues to differential diagnostic considerations.

- Some types of **arthritis** tend to have a rather pronounced osseous proliferation (e.g., psoriatic arthritis), which must be distinguished from marginal sclerotic transformation of erosions after arrest of the disease process.
- Even in early stages of **osteoarthritis,** osteophytic apposition takes place. This characteristically occurs at the bone–cartilage interface of the weight-bearing parts of the joint.

Mutilation and Ankylosis (Fig. 9.12)

Joint destruction can progress to mutilation and end in ankylosis with fibrous or osseous bridging.

- Some types of arthritis tend to have early mutilation (e.g., psoriatic arthritis). More often, mutilation and ankylosis occur in the later stages of the diseases.
- In **osteoarthritis,** except for the Charcôt joint, they are observed only after longstanding disease.

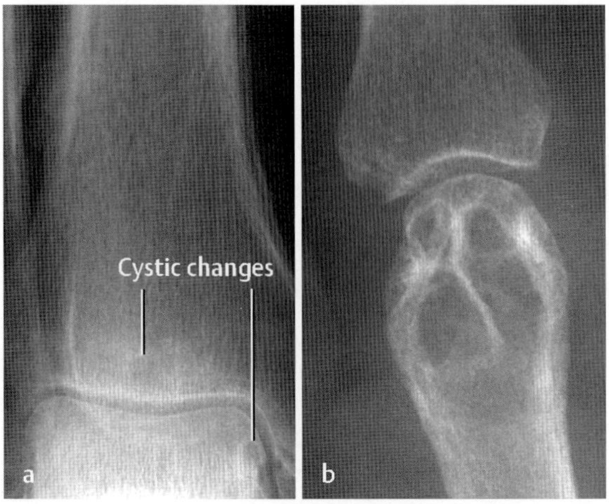

Fig. 9.7 Subchondral cysts of different sizes. These represent 'signal cysts' in both cases: **a** Psoriatic arthritis, **b** 'geode-type' rheumatoid arthritis.

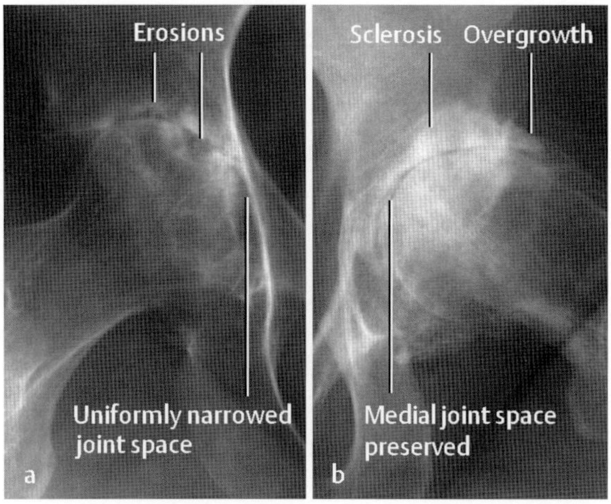

Fig. 9.8 Concentric (**a**) and eccentric (**b**) joint-space narrowing in longstanding juvenile rheumatoid arthritis (**a**) and osteoarthritis (**b**).

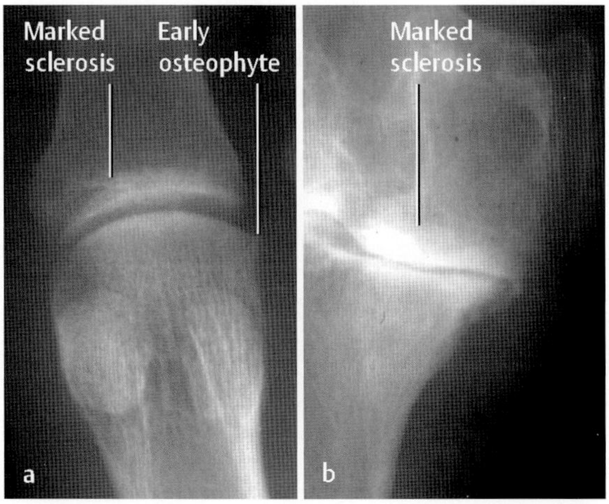

Fig. 9.9 Subchondral sclerosis indicates degenerative joint disease. **a** Preserved joint space, very subtle osteophyte formation. **b** Marked osteoarthritis of the knee.

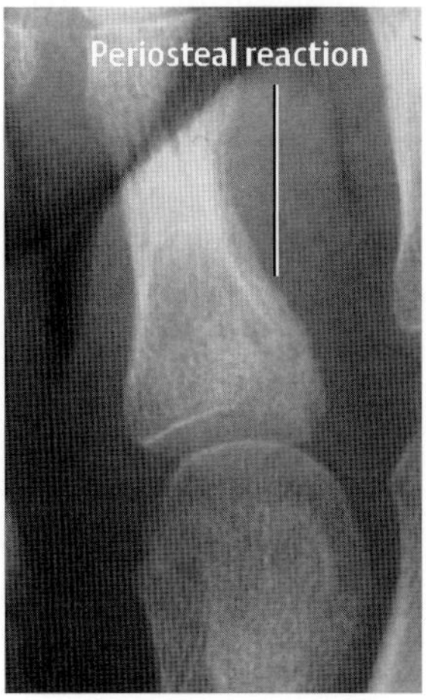

Fig. 9.10 Widening of the phalanges due to periosteal reaction in psoriatic arthritis.

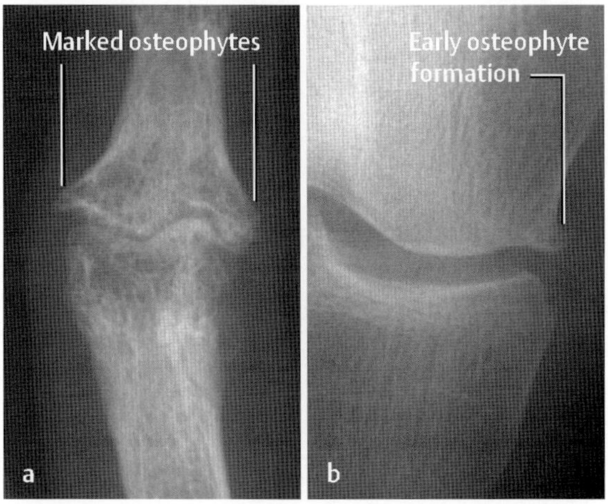

Fig. 9.11 Osteophytic overgrowth of different degrees at an interphalangeal joint (**a**) and knee (**b**).

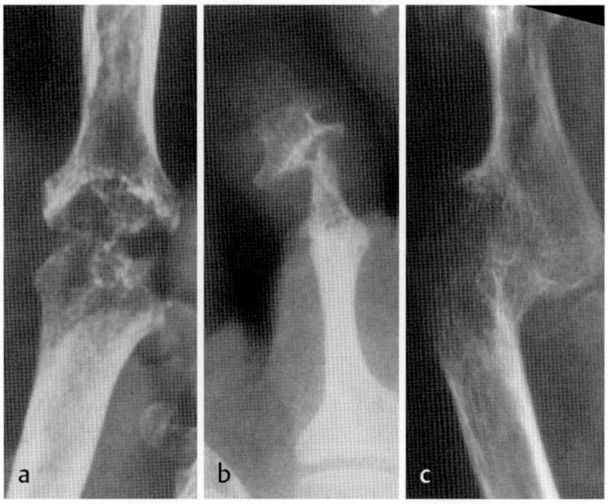

Fig. 9.12 **a, b** Mutilation. Typical 'pencil-in-cup' type in (**b**). **c** Osseous ankylosis of a proximal interphalangeal joint.

Radiographic Signs at Specific Joints

Spine

Anterior spondylitis (Romanus lesion): This represents the focal destruction of the anterior or posterior borders of the vertebral body and is similar to an erosion. The Romanus lesion is an early manifestation of an inflammation affecting the spine (Fig. 9.**14**). This defect is almost always surrounded by a broad sclerosis, producing a rather typical triangular sclerosis referred to as **shiny corner** sign (Fig. 9.**13**). It can occur with or without associated focal destruction.

Squared and rounded vertebra: Inflammatory destruction of the anterior surface of the vertebral body (anterior spondylitis) does not produce the classic Romanus lesion, but instead leads to loss of the anterior vertebral border. This results in squaring of the vertebral body due to flattening of its normally concave anterior **surface** (more often seen in the lateral than in the AP projection). Postinflammatory squaring can also develop differently; periosteal reaction with or without anterior spondylitis can fill the anterior concavity. Progression of anterior spondylitis causes destruction of the superior and inferior vertebral corner, resulting in a rounded vertebra (Fig. 9.**15**).

Andersson lesion, type A (inflammatory type): This is an inflammatory reaction with focal destruction of the disk and vertebral body. It is characterized by irregularities along the end plates, usually accompanied by extensive sclerotic zones. Differentiation from mechanically induced osteochondrosis (predilection for L4 – S1) is sometimes difficult.

Andersson lesion, type B (noninflammatory, pseudodegenerative type): This is a pseudarthrosis following a diskovertebral fracture of the demineralized and extensively ossified, stiff axial skeleton (as occurs in ankylosing spondylitis, Fig. 9.**119**).

Syndesmophytes: These are ossifications of the outer fibers of the anulus fibrosus, caused by a progressive **inflammatory process.** Initially, they are thin, vertical outgrowths along the contour of the disk. With progression, the syndesmophytes thicken and involve the anterior longitudinal ligament and paravertebral soft tissues. The end result is the 'bamboo spine'.

Spondylophytes: These are ossifications of the vertebral margins caused by disk **degeneration,** but might be secondary to an inflammation. The submarginal spondylophyte arises at the insertion of the anterior longitudinal ligament, several millimeters from the diskovertebral junction. Initially, it grows horizontally and then vertically (forming a hook). The marginal osteophyte merges horizontally with the end plate.

In addition to these major types – syndesmophyte secondary to an inflammatory process and spondylophyte secondary to degenerative alterations – numerous intermediate types are encountered.

Parasyndesmophytes are asymmetric ossifications that are thicker than syndesmophytes and not vertically oriented but are curved or comma-shaped and separated ('para-') from the margin of the vertebral body. They occur in three types: steer-horn type; paradiskal elongated, thin type; and paradiskal ossicle.

The term **mixed osteophyte** is applied by some authorities to an osteophyte constituting a mixture of syndesmophyte and spondylophyte.

Any interpretation of these special types is difficult, and in assigning an etiology one should always consider further radiographic findings (Fig. 9.**17**).

Block vertebra: This can be a developmental abnormality or the result of a preceding inflammatory process.

Sacro-iliac (SI) Joints

! Only the anteroinferior aspect of the SI joint is a synovial articulation. The posterior and superior portion (the fibrous retro-articular space) of the 'joint' is connected by ligaments and lacks articular cartilage.

Sacroiliitis is the hallmark of the seronegative and HLA-B27-positive spondyloarthropathies. Unilateral sacroiliitis can also occur on the basis of a bacterial infection. Seronegative spondyloarthropathies constitute a heterogeneous entity of clinically defined subcategories:
- ankylosing spondylitis,
- psoriatic arthropathies,
- reactive arthritis,
- enteropathic arthritis,
- undifferentiated spondyloarthropathy.

Radiographic signs of sacroiliitis (**'variegated picture' of Dihlmann,** Fig. 9.**16**):
- thinning of the subchondral bone plate,
- erosions (more severe on the iliac side than on the sacral side),
- joint-space widening (irregular),
- densification,
- osseous bridging, later osseous ankylosis,
- capsular and ligamentous calcifications.

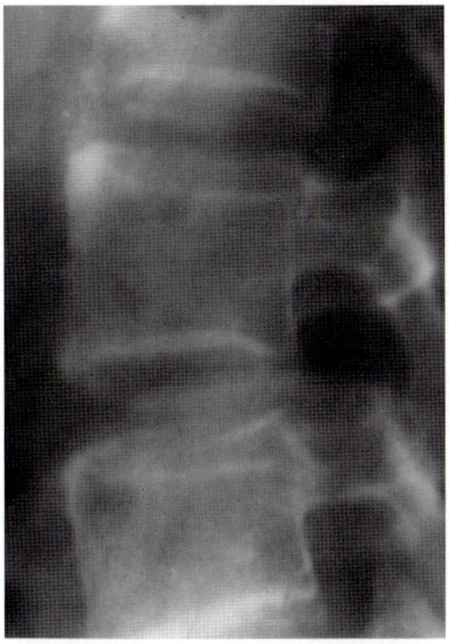

Fig. 9.**13** 'Shiny corner' in anterior spondylitis.

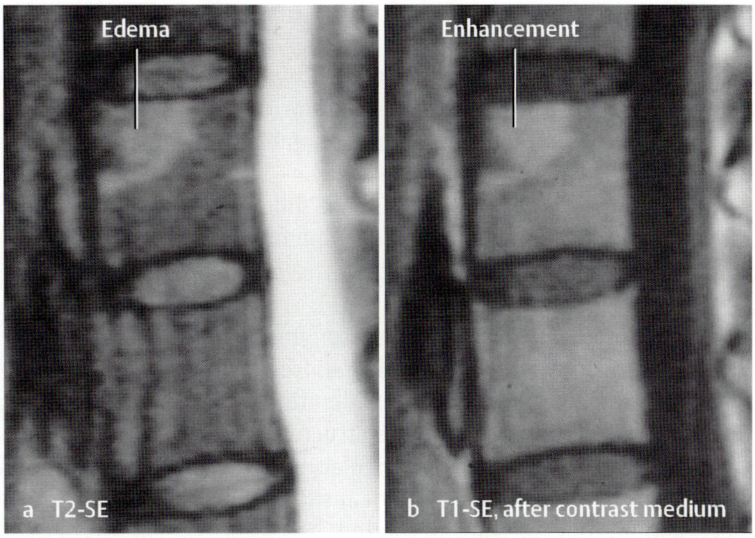

Fig. 9.**14** MRI of a Romanus lesion. **a** The T2-weighted SE sequence shows triangular edema at the anterior-superior corner of a vertebral body. Strong enhancement after the administration of contrast medium. **b** T1-weighted SE sequence.

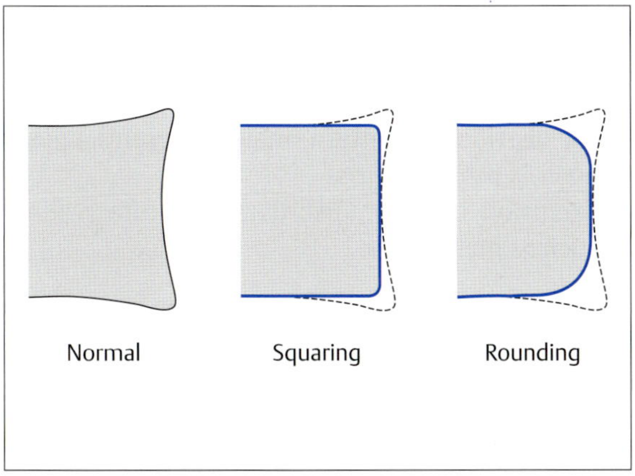

Fig. 9.**15** Squaring and rounding of the vertebral body due to anterior spondylitis.

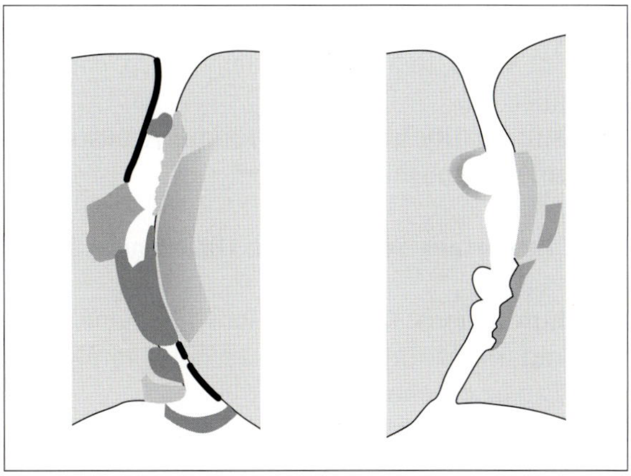

Fig. 9.**16** 'Variegated picture' of sacroiliitis.

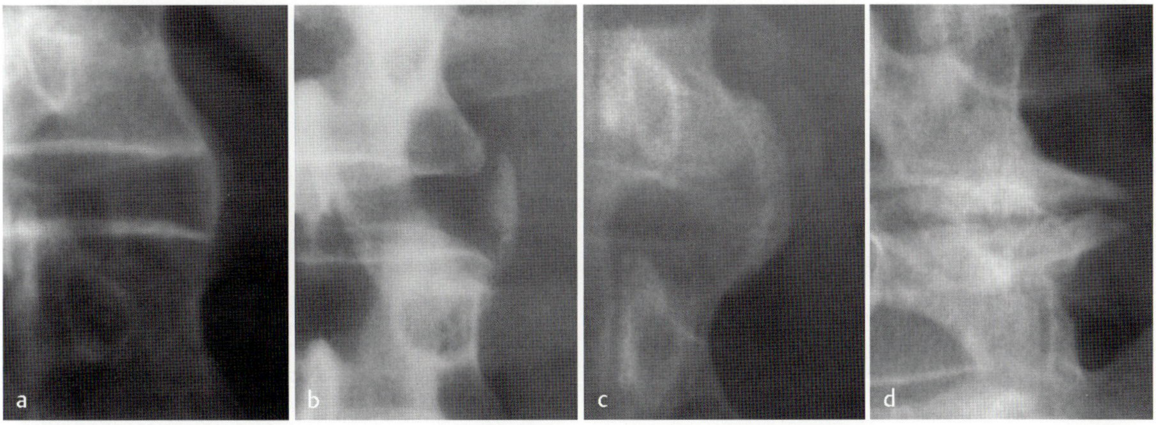

Fig. 9.**17** Comparison of the different ossifications between vertebral bodies. **a** Syndesmophyte, thin ossification, vertical growth. **b** Parasyndesmophyte, separated from the margin of the vertebral body. **c** Parasyndesmophyte of the 'Steer-horn type.' **d** Degenerative spondylophytes.

Sonography

Visualization of the joint requires probes with frequencies of 7 to 13 MHz. For examination of the strongly reflective structures of the neonatal hip, a frequency of 5 MHz is adequate.

The examination of each joint should follow an established protocol, which may be supplemented by additional sections, depending on the clinical question.

When tendons and muscles are examined, the acoustic anisotropy of the muscular and collagenous fibers must be taken into consideration. Due to the internal orientation of these structures, the echogenicity changes with the angulation of the probe. Differences in echogenicity caused by this effect should not be misinterpreted as lesions (Fig. 9.**18**).

Any report of sonographic findings should include the following aspects:

Location: Anatomic location and contact with neighboring structures.

Echogenicity: Anechoic, hypoechoic, hyperechoic.

Margin: Sharp, indistinct, partially sharp, partially indistinct.

Acoustic quality behind the lesion: Acoustic enhancement, acoustic shadowing.

Most Important Sonographic Differential Diagnoses:

Anechoic lesions: Cysts, ganglions, effusions.

Caution: Hematomas, abscesses, and, rarely, tumors can be anechoic.

Hypoechoic lesions: Hematomas, abscesses, granulation tissue, many lipomas (characteristic 'pennate' structures), many benign and almost all malignant tumors, many tendon tears. Some effusions or cysts can also contain echogenic fluid.

Echogenic lesions: Lipomas, tendon ruptures (reflecting interfaces), calcifications or ossifications (typical acoustic shadowing), defects at the bone surface (e.g., erosions, Hill-Sachs deformity).

! Hypoechoic lesions are nonspecific, and the differential diagnosis generally is determined by the clinical presentation and the findings of other imaging methods. Especially in synovial arthritis, the differentiation between hypoechoic effusion and pannus is very difficult or even impossible.

What Questions Can Be Answered by Sonography of Joints and Juxta-Articular Structures?

- Differentiation between intra-articular effusion and periarticular soft-tissue edema,
- Differentiation between effusion and tumor,
- Detection of a synovial cyst,
- Diagnosis of a tendon tear,
- Diagnosis of a tenosynovitis,
- Detection of osseous involvements (erosion) in arthritis,
- Detection of bursal involvement in arthritis.

Scintigraphy

The three-phase bone scan with Tc 99 m diphosphonate is performed with anterior and lateral views. The strength of bone scanning is that it provides an overview of disease manifestations in the skeleton, yielding information critical for the differential diagnosis. The most important indications are:

- In suspected rheumatoid arthritis patients who do not fulfill the American Rheumatology Association (ARA) criteria for rheumatoid disease and who have negative radiographic findings, to search for inflammatory foci and to determine the distribution pattern (major differential diagnosis is osteoarthritis),
- Exclusion of other disorders that affect bone, such as metastases.

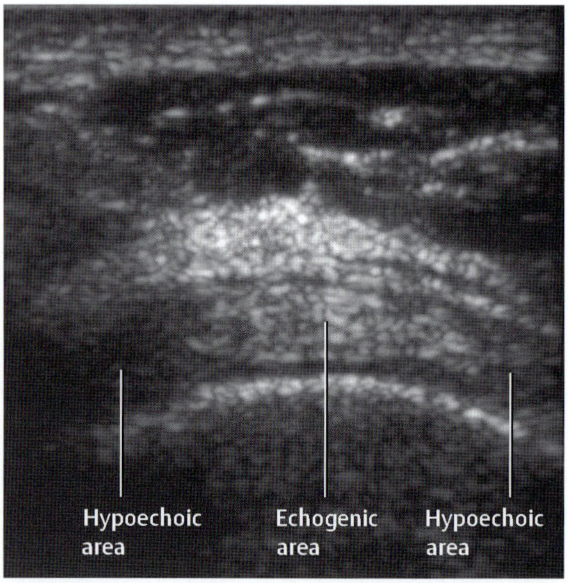

Fig. 9.**18** Because of acoustic anisotropy of fibers, the echogenicity of lamellated structures (here: normal rotator cuff) depends on the angle of the interrogating sound beam. This effect must be distinguished from pathologic differences in echogenicity.

MRI

Exquisite visualization of soft tissues and bone marrow has made MRI an examination of enormous value.

Examination technique:
To achieve good resolution, the use of suitable **superficial coils** is mandatory.

Examination protocols:
- T1-weighted and T2-weighted (fast) spin-echo sequences ('SE' or 'FSE'), possibly supplemented with 2-D or 3-D gradient echo sequences ('GRE') for visualization of the cartilage.
- Fat-suppression sequences: STIR ('short time inversion recovery') for the very sensitive visualization of edema and fluid of any origin, as well as T1-weighted SE sequences with frequency-selective fat suppression following administration of contrast medium.
- Contrast medium (gadolinium DTPA) can be administered **intravenously** to evaluate the extracellular distribution for tissue perfusion (as found in osteonecrosis or inflammation) or **intra-articularly** as MR arthrography to visualize the cartilage contour directly. Since intravenously administered contrast medium diffuses into the joint space, it also provides an arthrographic effect that can be used for visualizing the internal structures of the joint **(indirect arthrography).**

Image Analysis

Soft-tissue contrast is determined by the selected pulse sequences and is characteristic for each individual structure and for the joint content (Fig. 9.**19**).

Signal patterns of pathologic processes:
- lesions in the bone and bone marrow due to inflammation, tumor, or trauma: the signal intensity is decreased on T1-weighted images and increased on T2-weighted images,
- ossifications and calcifications: the signal intensity is decreased on T1-weighted and T2-weighted images,
- degeneration and tears involving tendons, ligaments, and fibrocartilage: the signal intensity is increased on T1-weighted and T2-weighted images,
- edema: the signal intensity is decreased on T1-weighted images and increased on T2-weighted images,
- tumor, synovitis, pannus, traumatic lesions after administration of contrast medium: enhancement with increased signal intensity on the T2-weighted images,
- tumors and inflammation enhance. Degenerative changes show no or only faint enhancement.

Which Questions Can MRI of the Joints and Adjacent Structures Answer?

- noninvasive diagnosis of cartilage/fibrocartilage defects (menisci),
- numerous questions after trauma,
- diagnosis of tendon ruptures, tenosynovitis, and synovial cysts,
- early diagnosis of subchondral osteonecrosis and insufficiency fractures,
- early diagnosis of synovitis/pannus,
- early detection of osseous involvement in arthritis,
- differentiation between intra-articular effusion and periarticular soft-tissue edema and synovitis/pannus,
- differentiation between septic arthritis and osteomyelitis,
- exact topographic display of the lesion (e.g., concomitant involvement of the joint or bursa in rheumatoid arthritis),
- diagnosis of joint tumor or articular involvement of bone tumors,
- diagnosis of compression of the spinal cord in rheumatoid arthritis of the upper cervical spine,
- early diagnosis of sacroiliitis.

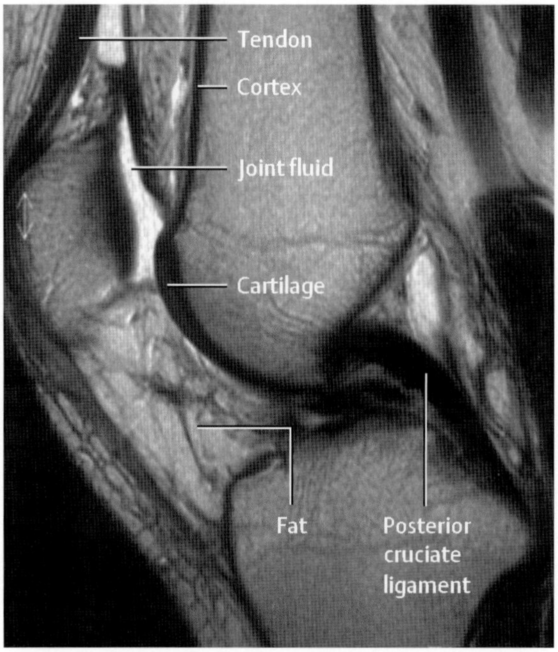

Fig. 9.**19** MRI of the knee. Normal sagittal plane of a T2-weighted TSE sequence.

Arthritis versus Osteoarthritis (Overview)

■ **Osteoarthritis** is a destructive joint disease, primarily caused by damaged cartilage – regardless of the nature of the cartilage damage. **Arthritis** is a destructive joint disease primarily caused by **synovitis** – regardless of the nature of the synovitis. ■

These basically different diseases are in reality inseparably intermingled, since damage of the cartilage plays the crucial role in both diseases.

'Primary' osteoarthritis invariably induces an inflammatory reaction of the synovitis due to faulty articulation and cartilaginous debris in the joint (secondary arthritis).

Likewise, the cartilage damage of 'primary' arthritis causes a secondary osteoarthritis.

These mechanisms explain why radiographically visualized joint changes represent a summation effect of the outcome of both disease processes. Conclusion: differentiating the signs of degenerative joint disease from those of arthritis is often difficult and sometimes impossible. However, the critical clinical relevance (i.e., totally different therapeutic approaches) demands that a differentiation should always be attempted, whether a disease is caused and maintained primarily by synovitis or by damaged cartilage.

Pathogenesis of Osteoarthritis and Its Radiographic Features

The cause of **osteoarthritis** is defective cartilage, with the cartilage in part damaged by mechanical or metabolic processes. In many cases, however, the etiology remains unclear (see page 308–312 for further details).

In the course of degenerative alterations, cartilage destruction leads to uneven mechanical loading, with overloading and subsequent destruction of still spared intact cartilage (Fig. 9.**20**).

The primary result of cartilage destruction is **narrowing** of the load-bearing zone of the **joint space.** The lack of the shock-absorbing cartilage increases the impact load of the subchondral bone, resulting in small areas of osteonecrosis, which become hypervascular toward the marrow space. The hypervascularity leads to increased osteoblastic activity and trabecular thickening, ultimately resulting in a **sclerosis.** Since the bone cannot withstand the continued overload, trabecular microfractures occur and, ultimately, the trabecular structures collapse. This leads to the formation of so-called **'detritic cysts',** which strictly speaking are not cysts, but are designated as such because of their radiographic appearance. It is still unresolved whether they are formed solely by subchondral compression fractures or by joint fluid extending into the trabecular space or both. A connection to the joint capsule can be detected only in some cases. The composition of the cyst contents (myxoid, proteoglycans, articular cartilage fragments, and metaplastically

Table 9.**1** Pathologic–radiologic correlations

Pathologic changes	Corresponding radiologic changes
Synovitis with joint effusion	Soft-tissue swelling, widened joint space
Hyperemia	Juxta-articular osteoporosis
Destruction of cartilage caused by inflammation or pannus	Joint-space narrowing
Destruction of subchondral bone and the 'bare area' caused by inflammation or pannus	Loss of the subchondral bone plate, marginal erosions, subchondral 'signal' cyst formation, mutilation
Extension of synovial fluid into the spongiosal space, subchondral compression fractures, and necroses	Subchondral 'detritic' cyst formation
Fibrosis and osseous ankylosis	Osseous ankylosis
Contractures of capsules, ligaments, and muscles	Deformities, subluxation, dislocation
Reactive osseous appositions, in part with fibrocartilage cover	Osteophytes
Reactive osteosclerosis forming a coarse, often disorganized meshwork of lamellar bone	Subchondral sclerosis

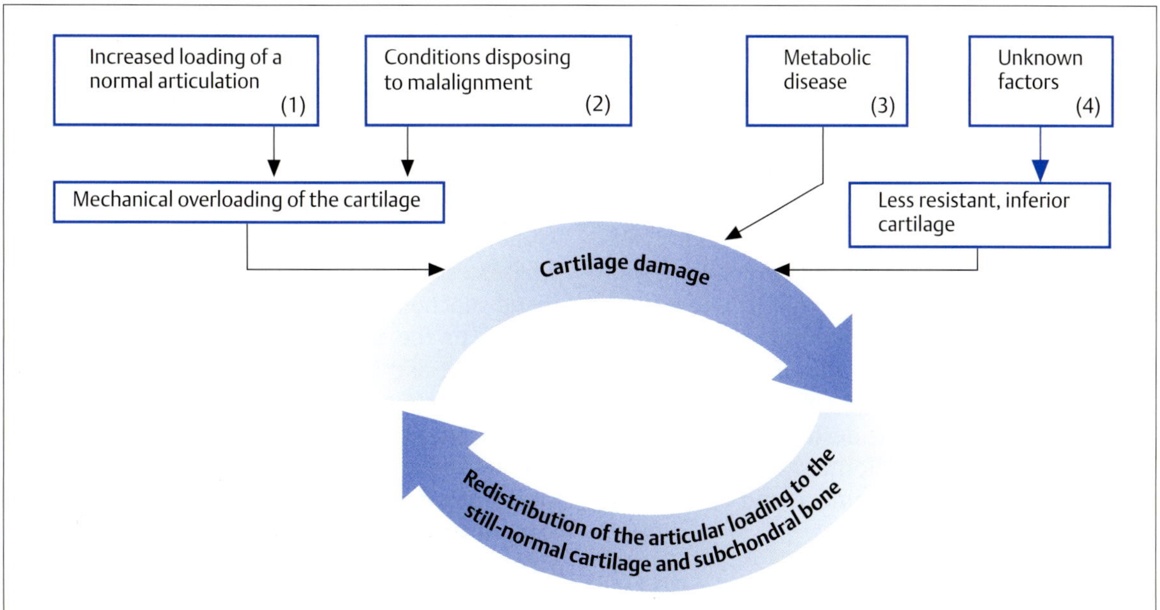

1 Overloading (obesity, sport, ...), neuropathy
2 Joint dysplasias, abnormal alignment of neighboring joints, post-traumatic, postinflammatory, damage of the subchondral bone (e.g., ischemia)
3 Crystal deposition disease
4 Genetic dispositions?

Fig. 9.**20** Conceptual overview of the pathophysiology of osteoarthritis.

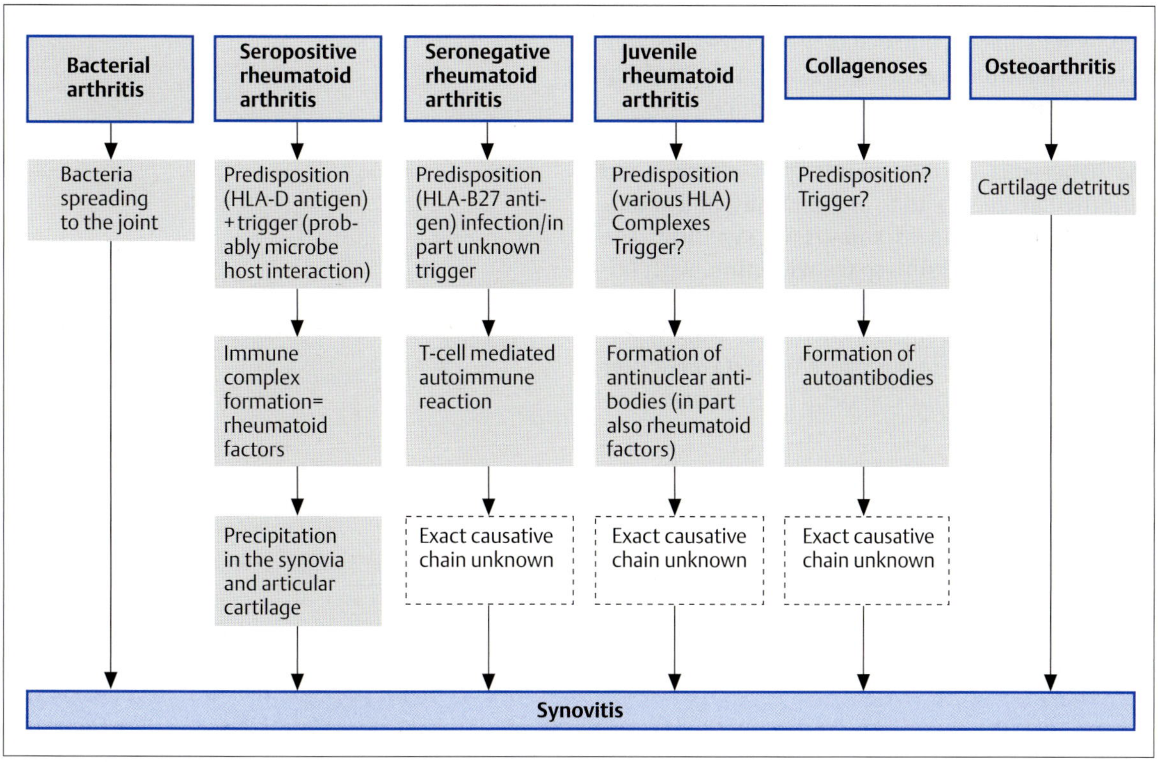

Fig. 9.**21** Conceptual overview of the pathophysiology of inflammatory arthritis.

formed cartilage) suggests a combination of both mechanisms. Within the cyst, vascularized fibrocartilage tissue can form and lead to enhancement on MRI. On conventional radiography, the subchondral cysts appear as localized osteolytic lesions that are more-or-less surrounded by a pronounced sclerotic rim (Fig. 9.**22**).

In contrast to the zones of increased compressive stress, the peripheral portions of the joint are subjected to less stress. Due to regional growth factors, enchondral bone formation produces **osteophytes.** This may be thought of as an attempt by the bone to broaden the load-bearing area of the joint.

With progression of the destructive and reparative processes, joint deformities increase over years, leading to misalignment and, ultimately, **mutilation.**

Pathogenesis of Arthritis and Its Radiographic Appearance

Arthritis has a vast number of causes (Fig. 9.**21**). They all have in common that they induce an inflammation of the synovial lining that is responsible for the disease process. This explains the similarity of the morphologic articular changes, regardless of the particular cause.

Any individual arthritis, in contrast, is characterized by its clinical course and age of onset, as well as by the distribution of the lesions in the skeletal system ('distribution pattern') and joints.

Synovitis with thickening of the synovial lining and hyperemia initially causes joint effusion and periarticular edema that are clinically and radiographically apparent as **soft-tissue swelling.** The effusion can cause **joint-space widening,** with potential damage to the joint capsule (e.g., due to recurrent inflammation). Furthermore, the hyperemia allegedly is a major cause of **juxta-articular osteoporosis** (arthritic collateral phenomenon).

Arising from the synovial lining as well as in the subchondral region, vessels and soft tissues proliferate and form granulation tissue ('pannus'). The pannus and inflammatory effusion erode joint cartilage and also bone not covered by the protecting cartilage layer ('bare area') adjacent to the capsular insertion, This leads to the formation of **erosions.** In the course of the disease, cartilage destruction progresses, and pannus extends from the peripheral and subchondral sites towards the joint, initially leading to the **destruction of the subchondral bone plate** and eventually to erosions and **osteolytic** defects (Fig. 9.**23**).

With progression of the disease process, cartilage and bone are further destroyed (resulting in **joint space narrowing**), eventually leading to complete **destruction** with **mutilation** and **misalignment.** This affects small joints quite frequently. With complete destruction of the joint, the disease arrests since the inflammation has subsided. In this stage, the reparative processes can produce an initially fibrous and later osseous bridging of the former joint resulting in **ankylosis.**

A long chronic process may show sclerosis around the erosions and cysts representing signs of repair. This enables differentiation between old and acute lesions.

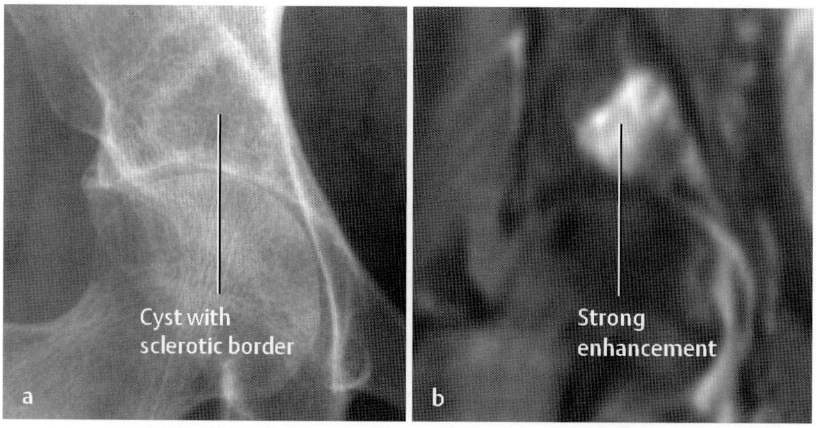

Fig. 9.**22** Large subchondral cyst in the acetabular roof in osteoarthritis of the hip. The radiograph shows a sclerotic rim around the osteolytic area.
b Strong contrast enhancement of the cyst content on MRI (T1-weighted TSE with fat suppression) indicates vascularized tissue.

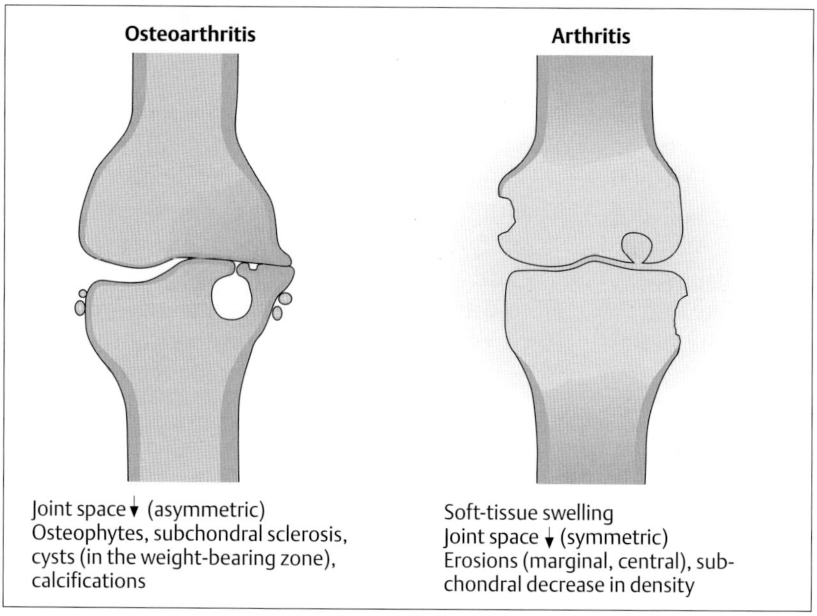

Fig. 9.**23** Schematic comparison of the most relevant signs of erosive osteoarthritis and inflammatory arthritis.

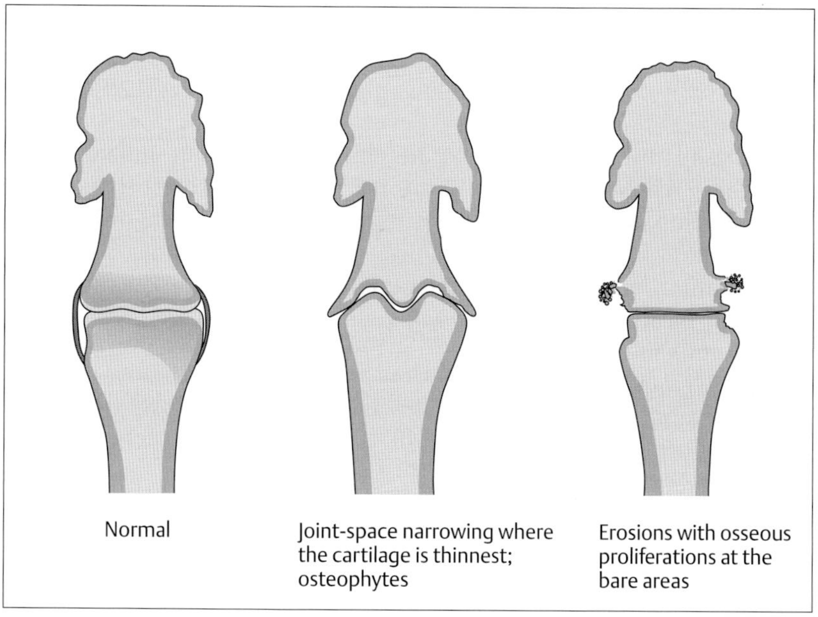

Fig. 9.**24** Schematic comparison of erosive osteoarthritis and psoriatic arthritis.

Enthesopathies (Fibro-ostosis and Fibro-ostitis)

■ Pathologic alterations at the osseous attachment of tendons, ligaments, and joint capsules are referred to as **enthesopathies.** They consist both of degenerative-reparative phenomena (fibro-ostosis) and inflammatory reactions (fibro-ostitis). Both processes can lead to hyperostosis with spur formation, as well as to osseous resorption. The corresponding osseous changes in the spine are referred to as syndesmophytes and parasyndesmophytes. ■

Anatomic Consideration: The epiphyseal and apophyseal insertions of the tendons, ligaments, and joint capsules lack periosteal coverage, and the fibers of the fibrous structures are not directly anchored to the underlying bone. Instead, a zone of **fibrocartilage** is interposed between the taut fiber bundles and bone. This fibrocartilage is mineralized along its interface with bone. At the diaphysis, in contrast, the fiber bundles extend fan-like into the covering periosteum, intertwine with the periosteal fibers, and only then penetrate into the osseous tissue. Thus, there are definite morphologic differences despite the identical functions of these tendinous, ligamentous, and capsular attachments (so-called 'stretch protection').

It should be kept in mind that the region of osseous insertion of fibers always preserves its potential of new bone formation. Trauma, degeneration, inflammation, and altered metabolism can act on this zone and induce new bone formation.

Fibro-ostosis

This is a traumatic or degenerative enthesopathy. It also occurs with sclerosis and acromegaly. An especially extensive manifestation is diffuse idiopathic skeletal hyperostosis (DISH).

Pathologic findings, clinical presentation, and imaging features depend on the duration, location, and extent of the change. Repetitive trauma induces 'inflammatory' tissue reactions with lymphocytic infiltration, edema, and resorptive changes at the bone. This can progress to calcifications and cystic bone defects.

Locations: Calcaneus (posterior and plantar calcaneal spur), greater trochanter, ischial tuberosity, olecranon, and iliac crest (Fig. 9.**26**). Other locations are less common.

CLINIC Fibro-ostosis is usually asymptomatic. Inflammatory reaction due to overuse can cause pain and swelling (e.g., 'epicondylitis' in tennis players, golfers).

X-RAY
- Irregular calcifications of the tendons and ligaments (Fig. 9.**25**).
- New bone formation at the tendon insertions (spurs, excrescence, Fig. 9.**26**).

Insertion defects are possible at the site of muscle insertions. These contour defects ('rarefying fibro-ostosis') occur in the region of the pubic bone, ilium, and sacrum, as well as in the region of the femoral neck and humerus (Fig. 9.**27**).

Fibro-ostitis

Two types of fibro-ostitis are distinguished:
- productive fibro-ostitis (new bone formation with specific radiographic features),
- rarefying fibro-ostitis (inflammatory insertion erosions, Figs. 9.**28**, 9.**29**).

Fibro-ostitis is a sign of inflammatory joint diseases, especially common in psoriatic arthritis, Reiter syndrome and ankylosing spondylitis.

CLINIC The clinical findings consist of localized swelling and pain.

X-RAY The productive fibro-ostitis produces new bone, which is irregularly outlined and has indistinct frayed borders.

The rarefying fibro-ositis is characterized by an indistinctly outlined osseous defect at the insertion of the tendon, ligament or capsule. Reactive sclerosis is common around the defect (Fig. 9.**29**).

DD 'Acute' fibro-ostosis with inflammatory tissue reaction and fibro-ostitis in rheumatoid diseases are not always distinguishable on imaging studies, since both conditions show evidence of inflammation on bone scan (increased activity) and MRI (edema).

! Enthesopathy in rheumatoid diseases can be detected on MRI quite early, before osseous changes are manifest (Fig. 9.**30**).

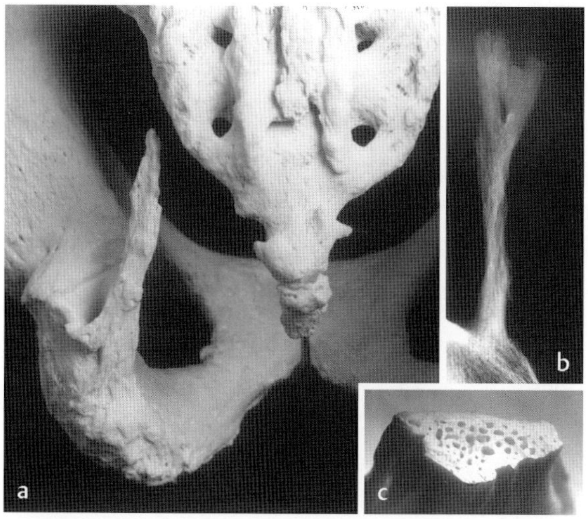

Fig. 9.**25** **a** Anatomic specimen of a calcified ischiosacral ligament. Radiograph of the specimen (**b**) and cross-section of the specimen (**c**) reveal the spongiosal texture.

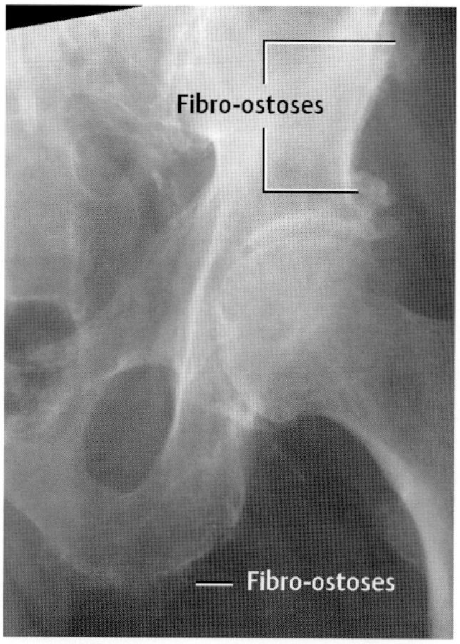

Fig. 9.**26** Extensive classic fibro-ostoses (enthesopathic change) within the pelvis.

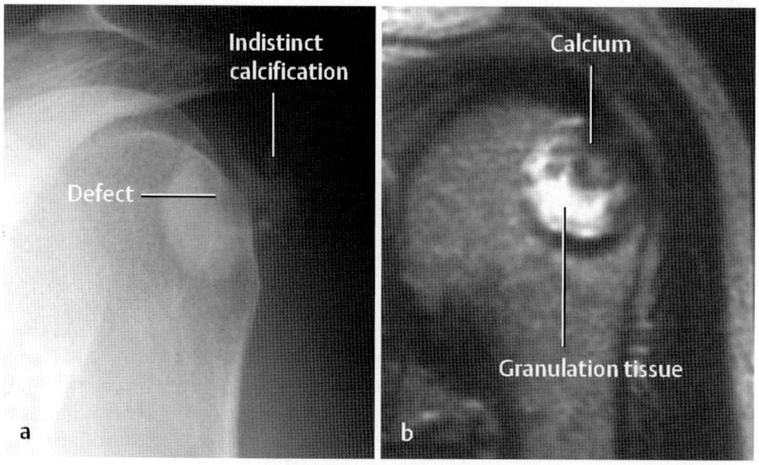

Fig. 9.**27** Chronic calcifying fibro-ostosis at the insertion of the infraspinatus muscle. **a** Oblique projection. The T2-weighted SE sequence (**b**) indicates absence of inflammation in the region of the tendinous insertion (no edema).

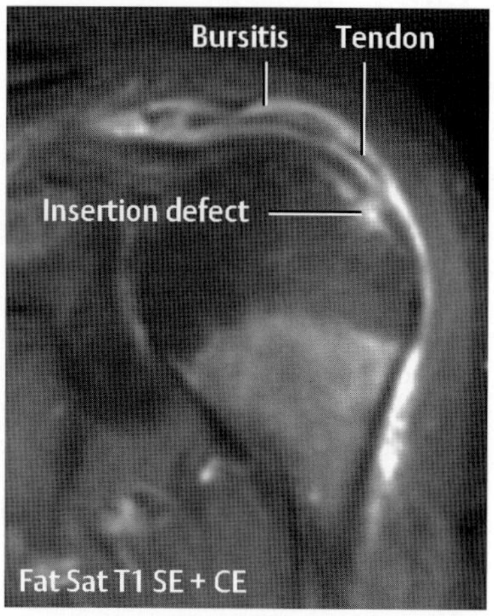

Fig. 9.**28** Enthesopathy (fibro-ostitis) at the insertion of the infraspinatus muscle in psoriasis.

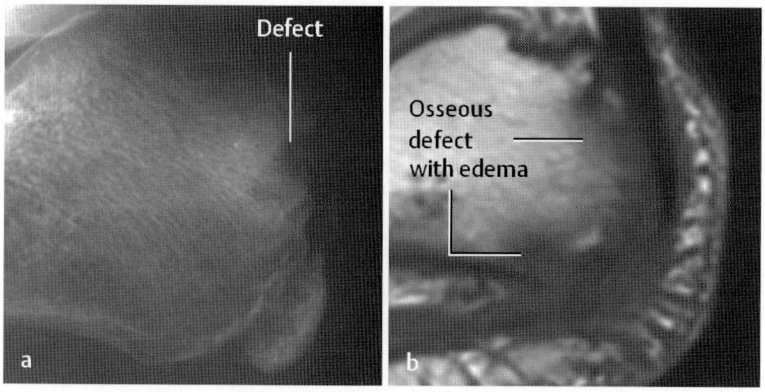

Fig. 9.**29** Rarefying fibro-ostitis at the calcaneal tuberosity in an 8-year-old boy with seronegative spondyloarthropathy. **a** Lateral view. **b** T1-weighted SE image.

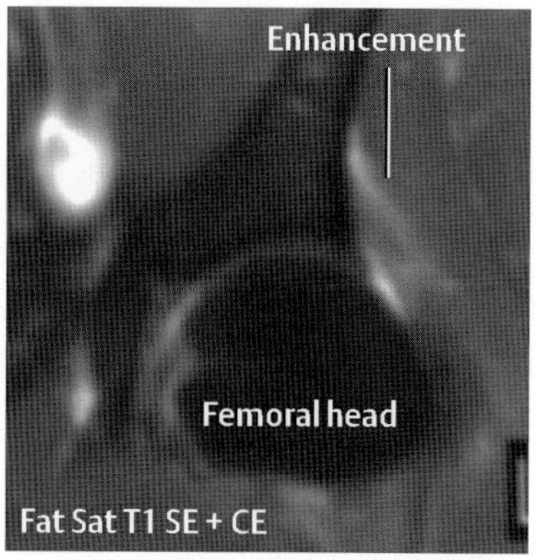

Fig. 9.**30** Enthesopathy without osseous involvement in seronegative spondyloarthropathy.

Degenerative Joint Diseases

Osteoarthritis of the Peripheral Joints

Degenerative joint diseases (= osteoarthritis) include many different conditions and often undetermined etiologies. They all have in common that they occur at an older age (in the fifth decade of life or later = **primary osteoarthritis**) or as **secondary osteoarthritis** following a pre-existing joint disorder. Secondary osteoarthritis can also occur early in life. Current scientific evidence indicates that primary osteoarthritis and aging are conceptually two separate processes. This is supported by both biochemical and histologic investigations.

PATH The etiology of joint degeneration is multifactorial. Misalignment, neuromuscular dysfunction, ligamentous loosening, repetitive local stress, and trauma are the commonest causes of articular overload. The compressible, noncalcified hyaline cartilage resists the increased mechanical stress at the articular surface for a relatively long time. The compressive force, however, is transmitted to the underlying calcified cartilage and subchondral bone plate. Both layers act as a functional unit that is barely compressible and more susceptible to damage by overloading. Whether the damage begins in the subchondral region or in the cartilage is undetermined. Both layers are connected by tiny channels, which are assumed to exchange fluid and to equalize the pressure between the subchondral region and cartilage. Many connecting channels are found in articular zones subjected to a high load, and correspondingly fewer channels in those zones are subjected to a lower load.

Distribution of Arthritic Changes

Primary osteoarthritic changes are found mainly in the spine and in the hip, knee, first metacarpophalangeal articulation, and interphalangeal articulations (Fig. 9.**31**). In contrast, the shoulder, elbow, foot, and ankle are infrequently involved. Osteoarthritic changes found in these joints should always be considered secondary in nature. Why primary arthritic changes rarely involve the ankles but commonly involve the hands is unknown.

Secondary osteoarthritic changes have preferred sites determined by the underlying joint disorder (see Table 9.**2**).

Table 9.**2** Preferred sites for secondary degenerative arthritic changes

Causes	Sites
Trauma	Knee, hip, shoulder, elbow, hand, ankle
Joint dysplasia	Hip
Osteonecrosis	Hip, knee, shoulder
Rheumatoid arthritis	Hand, foot, hip, knee
Acromegaly	Hand, foot, knee, shoulder
Gout	Hand, foot, knee, elbow

a) Damage to the Hyaline Articular Cartilage and Synovial Lining

Damage to the articular cartilage is called chondromalacia. The four stages in cartilage damage are:

I Cartilage edema (Fig. 9.**32**),
II Start of cartilage fragmentation with defects (Fig. 9.**33**),
III Cartilaginous fibrillation with large defects (Fig. 9.**35**),
IV Complete cartilage denudation.

In cartilage degeneration, the superficial zone of collagenous fibers is damaged first (in some cases accompanied by degradation of proteoglycans). The cartilage matrix, which consists mainly of hydrophilic proteoglycans, accumulates more water and becomes swollen, leading to **cartilage edema.** The resultant increased mechanical friction, together with the lost normal elasticity of the cartilage, leads to **fragmentation** of the cartilage substance with formation of defects.

Fragmentation and defect formation progress, producing the phenomenon known as **fibrillation.** This is the most frequently observed finding, since it also is the time when patients consult their physician because of increasing joint pain. Further progression leads to **denudation** of the articular surface (Fig. 9.**34**).

The synovial lining plays a major role in causing symptoms in osteoarthritis. Increased friction leads to mechanical and histochemical irritation **(synovitis)**, and with time a chronic effusion with its complications may develop (e.g., synovial cysts). Morever, nourishment of the cartilage supplied by synovial fluid is compromised. This can be followed by shrinkage of the joint capsule, adding joint deformities to the altered cartilage coat and cortical bone end.

b) Subchondral Damage

Continued overloading quickly leads to small areas of marrow edema, microhemorrhage and microfracture, and even focal osteonecrosis. Edematous areas can resolve within a few weeks without any residue. However, hyperemia, cellular infiltration, and proliferation of fibrovascular tissues might develop in the otherwise highly vascularized and nerve-rich subchondral bone. These changes can also be fully repaired, but might leave behind defects in the form of subchondral cysts (filled with liquid, myxoid, fibrous, or cartilaginous material) or reparative bone and subchondral sclerosis. These 'residues' (cysts, subchondral sclerosis) interfere with the fluid exchange between the subchondral region and cartilage. The radiolo-

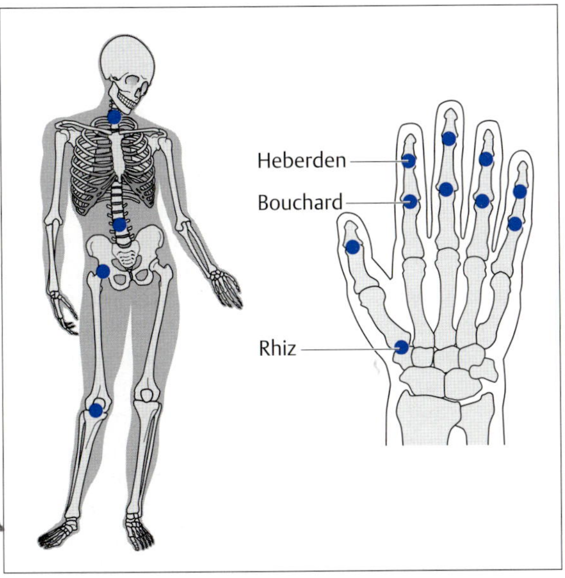

Fig. 9.**31** Distribution pattern of primary degenerative osteoarthropathy at the peripheral joints.

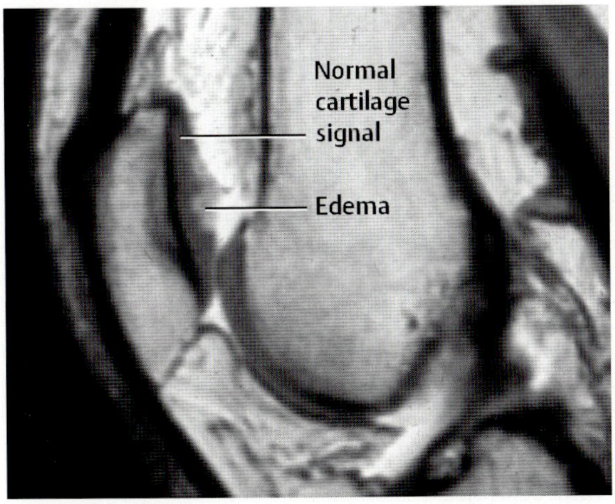

Fig. 9.**32** Sagittal MR arthrography of the knee, T1-weighted SE sequence. Cartilage edema along the retropatellar articular surface, indicating the first stage of damage to the articular cartilage.

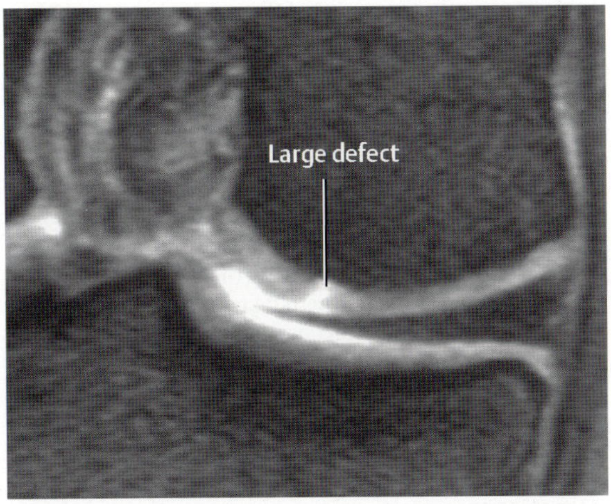

Fig. 9.**33** The start of cartilage fragmentation of the knee; indirect MR arthrography, gradient echo sequence. Stage II.

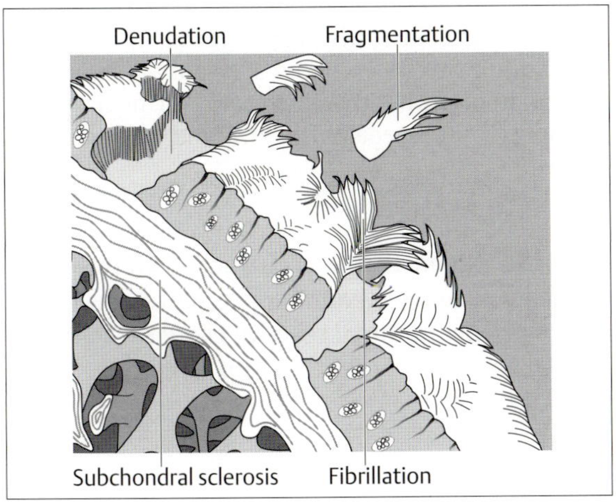

Fig. 9.**34** Degenerative changes of the cartilage and subchondral region.

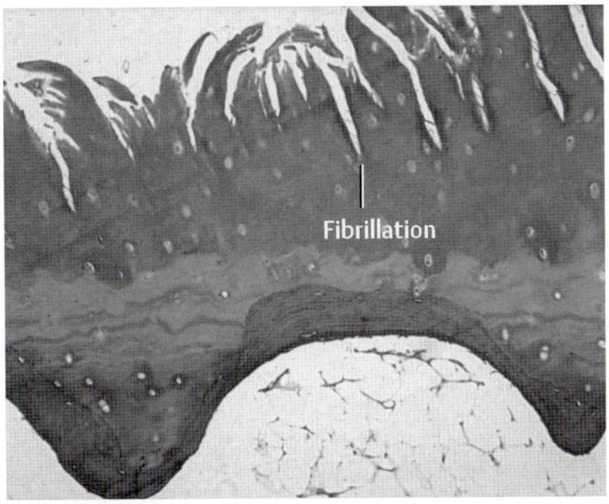

Fig. 9.**35** Histologic section through the articular cartilage. Stage III.

gic manifestations of these processes are local subchondral osteopenia, cysts, or sclerosis.

c) Cartilage Repair

Chondrocytes are highly specialized and cannot divide. If damaged, they become hypertrophied and develop increased nuclei to achieve increased production of matrix and collagenous fibers (= intrinsic repair). Subchondral damage can induce the formation of new cartilage, which arises from the depth of the subchondral region or from the edge of the articular cartilage to cover the defects in the cartilage or the denuded articular surface (= extrinsic repair). This 'reparative' cartilage contains more fibers than the original cartilage, and its surface is quite irregular and less compressible. This is why the repaired articular surface is less resistant to compressive forces.

d) Osteophyte Formation

Persistent overloading of a joint, especially if it is unstable, will produce new bone in the form of osteophytes by local activation of growth factors and by local tensile forces. The formation of osteophytes follows the same principle that underlies the formation of fibro-ostoses as metaplastic ossification of reparative connective tissue. By broadening the articulating surface, the marginal osteophytes reduce the local overload and improve stability. At the same time, they restrict joint motion, which further reduces any possible overload.

e) Meniscus and Disk Damage

Articulations can contain fibrocartilaginous structures in the form of menisci, as found in the knee, or disks, as found in the wrist, primarily to distribute the mechanical load more evenly across incongruent cartilage surfaces.

In the meniscus, the typical degenerative tear is horizontally directed. Such tears are found in 50%–70% of individuals 60 years old and older and are asymptomatic in the large majority. Meniscal damage is frequently associated with additional degenerative changes. Meniscal malformations (e.g., discoid meniscus) tend to accelerate degeneration. The typical degenerative tears in the triangular fibrocartilage of the wrist are on the radial side. An increased incidence of disk degeneration is observed with congenital ulnar minus variants.

Latent, Active, Erosive, and Atrophic Osteoarthritis

! A universally accepted terminology for degenerative alterations in joints does not exist. The most frequent, interchangeably used terms are **degenerative joint disease, (degenerative) osteoarthritis, (osteo)arthrosis,** and **arthrosis deformans**. The latter is the preferred term in the European literature. **Osteoarthritis,** which is widely accepted in the US, is the preferential term used in this book. Regardless of the unsettled nomenclature and arbitrary descriptive designations, a distinction between **latent** and **active** degenerative joint alterations is clinically relevant. Active joint degeneration is dominated by synovitis and produces joint symptoms perceived by the patient as signs of a disease process. There is often an associated effusion. In this setting, patients having primarily degenerative joint disease show typical symptoms of an inflammatory joint.

Erosive osteoarthritis (synonyms: inflammatory osteoarthritis, destructive osteoarthritis, Fig. 9.**38**) is a special form of osteoarthritis with swelling, redness and pain as found in synovial arthritis. The cardinal symptom is the radiographically detectable erosion. Distal and proximal interphalangeal joints are preferentially affected, but involvement of any joint is possible. An effusion (best shown by sonography) is always present. In destructive osteoarthritis, the erosions are more central than marginal and either progress to large cysts or become sclerotic.

! Erosive osteoarthritis also begins with a chondropathy, followed by synovitis. Consequently, it falls in the group of degenerative joint diseases. Erosive osteoarthritis is a diagnosis of exclusion. Conditions to be excluded are gouty arthropathy, psoriatic arthropathy, rheumatoid arthritis superimposed on osteoarthropathy, and infectious arthritis.

Atrophic osteoarthritis is characterized by loss of cartilage (leading to joint-space narrowing) with absent or only minimal reactive changes (sclerosis, osteophytes). It tends to involve the hands (Fig. 9.**47**).

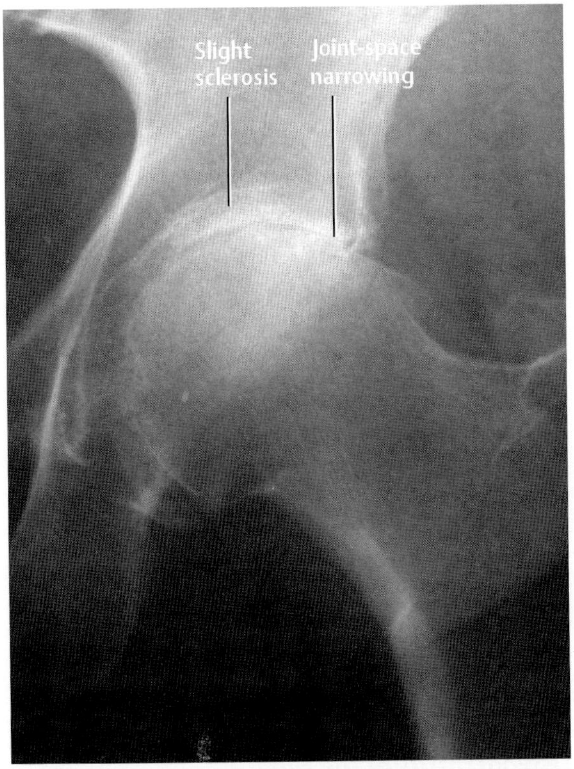

Fig. 9.**36** Signs of degeneration seen here in a representative case of moderately severe osteoarthritis.

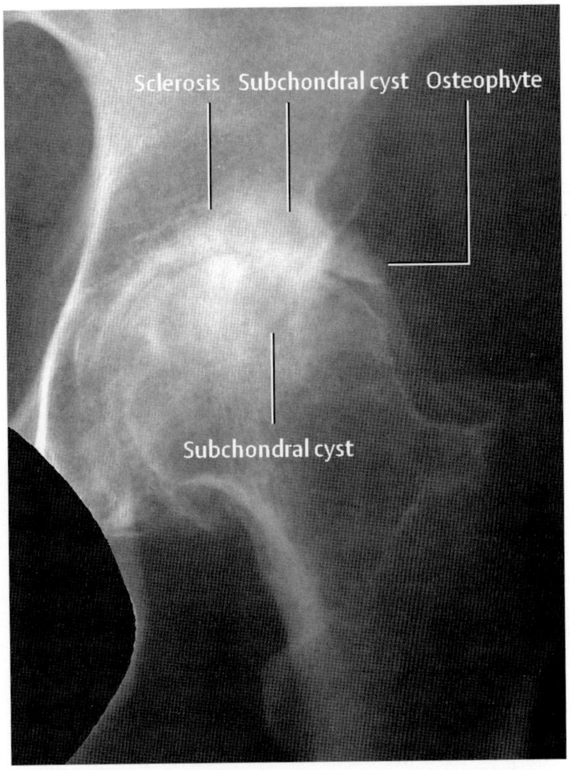

Fig. 9.**37** Signs of degeneration seen here in a representative case of an advanced osteoarthritis.

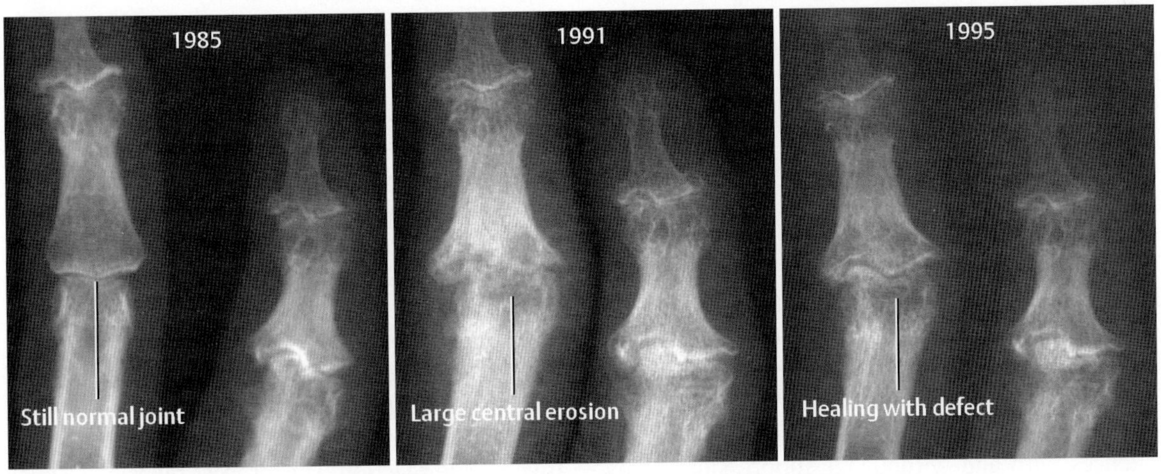

Fig. 9.**38** Resolution of a polyarthritis over 10 years. In 1985, the proximal interphalangeal joint of the middle finger is the only spared visualized joint. In 1991, an erosive arthritis with excessive erosions has developed here. Subsequently, the inflammatory component regresses, and a latent osteoarthritis has developed. The latent osteoarthritis of the remaining interphalangeal joints remains unchanged throughout the observation period.

CLINIC Typical signs of osteoarthritis are
- pain on weight bearing,
- limited range of motion,
- subluxation,
- subcutaneous soft-tissue nodules (Heberden nodes at the distal interphalangeal joints and Bouchard nodes at the proximal interphalangeal joints).

Imaging is used to confirm the diagnosis and to follow the clinical course. The radiographic findings often lag behind the clinical findings for years.

X-RAY **Technical consideration:** To detect alignment abnormalities, radiographic films have to be obtained under weight bearing (standing).

Primary and secondary osteoarthritic changes have the same basic manifestation (Figs. 9.**36**, 9.**37**; also compare with pages 294–296):
- joint-space narrowing, especially of the weight-bearing portions,
- subchondral sclerosis,
- subchondral cyst formation,
- osteophytes,
- joint deformity with misalignment,
- chondrocalcinosis (Fig. 9.**40**),
- loose intra-articular bodies ('joint mice'),
- insertional calcifications of ligaments, tendons, capsules.

Localized subchondral radiolucency, with or without joint-space narrowing, is an early diagnostic sign, but it is rarely encountered (Fig. 9.**39**).

NUC The three-phase bone scan shows increased uptake caused by increased regional perfusion (= early phase) and by increased bone turnover (= late phase) (Fig. 9.**42**). The role of the bone scan is determination of the distribution pattern, which frequently assists in discriminating between arthritis and (active) osteoarthritis.

MRI The pathologic changes of cartilage described above (cartilage edema, swelling, and fibrillation) can be visualized with MRI 'cartilage sequences' (T2-weighted gradient echo sequences with and without fat suppression) or by means of direct or indirect MR-arthrography of the major joints. Moreover, T2-weighted **turbo** (fast) spin echo sequences can also be used advantageously. The subchondral changes (microhemorrhages, microfractures, micronecrosis) are not well delineated because of their extremely small size.

See pages 108 and 316 for the MRI signs of the pathology of menisci and disks.

Osteoarthritis of Specific Joints

Osteoarthritis of the Knee

The knee is a common site of primary and secondary osteoarthritis. The latter is frequently associated with misalignment, instability, preceding severe trauma, osteonecrosis, and inflammation, as well as with neurogenic, metabolic, or hematologic disorders. Radiography can distinguish between:
- medial tibiofemoral,
- lateral tibiofemoral,
- patellofemoral

osteoarthritis of the knee (Fig. 9.**41**). To detect or exclude misalignments, views with the patient standing (with a vertically placed measuring device) are indicated. Degenerative meniscal changes are best detected with MRI.

DD **PVNS** (pigmented villonodular synovitis): This condition is dominated by large cystoid defects in the articular ends of the bone. In its early stages there is no joint-space narrowing.

Osteoarthritis of the Hip

In the hip, superolateral joint-space narrowing is more common than medioinferior narrowing (Fig. 9.**43**). Upright views of the hip show superolateral, superomedial or axial migration of the femoral head to the best advantage. Displacement of the femoral heads into the acetabulum with increasing depths of the acetabular cavity is referred to as acetabular protrusion. Besides dysplasias and other malformations (e.g., coxa vara and valgus), Paget disease and fibrous dysplasia should be added to the causes of secondary osteoarthritis already discussed.

An unusual variant of erosive osteoarthritis, the atrophic-destructive 'osteoarthritis' of the hip, leads to destruction of portions of the femoral head and, to a lesser degree, of the acetabulum, with relatively little reaction. This process takes place over months and mainly affects elderly women.

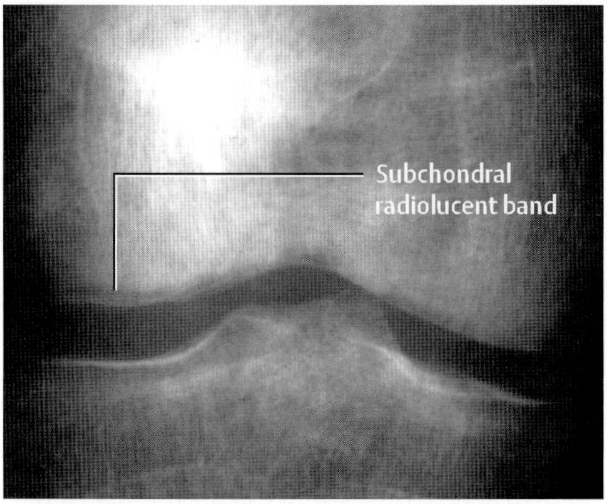

Fig. 9.**39** Osteoarthritis of the knee joint.

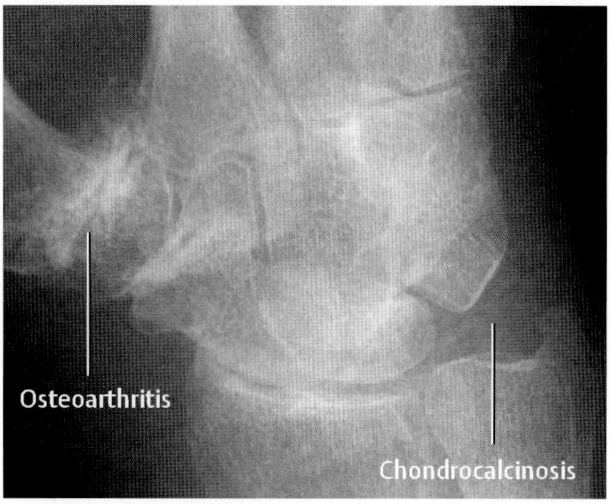

Fig. 9.**40** Chondrocalcinosis of the triangular fibrocartilage as part of degenerative joint disease.

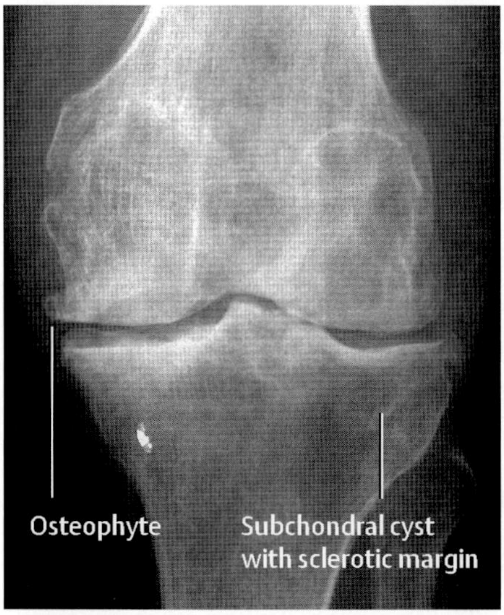

Fig. 9.**41** Osteoarthritis of the medial and lateral tibiofibular joints with a large subchondral cyst.

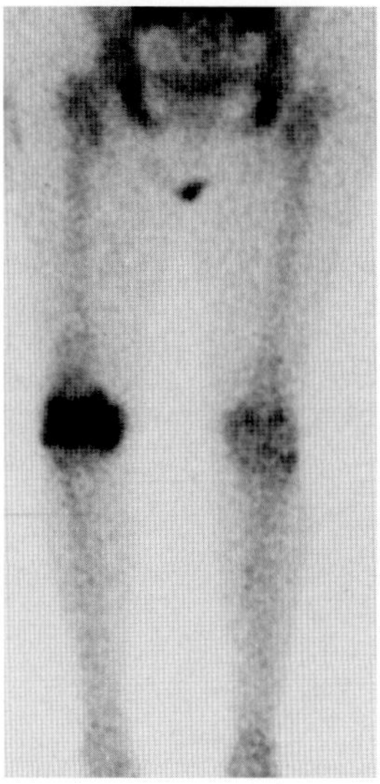

Fig. 9.**42** Three-phase bone scan (late phase). Active osteoarthritis involving both knees, the right more than the left. Typical increase in activity in the weight-bearing zones.

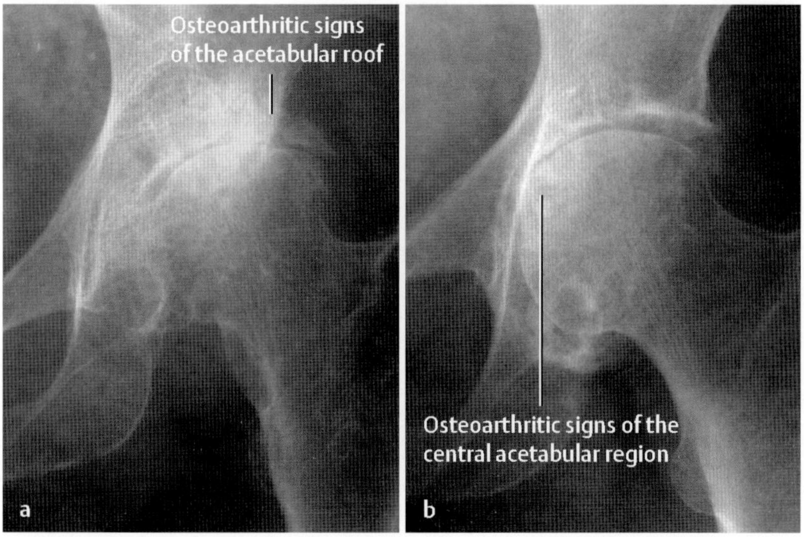

Fig. 9.**43** Osteoarthritis of the hips. (**a**) Superolateral narrowing with upward and lateral displacement of the femoral head. (**b**) Medioinferior narrowing.

DD Atrophic destructive osteoarthritis must be differentiated from **Charcot joint:** the neuropathic destruction also involves other joints of the affected extremity.

Infectious arthritis is diagnosed by analyzing the joint effusion after hip aspiration.

Osteonecrosis only in rare cases does involve the femoral head and the acetabulum at the same time. MRI can be used for further diagnostic evaluation of inconclusive cases.

Remember that circumferential osteophytes ('collar') can be mistaken for an impacted subcapital **fracture of the femoral neck.**

Osteoarthritis of the Shoulder

Primary osteoarthritis of the shoulder is rare. Secondary osteoarthritis (Fig. 9.**44**) develops on the basis of misalignment, trauma, Paget disease, dysplasias, acromegaly, and osteonecrosis, or as part of neurogenic, metabolic, and hematologic diseases. In the majority of cases, the glenohumeral and acromioclavicular articulations are equally involved. Acromioclavicular osteoarthritis can lead to the development of impingement syndrome with compression of the supraspinatus tendon.

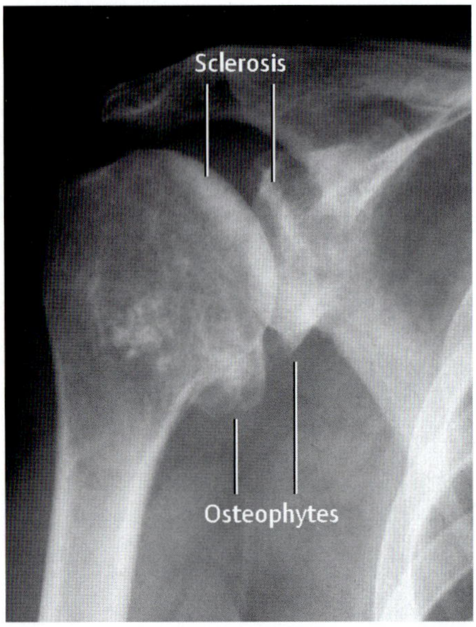

Fig. 9.**44** Osteoarthritis of the shoulder with deformity, osteophytes, and marked subchondral sclerosis.

Osteoarthritis of the Finger and Carpal Bones

Primary osteoarthritis of the distal (= Heberden) and proximal (= Bouchard) interphalangeal joints is the commonest osteoarthritis (Figs. 9.**45**, 9.**46**). The so-called 'Heberden and Bouchard nodes' are soft-tissue protuberances caused by underlying osteophytes. Osteoarthritis of the first carpal–metacarpal articulation frequently has an erosive component (Fig. 9.**48**). Osteoarthritis of the carpal bones mainly affects the scaphoid-trapezium-trapezoideum complex. A primary radiocarpal osteoarthritis is relatively rare.

In 1998, Dihlmann and Dihlmann described a subtype of osteoarthritis of the fingers, which they call **osteoclastic osteoarthritis** of the fingers. It is characterized by subchondral osteolytic areas that involve at least one-third of the length of the phalanx. These areas are larger than detritic cysts, which are confined to the articular end of the bone.

Secondary osteoarthritic changes can be observed together with chronic inflammatory conditions, acromegaly, and metabolic disorders such as hemochromatosis, diabetes mellitus, pseudogout (= CPDD).

DD Hemochromatosis leads to osteophytes with extensive cyst formation involving the metacarpophalangeal joints. This condition also often shows chondrocalcinosis.

Osteoarthritis of the Toes

The commonest causes of degenerative changes in the toe joints are malpositioned toes, especially the hallux valgus (Fig. 9.**49**). A striking finding of degenerative changes due to hallux valgus deformity is the often extreme hyperostosis and 'cystoid' osseous transformation in the first metatarsal head. Accompanying soft-tissue swelling (bursitis) is a frequent additional finding.

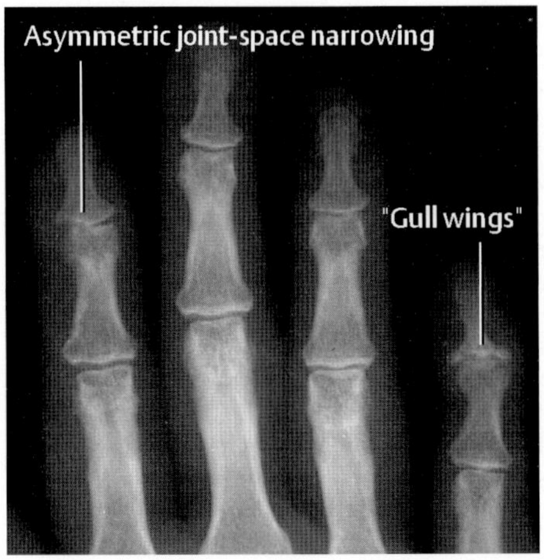

Fig. 9.**45** Interphalangeal osteoarthritis. The 'bird's wing' or 'seagull' appearance is caused by lateral osteophytes and central indentation.

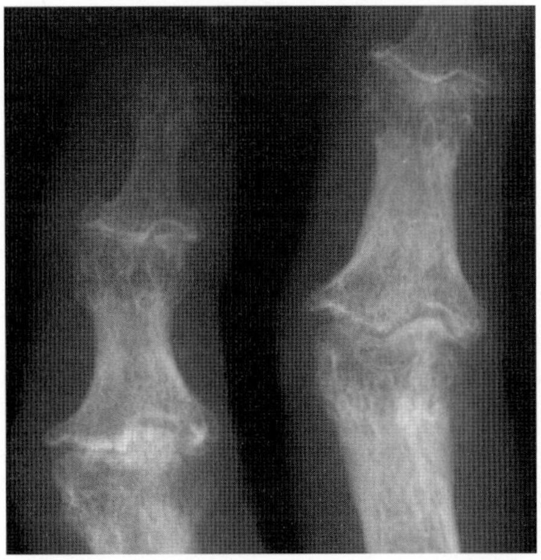

Fig. 9.**46** Prominent Bouchard osteoarthritis of the proximal interphalangeal joints, and also less pronounced Heberden osteoarthritis of the distal interphalangeal joints.

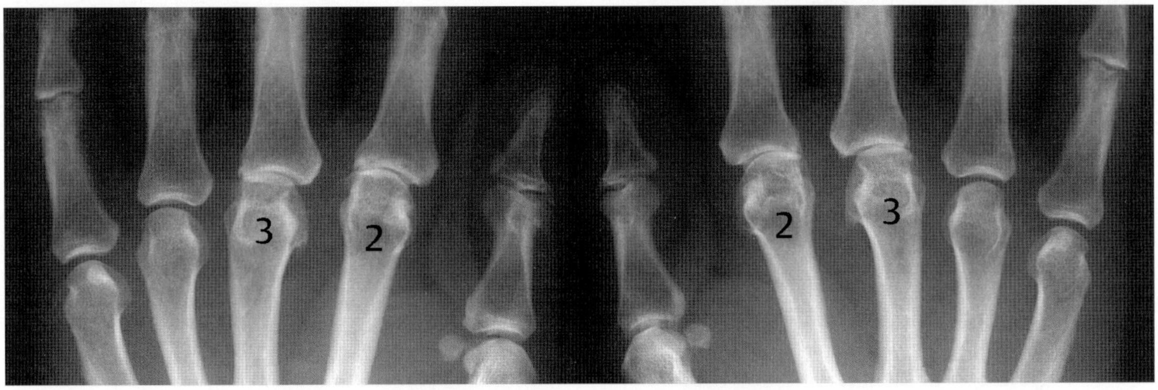

Fig. 9.**47** Rare form of atrophic osteoarthritis. The joint spaces are asymmetrically narrowed.

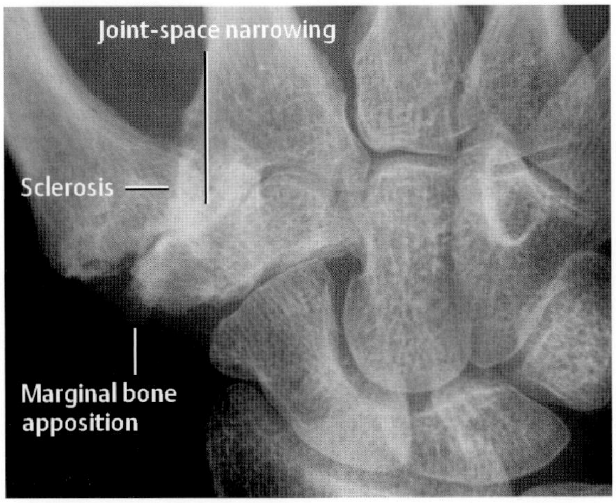

Fig. 9.**48** Osteoarthritis of the first carpometacarpal joint.

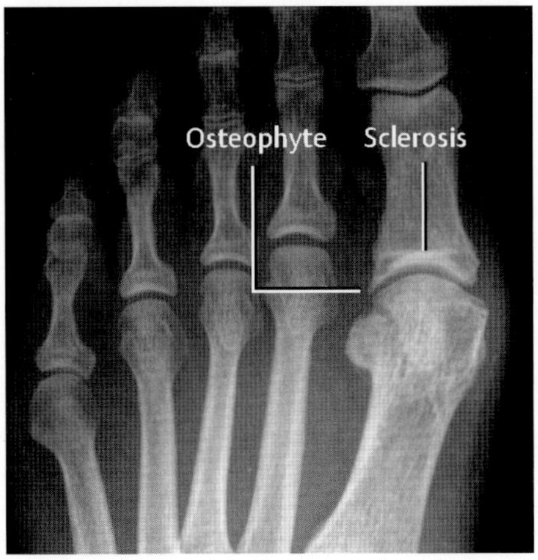

Fig. 9.**49** Hallux valgus with mild degenerative changes.

Degenerative Changes of the Spine

Degenerative disease of the spine is one of the most common clinical entities and affects the intervertebral disks, including apposing vertebral end plates, intervertebral (facet) articulations, and atlanto-axial articulation. Intervertebral and atlanto-axial articulations are genuine synovial articulations and consequently show the same basic abnormalities seen with degenerative disease of synovial articulations found at other sites in the body. The most severe primary spinal degenerative changes are found in the lower cervical and lumbar spine regions. Degenerative intervertebral joint disease can occur both separate from and together with degenerative disk changes. Secondary degenerative changes may result from articular misalignment, abnormal distribution of load-bearing following trauma, inflammations, congenital dysplasias or developmental malformations, metabolic and hematologic conditions, or osteonecroses.

Four basic manifestations of spinal degenerative changes are distinguished:

- spondylosis deformans,
- (osteo)chondrosis (intervertebral disk degeneration),
- apophyseal (facet) joint osteoarthritis and uncovertebral osteoarthritis,
- ligamentous calcifications and ossifications.

PATH

a) Changes of the Intervertebral Disk (Chondrosis)

The intervertebral disk consists of the nucleus pulposus, anulus fibrosus, and cartilaginous end plates (Fig. 9.**50**). Its major functions are to distribute axial loading and to keep surrounding ligaments taut. The degenerative process causes fissuring and fragmentation of the otherwise spirally intertwined collagenous fibers. The fibers might only partially withstand the high pressure of the nucleus pulposus (7 × atmospheric pressure). Repetitive overloading results most commonly in slowly developing herniation of the nucleus pulposus. However, acute herniations also rarely occur. In principle, the herniation can occur in any direction, but only posterior herniations are clinically relevant, since these are the only ones that compress the nerves or spinal cord, depending on whether the herniation is central or lateral in location.

Protrusion: Bulging of the disk (nucleus pulposus and anulus fibrosus). The nucleus pulposus extends into crevices of the inner zone of the anulus fibrosus and displaces fibers of the peripheral zone (Fig. 9.**52**).

Prolapse: Material of the nucleus pulposus leaves the anulus pulposus and extrudes through tears in the peripheral zone of the anulus fibrosus (Fig. 9.**53**).

Sequester: Displaced disk material is referred to as a sequestered fragment. This is usually accompanied by a tear in the posterior longitudinal ligament, but a sequestered fragment can remain subligamentous in location. Its differentiation from a prolapse is problematic, since it is only possible if discontinuation can be demonstrated between disk and sequester (rare) (Fig. 9.**54**).

Furthermore, disk material can herniate superiorly and inferiorly into the adjacent vertebral bodies. These herniations are called Schmorl's nodes.

In the process of degeneration, the disk loses water and decreases in height (Fig. 9.**51**). Furthermore, calcifications may be seen within the disk.

As the degenerative process progresses, reparative osseous processes involving the disk begin at the periphery, where there are no cartilaginous plates. This reparative osseous tissue grows into the disk and can lead to revascularization of the disk (the disk is partially vascularized until the fourth year of life). It is conceivable that this process removes pre-existing disk herniations.

> **!** Neurosurgical terminology distinguishes between 'hard' and 'soft' prolapses in the cervical spine. Since all types of spinal stenosis caused by calcified tissue (spondylophytes, calcified disks) are referred to as 'hard prolapses' this term is pathologically incorrect. However, classifying all of these conditions under a single term appropriately considers the presentation as a chronic encroachment of clinically undetermined cause.
> In contrast, the 'soft prolapse' corresponds to encroachment produced by tissues of soft-tissue consistency and generally presents clinically with acute symptoms.

b) Changes of the Vertebral End Plates

The intervertebral disk is avascular in adolescents and adults and is nourished by diffusion from adjacent bone marrow and bordering ligaments.

In the process of natural aging, the nucleus pulposus loses its water retention capacity, and its internal pressure decreases. This shifts weight bearing from the center to the lateral, leading to ligamentous loosening, and the limited elastic vertebral bone adjacent to the disk is subjected to increased compressive loads. This can result in microedema, microhemorrhage, microfractures, and micronecroses similar to the processes occurring in synovial joints.

This is followed by reactive changes with pseudo-inflammatory reactions in the subdiskal skeletal zones: hyperemia, and ingrowth of fibrovascular tissue. The outcome is subdiskal fibrosis and sclerosis as the bone attempts to counteract the increased axial pressure. The sclerotic bone is brittle and can collapse, resulting in tears and clefts and the formation of reparative connective tissue.

Instability with ligamentous loosening caused by the decreased pressure within the nucleus pulposus leads to reactive osseous proliferations, referred to as osteophytes, along the margin of the vertebral body (spondylosis deformans) and possibly to hypertrophy of the ligamenta flava. This process serves to counteract the instability. The same applies to the uncovertebral joints of the cervical spine (uncovertebral osteoarthritis or arthrosis). They prevent lateral displacement of the cervical vertebral bodies. The superiorly projecting uncinate processes are a peculiarity of the cervical spine and, in contrast to the dorsal and

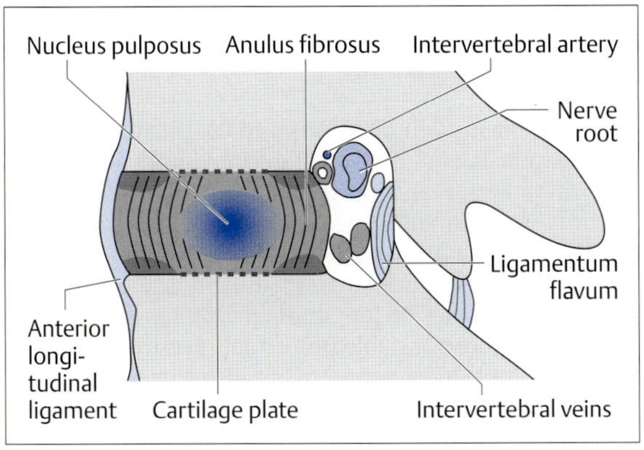

Fig. 9.**50** Schematic drawing of the intervertebral disk and intervertebral foramen.

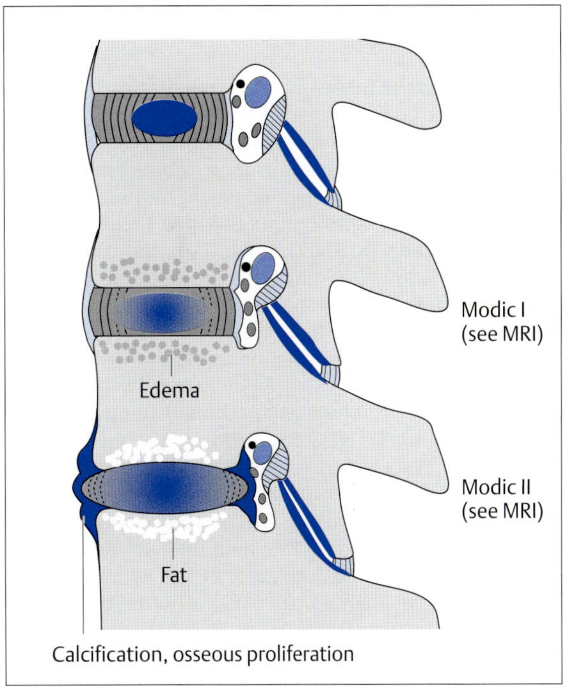

Fig. 9.**51** Schematic drawing of disk degeneration, skeletal changes along the disk, and increasing intervertebral degenerative changes. Modified after Gutmann.

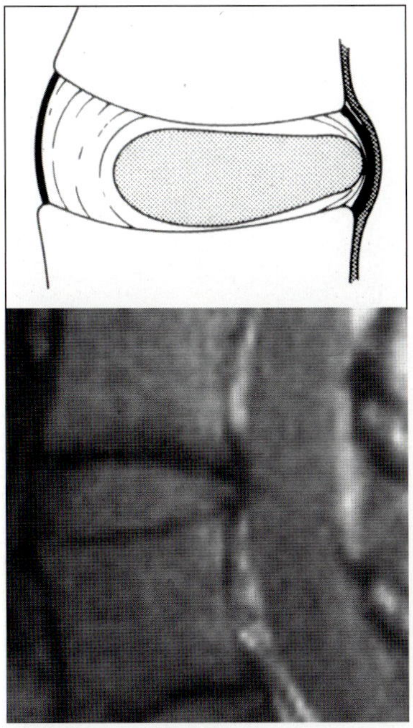

Fig. 9.**52** Disk protrusion (GE sequence).

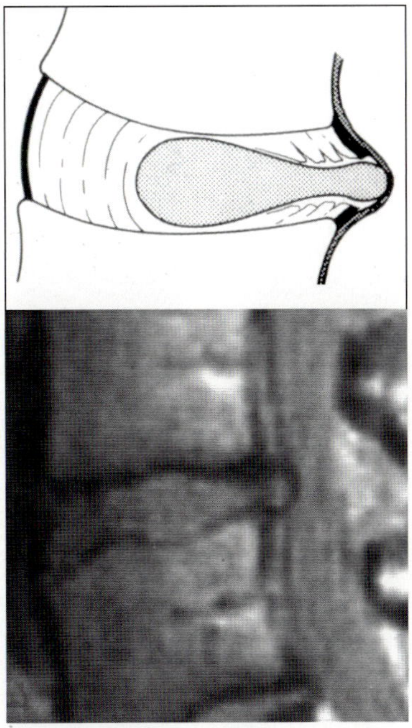

Fig. 9.**53** Disk prolapse (GE sequence).

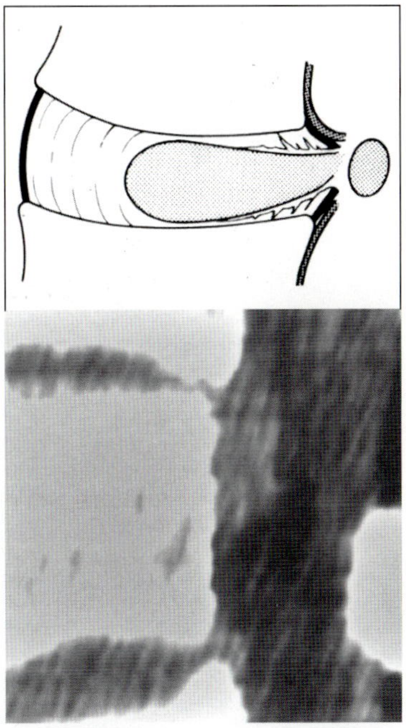

Fig. 9.**54** Disk prolapse with inferiorly dislocated sequestrum, sagittal CT reconstruction.

lumbar spine, form a vertical articulation. The uncovertebral joints are not synovial joints.

c) Changes to the Intervertebral Articulations

The basic pathophysiologic processes are the same as those that occur in other synovial joints. Neck and back pain frequently arise in the intervertebral articulations (synovial irritation, capsular and ligamentous laxity).

Degeneration of these joints is called **facet (apophyseal) joint osteoarthritis.** The atlanto-occipital and atlanto-axial joints are also subject to the same process. The pathologic findings correspond to those of osteoarthritis (cartilage damage, subchondral sclerosis, and cyst formation). Characteristic abnormalities are deformed articular surfaces and massive osteophytic overgrowth that can lead to clinically relevant encroachment upon the intervertebral foramina (Figs. 9.**55** – 9.**57**).

Synovial cysts consist of intraspinal, extradural protrusions of the joint capsule of osteoarthritically deformed intervertebral joints. They are invariably confined to the levels L3–S1 and contain joint fluid or, rarely, gas.

In the lumbar spine, especially at the L4/L5 segment, the degenerative changes can cause anterior gliding of a vertebra relative to its subjacent vertebra (degenerative or pseudospondylolisthesis, Fig. 9.**58**). This can cause spinal stenosis. In contradistinction, spondylolisthesis is caused by vertebral gliding because of a bilateral defect in the pars interarticularis (spondylolysis). Since in 'genuine' spondylolisthesis only the vertebral body glides, and the posterior vertebral arch, together with the spinal process, remains in place, the spinal canal is not narrowed. Etiologically, spondylolisthesis is generally congenital or traumatic (stress fracture).

d) Ligamentous Calcifications and Ossifications

Calcification and ossification of the longitudinal spinal ligaments (anterior and posterior ligaments, ligamentum flavum) are commonly encountered (Figs. 9.**59**, 9.**60**). Although this alteration increases after 50 years of age, it has a racial preference (increased incidence of calcifications in the posterior longitudinal ligaments in Asians) and shows quite a variable individual severity, suggesting not only simple 'degeneration' but also a genetic disposition. Diffuse idiopathic skeletal hyperostosis (DISH) has pathologic and radiographic findings that are identical to ligamentous calcifications and ossifications of other types, but it is nonetheless considered a distinct entity because of several unique features.

e) Stenosis of the Spinal Canal

In spinal stenosis, a distinction should be made between the central and lateral types. The lateral type involves lateral recess and intervertebral foramen. Congenital spinal canal stenosis is rare, and the acquired form is common.

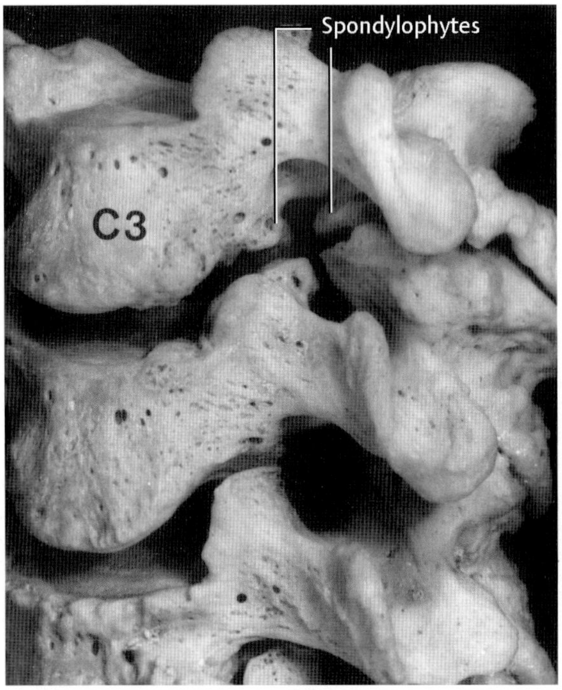

Fig. 9.**55** Massive narrowing of the C3–C4 intervertebral foramen by osteophytes of the facet joints and uncovertebral joints.

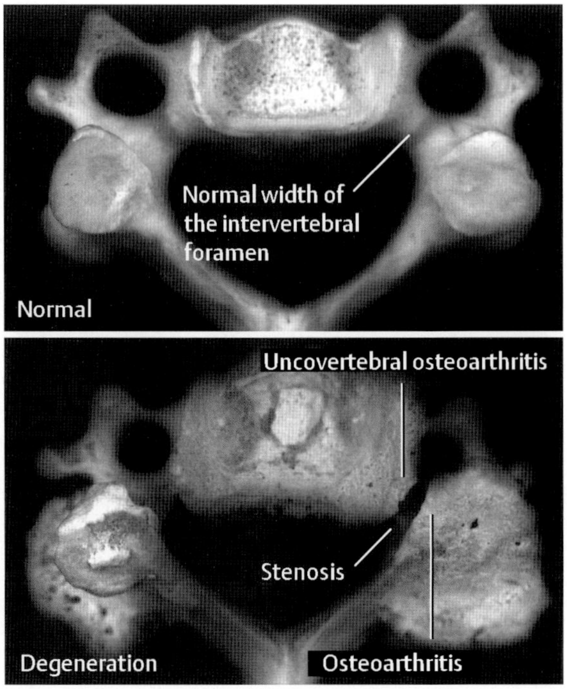

Fig. 9.**56** Specimen of a cervical vertebra with uncovertebral and facet joint osteoarthritis, compared with the specimen of a normal cervical vertebra.

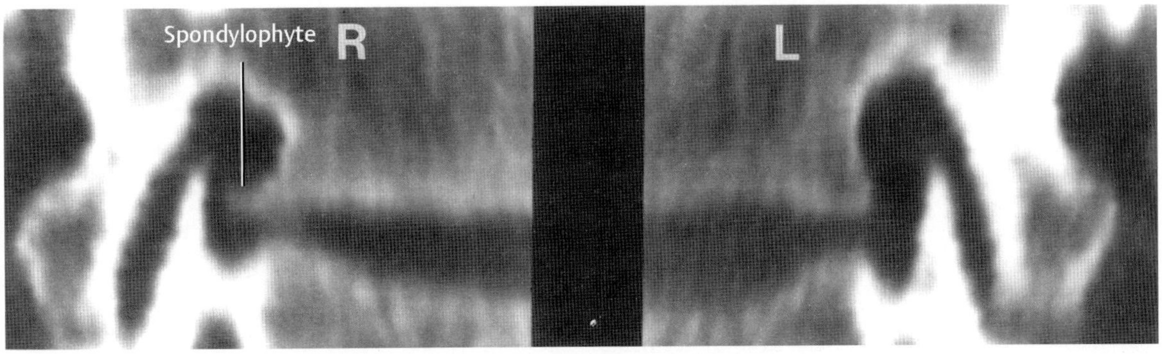

Fig. 9.**57** 2-D CT reconstruction of intervertebral foramina of both sides for comparison. The right intervertebral foramen is narrowed by a marginal osteophyte.

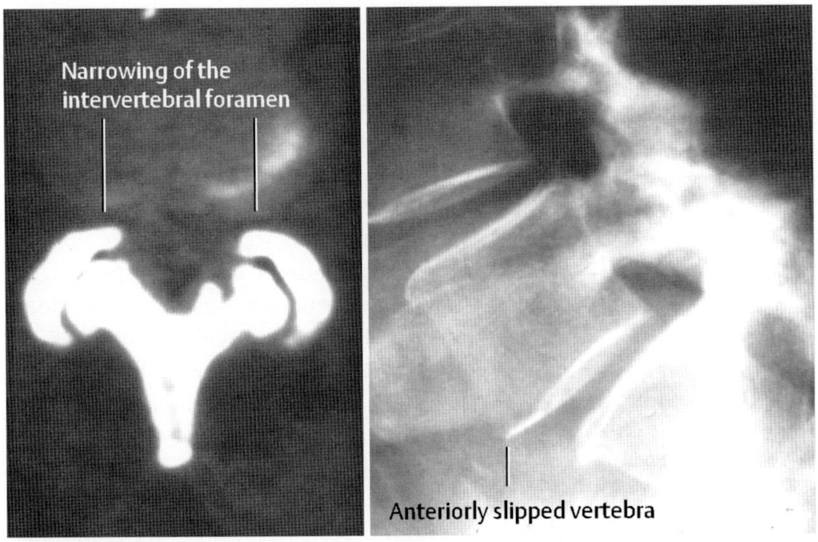

Fig. 9.**58** Marked degenerative changes of the facet joints.
In addition to narrowing of the intervertebral foramen, there is degenerative anterior slippage of the involved vertebrae (pseudo-spondylolisthesis).

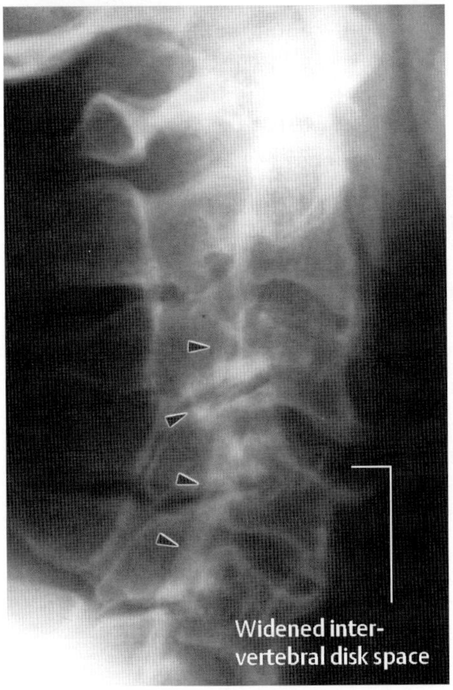

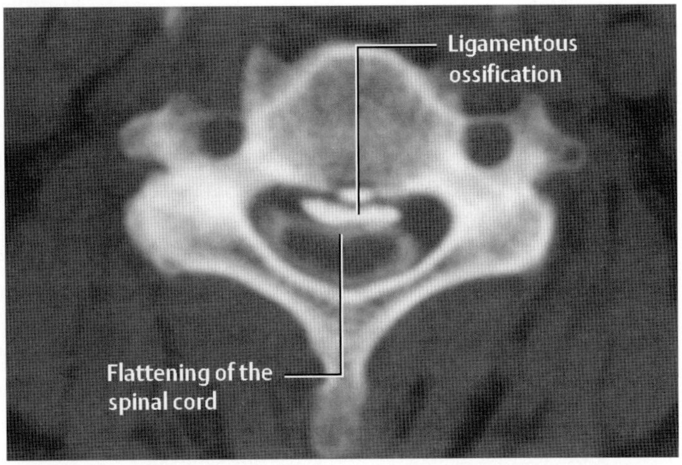

Fig. 9.**60** Ossification of the posterior ligament with indentation of the spinal cord (myelo-CT).

Left:
Fig. 9.**59** Ossification of the posterior ligaments (arrowheads) with fracture. The fracture is recognized by the discontinuity of the ligament and the widening of the disk space.

CLINIC A basic distinction must be made between
- the usually chronic and diffuse 'back pain', caused by spondylosis deformans, facet joint osteoarthritis, and uncovertebral osteoarthritis. As with osteoarthritis of peripheral joints, restricted motion and pain on weight bearing dominate the clinical presentation;
- the usually acutely presenting and often recurrent radicular pain syndrome.

Nerve root compression with radicular pain is caused by disk herniations, but also by osseous narrowing of the intervertebral foramina as part of facet joint osteoarthritis and uncovertebral osteoarthritis. The L3 to S1 segments are the most frequently involved. In general, the sensory deficits dominate in the form of radicular pain, hypoesthesia, and possible hypoalgesia. The strictly radicular distribution usually enables a precise clinical determination of the causative level (Table 9.**3**).

When correlating the radicular symptom complex with the expected radiographic findings, it should be kept in mind that the inferiorly extending lumbar roots begin medial to the cauda equina and then curve laterally to leave the spinal canal through the intervertebral foramen **below** the corresponding vertebral arch. This means that, for instance, L5 radicular pain can be caused by either a lateral or intraforaminal disk herniation at L5/S1 or a medial disk herniation at L4/L5. In the latter instance, a mixed symptom complex can be, but is not inevitably, present.

! Both skeletal and neurologic symptoms can have quite discrepant clinical and radiographic presentations. The clinical presentation is the deciding factor.

Table 9.**3** The most important radicular symptoms

Root	Sensory impairment	Motor impairment
L3	Anterior thigh	Quadriceps (weakened knee jerk)
L4	Anterior lower leg	Quadriceps and tibialis anterior (weakened knee jerk, impaired foot elevation)
L5	Lateral lower leg, extending obliquely to the anterior foot and first toe	Extensor hallucis longus (dorsiflexion of the first toe)
S1	Lateral thigh, posterior lower leg, lateral foot to the fifth toe	Peroneus brevis and triceps (tiptoeing and pronation impaired)

Disk Degeneration (Chondrosis, Osteochondrosis)

! The evaluation of disk herniation is still the subject of ongoing discussion, but the following conclusions can be drawn so far:
- Imaging for the evaluation of 'back pain' is frequently applied too uncritically and not selectively enough.
- Diffuse back pain as such is not an indication for indiscriminate imaging.
- Neurologic symptoms are a foremost indication for the use of imaging.

X-RAY The basic findings of disk degeneration are (Figs. 9.**61**, 9.**62**):
- disk-space narrowing (= chondrosis),
- subchondral sclerosis (rarely osteoporosis),
- Schmorl's nodes,
- spondylophytes,
- vacuum phenomenon,
- calcifications in the disk (nucleus pulposus).

The vacuum phenomenon is caused by the release of nitrogen into the degeneratively altered disk.

Osteochondrosis: The combination of altered vertebral end plates (band-like sclerosis, contour irregularities) and narrowed disk space.

The term 'erosive' osteochondrosis is used when the end plates show surface irregularities. 'Serrations' or contour defects ('erosions') are seen radiographically.

In these cases, differentiating this diagnosis from infectious spondylitis is difficult radiographically. A crucial discriminating criterion is the type of accompanying sclerosis: the subdiskal sclerosis is band-like in osteochondrosis and more focal in infectious spondylitis. Moreover, infectious spondylitis lacks other signs of disk degeneration. In cases of suspected infection superimposed on an (erosive) osteochondrosis, MRI is the preferred imaging modality.

Osteochondrosis and facet joint osteoarthritis of the cervical spine cause hypomobility, preferentially located at levels C5 to C7, frequently with hypermobility of higher cervical segments.

Hemispheric spondylosclerosis: This term coined by Dihlmann describes a **hemispheric** spongiosal sclerosis in the anterior or middle third of the vertebral body **above** an intervertebral disk that appears radiographically normal or narrowed. We consider this a special manifestation of the (normally band-like) subchondral sclerosis as frequently seen with disk degeneration. Awareness of this special manifestation is important for the differential diagnosis when the apposing subdiskal end plate fails to show a sclerosis in the presence of a normal disk space. The hemispheric spongiosal sclerosis must be distinguished from increased density caused by infectious spondylodiskitis (use MRI). Osteoblastic metastases (Fig. 9.**63**) pose difficulty only if the spine shows additional degenerative changes together with a solitary metastatic lesion (rare).

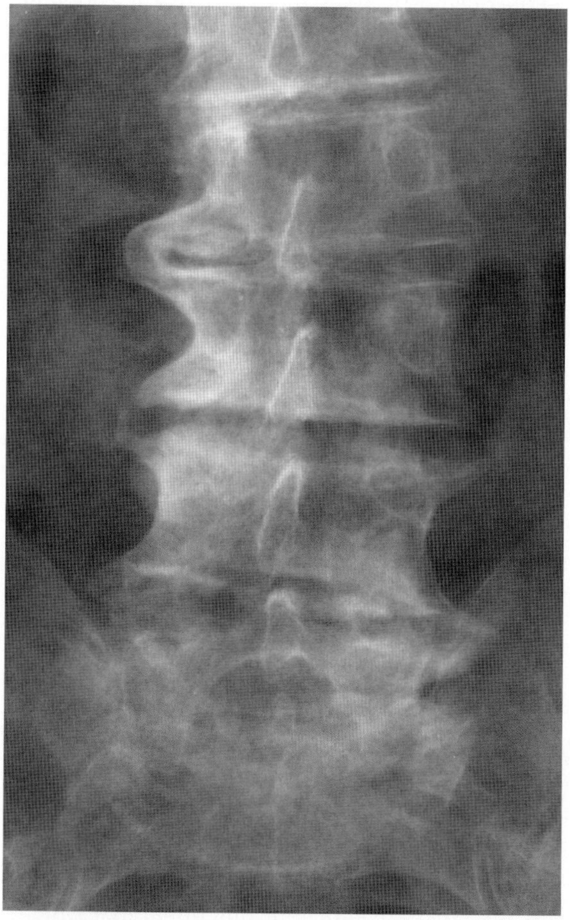

Fig. 9.**61** Degenerative changes of the lumbar spine with marginal osteophytes, end-plate sclerosis, and disk-space narrowing. The osseous appositions are most severe where the vertebral bodies show a decrease in height.

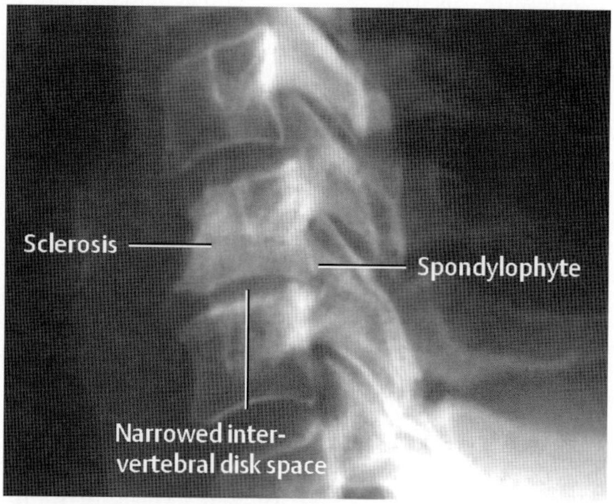

Fig. 9.**62** Degenerative changes of the cervical spine with disk-space narrowing and marked sclerosis along the vertebral end plates.

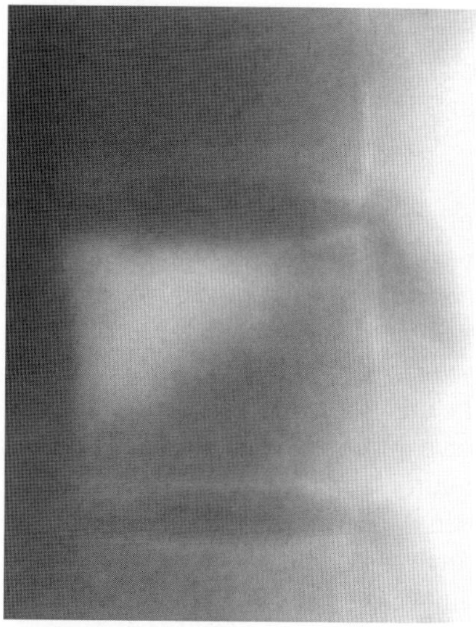

Fig. 9.**63** Osteosarcoma metastasis to the vertebral body in a 20-year-old patient. The adjacent vertebral body and the disk spaces are unremarkable.

CT

Technical consideration: The spinal segments to be examined are identified on the lateral scanogram. The gantry must be angled to be truly axial to the intervertebral disk space. The slice thickness should not exceed 3 mm in the lumbar spine and 2 mm in the cervical spine, and the intervertebral foramina must be completely included.

! In lumbarization of the first sacral segment and sacralization of the fifth lumbar segment and/or numeric variation of the ribs, the exact segmental assignment (referring to the exiting nerve root) can at times be achieved only by counting the vertebral segments all the way down from C1.

Cranial segmental regression: Cervical rib, sacralization of the fifth lumbar vertebra.

Caudal segmental regression: Shortened first rib, lumbarization of the first sacral vertebra, lumbar rib at L1.

Surgical planning based on faulty segmental assignment can have catastrophic consequences.

! When performing CT, vertebral segmentation variations must be looked for and expressly mentioned in the report. A supplemental radiographic view can also be helpful in planning the examination.

Protrusion: This is a symmetric and broad-based extension of disk material beyond the posterior vertebral border (Fig. 9.**64 a**).

Prolapse: This is a localized, variably shaped bulge that projects into the spinal canal, with loss of the overlying epidural fat. Any compression or displacement of the nerve roots is determined by the location (Fig. 9.**64**). The differentiation between protrusion and prolapse by means of CT is arbitrary, since CT does not visualize the underlying pathologic processes.
Caution: Massive prolapse with extensive compression of the dural sac eliminates the density differences between the dense prolapsed disk material and the normally less-dense dural sac, and this can lead to misinterpretation.

Calcifications are indicative of older diskogenic encroachments on the spinal canal. They may be difficult to separate from spondylophytes or ligamentous and capsular calcifications.

Synovial cysts (Fig. 9.**65**): These are easily diagnosed if the vacuum phenomenon is present, but are difficult to diagnose with CT if they are fluid-filled and isodense with the dural sac (use MRI, CT myelography).

Conventional and CT Myelography

Adding CT for the direct visualization of the dural sac has led to a renaissance of myelography. The CT sections are obtained through the area of interest after radiographic imaging following intrathecal installation of contrast medium through a lumbar puncture. By compensating for each method's limitations, this combination has an additive effect on the diagnostic assessment. The use of a nonionic water-soluble contrast medium that causes no meningeal irritation and is less neurotoxic has increased the safety of myelography by eliminating any side effects such as psychotic reactions and seizures. The smallest gauge needle feasible should be selected for the spinal tap. Changing the needle from 20 gauge to 22 gauge can decrease the incidence of postmyelography headache and neck pain by about half.
Technical consideration: The concentration and volume of contrast medium should be determined by the diagnostic needs, including the expected level of the pathologic findings. For lumbar spine myelography, a volume of approximately 10 ml of 200 mg iodine/ml is appropriate, and for the visualization of the cervical spinal canal, a volume of 20 ml is desirable. Cervical myelography following direct lateral puncture at C1/2 requires 10 ml of a higher iodine concentration.
Indications: Asymmetry or displacement of the nerve roots falls into the diagnostic domain of CT myelography. It is superior to conventional CT in differentiating the indirect signs of disk herniation from anatomic asymmetries, joined nerve root sleeves, and perineural cysts (Fig. 9.**66**).

Conventional myelography is not as accurate as CT in delineating the course of the nerve roots but has the great advantage of functional assessment. The compressive effect on the spinal canal can be deduced by the relative displacement of the vertebral bodies on weight bearing and in flexion and extension (Fig. 9.**67**). Another advantage is the simultaneous visualization of several disk space levels. Such an overview is especially important in patients with atypical complaints and consequently less-reliable clinical localization of the causative level. Finally, myelography with or without CT has kept its place for the evaluation of postsurgical findings. Metallic screws, plates, and other fixation devices barely interfere with the diagnostic evaluation. Adhesions, CSF leaks, and even epidural hematomas can also be easily diagnosed.

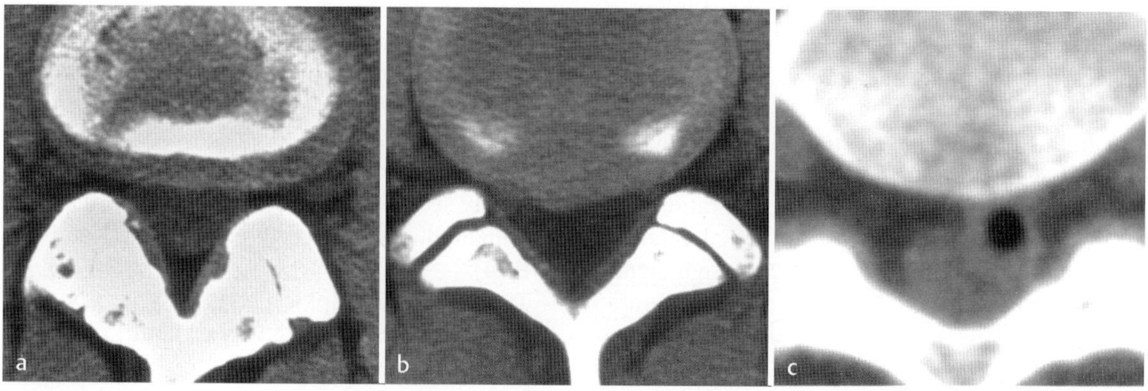

Fig. 9.**64** Different degrees of disk herniation as seen on CT. **a** Protrusion. **b** Medial prolapse: the epidural fat is displaced, the dural sac deformed. **c** Cranially sequestered prolapse with vacuum phenomenon.

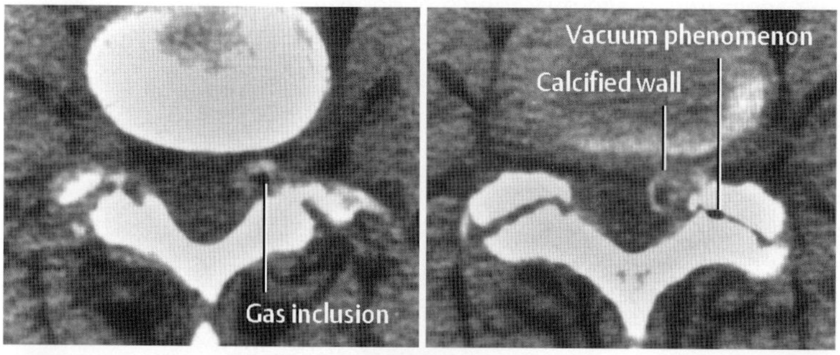

Fig. 9.**65** Synovial cyst with calcified wall and small air bubble. The intervertebral joint also exhibits a vacuum phenomenon.

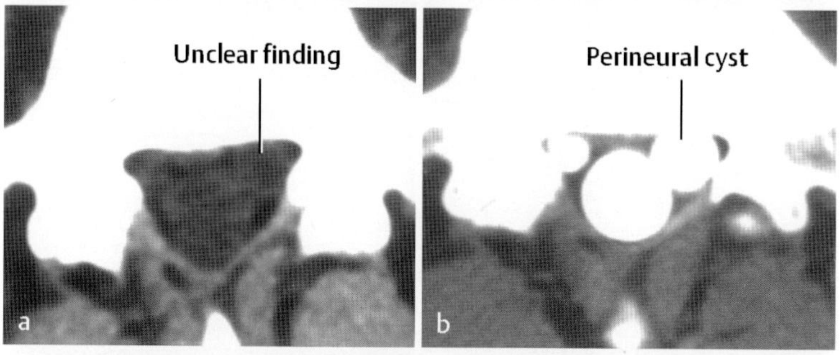

Fig. 9.**66** Unenhanced CT (**a**) and CT myelography (**b**) with visualization of a left nerve root cyst at the level of S1.

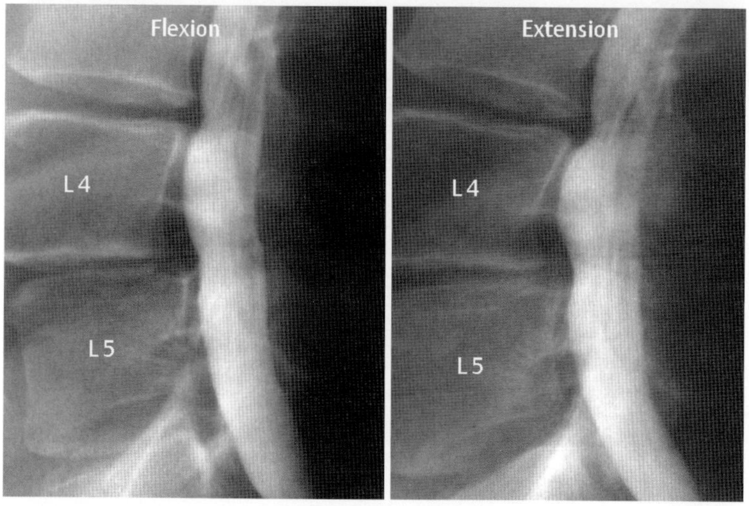

Fig. 9.**67** Lumbar myelography with functional views. Posterior displacement of L5. With flexion and extension, there is neither additional displacement of the vertebral bodies nor narrowing of the central canal.

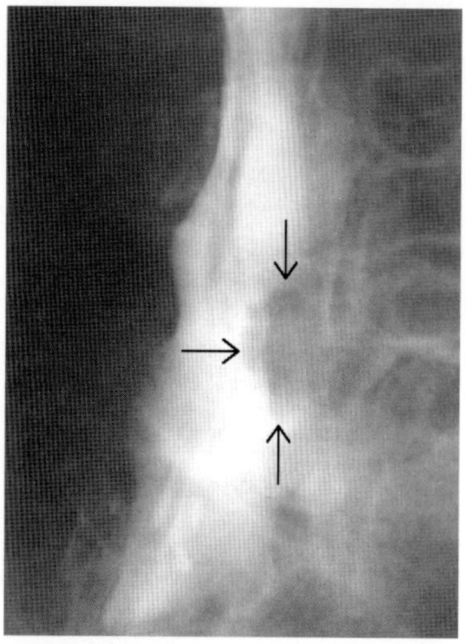

Fig. 9.**68** Lumbar myelography, oblique radiographic view. Intradural disk sequestrum at L4/L5.

MRI

Disk: The **nucleus pulposus** has increased signal intensity on T2-weighted images, but beginning at age 20 to 30 years, a stripe of decreased signal intensity develops centrally. The anulus fibrosus has decreased signal intensity on T1-weighted and T2-weighted images (Fig. 9.**69**). In the process of aging (degeneration), the entire disk shows a decrease in signal intensity and diminishes in height (Fig. 9.**71**). High-signal-intensity fluid can be found in the degenerated disk, and enhancement is seen after contrast administration (Figs. 9.**70**, 9.**71**). With progressive disk herniation, disk material, which is hypointense on T2-weighted images, extends posteriorly, anteriorly, inferiorly, or superiorly. The herniated material can remain connected to or become separated ('sequestered') from the original disk (Fig. 9.**73**).

Adjacent end plates: According to Modic, the marrow changes in the vertebral bodies adjacent to the end plates can be divided into three types:

- **Type I:** Pseudoinflammatory (sterile) edema, seen as increased signal intensity on T2-weighted images and enhancing after administration of contrast medium on T1-weighted images (Fig. 9.**72**).
- **Type II:** Fatty marrow replacement, characteristically seen as increased signal intensity on T1-weighted and T2-weighted images (Figs. 9.**72**, 9.**74**).
- **Type III:** Radiographically visible sclerosis, seen as decreased signal intensity on both T1-weighted and T2-weighted images.

Differentiating type I changes from an infectious process can be difficult. Other changes which favor degenerative disk disease, or extensive edema of the disk which is not seen with degeneration, can be helpful in the differential diagnosis (Fig. 9.**74**).

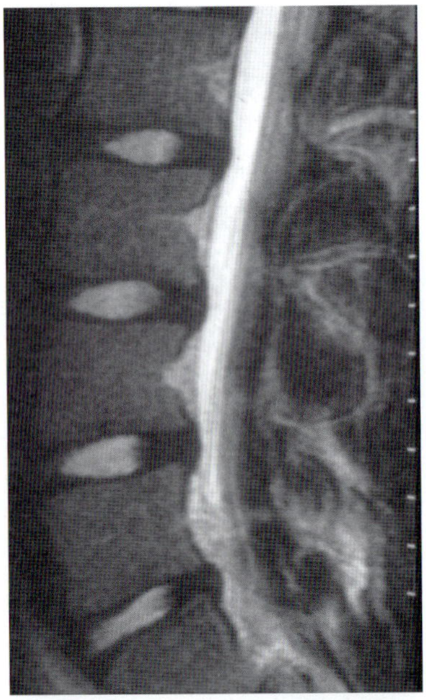

Fig. 9.**69** T2-weighted TSE image of a normal spine. The nucleus pulposus is clearly hyperintense and the anulus fibrosis hypointense.

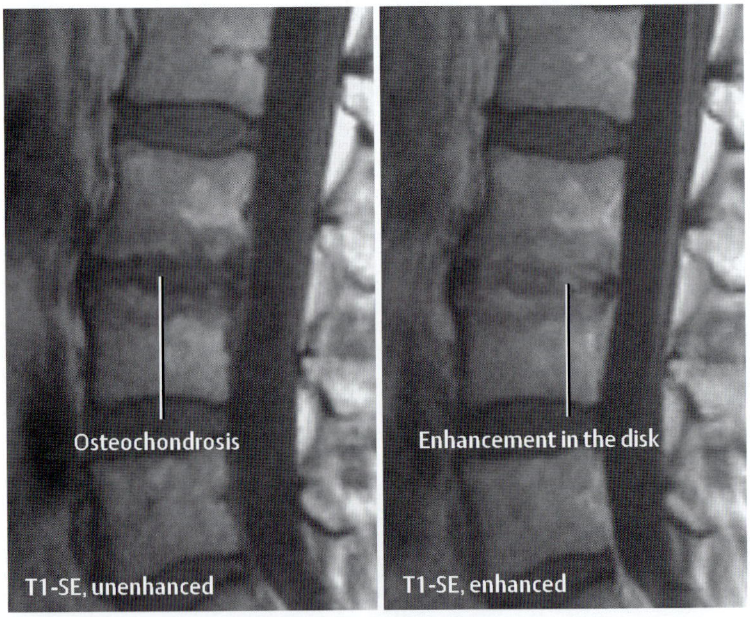

Fig. 9.**70** Extensive enhancement in the disk in osteochondrosis.

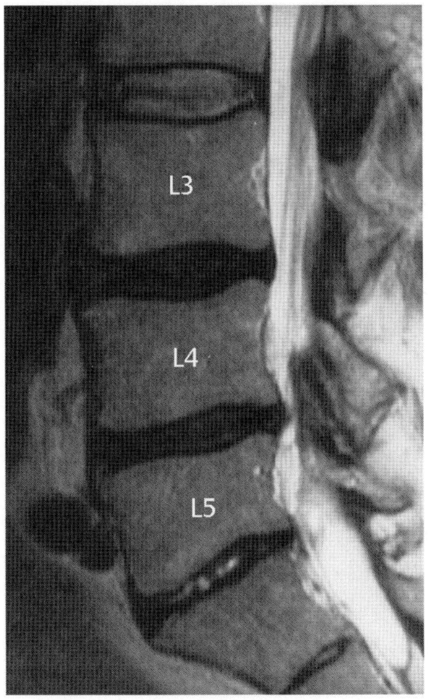

Fig. 9.**71** T2-weighted SE image at different stages of disk degeneration. L2/L3: normal disk; L3/L4 through L5/S1: decreased signal intensity due to dehydration and loss of height. The considerably degenerated disk at L5/S1 shows fluid within it.

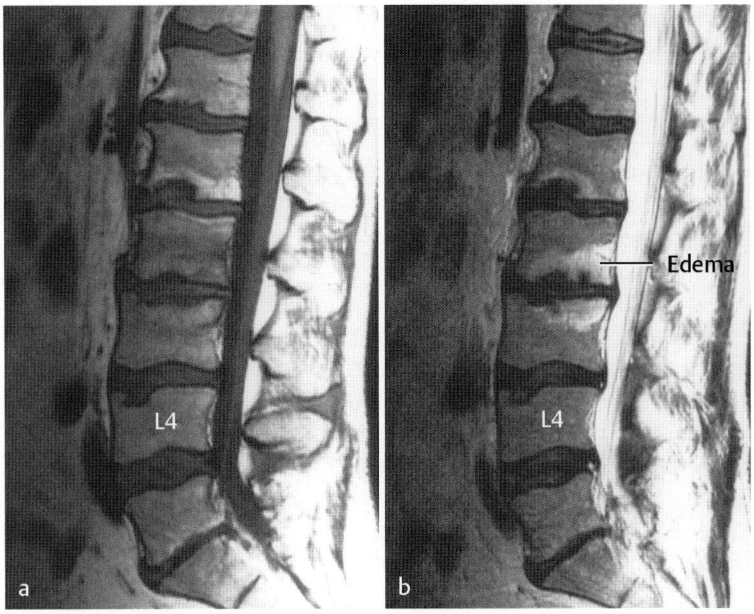

Fig. 9.**72** T1-weighted SE sequence (**a**) and T2-weighted TSE sequence (**b**) in disk degeneration and intraosseous disk herniations. The end plates along the L2/L3 segment are hyperintense on the T2-weighted image, corresponding to reactive edema (Modic I). The hyperintense zones in the other segments seen on the T1-weighted image correspond to marrow conversion (Modic II).

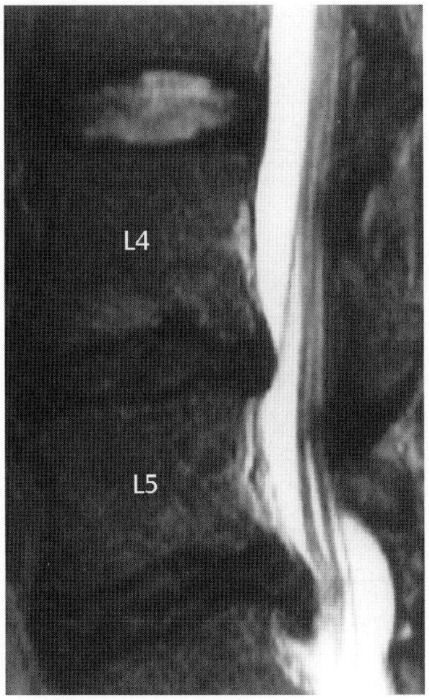

Fig. 9.**73** T2-weighted TSE sequence. Disk protrusion at L4/L5; disk prolapse L5/S1 with sequestration inferiorly and compression of the nerve roots (cauda equina).

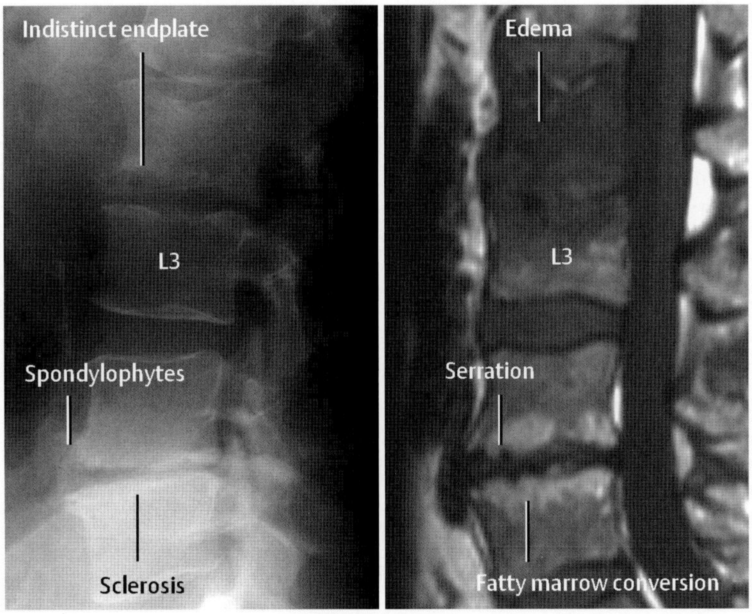

Fig. 9.**74** Co-existent spondylodiskitis at L2/L3 and osteochondrosis at L4/L5 on radiography and T1-weighted SE sequence. Typical features of intervertebral osteochondrosis with serration of the vertebral end plates and small erosions. In contradistinction to the spondylodiskitis, the adjacent areas of the vertebral body are hyperintense from fatty marrow conversion (Modic II changes).

Degeneration of the Intervertebral Articulations (Facet Joint Osteoarthritis)

X-RAY The cardinal findings are:
- joint space narrowing,
- subchondral sclerosis,
- marginal osteophytes,
- subchondral cyst formation,
- joint deformity.

In the upper lumbar spine, the facet joints are directed sagittally. They change direction superiorly and inferiorly, and assume an oblique direction in the lower lumbar spine and a frontal direction in the upper thoracic spine. Consequently, the AP projection displays the facet joints exclusively in the upper lumbar spine and the lateral projection exclusively in the upper thoracic spine.

Pseudospondylolisthesis is easily separable from spondylolisthesis in the lateral projection: the entire vertebral body slides anteriorly in the degenerative type, and the vertebral body alone moves, with posterior arch and spinous process left in place, in true spondylolisthesis. The spondylolysis of the true spondylolisthesis can be seen in oblique projections (Fig 9.**75**).

CT Extensive marginal osteophytes, reactive hypertrophy of the ligamentum flavum, possible ligamentous calcifications, and subchondral cysts are all well delineated on axial sections.
Spinal stenosis: Spinal stenosis is present if the lumbar spine measures less than 11 mm in sagittal diameter or the interpediculate distance is less than 16 mm. Slightly higher values fall into the 'gray area'. In general, the narrowing is most marked at the level of the intervertebral joints, with thickened ligamenta flava, osteophytes of the small vertebral joints, and disk material playing an important contributing role. The osseous component does not always prevail.

Encroachment (narrowing) of the recess and the intervertebral foramen should be assessed semi-quantitatively by comparison with the other side and the subjacent segment. A strictly quantitative assessment has not been proven useful.

MRI High-resolution MRI can directly visualize the articular cartilage with its characteristic degenerative changes as well as any accompanying joint effusion. Synovial cysts can be identified on the basis of their location and typical signal pattern (T1-weighted image: decreased signal intensity, T2-weighted image: increased signal intensity).

Direct visualization of the nerve, spinal cord, and articular outlines makes it possible to differentiate between compression of the spinal cord and of the nerves.

Advantages and Disadvantages of the Different Imaging Modalities in Degenerative Disease of the Spine with Neurologic Findings (Radiculopathy)

MRI

By taking advantage of multiplanar display (axial and sagittal) and by applying high-resolution coils and sequences that distinguish disk material from osseous structures, MRI can generally answer most questions concerning degenerative disk disease. It can also differentiate between scar tissue and recurrent prolapse. Therefore, this modality has become the primary diagnostic method today.

CT Myelography

Myelography combined with CT is comparable to MRI for diagnostic assessment of findings causing neurologic symptoms. Specific advantages are the direct visualization of spinal stenosis, nerve root compression, or indentation of the cord by osseous projections and soft-tissue masses. Moreover, if myelography is conducted as a functional test, any motion causing pain or other neurologic symptoms can be evaluated. Myelography with or without CT can be helpful by providing immediate diagnostic imaging, especially in the emergency situation.

CT

CT makes a valuable contribution to the morphologic evaluation of the spine and spinal canal even without intrathecal administration of contrast medium. However, artifacts can interfere with the clinical application of CT at the cervicothoracic junction. Any differentiation of the content of the spinal canal is limited.

Comments on Interpreting MRI, CT, and CT Myelography in Disk Diseases

- **No** morphologic criteria can differentiate between protrusion and prolapse. It is therefore preferable to refer to 'diskogenic narrowing' ('soft' material) as opposed to 'osseous narrowing' ('hard' material). This differentiation is also important from a therapeutic standpoint.
- It is a misconception that a sequestered fragment can invariably be detected or excluded.

The resolution of all imaging methods is still inadequate for this objective. In clinical practice it is adequate to suggest sequestered disk material above or below the level of the intervertebral disk space or within the intervertebral foramen.

- The location of the prolapse and sequestered fragment should be stated (Fig. 9.**76**):
  central,
  centrolateral,
  lateral (in the recess),
  intraforaminal/extraforaminal.
- The clinical findings, especially the level of the neurologic symptoms, should be known. Correlation between clinical (root) symptoms and the radiologic findings should be attempted, and the interpretation should address which root is 'compressed' or even obliterated by diskogenic or osseous tissue.
- The important differential diagnosis of a spinal tumor (especially since neurinomas and meningioma can be mistaken for a herniated disk) must be kept in mind. Above all, atypical clinical findings or an unusual nerve root level should always be considered suspect.

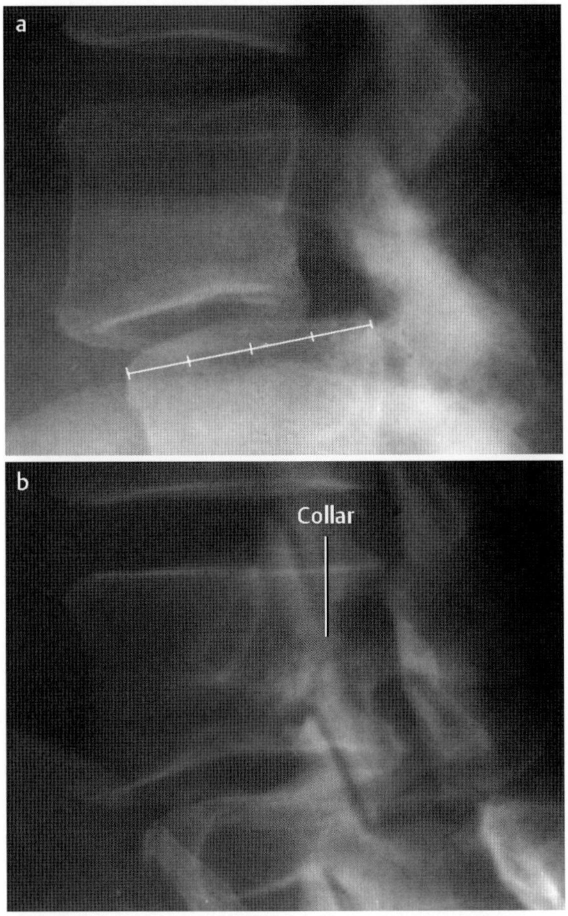

Fig. 9.**75** 'True' spondylolisthesis (spondylolysis with vertebral displacement). On the lateral radiograph (**a**), the degree of spondylolysis can be categorized (according to Meyerding):
The end plate of the vertebral bodies below the displaced vertebral body is divided into quarters. The anterior displacement of less than one quarter corresponds to Grade 1,
of ¼ to ½ to Grade 2,
of ½ to ¾ to Grade 3, and
of ¾ to 1 to Grade 4.
The oblique radiograph (**b**) shows the vertebral arches and displays the pars interarticularis defects ('collar around the neck of the Scotty dog').

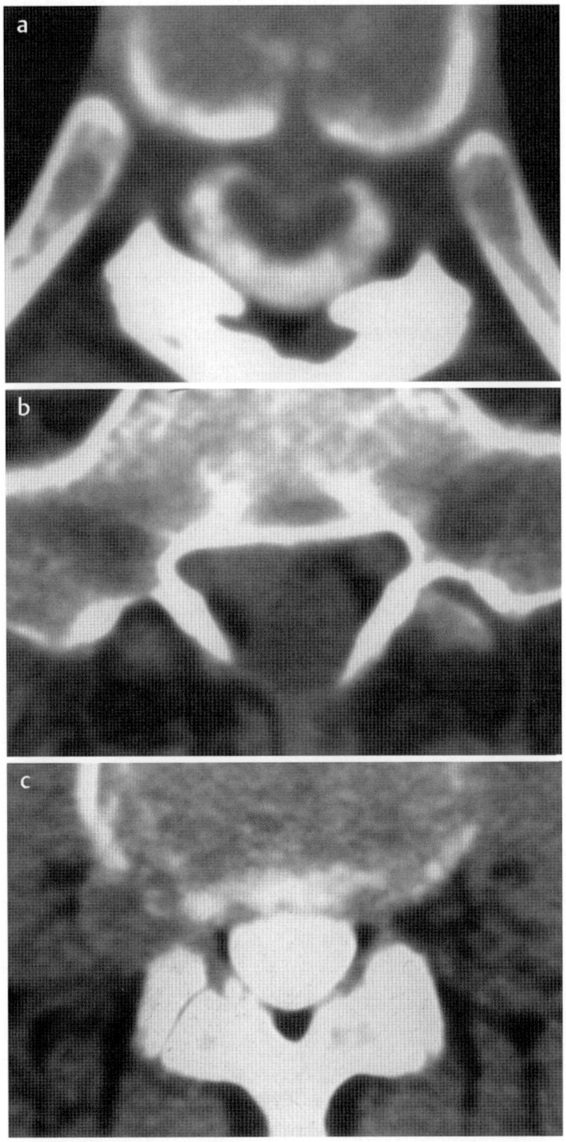

Fig. 9.**76** Locations of disk herniations. **a** central, **b** centrolateral, **c** extraforaminal, in this case with prolapse and liquefaction.

Diffuse Idiopathic Skeletal Hyperostosis (DISH, Forestier Disease)

■ According to Resnick, the following criteria have to be fulfilled to suggest a diagnosis of DISH:
- Flowing ossification, primarily involving the anterior longitudinal ligament, extending over at least four segments,
- No marked disk changes (osteochondrosis, prolapse),
- No significant osteoarthritis of the intervertebral and iliosacral joints. ■

CLINIC Patients are usually more than 50 years old and complain of progressive restricted motion of the cervical and lower thoracic spines. As with osteoarthritis, a striking discrepancy can exist between the severity of the clinical findings and radiographic features.

PATH The etiology of the skeletal changes is quite variable (diabetes mellitus combined with hyperinsulinemia, fluorosis, vitamin A excess, etc.). Characteristically, calcification and ossification occur in the region of the anterior longitudinal ligament (Fig. 9.**78**). About 30% of all patients with DISH show additional marked osteophytes at the peripheral joints and calcifications in the ligaments and tendons.

X-RAY There is extensive 'flowing' hyperostoses involving the anterior surface of at least four contiguous vertebral bodies, most commonly in the lower cervical spine and thoracolumbar transitions (Figs. 9.**77**, 9.**79**). Occasionally, a radiolucent line is seen between the ossification and the vertebral bodies, differentiating DISH from osteophytes. The intervertebral disks, sacroiliac joints, and intervertebral joints are generally unremarkable.

Complications of DISH

Myelopathy: Deformity and narrowing of the spinal canal produced by the ligamentous ossifications (posterior longitudinal ligament, ligamenta flava) can cause myelopathy. Although compression of the spinal cord can be directly visualized by CT, direct visualization of the myelopathy requires MRI (increased signal intensity on T2-weighted images and enhancement).

The ligamentous ossifications render the spine rigid and make it vulnerable to trauma. These ligamentous ossifications can fracture.

Glossary

Scoliosis: This is a **fixed** axial deviation of the spine in the frontal plane with rotational component and is a **clinical** diagnosis. Radiographically, this finding should only be referred to as 'scoliotic deformity'.

The idiopathic type of scoliosis predominates and is divided into infantile, juvenile, and adolescent types. A number of other secondary causes (e.g., spinal cord damage, rheumatic diseases, infections) need to be distinguished from these types.

Scoliosis is measured clinically and radiographically (curvature angle according to Cobb and rotation angle according to Nash and Moe; see the orthopedic literature for further details).

Kyphosis: Kyphosis is a dorsal convex deviation of the spine in the sagittal plane in excess of the normal curvature. Measurement methods have been proposed to quantify kyphosis. Besides Scheuermann disease, most kyphoses are caused by trauma, osteoporosis, or inflammation.

Scheuermann disease (Synonyms: adolescent kyphosis, juvenile kyphosis): The cardinal feature of Scheuermann disease is kyphosis of the thoracic spine. It is not known why the kyphosis develops in children and adolescents (< 5%). Dihlmann assumes a constitutional vertebral deficiency of the cartilaginous end plates and disk. Only about one-third of patients complain of back pain. Radiographic features (Fig. 9.**81**):
- kyphosis of the thoracic spine,
- wedge-shaped vertebral bodies with or without shortening of the sagittal diameter,
- irregular end plates with or without Schmorl's nodes, which occur in the center or anterior portion of the end plates,
- compensatory hyperostosis adjacent to Schmorl's nodes (in Europe known as 'Edgren-Vaino sign'),
- anterior loss of height of the intervertebral disk space.

! Schmorl's nodes occur in the center or in the anterior aspect of the end plate. The so-called cord remnant (= normal variant, Fig. 9.**82**) is located posteriorly and exhibits a shallower indentation.

Retromarginal disk prolapse ('limbus vertebra'): Before fusion of the osseous ring epiphysis, disk material can extend between it and the vertebral body. Thus, the retromarginal disk prolapse is a Schmorl's node at a different location.

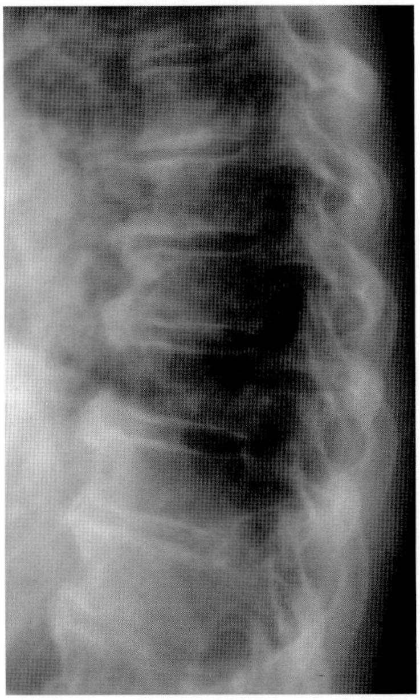

Fig. 9.77 Lower thoracic spine with anterior osteophyte formation in DISH. The disk spaces are unremarkable.

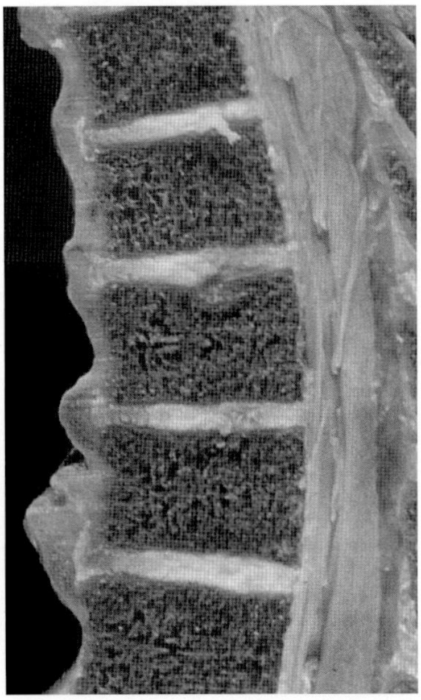

Fig. 9.78 Anatomic specimen. Anterior longitudinal ligament ossification in DISH.

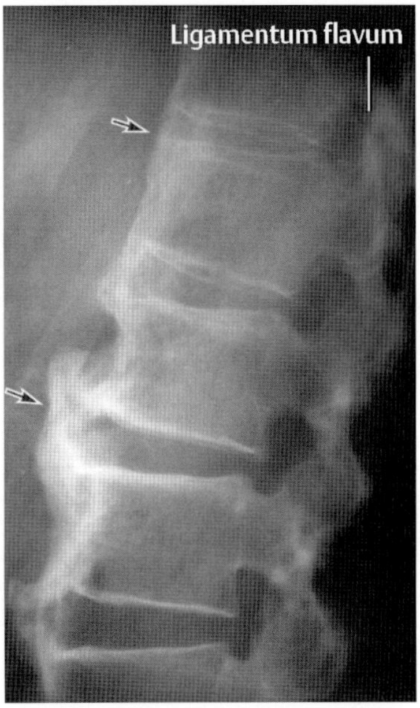

Fig. 9.79 Thoracolumbar transition. Aside from anterior osteophyte formation in DISH, calcification of the ligamenta flava.

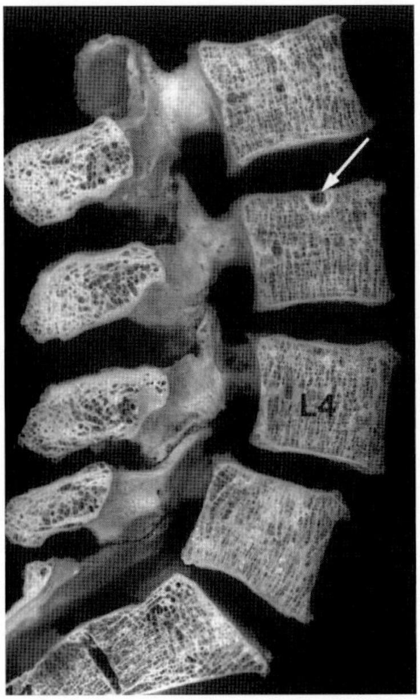

Fig. 9.80 Anatomic specimen of a typical centrally located Schmorl's node. In addition, anterior displacement of the entire L4 vertebra on L5 (pseudospondylolisthesis), Grade I.

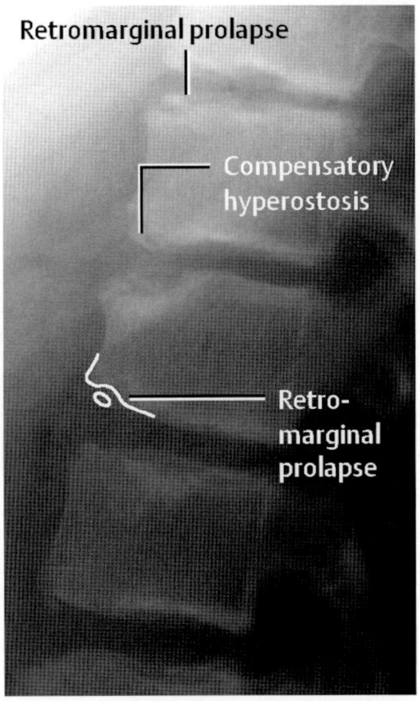

Fig. 9.81 Scheuermann disease with multiple anteriorly located Schmorl's nodes and subtle wedge deformity of the lower thoracic vertebral bodies.

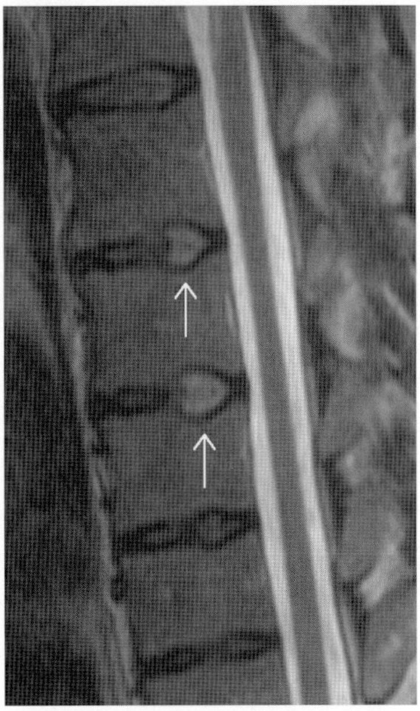

Fig. 9.82 Incomplete evolution of the chorda ('cord remnant'), T2-weighted TSE sequence. The defects are in the dorsal aspect of the vertebral end plates and are shallower than Schmorl's nodes.

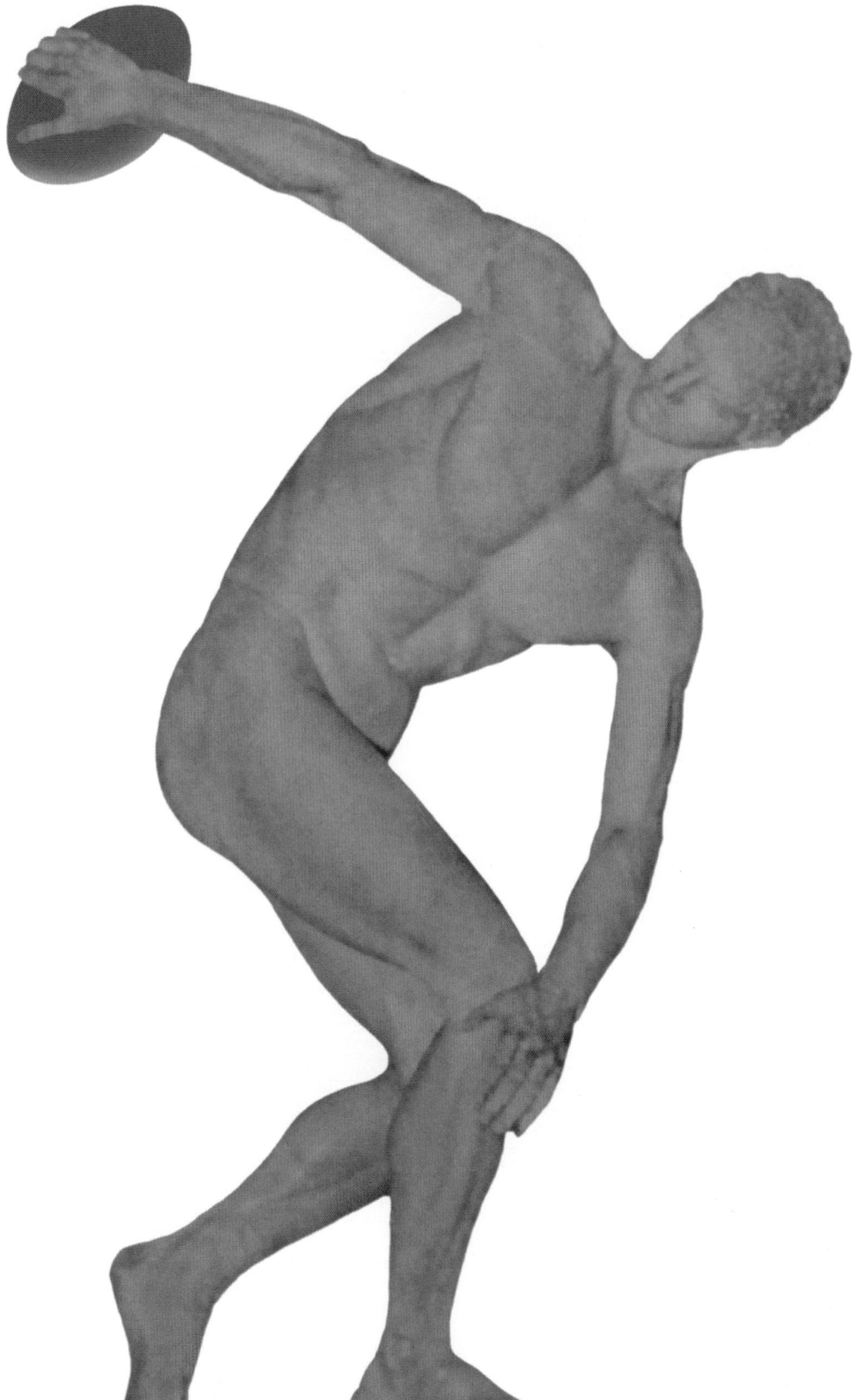

Inflammatory Joint Diseases

Classification of the Arthritides

The exact etiology of the various forms of arthritis is still unknown and is reflected in an incoherent and often confusing nomenclature and classification. Furthermore, the assignment of clinical findings to a disease entity, especially in early stages, is often quite conjectural. What has been established is the differentiation between infectious (e.g., 'bacterial,' 'pyogenic,' 'septic') arthritis and arthritis caused by inflammation as a manifestation of an immunopathologic process without detectable causative organism (e.g., rheumatoid arthritis and related diseases). Based on the current scientific and empirical state of the art, the following categorization is used:

1. **Infectious Arthritis and Spondylitis (Diskitis)**
   The inflammation is caused by organisms (usually bacteria) that enter the joint from perforation of the skin, from direct spread from soft-tissue infection, or from the blood.
2. **Rheumatoid Arthritis**
   This is a systemic inflammatory disease of the connective tissue consisting primarily of a polyarthritis, but also has extra-articular manifestations such as inflammations of the bursae, tendon sheaths, vessels, and internal organs. In more than 70%–80% of cases the serum rheumatoid factor is present ('seropositive rheumatoid arthritis').
3. **Seronegative Spondyloarthropathy**
   This is an inflammatory condition with characteristic involvement of the axial skeleton, peripheral arthritis, and various extra-articular manifestations. The rheumatoid factor is not present, but there is a strong association with the HLA-B27 antigen. The group of seronegative spondyloarthropathies includes:
   - ankylosing spondylitis (Bekhterev disease),
   - reactive arthritis (special type: Reiter syndrome),
   - psoriatic arthropathy,
   - enteropathic arthropathy.

   In addition to the arthritic changes, these conditions are characterized by **enthesopathies** with often characteristic radiographic features.
4. **Inflammatory Systemic Connective Tissue Diseases**
   This is a group of diseases associated with noninfectious inflammation of the connective tissues. Articular involvement is one of many clinical symptoms and often is a minor feature. This group of diseases includes:
   - systemic lupus erythematosus,
   - progressive systemic sclerosis (scleroderma),
   - polymyositis and dermatomyositis,
   - vasculitis (above all, polyarteritis nodosa),
   - mixed collagenosis,
   - nonclassifiable overlapping syndromes.

! There is believed to be a genetic predisposition to these noninfectious forms of arthritis because of the presence of certain tissue antigens (HLA antigens). An infection is suspected to initiate the disease in many of these patients (= 'promoter effect' of the infection acting on the respective genetic disposition).

Special Problems

Juvenile Chronic Arthritis

This arthritis, found in childhood and adolescence, cannot be classified with the groups mentioned above. Juvenile rheumatoid arthritis and juvenile spondyloarthropathy are to be considered separate entities.

Lyme Arthritis

This arthritis follows a tick bite and is caused by an indolent infection with *Borrelia.* The organism can often be detected in joint fluid and the periarticular tissues. The joint damage caused by the organism is pathogenetically less toxic than the autoimmune reaction that is induced. There is no association with the HLA-B27 antigen.

Rheumatic Fever

This is an autoimmune disease of childhood that occurs 2 to 4 weeks after a streptococcal infection. The cardinal sign of this disorder is a polyarthritis with large joint involvement, although endocarditis, subcutaneous nodules, and, less frequently, erythema nodosum and chorea minor may be present. Typically, the arthritic location is fluctuating, but the legs are usually involved first. The exact pathologic mechanism of the disease is still undetermined.

HIV-associated Arthritis

HIV infection can cause an arthritis in several ways: organisms within the joint, associated autoimmune reaction, or opportunistic infection with septic arthritis.

Infectious Arthritis, Spondylitis, and Spondylodiskitis

Bacterial Arthritis

PATH The infection results from intra-articular organisms that can enter the joint through various routes:
- penetration (injection, surgery, injury),
- direct spreading from soft-tissue infection or osteomyelitis, or
- hematogenous seeding in bacteremia.

Direct spreading of infection from metaphyseal osteomyelitis is extremely rare during the growth period, since the cartilage growth plate acts as an effective barrier to bacterial spreading. In infancy and adulthood after closure of the growth plate, however, epiphyseal vascular connections exist, and these may facilitate intra-articular extension of the infection.

! Intra-articular injection is the commonest cause of bacterial arthritis.

The most common infecting organism is *Staphylococcus aureus* (more than 60%), followed by *Pseudomonas* (15%), streptococci, enterococci, salmonellae, and *Haemophilus influenza.* Fungal and viral arthritis is rare.

Patients with rheumatoid arthritis, diabetes mellitus, peripheral neuropathy, or peripheral vascular disease, as well as patients with an immune defect, are predisposed to bacterial arthritis. In the immunocompromised host the entire spectrum of opportunistic infection may be seen.

CLINIC **Symptoms:** The typical findings of an acute localized arthritis (redness, heat, swelling, pain, and restricted range of motion) are commonly seen. Signs of sepsis (general malaise, fever, chills, obtundation) may also be observed. When several joints are involved, the symptoms generally appear sequentially, a fact that is relevant in the differential diagnosis.

Distribution pattern: This disorder is generally monoarticular but rarely can be oligoarticular. Any joint can be involved.

Course and prognosis: Septic arthritis will rapidly cause massive joint destruction if not treated promptly.

X-RAY Osseous changes are not to be expected in the early stage of infectious arthritis. The major radiographic findings are confined to soft-tissue swelling (Fig. 9.**83**) and possible joint-space widening (effusion). Juxta-articular osteoporosis can be detected about 10 to 14 days later and is followed by joint-space narrowing (Fig. 9.**85**).

The subsequent course brings out the classic arthritic changes, such as erosions and subluxation, which are described on pages 294–298. The distinctive feature of a bacterial arthritis is the unusually rapid progression of massive destruction of osseous structures of the joint. The final stage is ankylosis.

SI Joints:

The cardinal feature is joint-space **widening** in the presence of **indistinct** articular contours.

Caution! In childhood, the SI joints are physiologically wide, and looking for any asymmetry is crucial. Cross-sectional imaging (CT, MRI) is especially valuable.

SONO The cardinal finding is an effusion that can be echo-free, but can also be hyperechoic in empyema, which may also exhibit air bubbles (Fig. 9.**84**).

! Depending on the echogenicity, effusion and thickened synovial linings often are indistinguishable. The use of Doppler ultrasonography may be helpful in this situation.

Sonography can also be used to guide joint aspiration.

CT Erosions can be detected on both sides of the joint with a high degree of sensitivity and can confirm the diagnosis of an advanced articular process. The definitive diagnosis of an **infection** can be made if:
1. an abscess is detected,
2. **all** of the osseous structures of the joint are 'equally' affected (e.g., sacroiliac joint).

Special target areas for CT: sternoclavicular joint, temporomandibular joint, sacroiliac joint.

MRI The cardinal findings are an effusion and a strongly enhancing synovial lining (Figs. 9.**83**, 9.**84**). On MRI, the adjacent subchondral bone marrow shows edema, especially on the STIR sequence, very early in the disease process (Fig. 9.**87 b**).

! Remember that edema in the adjacent bone does not prove osteomyelitis.

MRI is especially valuable for anatomic sites with a complex topography (temporomandibular joint, sternoclavicular joint, sacroiliac joint, tarsal joints). Moreover, it can detect accompanying abscesses.

DD There are no radiographic features that prove the **infectious** origin of an arthritis.

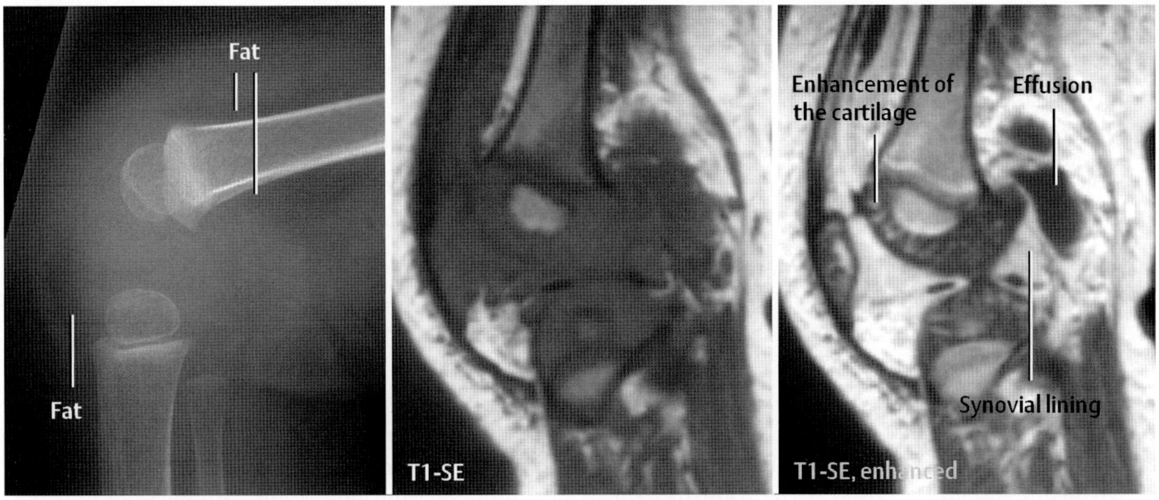

Fig. 9.**83** Tuberculosis of the knee in a 1-year-old child. The radiograph shows pronounced soft-tissue swelling around the joint. MRI (T1-weighted SE sequence before and after administration of contrast medium) allows the differentiation between massively thickened synovial lining and joint effusion.

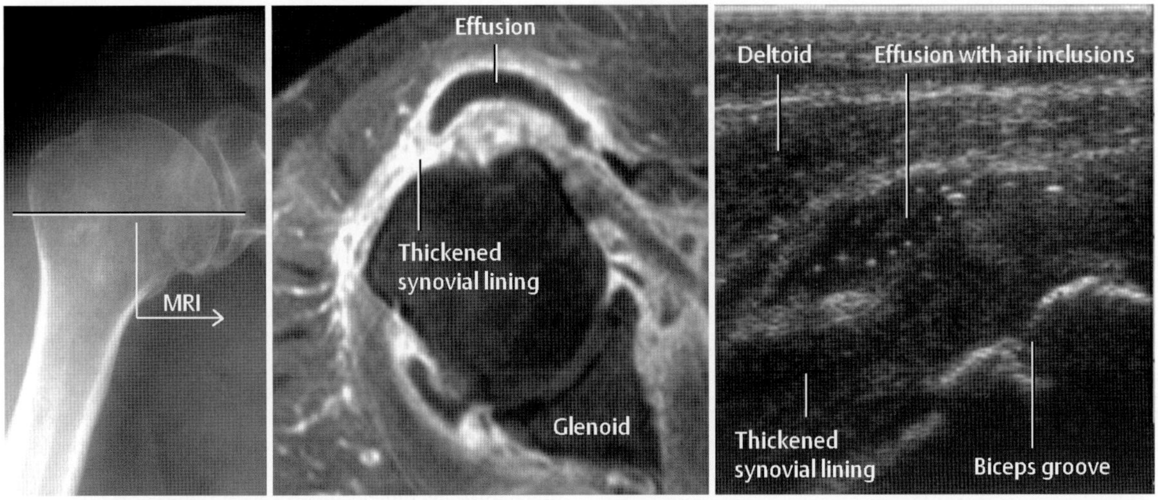

Fig. 9.**84** Empyema of the shoulder. The comparison between axial MRI (T1-SE sequence with fat suppression, after administration of contrast medium) and sonography reveals the relatively poor sonographic discrimination between effusion (with air bubbles) and pannus. The effusion here is relatively small in comparison to the massive synovial proliferation.

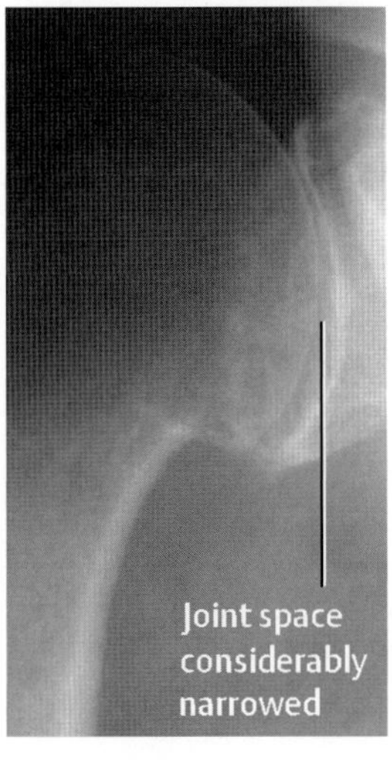

Fig. 9.**85** Shoulder joint of the patient of Fig. 9.**84** 4 weeks later. Marked joint-space narrowing is due to cartilage destruction.

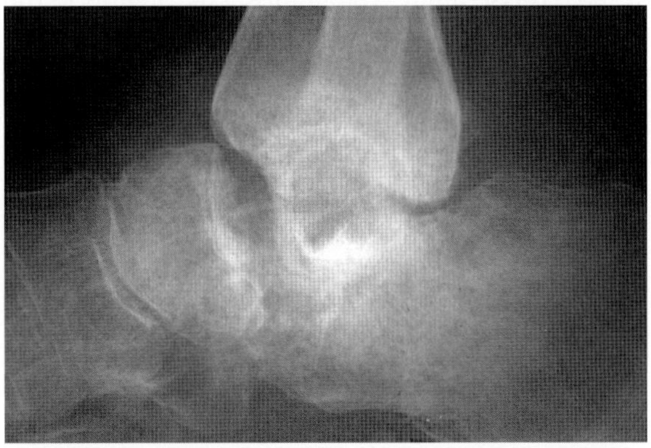

Fig. 9.**86** Tuberculous arthritis of the tibiotalar articulation. Note the complete destruction of the joint.

! Any acute monoarthritis should initially be suspected to be bacterial in origin. Since it is mandatory to initiate therapy before osseous changes become apparent, a diagnostic aspiration of any suspicious joint should be performed immediately.

- Acute monoarthritis quite frequently is the first manifestation of gout in males. The typical location and laboratory parameters will generally provide clues to this diagnosis.
- Special diagnostic problems are caused by bacterial arthritis superimposed on a preceding joint disease, in particular rheumatoid arthritis. The suspicion should be raised if the joint destruction is disproportionately rapid, or if the clinical and radiologic findings are confined to one joint and do not match the overall disease pattern. Again, the joint must be aspirated early.
- The question is frequently raised as to whether osteomyelitis or septic arthritis is present in a joint. Osteomyelitis arises in a **single** bone; therefore, if **one** of the joint-forming bones is heavily destroyed and the other is unremarkable, then osteomyelitis is likely. Septic arthritis, in contrast, destroys both articulating bones more-or-less simultaneously.
- The differential diagnosis of the symptomatic hip in children or adolescents includes:
  transient synovitis ('coxitis fugax', usually differentiated from bacterial arthritis clinically or by the aspirated joint fluid),
  traumatic hemarthrosis (puncture),
  early stage of Legg-Calvé-Perthes disease (differentiation with MRI).

Special Manifestation: Tuberculous Arthritis

Skeletal tuberculosis has a predilection for the spine (tuberculous spondylitis, see below), the weight-bearing joints (knee, hip and ankle, Figs. 9.**83**, 9.**86**), and, with moderate frequency, the carpal and tarsal joints. In contrast to bacterial arthritis, tuberculous arthritis follows a protracted course and develops radiographic changes over months.

The radiographic differentiation of tuberculosis from septic bacterial arthritis is difficult (Table 9.**4**). Occasionally, extensive 'cyst formation' from granulomas occurs in the juxta-articular osseous structures. In fact, in the hand, the radiographic features may resemble the cystic type of sarcoidosis. Sarcoidosis, however, has a preference for metacarpal and phalangeal involvement.

Table 9.**4** Pyogenic versus tuberculous arthritis. Unreliable (!) differentiating criteria

	Tuberculous	Pyogenic
Clinical course	slow	acute
Juxta-articular osteoporosis	+++	+
Joint-space narrowing	+ (late)	+ (early)
Erosions	+ (late)	+
Juxta-articular osteosclerosis	(+)	+

Special Type: Echinococcal Arthritis

This arthritis is dominated by large cystic lesions in the joint-bearing bones, which may contain calcifications. *Echinococcus* should be considered in patients from sheep- and cattle-raising areas, especially in patients from countries around the Mediterranean (Fig. 9.**90**).

Infectious Spondylitis and Spondylodiskitis

Synonym: Pott disease = tuberculous spondylitis.

PATH The route of infection is usually hematogenous but less frequently iatrogenic in origin. As in the peripheral skeleton, infections in the spine are most frequently caused by staphylococci and gram-negative organisms. However, tuberculosis is also a common organism in the spine. In patients with sickle cell anemia and diabetes, salmonellosis must also be considered. The infection begins at the anterior and lateral aspect of **one** vertebral body adjacent to the end plate. In this stage **('spondylitis'),** the avascular disk is excluded from the inflammatory process. The process then extends to the disk **('spondylodiscitis')** and adjacent vertebral body. The mechanism by which the process progresses is not entirely understood. Based on our own observation, this process depends to a large extent on the disk and whether it is intact or degenerate (osteochondrosis). The revascularization found in degenerative disks may be the route of spread (Fig. 9.**91**).

Because the vascular supply in children is different, the primary site of infection in this setting can be both in the disk ('diskitis') and in the bone as a primary spondylitis (Fig. 9.**88**).

CLINIC In the acute setting, the major the complaint is local spinal pain (often as dull pain, mostly at night) with corresponding spinal rigidity and generalized malaise and fever. However, the condition may follow a chronic course with less severe systemic symptoms. These cases often are diagnosed late, since the clinician has to take into consideration the entire spectrum of diseases that are associated with spinal pain. Tuberculous spondylitis, in particular, progresses for months to years and is often detected late in its course. Abscess formation or collapse of the affected vertebrae can produce neurologic deficits and even paraplegia.

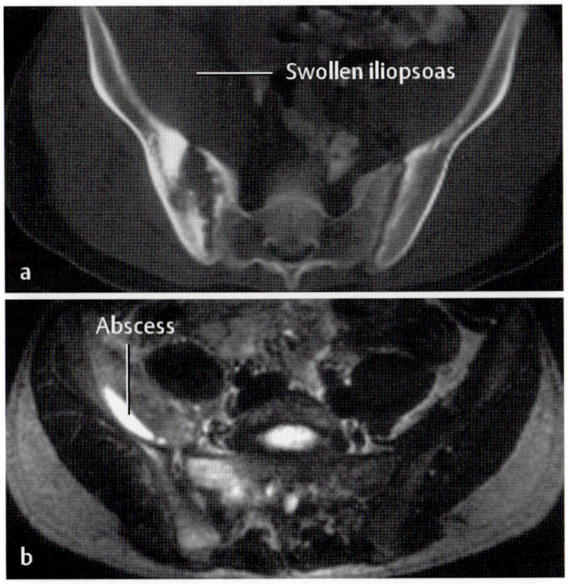

Fig. 9.**87** Sacroiliitis on the left with considerable osseous destruction. **a** CT. **b** MRI (T2-weighted SE sequence) shows the accompanying bone marrow edema and a joint effusion.

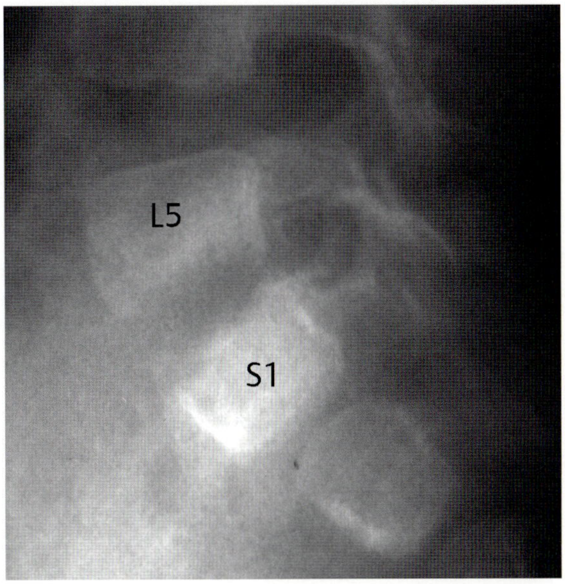

Fig. 9.**88** Spondylodiskitis at L5/S1 in a child. The markedly indistinct end plates indicate a rather advanced state.

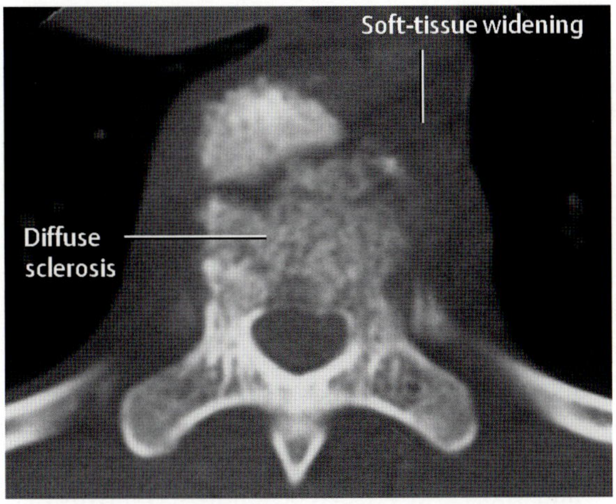

Fig. 9.**89** Tuberculous spondylodiskitis with destruction of the T9 vertebral body. Notice the severe paraspinal soft-tissue widening.

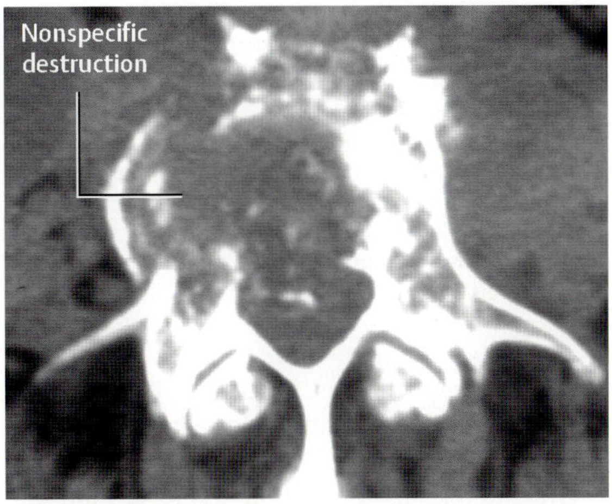

Fig. 9.**90** Echinococcosis. The 'cystic' aspect is absent, and the finding is nonspecific.

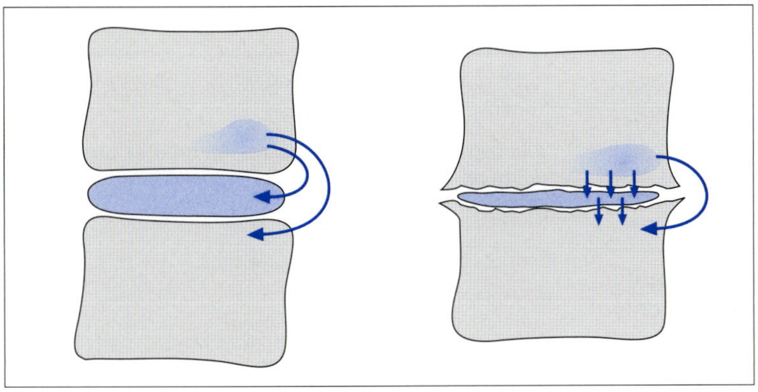

Fig. 9.**91** Bacterial spreading in spondylitis related to the degree of disk degeneration: in contrast to the degenerate disk, the healthy disk may represent a barrier.

Distribution pattern: The entire spine can be affected, but **bacterial** spondylitis tends to involve the lumbar spine and **tuberculous** spondylitis the lower thoracic spine.

X-RAY In the early stages, spinal infection might cause changes only in the soft tissue, and it is therefore crucial to evaluate the paravertebral lines and psoas margin.

Radiographic signs are detected only 3 – 8 weeks after the onset of clinical findings and the younger the patient, the earlier:
- indistinct vertebral end plates,
- narrowing of the intervertebral disk space,
- contour defects of the end plates,
- vertebral destruction followed by collapse,
- reactive sclerosis,
- gibbus formation (secondary finding).

! Narrowing of a single intervertebral disk space without accompanying reactive changes is suspicious for a spondylitis. This is especially applicable to children and adolescents, since other causes of disk-space narrowing (especially degeneration) are extremely unusual in this age group.

NUC The three-phase Tc 99 m bone scan shows very intense uptake. Though this is a nonspecific finding, it supports the diagnosis when a solitary focus involves only one vertebral segment. The bone scan is very sensitive, and determining the anatomic location can be improved with the help of single photon emission computed tomography (SPECT).

CT The changes correspond to the radiographic findings described above and are easily recognized on sagittal reformation. Additional findings can be:
- circumferential granulation tissue around the vertebral body with enhancement,
- paravertebral abscesses,
- extension of inflammatory tissue into the epidural space,
- hypodense disk.

! A vacuum phenomenon (classic sign of degeneration) does not by itself exclude infection.

! CT-guided biopsy is the best method to identify the causative organism, but it is successful in only about 50% of cases.

MRI MRI has become the method of choice for timely diagnosis, for differentiation of infection from other pathologic processes (osteochondrosis, tumors), and for planning the therapeutic approach (conservative versus surgical intervention).

MRI may show any of the following findings (Figs. 9.**92** – 9.**94**):
- edema in one or several vertebral bodies, less frequently also in the disk (STIR sequence, T1-weighted SE sequence).
- inflammatory tissue enhancement (exception: abscesses).
- abscesses (epidural, paravertebral, intradiskal) show increased signal intensity (T2-weighted FSE sequence) and enhancement only of the surrounding rim.
- depending on preceding damage, the disk is irregular in signal intensity.

! Detection (or exclusion) of an epidural abscess is critical, since an epidural abscess, depending on size, is an indication for surgical intervention.

DD
- Involvement of more than two adjacent vertebral bodies is suggestive of tuberculosis. A definitive differentiation between tuberculous and bacterial spondylitis, however, is not possible by imaging (Table 9.**5**).
- Disk involvement occurs late in metastasis since the tumor spreads to the soft tissues. Tumor exerts a well-differentiated 'space-occupying' effect, while infection causes a more 'diffuse' effect.
- Differentiating osteochondrosis type 1 from spondylodiskitis is difficult with radiography and MRI. However, osteochondrosis is always associated with a narrowed intervertebral disk space and sclerosis of the end plates.

Table 9.**5** Findings suggesting tuberculosis as cause of a spondylodiskitis

- Large paravertebral abscess (with or without calcifications)
- Subligamentous extension across more than one disk segment
- Thoracic involvement
- Spondylitis without disk involvement
- Kyphosis (gibbus deformity)
- Diffuse osteosclerosis ('eburnation') of the vertebral body with concomitant osteolytic destruction

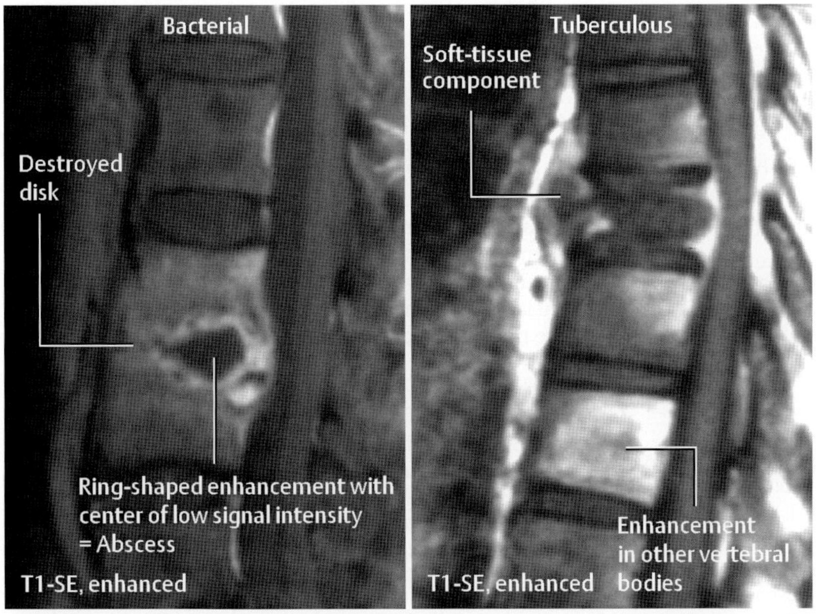

Fig. 9.**92** Comparison of a bacterial (left, **lumbar**) and a tuberculous (right, **thoracic**) spondylodiskitis. The bacterial type is confined to two adjacent vertebral bodies and includes the destruction of the intervening disk. In this particular case, an abscess is also present. The tuberculous spondylodiskitis affects several vertebral bodies, and the disk spaces are almost preserved. There is typically a large soft-tissue component.

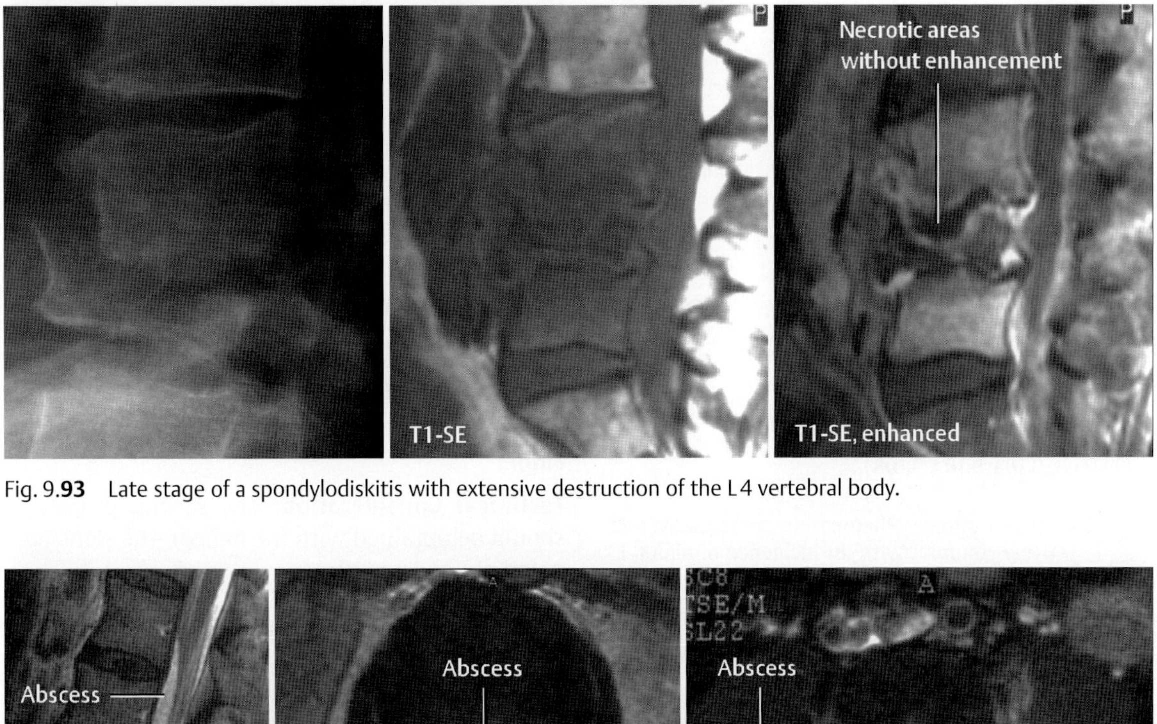

Fig. 9.**93** Late stage of a spondylodiskitis with extensive destruction of the L 4 vertebral body.

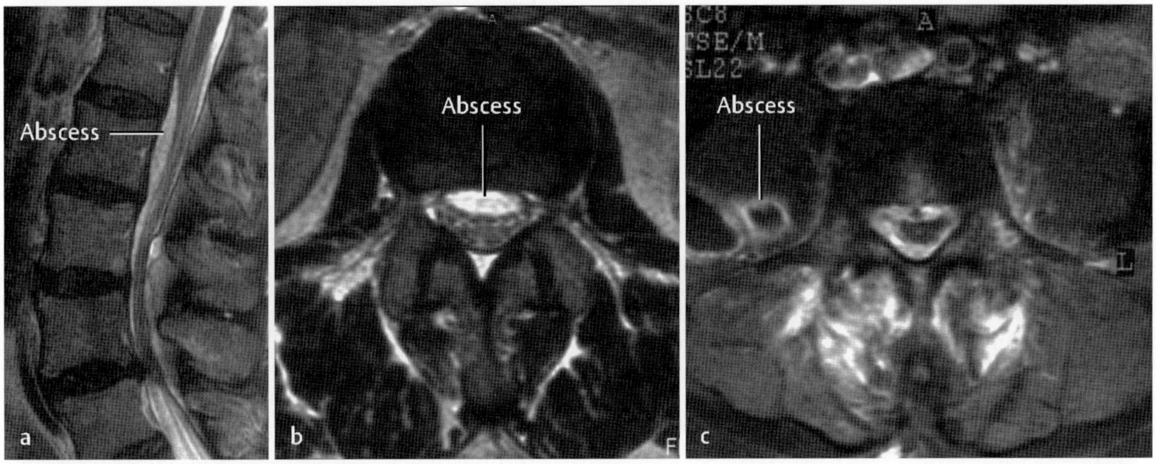

Fig. 9.**94** Complication of spondylodiskitis: epidural and psoas abscesses (**a**, **b** sagittal and axial T2-weighted TSE images, **c** T1-weighted TSE image with fat suppression after administration of contrast medium).

Rheumatoid Arthritis

Synonym: Chronic polyarthritis.

Rheumatoid arthritis is clinically and histologically an inflammatory systemic connective tissue disease of undetermined etiology, with chronic joint involvement (synovitis), systemic symptoms and frequent involvement of tendon sheaths, bursae, vessels, serous membranes, eyes and internal organs. Manifestations of individual organs characterize special forms of rheumatoid arthritis.

PATH In the presence of a susceptible genetic predisposition (HLA-D antigen), contact with arthrotropic organisms (parvoviruses and lentiviruses have been identified so far) induces proliferation of the T4 helper cells and a cytokine-mediated oligoclonal B cell stimulation with release of IgG and IgM autoantibodies – the so-called **rheumatoid factors.** These primarily initiate the synovitis – mediated, among other interactions, by complement activation.

The reactive pannus creeps across the cartilage and undermines it. The result is a more severe destruction than seen in other forms of arthritis ('tumor-like').

Synovial cysts and sinus tracts:
These are caused by increased intra-articular pressure. Joint decompression can occur through three potential pathways (Fig. 9.**95**):

1. Extension through the subchondral bone plate with formation of subchondral cysts,
2. Herniation of the synovial membrane with the formation of synovial cysts,
3. Extension through the synovial membrane with the formation of cutaneous joint sinus tracts.

Synovial cysts arise most frequently at the knee (Baker cyst), but are also found at the shoulder, hip, elbow, and ankle (Figs. 9.**103**, 9.**107**, 9.**108**).

CLINIC **Epidemiology:** Rheumatoid arthritis is relatively common with an incidence of about 1% of the population. It usually begins between the ages of 25 and 55 and women are affected three times more often than men. The reason for this female predilection is unknown.

Symptoms: The onset is insidious in about 70% of cases and occurs over weeks to months. The major prodromal symptoms are fatigue, weight loss and subfebrile temperature elevation. In 30% of cases, an acute or subacute onset follows within several days to weeks.

Subsequently, specific symptoms of rheumatoid arthritis occur, but the clinical course may be quite variable. Because of this difficulty, diagnostic criteria have been proposed by the American Rheumatology Association (ARA Criteria, Table 9.**6**).

Distribution Pattern: The disease generally begins symmetrically at several metacarpophalangeal and metatarsophalangeal joints and at the proximal interphalangeal joints of fingers and toes. Carpal articulations and tendon sheaths are also involved early. A typical finding is the synovitis of the extensor carpi ulnaris, which often produces an indolent swelling along the ulnar aspect of the wrist.

Rheumatoid arthritis can be confined to the peripheral joints for a long time, but sooner or later a **centripetal spread** results and involvement of the larger joints (ankle, knee, elbow, shoulder and hip), spine and the articulations of the occipito-cervical transition develop.

Rheumatoid arthritis frequently involves the **cervical spine** (30%) and is predominately present in the cranial segment. In about 40 – 60% of cases, neurologic symptoms occur, primarily pain, stiffness, paresthesias and palsies. Quadriplegia and death secondary to respiratory arrest are rare but reported complications.

Course and Prognosis:
- In 10 – 15% of patients the course is mild with partial or complete remission.
- In 70 – 80% of patients a more or less rapid progression occurs, without intermittent remission, up to severe immobilization,
- In 10 – 15% of patients the disease process is very severe and rapidly destructive.

Special Clinical Course of the Disease with Onset after the Age of 60.
Joint stiffness is considerably more pronounced and patients often become totally immobile within a short period. The clinical onset resembles polymyalgia rheumatica and is observed four times more frequently than in young patients. However, the disease tends to follow a milder course and, despite the immobility, the mutilating joint changes are less frequent. Moreover, rheumatoid nodules occur less frequently.

X-RAY The common radiographic features of arthritis were presented on pages 293 – 297. The following sections address the manifestation of rheumatoid arthritis at specific locations.

Finger

Technical Consideration: The second projection should be obtained with the hand in the semi-pronated oblique position.

Early abnormalities:
- Involvement of the **metacarpophalangeal** articulations (in particular, radial aspect of the second and third rays) and the **proximal interphalangeal** articulations (in particular, radial and ulnar aspects of the third rays) with later and less severe involvement of the distal interphalangeal articulations.

Late abnormalities:
- Characteristic deformities caused by inflammatory damage of the ligaments: **ulnar deviation** of the metacarpal-phalangeal articulation, **boutonnière deformity** (flexion of the proximal interphalangeal articulation and hyperextension of the distal interphalangeal articulation, Fig. 9.**96**), **swan-neck deformity** (flexion of the metacarpophalangeal and distal interphalangeal

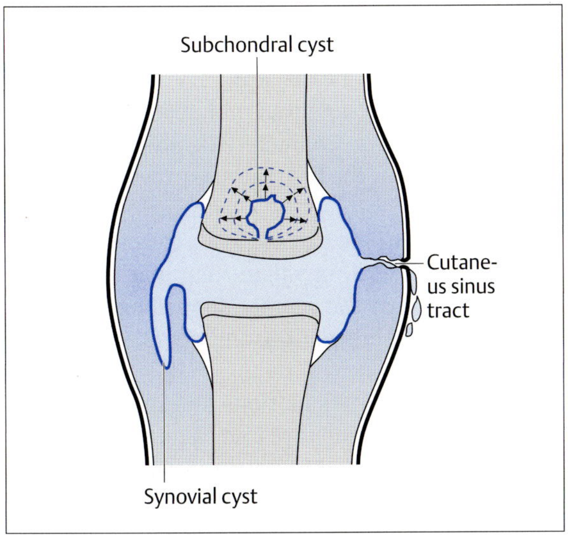

Fig. 9.**95** Mechanism of decompression of synovial joints with increased intra-articular pressure (according to Resnick).

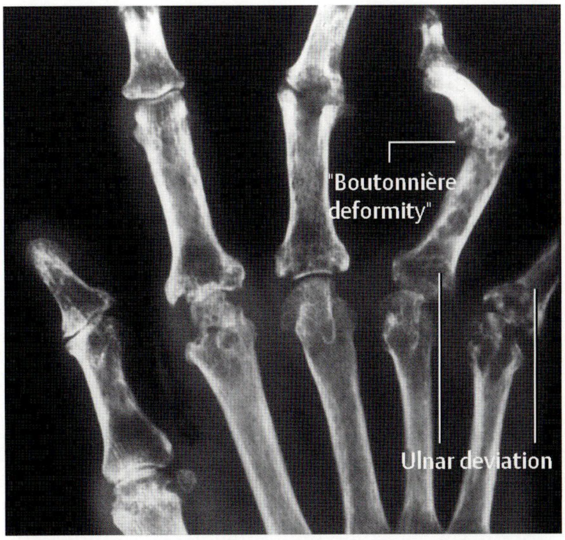

Fig. 9.**96** Late stage of hand involvement in rheumatoid arthritis with predominant involvement of the metacarpal-phalangeal joints.

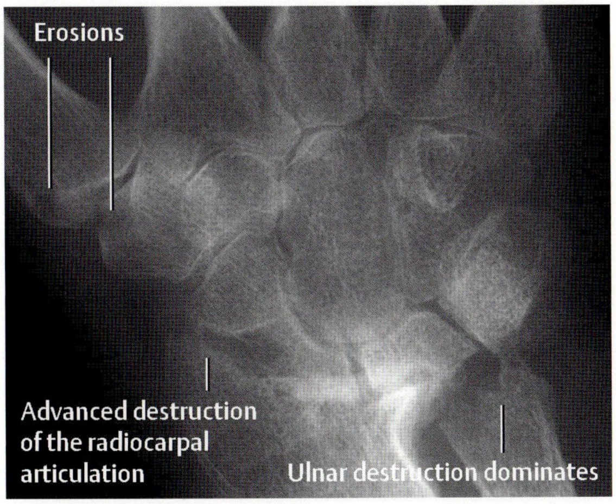

Fig. 9.**97** Destruction of the wrist in rheumatoid arthritis: the most severe involvement of the ulnar styloid process is typical. Early destruction involving other carpal bones.

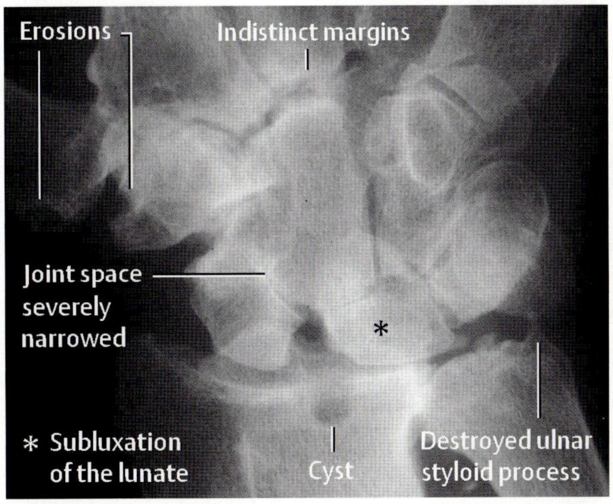

Fig. 9.**98** Advanced destruction in the radiocarpal and ulnocarpal joints and early development of a carpal mass (os carpale).

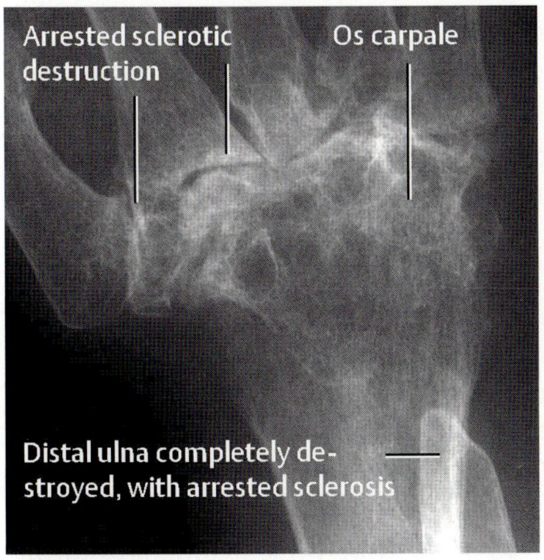

Fig. 9.**99** 'Burned out' rheumatoid arthritis with complete carpal mass (os carpale) and destroyed distal ulna. Since the synovial lining is destroyed, the disease is arrested.

Table 9.**6** Shortened list of acute rheumatoid arthritis criteria

1. Morning stiffness
2. Oligo-/polyarthritis in three or more joints or several joint groups
3. Arthritis of the hands
4. Symmetric arthritis
5. Rheumatic nodules
6. Serum rheumatoid factors
7. Radiologically visible changes of the hand (erosions and juxta-articular demineralization

To diagnose rheumatoid arthritis, four of the seven criteria must be met, whereby criteria 1 – 4 must be present for at least 6 weeks.

articulations combined with hyperextension of the proximal interphalangeal articulation), and **Z-deformity** of the thumb (flexion of the metacarpophalangeal articulation and hyperextension of the interphalangeal articulation, also referred to as 'hitchhiker deformity').

Wrist

Technical consideration: The central ray must be centered on the wrist for optimal imaging evaluation.

Early abnormalities:

- Erosions of the distal end of the ulna, especially along the ulnar styloid process (Figs. 9.**97**–9.**99**). This indicates involvement of the three compartments of the distal radioulnar articulation: the saccular radioulnar recess erodes the ulnar side of the radius; the prestyloid recess erodes the tip of the styloid process; if the extensor carpi ulnaris tendon sheath, which borders the ulna laterally, is inflamed, it erodes the laterodorsal ulnar circumference.
- Involvement of the radiocarpal articulation causes corresponding erosions at the distal radius (radial styloid process) and bordering scaphoid (Fig. 9.**97**).
- The triquetrum (typically its medial side) and the pisiform are often involved.

Late abnormalities:

- All compartments of the radiocarpal, intercarpal, and carpometacarpal articulations can participate in the inflammatory process **('pancompartmental distribution').** In the extreme case, fibrous and osseous fusion of the carpal bones can form a single **os carpale** (Figs. 9.**98**, 9.**99**).
- Misalignment caused by ulnar and **palmar deviation** of the proximal carpal row. Characteristic radiographic features: the lunate extends beyond the distal radial end; the ulna is displaced posteriorly; the distal radioulnar articulation is widened. The corresponding clinical finding is the 'caput-ulnae syndrome' with pain, restricted motion, and posterior prominence of the distal ulna.

Elbow and Shoulder

- Involvement of both joints is relatively common. Radiographs frequently underestimate the erosions, which are best demonstrated by sonography or MRI. **Rotator cuff atrophy or tear** is a common complication of long-standing rheumatoid arthritis of the shoulder, characterized by elevation of the humeral head.

Forefoot and Middle Foot

- The metatarsal heads are very commonly involved and are the initial manifestation in about 20% of patients. Characteristically, the involvement begins at the fifth ray and progresses medially.
- Progression of the disease leads to deformities of the forefoot (hallux valgus, hammer toe, lateral subluxation of the metatarsophalangeal articulations, lateral deviation, and dorsiflexion of the toes).
- The intertarsal articulations and metatarsophalangeal articulations are also frequently involved but are difficult to see on standard radiographic views.

Heel and Ankle (Fig. 9.**108**)

- The relatively common **retrocalcaneal bursitis** produces a soft-tissue density in the pre-Achilles fat pad, a focal osteoporosis, and possibly erosions at the neighboring calcaneus.
- **Achilles tendinitis** leads to widening and indistinctness of the Achilles tendon.
- **Plantar fasciitis** might induce a plantar calcaneal spur.
- The subtalar articulation is more frequently involved than the tibiotalar articulation.

Knee

- The knee is frequently involved, and the lateral compartment is more often affected. Longstanding disease typically leads to **valgus deformity.**
- Damage to the joint capsule frequently leads to the formation of synovial cysts in the popliteal fossa.

Cervical Spine

Technical consideration: In known rheumatoid arthritis, a complete examination consists of AP and lateral films of the entire cervical spine, open-mouth AP view of the dens, and lateral films in flexion and extension.

> **!** Conventional tomography, if available, remains a very reliable method for the assessment of bone destruction and subluxations in the cervical spine. However, in most departments this modality has been replaced by MRI or spiral CT.

- Destruction of the transverse ligament of the atlas leads to **anterior atlanto-axial subluxation.** In this setting, the lateral view will show more

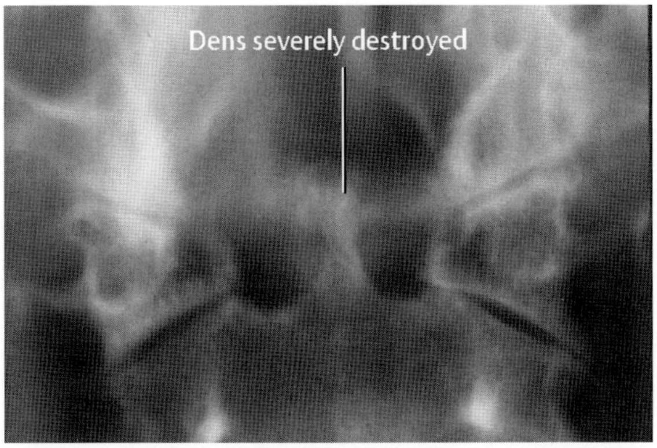

Fig. 9.**100** AP conventional tomography of the dens shows severe destruction as manifestation of rheumatoid arthritis.

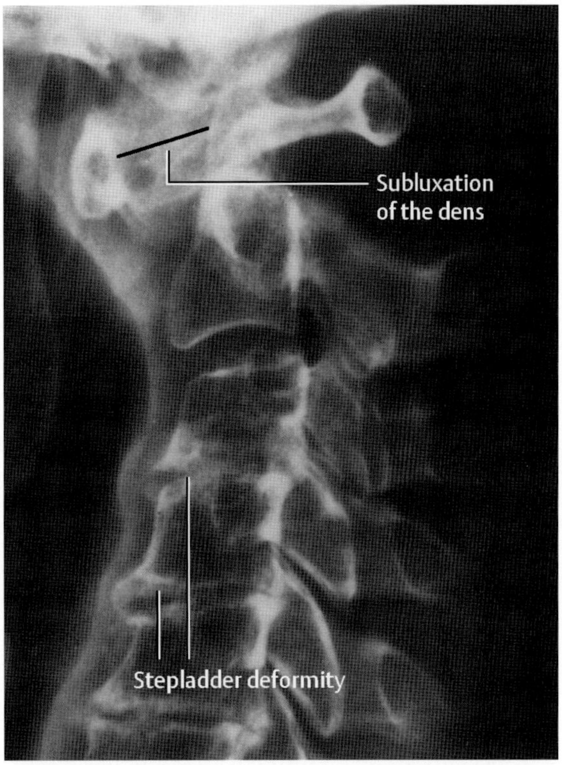

Fig. 9.**101** Destruction of the transverse ligament of the atlas causes posterior subluxation of the dens and the risk of spinal cord compression. The mid-cervical spine shows a typical 'stepladder' deformity due to a posterior displacement of the vertebral bodies.

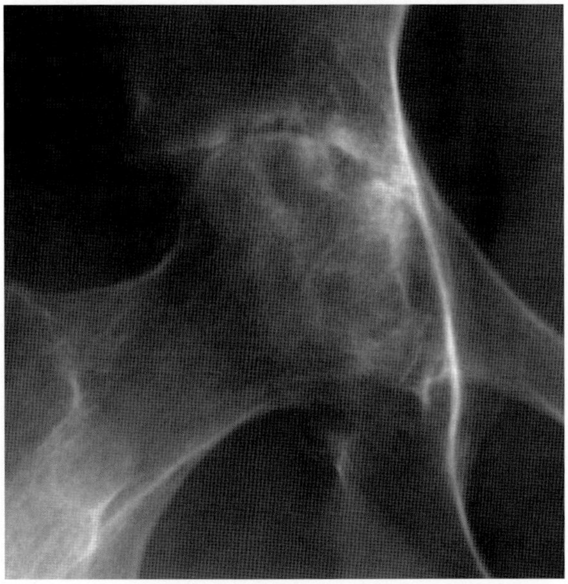

Fig. 9.**102** Massive joint destruction in longstanding rheumatoid arthritis. The joint space is obliterated and large portions of the femoral head destroyed.

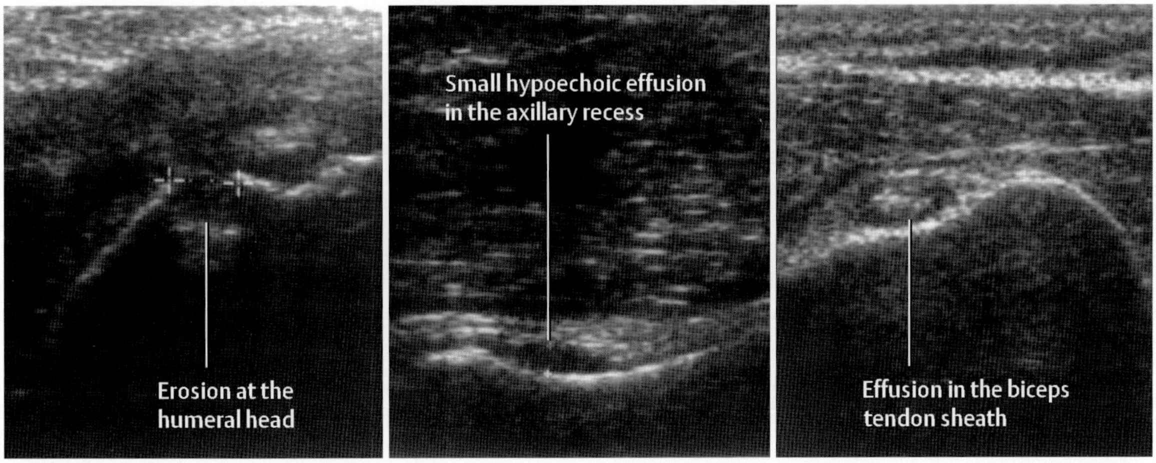

Fig. 9.**103** Sonography of the shoulder. Erosion of the humeral head, effusion, and tenosynovitis of the biceps are indicative of an inflammatory joint disease.

than 2.5 mm of separation between the anterior arch of the atlas and dens (Fig. 9.**101**). It should be kept in mind that the subluxation might be visualized in flexion only.

- Loss of height and anterior gliding and angulation of the atlas can produce **basilar invagination** and may lead to neurologic complications. Basilar invagination is present if the tip of the dens projects more than 5 mm above the McGregor line on the lateral view (Fig. 9.**105**).
  Lateral atlanto-axial subluxation results from severe osseous destruction of the atlas and dens and is identified by the asymmetric position of the dens relative to the lateral masses of the atlas.
- **Erosions** of the dens are observed in about one-third of patients with rheumatoid arthritis. They initially involve the anterior surface of the dens and later the posterior surface and tip (Figs. 9.**100**, 9.**104**, 9.**105**). Pathologic fracture of the dens can occur, especially in patients who have subluxation in addition to extensive erosions.
- Ligamentous laxity can cause a **retrolisthesis,** especially at the C3 through C5 segments. If multiple segments are involved, the cervical spine assumes a **'stepladder' appearance** (Fig. 9.**101**). Inflammatory changes are also found in the **facet joints.**

SONO Using sonography in rheumatoid arthritis is especially helpful

- to look for articular or periarticular soft-tissue swelling (effusion?) and to guide aspiration, especially of the small joints.
- to detect erosions of the humeral head, femoral condyles, and tibial plateau,
- to confirm the clinical suspicion of tenosynovitis,
- to detect rotator cuff tears of the shoulders.

MRI The general statements on page 293 apply. Though a clinical routine has not yet been established, MRI has been found useful in rheumatoid arthritis for the evaluation of:

- the shoulder (synovitis? effusion? erosion? rotator cuff tear?) (Fig. 9.**106**),
- the subtalar articulation (for the improved detection of the frequently extensive erosions) (Fig. 9.**108**),
- the wrist (to improve the detection of erosions).

! So far, the only standard indication for MRI is the evaluation of the upper cervical spine to delineate the relationship between pannus and spinal cord. The best technique is the T2-weighted FSE sequence with the neck in flexion and extension.

DD Osteoarthritis with its involvement of multiple joints is usually easily distinguishable by the different distribution pattern and the sclerotic changes (see pages 302 – 305, arthritis versus osteoarthritis).

Isolated infectious monoarthritis is suspected by clinical history, location, and regional findings, but its diagnosis ultimately depends on aspiration of joint fluid. It is extremely difficult to detect bacterial arthritis superimposed on rheumatoid arthritis (e.g., after corticosteroid injection). In this situation, also, it is solely the diagnostic joint aspiration that provides the answer.

The most difficult task often is to differentiate rheumatoid arthritis from the seronegative spondyloarthropathies.

Findings favoring rheumatoid arthritis are:

- absence of proliferative (periosteal) reaction,
- extreme osteoporosis,
- predilection for the synovial joint; enthesopathies are less frequent and severe in rheumatoid arthritis.

Glossary

Special Manifestations of Rheumatoid Arthritis

Felty syndrome:
Hematologic involvement (granulopenia, splenomegaly, lymphadenopathy) in longstanding rheumatoid arthritis and secondary infections.

Kaplan syndrome:
Association of rheumatoid arthritis and pulmonary silicosis.

Seronegative 'rheumatoid' arthritis:
Seronegative rheumatoid arthritis can be divided into two groups:

- typical rheumatoid arthritis negative for rheumatoid factor. Although this group once constituted 25% of all forms of rheumatoid arthritis, modern laboratory methods find rheumatoid factor in more than 90% of patients. Also, some patients will become seropositive within 2 years. Furthermore, patients who are initially seropositive may become seronegative as a result of successful therapy;
- other forms of arthritis with several features that distinguish them from rheumatoid arthritis, such as asymmetric, osteosclerosis, osseous proliferations, and osseous ankylosis. They can evolve into other entities (e.g., systemic lupus erythematosus, psoriasis).

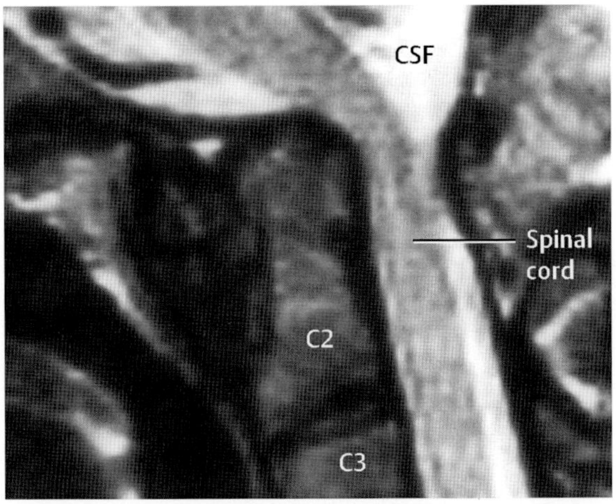

Fig. 9.**104** Classic MRI finding (T2-weighted SE sequence) of rheumatoid arthritis in the cervical spine with pannus formation and compression of the spinal cord.

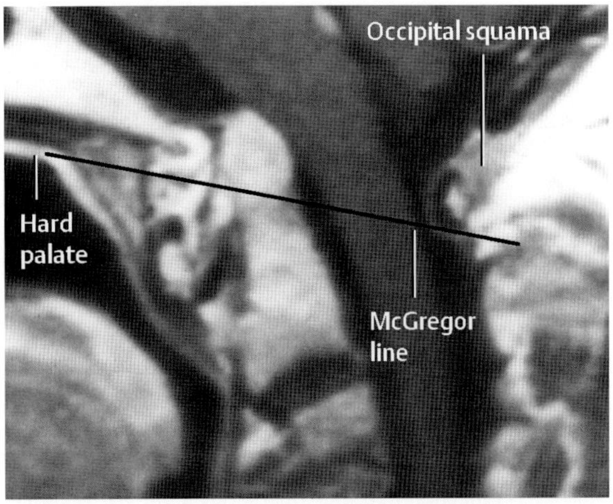

Fig. 9.**105** Basilar invagination due to vertical atlanto-dental subluxation. The tip of the dens projects more than 5 mm above the McGregor line (line connecting the superior margin of the hard palate and the lowermost point on the occipital squama).

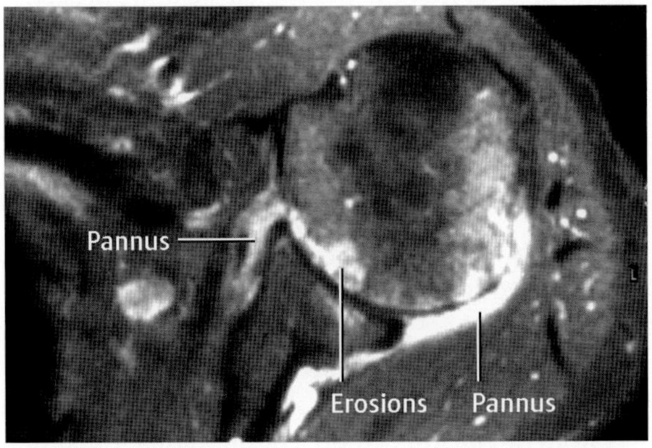

Fig. 9.**106** Axial MRI of the shoulder, T1-weighted TSE image with fat suppression and after intravenous administration of contrast medium. Strong enhancement of the pannus.

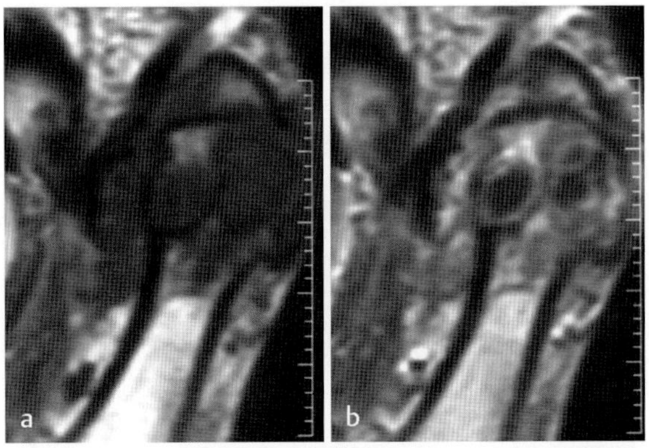

Fig. 9.**107** Rheumatoid arthritis of the metatarsophalangeal joint of the first ray with extensive pseudocyst (geode) formation. T1-weighted TSE sequences before (**a**) and after (**b**) administration of contrast medium. The peripheral enhancement is clearly visible.

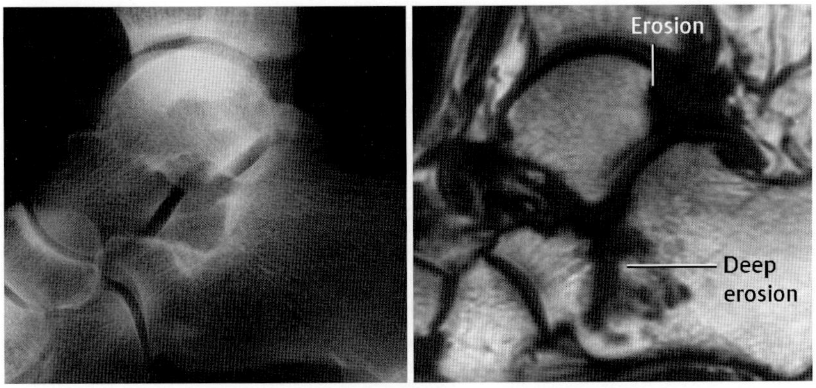

Fig. 9.**108** Rheumatoid arthritis of the tibiotalar and talocalcaneal joints. The radiographs show only discrete sclerotic zones above the normal radiolucency. MRI (T1-weighted TSE image) reveals considerable destruction of the tibiotalar and talocalcaneal joint.

Juvenile Rheumatoid Arthritis (Juvenile chronic arthritis)

Synonyms: Still disease: systemic manifestation of juvenile rheumatoid arthritis.

> Juvenile rheumatoid arthritis is the most common connective tissue disease in childhood. It can be divided into three major groups, of which the oligoarthritic variant is most common. The histologic findings resemble those found with rheumatoid arthritis in adults.

PATH As in all other types of immune arthritis, juvenile rheumatoid arthritis has a genetic disposition. There is evidence to suggest that it may be triggered by a latent infection with the rubella virus.

More than 90% of cases are negative for rheumatoid factor. The rare seropositive polyarticular diseases used to be subsumed under the term **'Juvenile Onset Adult-Type Rheumatoid Arthritis'.** Since these diseases are neither pathologically nor clinically different from seronegative diseases, such differentiation does not seem meaningful.

Although the rheumatoid factor plays a minor role, **antinuclear antibodies** (ANA) are frequently found.

CLINIC The peak incidence for juvenile rheumatoid arthritis is between the first and third years, and it is three times more frequent in girls than in boys. With increasing age, the incidence decreases and the gender distribution equalizes.

The early symptoms are morning stiffness as well as pain at night and after inactivity. Pain, however, might not be experienced, and the parents might notice solely an increasing unwillingness of the child to walk or that the child tires easily. Systemic symptoms, such as subfebrile temperature, weight loss, and delayed growth may also be present. Because of the vague clinical manifestation, the diagnosis is frequently delayed.

Three major groups (Table 9.**7**) are distinguished by their clinical course and prognosis.

Growth disturbances: The acute phases of the disease usually cause growth arrest. Permanent involvement confined to one region may cause asymmetric growth due to overgrowth of the affected sites caused by hyperemia. However, if this leads to early epiphyseal closure (epiphyseal collapse), the longitudinal growth of the affected side is delayed.

X-RAY In contrast to other forms of arthritis, juvenile rheumatoid arthritis is associated with frequent periosteal reaction. Depending on the location, the following specific abnormalities are found:

Large Peripheral Joints

In localized disease the effect of inflammation is to enlarge the epiphysis (growth activation). This 'ballooning' effect is most marked at the knee and ankle (Fig. 9.**110**).

Cervical Spine

The characteristic findings are similar to those of rheumatoid arthritis:
- erosions of the dens,
- atlanto-axial subluxation (in a child, the atlanto-dental distance in flexion should not exceed 4 mm),
- ankylosis of the facet joints,
- decreased height of the corresponding vertebral bodies.

Mandible

Involvement of the temporo-mandibular joints is typical and can lead to micrognathia and antegonial (pre-angular) notching along the undersurface of the mandible. These changes must be distinguished from malformations of the mandible as part of the various malformation syndromes.

Hands, Wrists and Elbows (Fig. 9.**109**, 9.**111**)

The distribution pattern coincides to a large extent with the adult-onset type except for three unique features:
- the **distal interphalangeal joints** are commonly involved,
- **radial deviation** is more common than ulnar deviation,
- **periosteal new bone formation** causes widening of the phalanges.

DD
- Arthritis in **systemic lupus erythematosus:** generally not erosive or destructive.
- **Juvenile spondyloarthropathy:** older mean age of onset, family history, HLA-B27 antigen. Like the adult type, evidence of enthesopathies.
- **Rheumatic fever:** this is a nonerosive, reactive oligoarthritis or polyarthritis. Clinically, the cardiac findings dominate.
- **Hemophilia:** in the large joints, the radiographic picture may be identical to juvenile rheumatoid arthritis. There is less frequent involvement of the small joints, however. Hemophilic arthropathy is easily diagnosed, since the patient knows the diagnosis.

Table 9.7 Major types of juvenile rheumatoid arthritis

	Polyarthritis	Mono-/oligoarthritis	Systemic types
Affected joints	At least five joints, especially large joints of the upper extremity. Cervical spine involvement in 50%	At most four joints; knee and ankle are most frequently involved	
Relative frequency	30%	60%	10%
Distribution (m:f)	1:3	1:5	1:1
Rheumatoid factors	15%	Rare	Rare
Antinuclear bodies (ANA)	40%	85%	10%
Chronic uveitis	5%	20%	Rare
Other extra-articular symptoms	Mild	None	Febrile episodes, exanthema, hepatosplenomegaly, lymphadenopathy, pericarditis, rarely CNS involvement
Clinical course	Continuing joint complaints dominate	Uveitis is clinically dominant	Systemic disease often self-limited, in part destructive arthritis
Prognosis	In 70%–89% healing	Very good [1]	Moderate
Unfavorable prognostic factors	Positive rheumatoid factor, late onset of the disease, early involvement of the small joints	ANA-positive subtype. Severe course of the uveitis, especially in ANA-positive girls	Polyarthritic joint involvement

[1] Caution: In 5%–10% of older, HLA-B27-positive children, the disease progresses to ankylosing spondylitis.

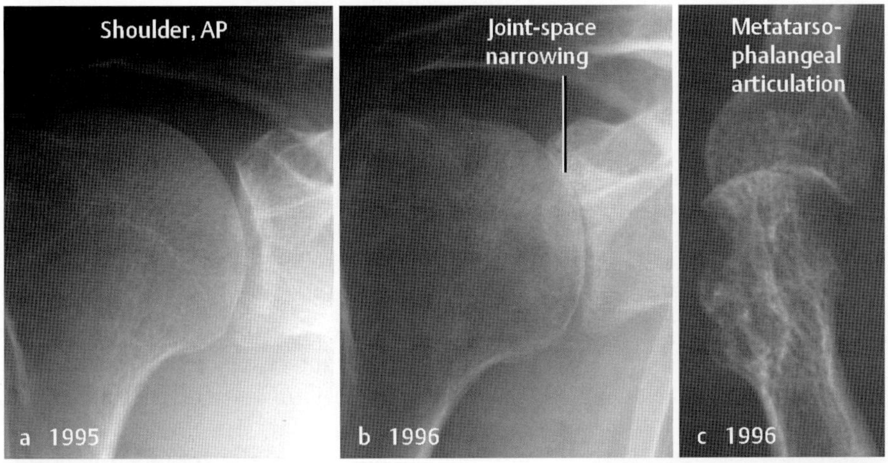

Fig. 9.**109** Juvenile rheumatoid arthritis, polyarthritic type. Late onset and rapid progression of the disease (see Table 9.**7**) as indicated by the considerable destruction of the metatarsophalangeal joints, which was unremarkable in 1995.

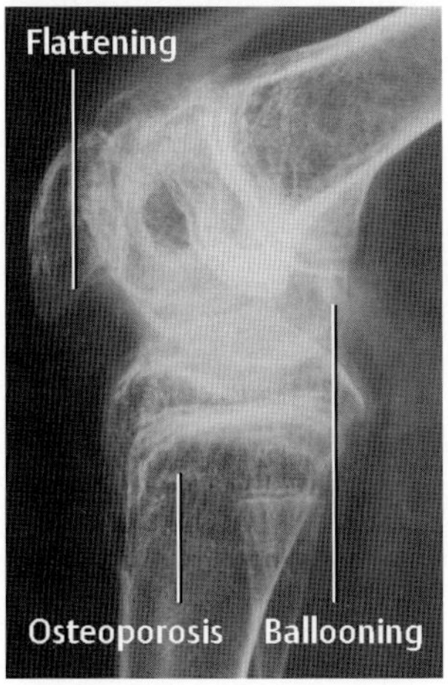

Fig. 9.**110** Osteoporosis and metaphyseal/epiphyseal 'ballooning'. Note the joint-space narrowing and flattened inferior patellar pole. The major differential diagnosis is hemophilic arthropathy.

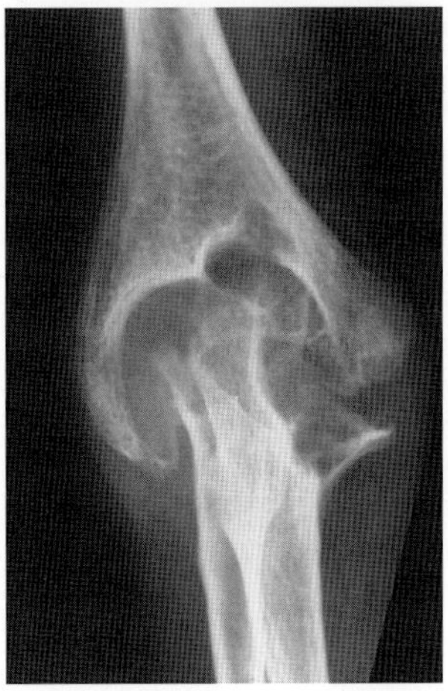

Fig. 9.**111** Inflammatory destruction of the elbow joint at the mutilation stage.

Ankylosing Spondylitis

Synonym: Bekhterev disease.

■ Ankylosing spondylitis is a seronegative spondyloarthropathy that primarily affects the joints of the axial skeleton, including the articular junctions of the pelvis and thorax. Concomitant destruction, subchondral sclerosis, and osseous ankylosis lead to the typical 'variegated picture' of this disease. ■

PATH The **entheses** (sites of tendon and ligament attachments to bone) are the **target tissue** of the inflammation in ankylosing spondylitis, and synovitis plays a secondary role. This phenomenon explains the formation of the characteristic features of syndesmophytes, squaring of the vertebral bodies, diskovertebral destruction, and Achilles tendinitis.

Exudative enthesitis as well as peripheral arthritis leads to the **combination of fibrosis and osteolysis** and later to metaplastic new bone formation and osseous **ankylosis.**

CLINIC **Epidemiology:** The disease is considerably less common than rheumatoid arthritis. Men are more frequently affected than women, and approximately 10% of the patients who are HLA-B27 positive develop the disorder.

The 1984 modified version of the New York criteria is generally used to confirm the diagnosis of ankylosing spondylitis (Table 9.**8**).

In 70% of the patients, the disease begins with **low back pain and dull gluteal pain,** associated with morning stiffness and improved with activity. **Permanent bilateral pain** develops within several weeks. Additional pseudoradicular lumbar pain is mentioned by about 10% of patients and is associated with painful tenopathy in an additional 10%. Progression of the disease is upward, especially affecting the **costovertebral articulations.** The initially 'pleuritic' chest pain later advances to restricted respiratory excursions.

The complete picture of ankylosing spondylitis leads to a painful stiffening of the entire spine, severe thoracic kyphosis, and a rigid thorax.

Additional extra-axial articular manifestations are found in about one-third of all patients and are the initial manifestation in about half of those patients.

In rare cases, the disease begins simultaneously at the SI joints and cervical spine ('bipolar type').

Extraskeletal manifestations: Iridocyclitis occurs in about 25%–30% of all patients and cardiovascular involvement, especially aortitis which can be clinically silent, in about 10%. Involvement of the lung is rare and delayed, presenting as slowly progressing upper lobe fibrosis. Neurologic symptoms primarily are secondary to cord compression after fracture and inflammation. The most frequently involved levels are the C5–6 and C6–7 segments, as well as the lumbosacral nerve roots (cauda equina syndrome).

Distribution pattern: Most common is symmetric involvement of the SI joints and thoracolumbar junction. The most commonly affected peripheral joints are the hips, shoulders, and knees, which are often symmetrically involved. Manubriosternal joint involvement generally occurs in patients with longstanding disease.

Prognosis and course: The clinical course of ankylosing spondylitis is extremely variable and unpredictable.

X-RAY The different locations of the disease – SI joints, spine, peripheral joints, and entheses – have quite characteristic radiographic features.

1. **Sacroiliitis** of the 'variegated picture' type (Figs. 9.**112**–9.**114**, see also page 299). This is the initial radiographic finding in over 95% of patients. In about 10% of cases, the sacroiliitis begins unilaterally.
2. In the **spine** (see page 299):
   - Anterior spondylitis (Romanus lesion),
   - 'Shiny corner' sign,
   - Squared vertebral bodies,
   - Andersson lesion (Fig. 9.**119**),
   - Syndesmophytes (Fig. 9.**115**). In about two-thirds of patients with ankylosing spondylitis, the syndesmophytes are first detected in the thoracolumbar junction.
   - Linear or circular **disk calcifications.** They are particularly apparent with osteoporosis in the neighboring vertebral bodies.
   - Costovertebral ankylosis (especially in patients with mild sacroiliitis) is important diagnostically and contributes more to the stiffening of the spine than the syndesmophytes, especially in adolescents. The AP radiograph shows the **'trolley track sign':** three vertical radiolucent lines corresponding to the ossified supra- and interspinal ligaments and the osseous ankylosis of the costovertebral and costotransversal joints (Fig. 9.**116**).
   - Though ossification of the anterior and posterior longitudinal ligaments is the hallmark of ankylosing spondylitis, it occurs only in the late stages of the disease ('bamboo spine').

Table **9.8** Diagnostic criteria of ankylosing spondylitis (modified New York classification 1984)

The diagnosis of ankylosing spondylitis is based on radiographic signs of unilateral or bilateral **sacroiliitis** and **clinical criteria**:

1. Previous or acute **pain** in the region of the thoracolumbar transition or lumbar spine
2. **Limited motion** of the lumbar spine in all three planes
3. **Limited chest expansion** (< 2.5 cm measured at the level of the fourth intercostal space)

Ankylosing spondylitis is **definitely** present in cases with:
- bilateral sacroiliitis grade 3 – 4 and at least one of the clinical criteria
- unilateral sacroiliitis grade 3 – 4 with clinical criterion 1 or clinical criteria 2 and 3
- bilateral sacroiliitis grade 2 with clinical criterion 1 or clinical criteria 2 and 3

Ankylosing spondylitis is **probably** present in cases with bilateral sacroiliitis grade 3 – 4 without clinical criteria

Gradation of the radiologic findings of the SI joint:

Grade 0:	Normal finding
Grade 1:	Questionable erosions
Grade 2:	Erosions with subchondral sclerosis, beginning osseous bridging
Grade 3:	Pseudo-widening of the joint space, erosions, sclerosis, and osseous bridging
Grade 4:	Ankylosis

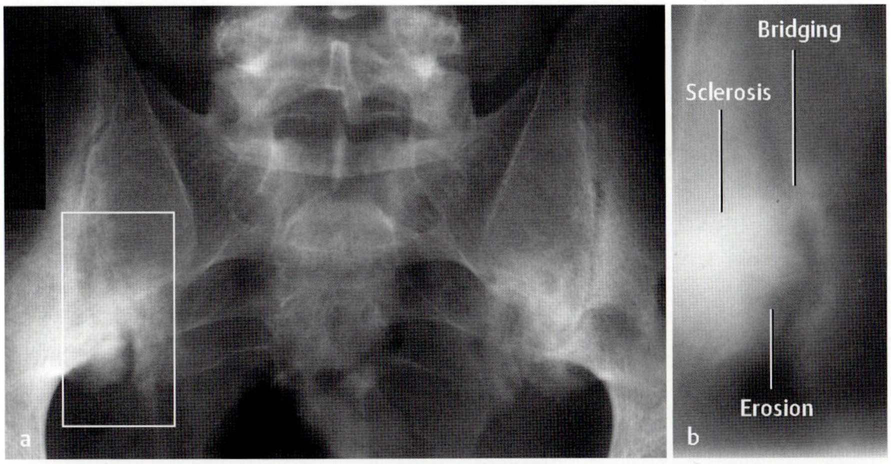

Fig. 9.**112** Sacroiliitis shown by radiography. The inferior aspect of the sacroiliac joint is indistinct and shows increased sclerosis. Conventional tomography (**b**) reveals large erosions.

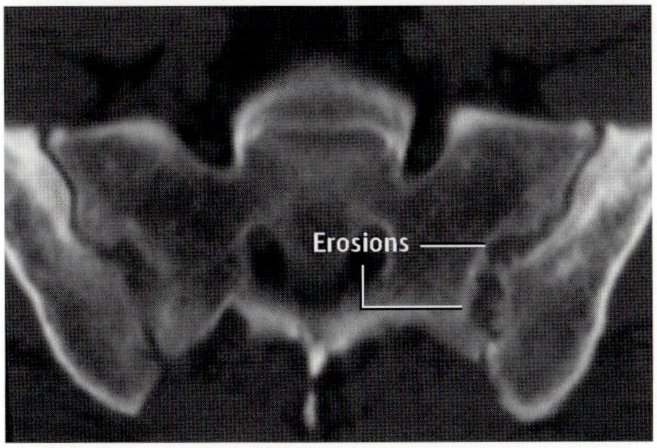

Fig. 9.**113** Severe sacroiliitis on the left on axial CT. The right sacroiliac joint also shows mild inflammatory changes.

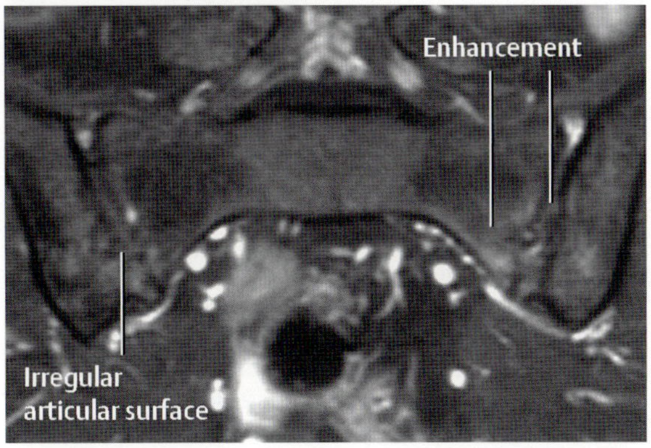

Fig. 9.**114** Mild sacroiliitis as seen on T1-weighted SE sequence with fat suppression and after administration of contrast medium. Enhancement is seen both within and adjacent to the joint.

3. **Extravertebral joints:**
   Clinically diagnosed peripheral arthritis often fails to show corresponding radiographic changes, but may show abnormalities on MRI. This indicates a good prognosis. Very young patients can develop destructive, inflammatory ankylosing monoarthritides and oligoarthritides. Even nonerosive arthritic episodes can damage the articular cartilage and predispose the patient to developing osteoarthritis (Fig. 9.**117**).
   - In contrast to rheumatoid arthritis, **ankylosing spondylitis** more frequently affects the proximal appendicular joints (hips, shoulder, sternomanubrial joints, Figs. 9.**117**, 9.**118**) and the joints of the lower extremities.
   - Since osseous proliferations prevail over erosions, accompanying periosteal reactions and, late in disease, ankylosis are common.
4. **Rarefying and productive fibro-ostitis:**
   This is a manifestation of a typical enthesopathy. Most common locations are
   - ischium,
   - iliac crest just above the SI joints,
   - calcaneus (rheumatic calcaneopathy), and
   - other muscle insertions, primarily in the foot.

   Radiographically, these enthesopathies appear as whisker- and blister-like calcifications (fibro-ostoses) and serrated contour irregularities. Erosions at the entheses are not infrequent (especially at the insertion of the supraspinatus and Achilles tendons, Fig. 9.**120**).

CT Except for MRI, CT is the method of choice and has replaced conventional tomography. It should be performed in all cases with unclear radiographic findings, since it can reveal discrete morphologic changes earlier and with more clarity (Fig. 9.**113**). In addition, it can detect spinal complications, such as vertebral fractures, spinal stenosis, and segmental instabilities.

NUC This imaging method adds no additional relevant information to the diagnosis of early disease, since the bone turnover in SI joints is physiologically high and shows increased uptake. Even quantification by determining a threshold value is fraught with errors because of the wide physiologic range. In individual cases, determining the distribution pattern can provide diagnostic clues.

MRI This is the method of choice for the early diagnosis of sacroiliitis and spondylodiscitis (Fig. 9.**114**, see also pages 334 – 337).

DD
- **Spondylosis deformans:** Spondylophytes (marginal osteophytes) are beak- or hook-shaped in contrast to syndesmophytes. Furthermore, sacroiliitis is absent. Degenerative changes of the SI joints frequently cause ossification of the anterior joint capsule. This does not usually occur in ankylosing spondylitis, but if it does, it occurs late in the disease when there are superimposed degenerative changes, best demonstrated by CT.
- **Diffuse idiopathic skeletal hyperostosis** (DISH, Forestier disease): This condition causes hyperostotic spondylophytes that spread to the longitudinal ligaments, anulus fibrosus, and paraspinal connective tissue. The 'shield-like' osseous appositions are predominantly along the thoracic spine and extend over four vertebral bodies. The intervertebral disk space is usually normal or may be slightly narrowed. The facet joints and SI joints are normal.
- **Reactive arthritis, psoriatic arthropathy:** Parasyndesmophytes have a different configuration than syndesmophytes have (see page 298).
- **Bacterial spondylitis and spondylodiskitis:** In the presence of an Andersson lesion, the radiographic differentiation is only possible if syndesmophytes coexist.
- **Rheumatoid arthritis:** Different distribution pattern. Involvement of the SI joints is rare.

Glossary

Juvenile-onset ankylosing spondylitis: As in the adult-onset type, the most severe pathologic changes are at the tendon and ligament insertions (enthesopathies). Boys are about twice as often affected as girls. The peak age of onset is 7 – 9 years. More than 90% of children with juvenile ankylosing spondylitis are HLA-B27-positive, and a familial history is common. The radiologic features of the juvenile-onset type are completely identical to those found in adulthood.

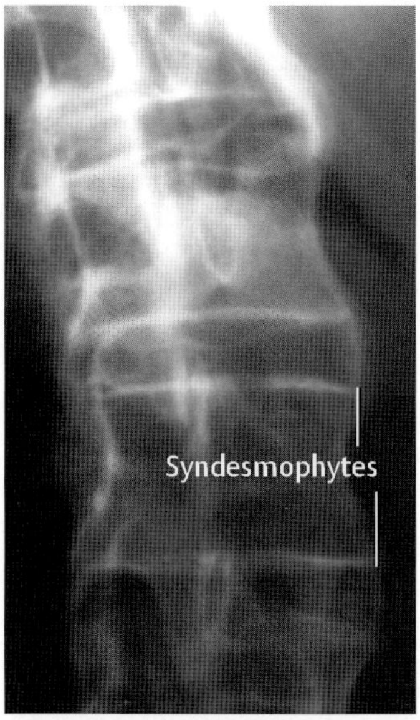

Fig. 9.**115** Syndesmophytes at the thoracolumbar transition (oblique view).

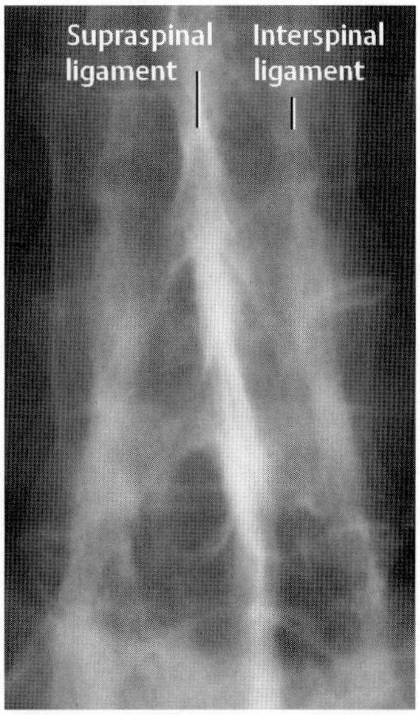

Fig. 9.**116** 'Burned out' spondylitis with osseous ankylosis of the vertebral bodies and facet joints. The ligamentous ossifications produce radiodense lines ('trolleytrack' sign).

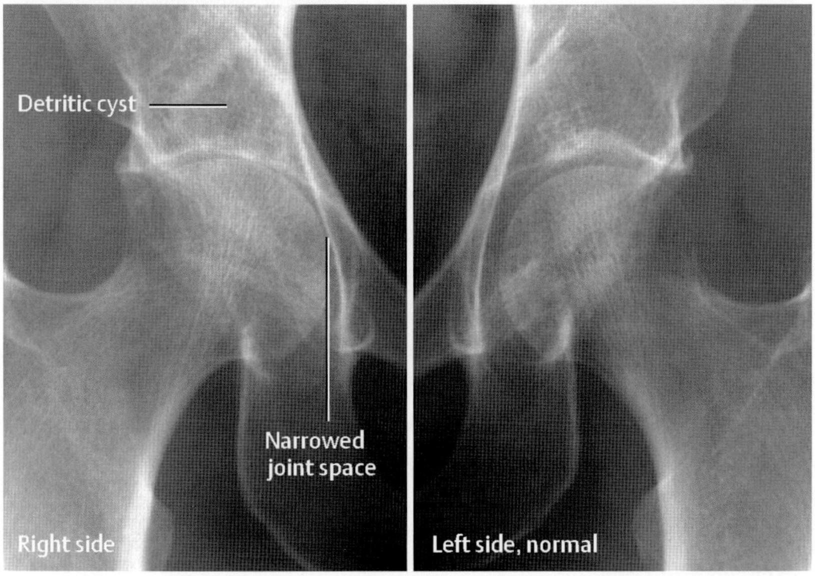

Fig. 9.**117** Patient with known ankylosing spondylitis. There is degenerative change in the right hip with articular space narrowing and without osseous overgrowth. This results from cartilage damage. The contralateral hip is unremarkable.

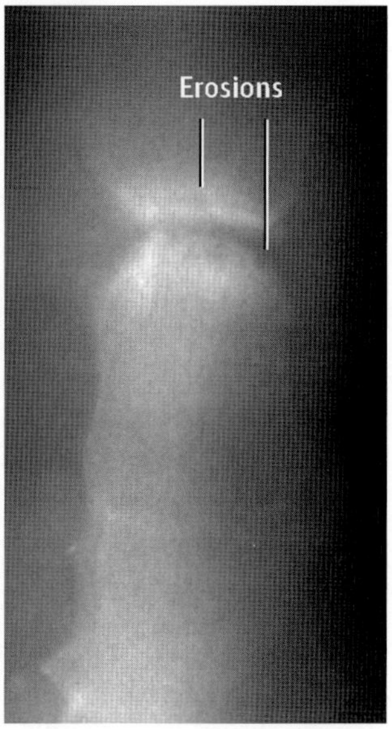

Fig. 9.**118** Erosive changes of the manubriosternal joint (conventional tomography).

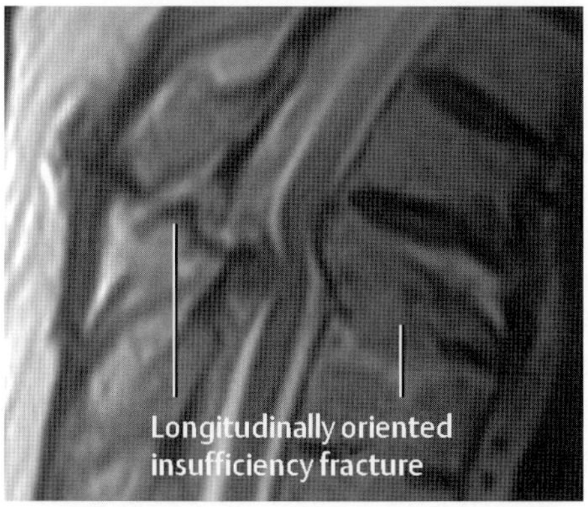

Fig. 9.**119** MRI of a noninfectious Andersson lesion, T2-weighted FSE sequence.

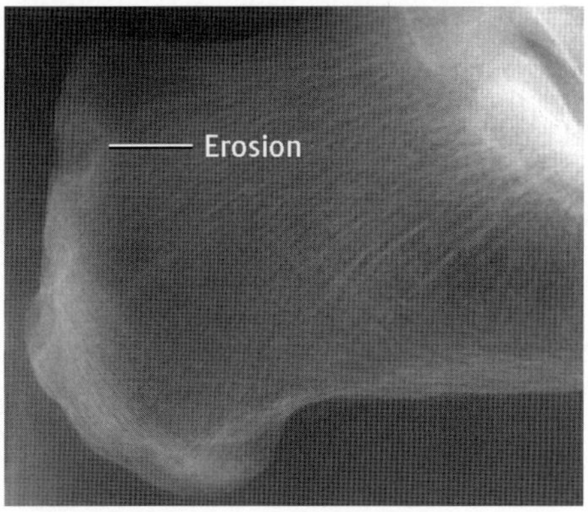

Fig. 9.**120** Erosive enthesopathy of the Achilles tendon.

Reactive Arthritis

■ Reactive arthritis occurs days to weeks after a distant infection and is associated with several other disease manifestations. It is characterized by bilateral, though asymmetric, oligoarthritic involvement, predominately in the lower extremity. **Reiter syndrome** is a special form of reactive arthritis following urogenital or gastrointestinal infections and consists of the triad of arthritis, urethritis, and conjunctivitis. ■

PATH Reactive arthritis has a genetic predisposition, and the HLA-B27 antigen is present in 80% of affected patients. The exact pathogenetic mechanism of the disease is still unknown.

Reiter Syndrome

As the representative and most important reactive arthritis, Reiter syndrome will be described in some detail. It follows either a sexually transmitted infection, presumably caused by chlamydiae, or an intestinal infection with Yersinieae, campylobacters, shigellae, or salmonellae.

CLINIC **Epidemiology:** Reiter syndrome is about 100 times less common than rheumatoid arthritis. Typically occurring in patients between 20 and 40 years of age, it is much more common in men than in women, since the more frequent sexually transmitted type almost exclusively affects men.

Symptoms: In most cases, the initial manifestation is an abacterial **urethritis** or balanitis. In cases conforming to the typical course of Reiter syndrome, these symptoms appear 7–14 days after sexual exposure or dysentery. The urethritis is less painful and has less purulent discharge than gonorrhea and can be accompanied by hemorrhagic cystitis or prostatitis. In women, urethritis and cervicitis can have few symptoms (with dysuria or minimal vaginal burning) or can be completely asymptomatic, making assignment of the diagnosis difficult.

Usually within a few weeks, moderate **fever, conjunctivitis,** and **arthritis** develop. Conjunctivitis, the most common ocular manifestation, is generally mild, unless keratitis or uveitis develops. The articular symptoms can be mild or severe when compared to the attacks of other arthritic conditions.

Enthesopathy (inflammation at the osseous insertion of tendons and ligaments) is common. The cardinal findings are plantar fasciitis, digital periostitis, and Achilles tendinitis.

Mucocutaneous lesions, which are small, painless superficial ulcerations outlined by a map-like border, occur in 5%–30% of all patients. They are located mostly on the buccal mucosa, tongue, and glans of the penis. Furthermore, hyperkeratotic skin lesions are common, and are mainly found on the palms of the hands and soles of the feet and around the nails.

Cardiovascular involvement, with aortitis, aortic insufficiency, and conduction disturbances, may occur but is rare.

Distribution pattern: In general, the involvement is asymmetric, monoarticular to oligoarticular, but rarely also polyarticular. The knee and ankle are most commonly involved initially, followed by involvement of the metatarsophalangeal articulations and calcaneus. Characteristically, the first metatarsophalangeal articulation and the interphalangeal articulation of the first toe are most severely involved.

In more severe cases, the SI joints and lumbar spine can be affected. The joints of the upper extremities, especially the shoulders, can show relatively late and variable involvement.

Course and prognosis: In the typical cases, the initial manifestation resolves within 3 to 4 months, but about 50% of patients have recurrent arthritis or other symptoms of Reiter syndrome for a period of several years. The recurrent or chronic manifestations may result in joint deformities, ankylosis, sacroiliitis, and spondylitis.

In principle, the post-dysenteric type follows a more favorable course than the post-venereal type and tends to be chronic less often. For instance, in patients with Reiter syndrome following *Yersinia* infection, recurrent arthritis was found in 5% and chronic arthritis in 2.5%. Also in *Salmonella* enteritis, the frequency of the chronic Reiter syndrome is under 25%, in contrast to a frequency of 60% after *Chlamydia* infection.

X-RAY Radiographically detectable articular changes may be observed in 60%–80% of patients. As in other seronegative types of arthritis, they are in part attributable to enthesitis.

Peripheral Joints

! The foot (metatarsophalangeal joints, calcaneus) is preferentially involved. Erosive changes predominate over osteoproliferative changes.

- In the toes and fingers, **soft-tissue swelling** associated with the acute phase is not only confined to the articular region, but also uniformly involves the entire shaft. This causes **sausage-like toes** or **sausage-like fingers.** Aside from Reiter syndrome, sausage-like swelling along an entire digit is also observed in psoriatic arthritis and is crucial in its differentiation from rheumatoid arthritis.
- Characteristically, the **simultaneous osteodestructive** (especially erosions) **and osteoproliferative changes** appear early. The osteoproliferative changes appear as accompanying periosteal reaction in the form of a delicate periosteal lamella along the metadiaphyseal transition,

and as fibro-exostoses at the calcaneus (Fig. 9.**121**), tibial tuberosity, ischial tuberosity, and trochanters. In the chronic type, they appear as periosteal ossifications (with thickening of the diaphyseal cortex) and as osseous appositions (whiskering) near the articular end of the bone.

- Juxta-articular osteoporosis develops later and is not as severe as in rheumatoid arthritis. In some cases it might be totally absent.

SI Joints

Inflammatory changes are observed in 5%–10% of patients during the early phase of Reiter syndrome and are characteristically **unilateral.** In the chronic manifestation, the frequency of sacroiliac involvement increases up to 70%. These changes are bilateral but asymmetric and resemble the 'variegated picture' of sacroiliitis in ankylosing spondylitis (Fig. 9.**122**).

Spine

In the chronic manifestation, axial skeletal involvement invariably occurs. **Parasyndesmophytes** develop and, because of their predominant location along the thoracolumbar transition, may mimic a spondylosis deformans.

Moreover, patients with Reiter syndrome can develop syndesmophytes and, in its full expression, a bamboo spine, though this occurs less frequently than in ankylosing spondylitis.

Other typical findings are **fibro-ostoses,** most common at the ischial tuberosities, trochanters and **calcaneus.** When the calcaneus is involved, retrocalcaneal bursitis should be excluded.

DD Reiter syndrome must be differentiated from gonococcal arthritis as another **post-venereal arthritis,** especially in view of the frequent simultaneous infections with gonococci and chlamydiae. Gonococcal arthritis usually is a purulent monoarthritis of sudden onset. The extra-articular manifestations, especially the cutaneous changes, often enable the clinical differentiation.

Psoriatic arthritis generally has a distinct distribution pattern, but can present with findings identical to those of Reiter syndrome. Psoriatic arthropathy mainly involves the hands, and the Reiter syndrome mainly the feet or knees.

Ankylosing spondylitis is clinically and radiographically dominated by the sacroiliac joints, unlike Reiter syndrome.

Rheumatoid arthritis usually has positive rheumatoid factors and primarily involves the hands.

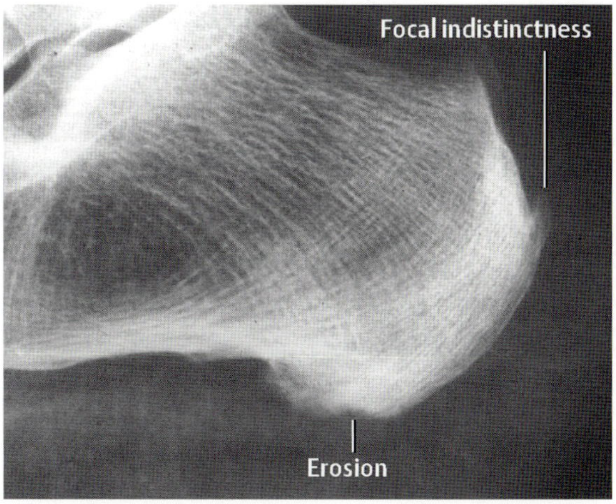

Fig. 9.**121** Erosive tenopathy of the plantar aponeurosis. Focal erosive changes are also seen at the insertion of the Achilles tendon.

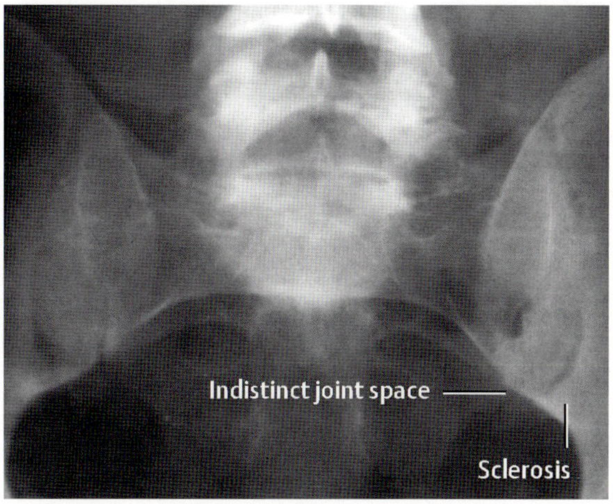

Fig. 9.**122** Asymmetric sacroiliitis.

Psoriatic Arthropathy

Synonym: Psoriatic arthritis.

■ Psoriatic arthritis is characterized by the coexistence of erosive destructive articular changes and proliferative osseous changes. It predominantly affects the bones of the hands and feet, as well as the SI joints and spine. ■

PATH Psoriatic arthritis is a seronegative spondyloarthropathy, and its exact pathogenesis is unknown.

CLINIC **Epidemiology:** The incidence of psoriatic arthritis is about 1% based on the 2%–4% incidence of common psoriasis and a concomitant arthritic involvement of 7%–40% (the stated estimates are quite variable). There is no gender bias, and the average age of onset is before 40 years.

In most cases, psoriatic arthropathy appears 5–15 years after the onset of psoriatic skin changes, but it can occur before the appearance of any skin lesions in about 10%–20% of patients.

Distribution pattern: It usually is a polyarthritis of the small joints of the hands and feet. Less commonly it may be an oligoarthritis or monoarthritis. The following types are distinguished:
- the transverse type (20%–35%), with isolated involvement of the distal interphalangeal articulations of the hands and feet, and
- the axial type (10%), with involvement of the distal interphalangeal, proximal interphalangeal, and metacarpophalangeal, or, respectively, metatarsophalangeal articulations of a single ray.

The remaining cases show a combined, usually asymmetric involvement of the distal interphalangeal, proximal interphalangeal, and metacarpophalangeal or, respectively, metatarsophalangeal articulations. In about 15% of cases, the skeletal manifestation is indistinguishable from rheumatoid arthritis.

A sacroiliitis and spondylitis develop in 20%–40% of patients, affecting mainly older men.

The hips and shoulders are rarely affected.

Course and prognosis: It is typical for psoriatic arthropathy to follow an intermittent course. Severe arthritic attacks alternate with longstanding remissions.

Destructions are observed in one-third of patients with an oligoarthritic pattern and in two-thirds with a polyarthritic pattern. In about 5% of patients, psoriatic arthritis follows a severe course, and mutilations appear early. Women, young patients, and patients with severe arthritic attacks tend to have a particularly severe clinical course.

X-RAY It is characteristic of psoriatic arthritis to show a **combination of destructive and proliferative changes** (Fig. 9.**123**).

Peripheral Joints

In addition to the general signs of arthritis, signs of destructive processes are also evident:
- very extensive erosions involving the 'bare areas', producing the appearance of **'mouse ears'** (Fig. 9.**124**),
- extensive mutilations in the final stage. This produces the **'pencil-in-cup'** or **'pencil-to-pencil'** appearance and, later, an ankylosis (compare with Fig. 9.**12** on page 297),
- occasionally, osteolysis and destruction affect the tuft of the distal phalanges and give it a frayed appearance **('tuft resorption').** The changes are invariably associated with diseased nails.

Signs of **osteoproliferative processes** are:
- **irregular** (spiculated) **ossifications** ('protuberances') at the sites of tendon and ligament insertions secondary to tendinitis. They are located at the metaphysis and diametaphysis of the short tubular bones (especially at the bases of the distal phalanx), calcaneus, talus (Fig. 9.**123**), trochanters, and ischial tuberosity;
- lamellated-undulated **periosteal ossification** (Fig. 9.**126**) secondary to the typical periostitis of the initial phase of psoriatic arthritis, often associated with soft-tissue swelling ('sausage-like fingers and toes'); the phalanges thus become more radiodense ('ivory phalanx,' Fig. 9.**125**).

SI Joints

The SI joints are involved in approximately 30%–50% of patients, and the changes are predominately **bilateral** and **symmetric.** The articulating surfaces and subchondral osseous structures are indistinct and represent destructive processes. Bone proliferations appear as subchondral sclerosis and fibroostosis at the iliac crest and ischial tuberosities.

Spine

As in Reiter syndrome, **parasyndesmophytes** are a typical finding (Fig. 9.**127**). Syndesmophytes also occur, but, compared to those of ankylosing spondylitis, they are frequently asymmetric and, furthermore, characteristically involve the middle and lower lumbar spine more often than the thoracolumbar transition. Atlanto-axial subluxation and involvement of the upper cervical spine (as in rheumatoid arthritis) are rare.

DD The most conspicuous signs of psoriatic arthritis are:

- asymmetric distribution pattern,
- osteoproliferative changes,
- often absent juxta-articular osteoporosis.

These findings generally enable differentiation from rheumatoid arthritis.

The most problematic differential diagnosis is **Reiter syndrome** since both conditions show a combination of osteodestructive and proliferative disorders. Furthermore, patients with Reiter syndrome can have psoriasis-like skin and nail changes.

The following findings can help with the differential diagnosis:

- Psoriatic arthritis shows equal involvement of the hands and feet, with an emphasis on the distal interphalangeal articulation. Reiter syndrome predominately involves the lower extremities and has a predilection for the metatarsophalangeal articulations.
- The paraspinal ossifications are less plump than in Reiter syndrome.

In **ankylosing spondylitis,** syndesmophytes, not parasyndesmophytes, dominate in the spine. Involvement of the distal extremities is considerably less common than in psoriatic arthritis. Involvement of the SI joints does not enable a differentiation between the conditions.

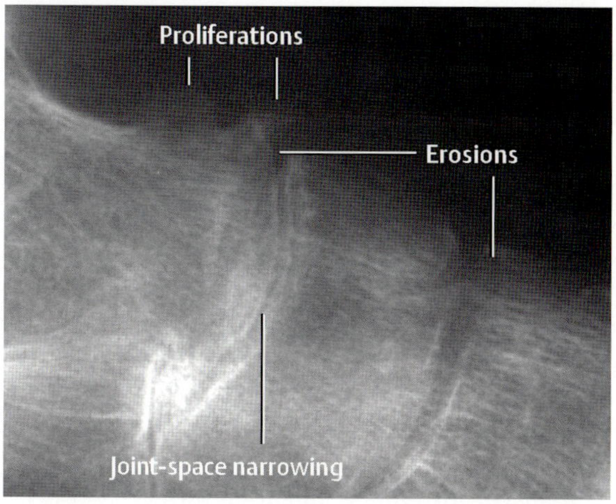

Fig. 9.**123** There are osseous proliferations and erosive changes at the talonavicular joint. The osseous apposition at the talar neck is not degenerative, but the osseous overgrowth along the articular margin could represent secondary degenerative changes.

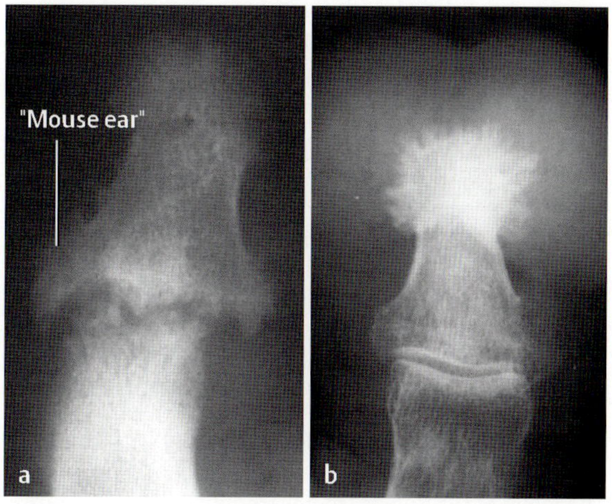

Fig. 9.**124** **a** Resorption and proliferation at the distal interphalangeal joint, beginning formation of 'mouse ears.' In contrast to erosive osteoarthritis, subchondral sclerosis is absent. **b** Periosteal proliferation along the phalangeal tuft with soft-tissue swelling ('psoriatic morning star' – named after the spiked medieval cudgel).

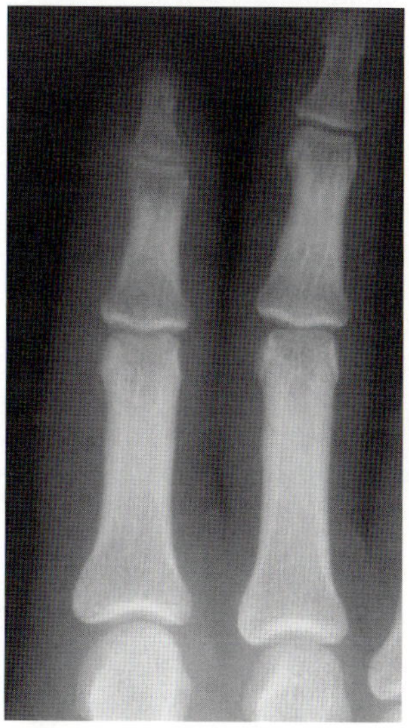

Fig. 9.**125** 'Sausage-like finger' (left) and 'ivory phalanx' (right).

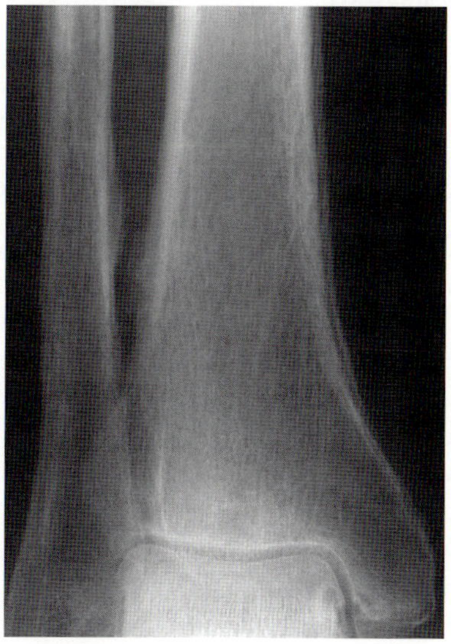

Fig. 9.**126** Periosteal reaction.

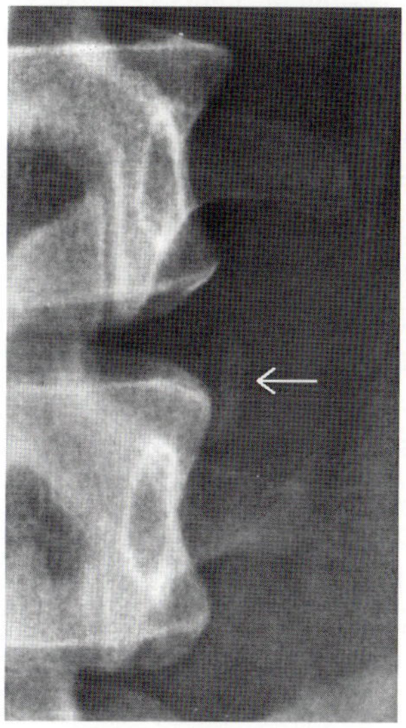

Fig. 9.**127** Discrete parasyndesmophyte (arrow).

Enteropathic Arthropathies

■ Enteropathic arthritis and spondylitis are disorders that follow inflammatory intestinal diseases. ■

The arthritis associated with **ulcerative colitis** and **Crohn disease** are the most important conditions in this group.

Other less-important intestinal disorders associated with arthritis are:
- gluten-sensitive enteropathy (celiac disease),
- Whipple disease (intestinal lipodystrophy),
- intestinal surgeries with blind loop,
- primary biliary cirrhosis,
- collagenous colitis, and
- nonclassifiable overlapping syndromes.

CLINIC **Epidemiology:** The incidence of arthropathy is about 10% for Crohn disease and somewhat lower for ulcerative colitis.
Symptoms: Whereas ulcerative colitis is characteristically associated with the acute onset of a monoarthritis or oligoarthritis, Crohn disease frequently is associated with an insidious migratory arthritis. The arthritis generally appears together with or after the intestinal symptoms, but in ulcerative colitis it can precede the intestinal manifestations in about 10%–15% of cases.
Distribution pattern: In both conditions, the most frequently involved joint is the knee, followed by the ankle. The joints of the fingers (metacarpophalangeal and proximal interphalangeal articulations) are occasionally involved in ulcerative colitis, but almost never in Crohn disease. In about 15% of cases, sacroiliitis or spondylitis develops.
Course and prognosis: The disease is generally transient, and articular destruction is rare. Interestingly, involvement of the peripheral joints correlates with intestinal symptoms, whereas involvement of the spine does not.

X-RAY **Peripheral Arthritis:**
The articular changes are nonspecific and usually confined to soft-tissue swelling and juxta-articular osteoporosis. Destructive changes (erosions, cysts) and joint-space narrowing are extremely rare, and are relevant in the differential diagnosis.
Sacroiliitis and Spondylitis:
The radiographic features are identical to those found in ankylosing spondylitis. The involvement of the SI joints is symmetric, and all features of the 'variegated picture' are present. In the spine, the vertebral bodies show erosions, deformities, and syndesmophytes. Even the bamboo spine can be observed in the late stages of either ulcerative colitis or Crohn disease.

Caution! Asymmetric involvement of the SI joints may represent septic arthritis from direct extension of the inflammatory process (especially with psoas abscesses).

DD The radiographic features are indistinguishable from those of ankylosing spondylitis. In the majority of patients, however, a chronic inflammatory intestinal disease is already known.

Articular Changes in Inflammatory Systemic Connective-tissue Diseases

■ This is a group of diseases characterized by abacterial inflammation of the connective tissue with swelling of the intracellular substance. They present as a monoarthritis, oligoarthritis, or a polyarthritis primarily involving the wrist. In contrast to rheumatoid arthritis and seronegative arthritis, they are frequently associated with soft-tissue calcifications, skin changes, and neurologic symptoms. ■

These conditions include:
- systemic lupus erythematosus (SLE),
- scleroderma,
- dermatomyositis/polymyositis,
- polyarteritis nodosa and other forms of vasculitis, and
- overlap collagenosis ('Sharp syndrome,' 'mixed connective-tissue disease').

PATH These inflammatory systemic connective-tissue disorders are autoimmune diseases whose pathogenesis is still not fully understood. They develop in patients with a genetic predisposition, and the onset of the disease is believed to be triggered by environmental factors (UV radiation, nutrients, medications) and infections.

Several types can be diagnosed by means of specific immunologic laboratory tests (ANA = antinuclear antibodies against DNA, RNA, and others). Confirmation of the diagnosis requires the entire armamentarium of imaging, laboratory, and histologic techniques.

CLINIC The diseases are characterized by an extreme variability of symptoms and course.

Systemic Lupus Erythematosus (SLE)

CLINIC **Epidemiology:** The disease is rare, but the incidence varies regionally and between cultures. There has been a recent increase in incidence, and women make up 90% of all patients.
Symptoms: The disease begins with nonspecific symptoms: abrupt onset with fever and malaise (as in an acute infection) or insidious onset over months with febrile episodes. Articular symptoms (arthralgias) up to the complete clinical picture of chronic polyarthritis develop in 90% of patients, and cutaneous findings are seen in up to 70%. Organ involvement is variable.
Distribution pattern: The articular involvement of systemic lupus erythematosus is symmetric, primarily affecting the joints of the hand and wrist, the knee, and the shoulder.
Course and prognosis: The course is chronic and progressive, typically with intermittent acute bouts. With early diagnosis and therapy, the 10-year survival rate is 90%–100%. Renal involvement, septic complications, and CNS involvement determine the prognosis.

X-RAY In most cases, the radiographic findings are limited to soft-tissue swelling and juxta-articular osteoporosis. Destructions of the cartilage and bones are **rare.** Also rare, in contrast to other collagenosis, are soft-tissue calcifications and acro-osteolyses.

Longstanding disease with recurrent arthritic attacks can lead to deforming nonerosive arthropathy (Jaccoud arthropathy). Ligamentous abnormalities cause the same typical deformities observed in rheumatoid arthritis (swan-neck deformity, boutonnière deformity).

DD The discrepancy between clinical findings identical to those seen in rheumatoid arthritis and radiographic findings without detectable erosive articular changes is typical for systemic lupus erythematosus (Fig. 9.**131**).

Because of the altered humoral immunity and the long-term corticosteroid therapy often required, patients are susceptible to bacteremia and, as a result, septic arthritis, and to bone infarcts. This should be considered in the differential diagnosis.

Progressive Systemic Scleroderma (PSS)

CREST syndrome: special manifestation of PSS: acral type, associated with **c**alcinosis, **R**aynaud symptoms, **e**sophageal dysfunction, **s**clerodactyly, and **t**elangiectases.

CLINIC Progressive systemic scleroderma usually begins with Raynaud syndrome, edematous swelling of the distal extremities including skin thickening, and polyarthralgias.

The skin induration is symmetrical. Based on the extent and progression of the disease, three types are distinguished:
Type I: Cutaneous sclerosis from the fingers to the wrist,
Type II: Cutaneous sclerosis from the wrist up the arms to the torso,
Type III: Cutaneous sclerosis of the torso and extending from there to the extremities.
The skin is taut, glassy, and hyperpigmented. The face is mask-like. Trophic ulcers (rat-bite lesions) can appear, especially at the fingertips.

The primary visceral manifestations include esophageal dysfunction, intestinal dysfunction with malabsorption, saccular herniations of the colon (due to atrophy of the smooth musculature), pulmonary fibrosis, cardiac insufficiency, and renal failure.
Distribution pattern: The radiologic changes are most pronounced at the hands, followed by the knee and ankle.
Course and prognosis: The course of scleroderma is variable, and progression is often slow. The prognosis is determined by the development of cardiac, pulmonary, and renal complications.

X-RAY **Soft Tissues:**
- initially thickening, later thinning of the soft-tissue mantle around the distal phalanges (chronic thinning: 'sugar loaf sign'),
- extensive subcutaneous extra-articular and sometimes also intra-articular calcifications.

Bone:
- osteoporosis (generalized or juxta-articular),
- in 40%–80%, osteolysis without productive changes involving the distal phalanges and middle phalanges (acro-osteolysis syndrome); in severe cases, complete destruction of the distal phalanges (Fig. 9.**128**),
- sclerosis of the distal phalanges (Fig. 9.**128**, 9.**129**),
- erosions of the first carpometacarpal articulation, with radial subluxation of the first metacarpal bone.

Joints:
- joint-space narrowing occurs but is rare.

See page 284 for the differential diagnosis of soft-tissue calcifications.

Polymyositis, Dermatomyositis

CLINIC The onset of the disease can be acute or insidious. In general, it begins with weakness of the musculature of the proximal extremities, polymyalgia, polyarthralgias, skin rashes, and Raynaud syndrome. The muscle weakness is primarily apparent when raising the arms, climbing stairs, and getting up from the supine position (neck flexor). Involvement of the pharynx and tongue musculature (dysphagia) occurs later. Hands, feet, and facial musculature are spared.

Skin involvement plus muscular findings (polymyositis) is referred to as dermatomyositis. Typical skin mani-

festations are dark erythematous rash on the face, and periorbital edema with discolorations (pathognomonic).
Caution: Both diseases can be paraneoplastic and require a tumor search when first detected.
Course and prognosis: With therapy, the 5-year survival rate exceeds 80%.
- Soft tissues: initially edematous swelling, later interstitial calcinosis as found with scleroderma.
- Joints: usually no radiologic changes, occasionally juxta-articular osteoporosis.

Polyarteritis nodosa

CLINIC Since the underlying necrotizing inflammation of the media and adventitia can affect almost any artery, the clinical presentation of polyarteritis nodosa is quite variable. The initial systemic complaints (fever, diffuse abdominal pain, weakness, weight loss) are followed by organ-related symptoms, with the clinical symptoms and signs determined by the affected organ. Polyarthralgias occur in 50% of patients.
Course and prognosis: Without therapy, two-thirds of the patients die within 1 year. Even with therapy, the 5-year survival rate is only 60%. Cardiac decompensation, renal insufficiency, and massive intestinal necrosis are the commonest causes of death.

X-RAY The arthralgias rarely show corresponding morphologic features. A diffuse osteoporosis is possible.

Mixed Collagenosis

Synonyms: Sharp syndrome, mixed connective-tissue disorder (MCTD).

Mixed collagenosis shows overlapping features of scleroderma, systemic lupus erythematosus, polymyositis, and rheumatoid arthritis.

The overlapping nature is also reflected in the radiographic manifestations:
- acral and marginal articular osteolysis, especially involving the distal interphalangeal joints as in scleroderma,
- erosions and juxta-articular osteoporosis as in rheumatoid arthritis,
- deformities as in systemic lupus erythematosus and rheumatoid arthritis,
- interstitial calcinosis (Fig. 9.**130**).

HIV-associated Articular Disease

There are three proposed mechanisms that lead to the arthritis associated with HIV infection:

1. Idiopathic AIDS-associated Arthralgia/Arthritis:

PATH It is still unknown whether the intra-articular presence of the virus alone can induce arthritis. So far, cultivating the human immunodeficiency virus in fluid aspirated from an affected joint has been successful in only a few cases. It has been suggested that the arthralgia may be related to the high incidence of avascular necrosis.

CLINIC The following clinical findings can be observed in AIDS arthritis:
- Arthralgias, primarily involving the joints of the lower extremities (knee, ankles), as well as elbow and shoulder; 10% of all AIDS patients develop articular attacks with severe tenderness and pain with motion; mild arthralgias are observed in an additional 30% of patients.
- Additional inflammatory signs are joint swelling and redness, primarily observed during self-limiting severe articular pain.
- Finally, idiopathic myalgias can occur, possibly as a manifestation of a 'subclinical myositis', as can symmetrical peripheral neuropathy; both are characterized by severe pain.
- Both radiographic and scintigraphic findings are generally unremarkable.

2. Associated Rheumatoid or Autoimmune Arthritis:

A higher incidence of a reactive arthritis similar to an incomplete Reiter syndrome has been observed in HIV infection. In the majority of cases, it occurs only in the late stages of AIDS, but in individual cases it can precede the onset of AIDS. Therefore, patients who are at risk for AIDS and are newly diagnosed with Reiter syndrome should be screened for HIV titers. This is especially important in view of reports that the immunosuppressive therapy of Reiter syndrome can promote AIDS in the presence of an unsuspected HIV infection. The disease then follows a very aggressive course, with early development of Kaposi sarcoma.

3. HIV-associated Septic Arthritis:

There is a slightly increased incidence of musculoskeletal infection in HIV-infected patients. In view of the increasing life expectancy of AIDS patients, this complication can be expected to play a major role in the future. Bacterial arthritis, bursitis, and pyomyositis, as well as opportunistic infections of the joints and bones, all occur.

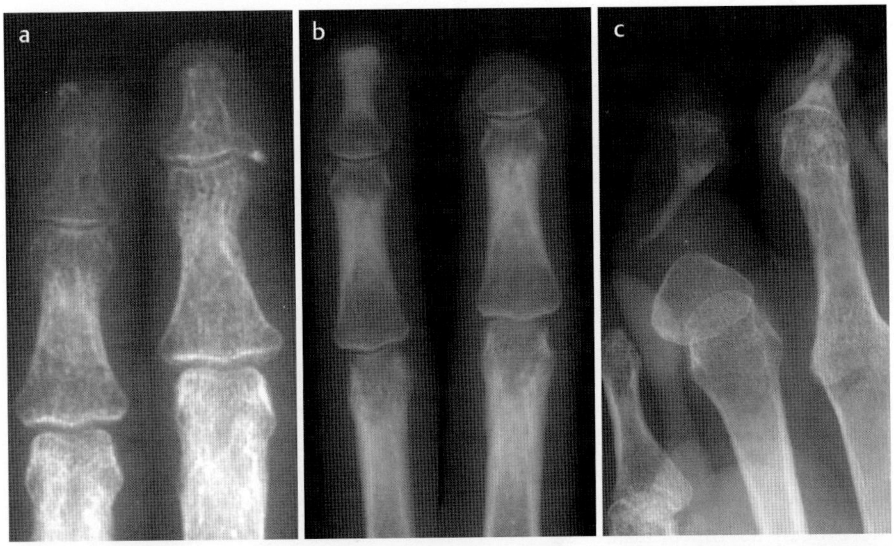

Fig. 9.**128** Several manifestations of scleroderma in the hand. Osteoporosis dominates in (**a**) and phalangeal sclerosis in (**b**). All cases show osteolytic destruction of different degrees, leading to complete phalangeal destruction (**c**) in severe cases.

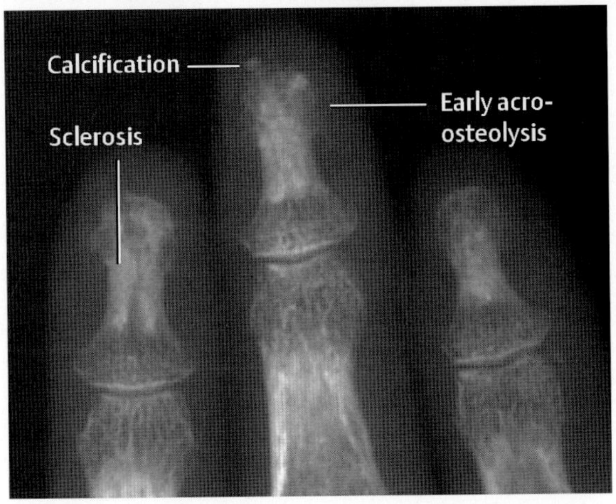

Fig. 9.**129** Mixed collagenosis (Sharp syndrome). Early radiographic changes manifested as soft-tissue calcifications, acro-osteosclerosis, and acro-osteolysis.

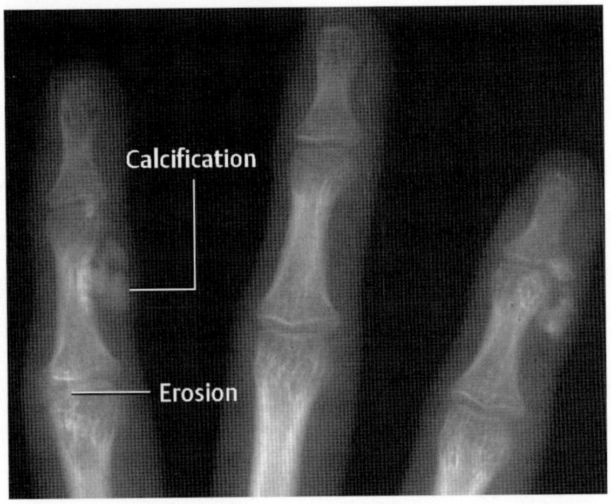

Fig. 9.**130** Sharp syndrome in a 14-year-old female patient. Besides soft-tissue calcifications, erosions are seen at the proximal interphalangeal joint of the fourth ray.

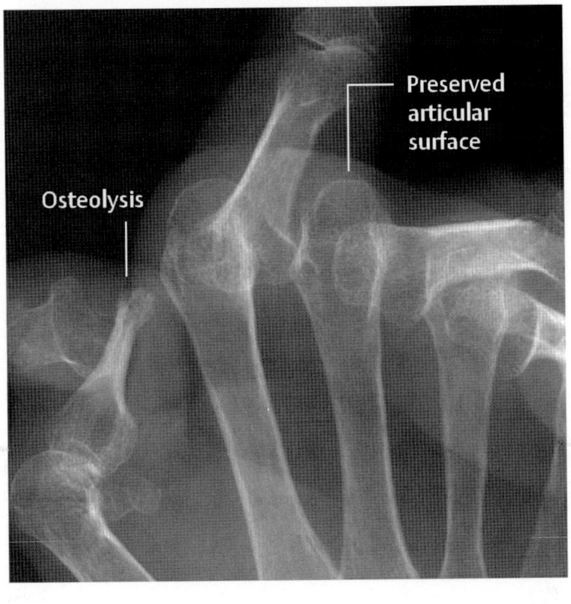

Fig. 9.**131** Systemic lupus erythematosus. The clinical picture could not be distinguished from rheumatoid arthritis. Radiographically, the metacarpal heads are misaligned, but the articular surfaces are intact. This discrepancy is typical of systemic lupus erythematosus. Marked resorptions, as seen here at the proximal phalanx of the thumb, are less frequent.

Differential Diagnosis of Arthritis

Even with the help of all of the imaging modalities, analyzing the imaging features of one joint will not succeed in distinguishing among the various factors that have caused the arthritis. The evaluation must always include the **clinical aspects** and relies on the close cooperation of the radiologist and the rheumatologist. Especially important are:

- The patient group: Age, gender, known underlying diseases, family history, risk factors,
- Acute complaints: Morning stiffness? Is the arthritis active? Systemic symptoms or 'only' arthritis? Skin changes?
- Course of the disease: Where was the initial manifestation? How long have the symptoms been present? Have there been asymptomatic intervals?
- Distribution pattern: Which joints are involved? Is the articular involvement symmetric? Is the central skeleton involved?

! The distribution pattern is the most important criterion in the differential diagnosis of articular diseases.

Analysis of the imaging studies should answer the following questions:

- Does the disease really arise from the joint, from the soft tissue, or from the juxta-articular bone?
- Which radiographic features dominate? Are they the result of synovitis or alterations in cartilage (compare with pages 294–304)?
- Are there signs of enthesopathy? Do these signs dominate? Do these signs precede the signs of synovitis, or did they develop later?
- Do the radiographic signs reflect acute or chronic (old) changes, or are they a combination of both?
- Is there reactive osseous change (periosteal reaction)?

! The more advanced the arthritis, the more difficult the interpretation of an image becomes. To answer these questions, images obtained at the earlier stage of the disease should be compared to current radiographic studies.

The differential diagnosis of the many forms of arthritis is easier once all of the clinical and radiologic findings are known. A summary of the most important discriminating criteria is presented in Table 9.**9**.

Table 9.**9** Synopsis of the important differentiating criteria of arthritis

	Septic arthritis	Rheumatoid arthritis	Juvenile rheumatoid arthritis	Ankylosing spondylitis	Reactive arthritis	Psoriatic arthritis	Enteropathic arthritis	SLE, PSS, polymyositis and others
Distribution pattern	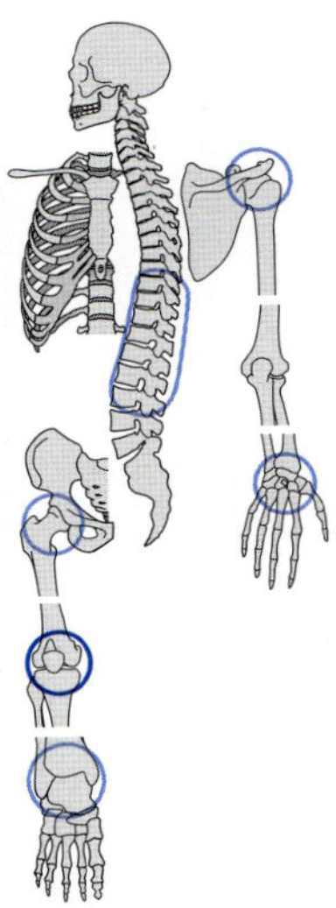	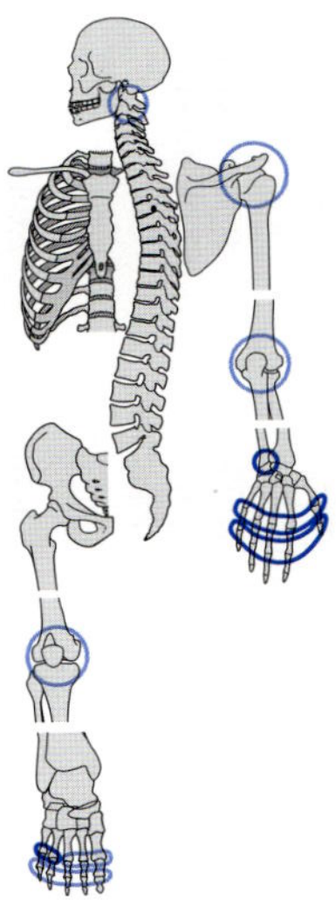	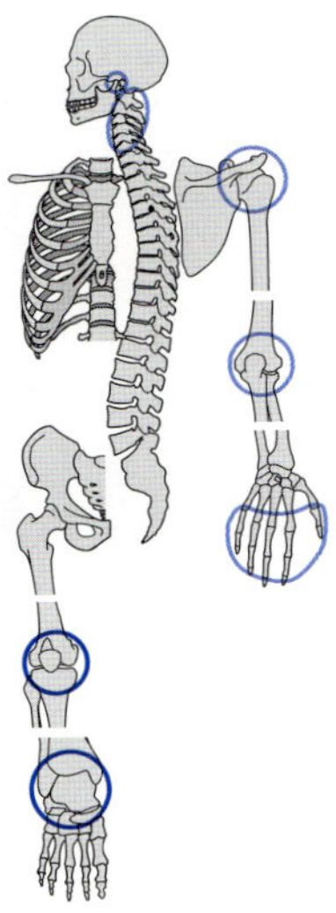	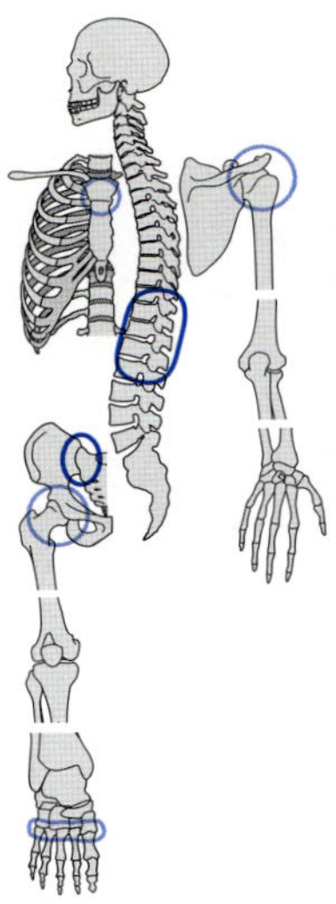	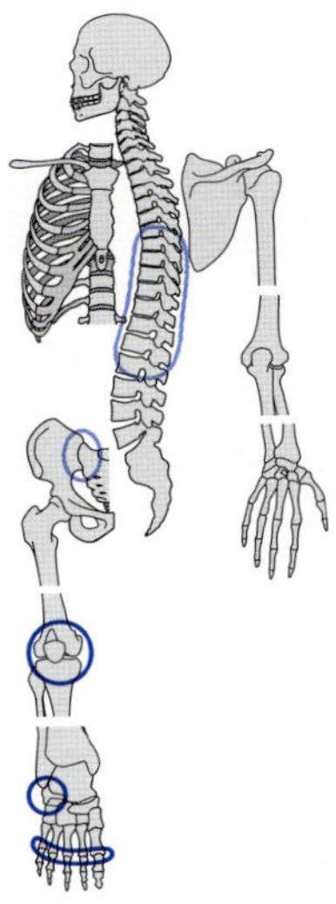	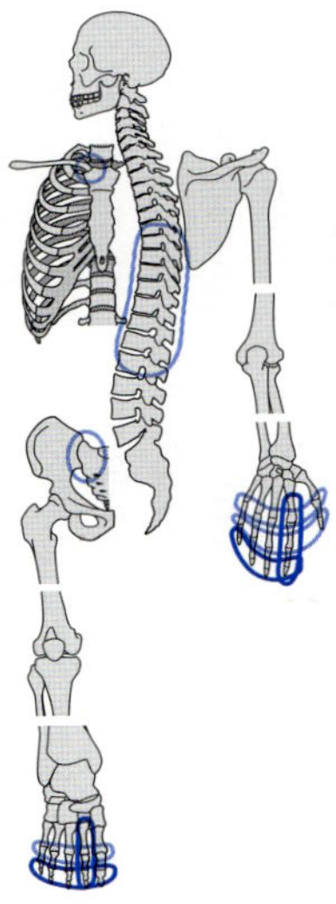	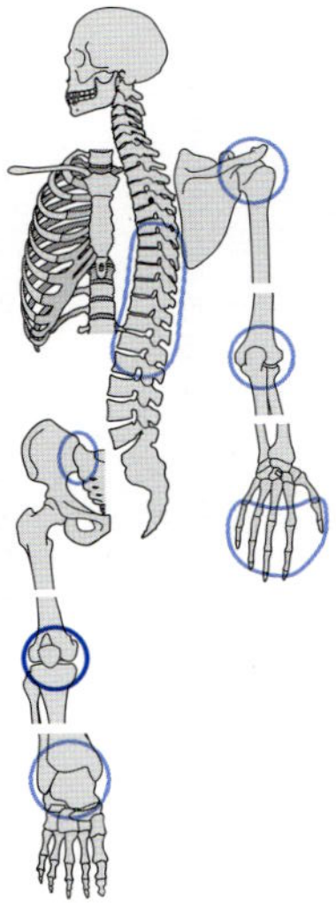	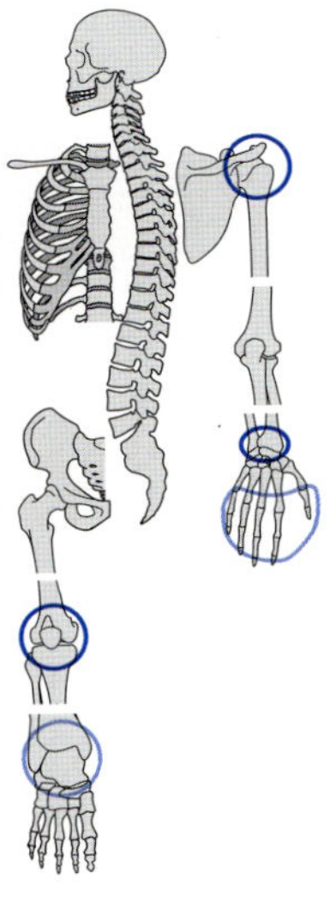
Symmetry?	No	Yes	Yes	Yes	No	No	No	Yes
Juxta-articular osteoporosis	++	+++	++	+/–	+/–	+++	+	++
Destructive changes	+++	+++	++	+	+	+++	+/–	++
Proliferative changes	–	–	+	++	+++	+++	++	
Special features	Rapidly progressing joint destruction	Almost always ulnar styloid process involvement, later involvement of the DIP joints, finger deformities, cervical spine often also involved	Periosteal reaction, involvement of the TM joint, ballooning	'Variegated picture' of sacroiliitis, syndesmophytes, fibro-exostoses, involvement of the manubriosternal articulation	Periosteal reaction, sausage-like fingers, parasyndesmophytes, fibro-exostoses	'Mouse ears', 'sausage-like fingers', parasyndesmophytes, fibro-exostoses	Only ra destruc	

Neuroge
Hemat

Ne

…nic, Metabolic, and …ologic Joint Diseases

…urogenic Osteoarthropathy (Charcot Joint)

■ Neurogenic osteoarthropathy is a disease of the joint, bone, and soft tissue representing excessive destruction caused by deficient innervation. There are many causes (Table 9.**10**). ■

The initial disease entity described by **Charcot** was caused by tabes dorsalis (Fig. 9.**135**), but the most frequent type encountered today is diabetic osteoarthropathy of the foot. The changes caused by neurogenic osteoarthropathy have nothing in common with those caused by paralysis or spasticity, which lead to hypoplasia or atrophy of the affected musculoskeletal region, disuse osteoporosis, or deformity of the joint-forming bone.

PATH A joint relies on neural feedback to maintain its integrity. This feedback assures the correctly balanced mechanical loading of the joint (corresponding to the regulatory circuit that controls the muscular system) and adapts the blood supply exactly to the needs of the various tissues.

If this feedback system is interrupted by neuropathy, the joint no longer can withstand the daily weight-bearing strain, and this results in articular destruction that ultimately far exceeds 'normal' osteoarthritic changes.

Based on the neuropathic joint destruction observed in bedridden patients, it is now assumed that neural and vascular aberrations ('neurovascular theory') contribute more to this destruction than unequal mechanical loading ('neurotraumatic theory'). However, the pathogenesis is still not fully understood.

CLINIC Superficial soft-tissue changes, such as edema, fistulae, and painless ulcers are clinically suspicious findings. Because of the hyposensitivity, a marked discrepancy almost always exists between the minor subjective complaints and the impressive abnormal radiographic findings.

X-RAY The variably severe destructive changes of the joints and bones, often reaching bizarre proportions, are appropriately called the 'anarchic' radiographic picture. The changes can be atrophic (osteolytic), hypertrophic (sclerotic), or a combination of both (Table 9.**11**, Figs. 9.**132**–9.**135**).

Other imaging modalities do not play a major role in diagnosing neurogenic osteoarthropathies but do help to exclude other conditions (e.g., infections).

DD Excessive joint destruction from other causes must be distinguished from neuropathic arthropathy. Important are:

- destructive osteoarthrosis (insufficiency fractures, fragmentations, and exuberant callus formation are absent),
- infectious and other forms of arthritis (signs of hypertrophy and insufficiency fractures are absent).

Table 9.**10** Causes and sites of neurogenic osteopathies and arthropathies

Causes	Typical sites
Metabolic	
Diabetes mellitus	Foot
Cushing syndrome	Hip, knee, shoulder
Amyloid neuropathy	Ankle and foot joints
Inflammatory	
Leprosy	Variable
Tabes dorsalis	Knee, hip, foot
Congenital	
Spinal syringomyelia	Shoulder, elbow
Dysraphism	Ankle and foot joints
Trauma	Depending on nature of trauma
Idiopathic	Variable

Table 9.**11** Synopsis of radiographic features in neurogenic osteoarthropathy

Atrophic changes	Hypertrophic changes
Juxta-articular demineralization to osteolysis, (marginal) erosions. Final stage: 'sucked-on' appearing bone	Sclerotic spongiosa, periosteal reaction, 'column-like' metatarsals
Insufficiency fractures: fragmentation, disintegration	Exuberant callus formation, pseudarthrosis
Dislocations	Synostoses
Soft-tissue swelling, possibly with gas in soft tissues	Heterotopic soft-tissue calcifications

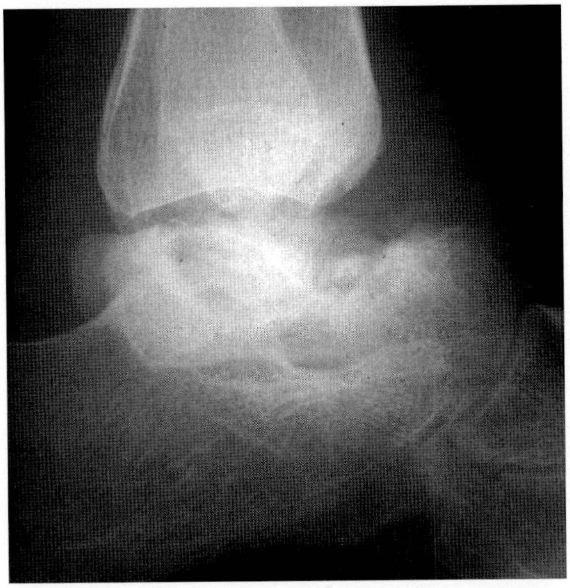

Fig. 9.132 Female patient with spinal dysraphism. The radiograph shows evidence of osteoarthropathy dominated by structural collapse of the talus.

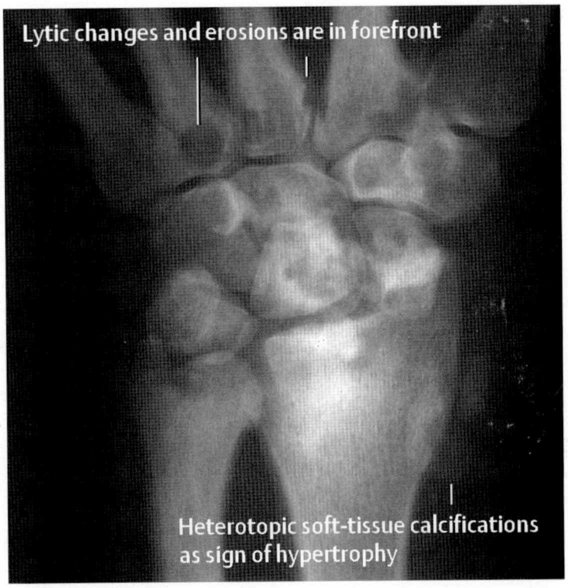

Fig. 9.133 Patient with syringomyelia. Atrophic type of neurogenic osteoarthropathy.

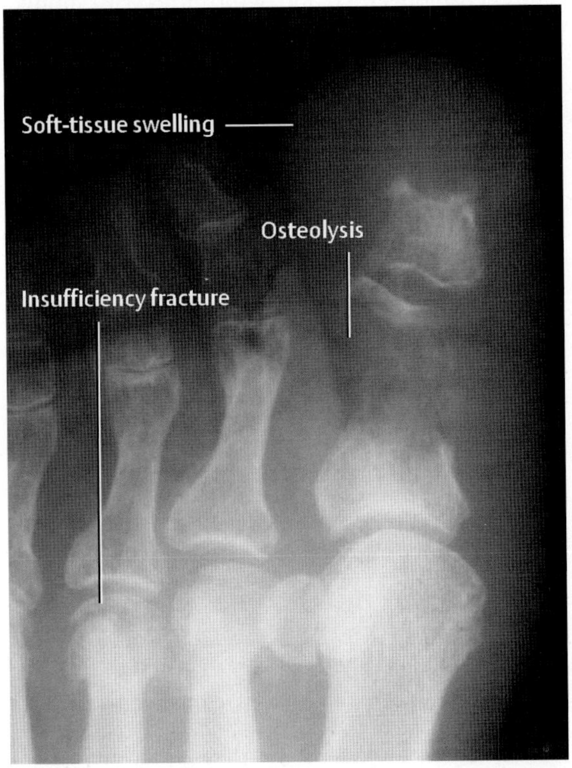

Fig. 9.134 Neurogenic osteoarthropathy due to traumatic neural damage (war injury): typical radiographic features. Diabetes mellitus could be excluded.

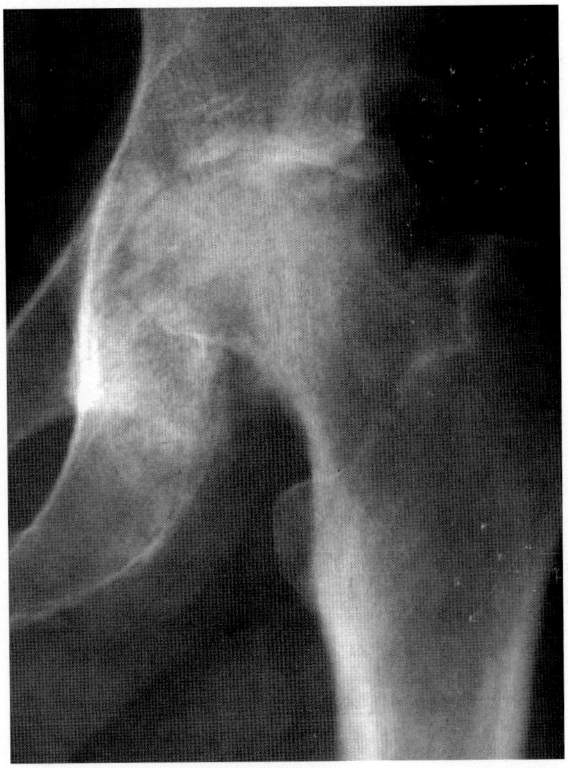

Fig. 9.135 Classic Charcot joint in a 66-year-old female patient with tabes dorsalis. The femoral head is beginning to 'melt away'. There are soft-tissue calcifications. Differentiating this from a destructive osteoarthritis was possible because of the additional involvement of the knee joint and feet.

The Diabetic Foot

■ The term 'diabetic foot' refers to soft-tissue and bone changes in diabetes mellitus caused by neuropathy and the resultant unequal mechanical loading, angiopathy, and arterial superinfection (immunopathy). Furthermore, fluctuating blood insulin levels and hyperglycemias promote periosteal new bone formation and sclerosis and might even lead to complete arrest of bone turnover ('freeze' effect). ■

PATH Neuropathy (caused by metabolic damage of the peripheral nerves and a microangiopathy of their nutrient vessels) is viewed as the most important cause of the potential pathogenic factors. The exact interaction of the factors causing diabetic neuropathy and angiopathy is still not known.

CLINIC Important cardinal symptoms are hypoesthesias, reflex anomalies, burning pain, later ulcerations, and soft-tissue swelling.

X-RAY Radiographs show a severe decrease in bone density of the entire skeleton and osteolysis of the metatarsal heads with concomitant decrease in the diameter of the metatarsal shafts. Otherwise, the general radiographic signs of neurogenic arthropathy are found (Figs. 9.**137**–9.**139**). The pedal arteries show media calcifications, and this helps in the differentiation from other types of neurologic osteoarthropathy.

The tarsal bones are the most commonly affected location, followed in incidence by the tarsometatarsal and metatarsophalangeal articulations.

Radiographic signs of a superinfection are:
- rapid appearance of erosions without evidence of bone production,
- rapid disintegration of the bone,
- gas in the soft tissues.

Caution! Definitive radiographic signs of a superinfection do not exist.

MRI The transformation caused by the neuropathy or angiopathy and infectious changes both produce a nonspecific increase in signal intensity, especially in the soft tissues. If a fracture has occurred, these changes also involve the bones (T2-weighted SE images or STIR sequence, Fig. 9.**140**). For differentiation from a superinfection, it is helpful to detect a contiguous extension of the infection along a compartment, from skin ulcers, soft-tissue edema, and abscesses, as well as osseous involvement (Fig. 9.**136**).

It is the goal of the radiographic examination to assess the extent of the disease process and, as far as possible, to determine the effects of the four pathogenetic factors. Radiographs can differentiate between an atrophic (early, active phase; 'decompensated foot') and a hypertrophic (later, reparative phase; 'stabilized foot') type. For therapy planning (especially targeted surgical abscess drainage or excision), the extent of the infection is best appreciated on MRI. Microangiopathy can also be detected angiographically.

Corticosteroid-induced Neuropathic-like Alterations (Pseudo-Charcot Joint)

Systemic application of corticosteroids interferes with the **protective joint sensibility** and causes hypoesthesia. In addition, it induces epiphyseal vascular occlusion and **osteonecrosis.** Finally, collagen damage leads to degeneration and **rupture** of ligaments and joint capsules.

Signs of osteonecrosis and deformities with subluxations and dislocations are observed radiographically. The impaired protected mechanisms can lead to massive destruction. Involvement of the hip and knee is most common.

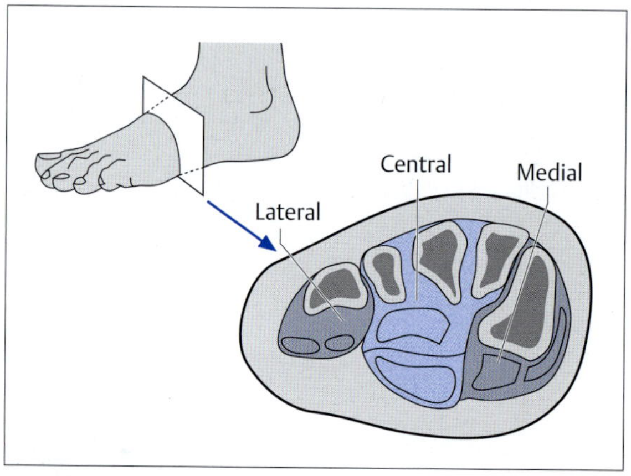

Fig. 9.**136** Compartments of the foot and their influence on the spread of infections: the intercompartmental septa are effective barriers to the flow of fluids. In contrast, the septa dividing the central compartment show disruptions (modified after Goodwin et al., 1995).

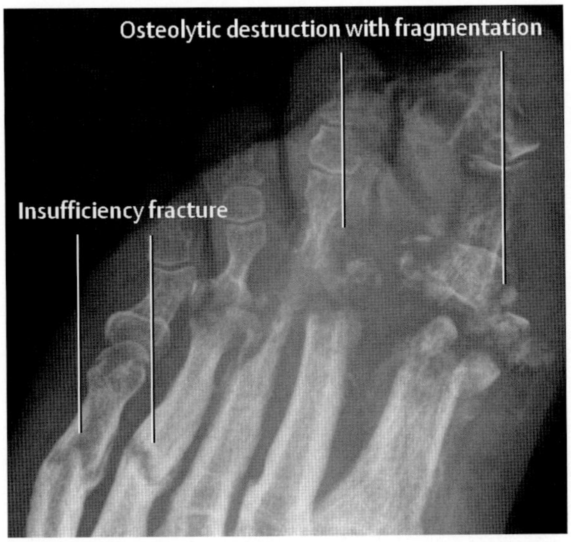

Fig. 9.**137** Diabetic osteoarthropathy.

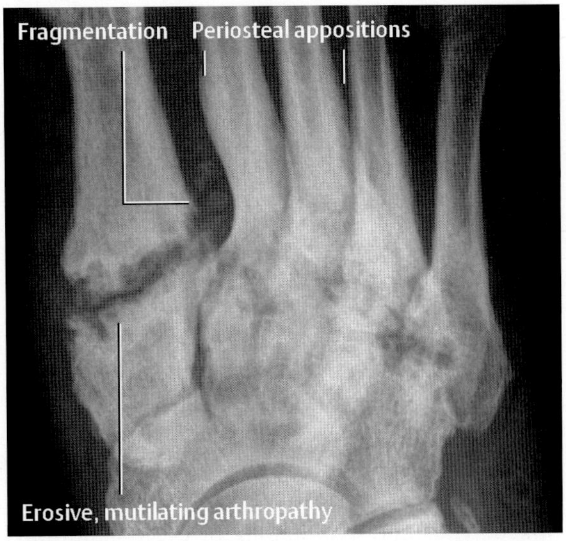

Fig. 9.**138** Diabetic osteoarthropathy with diffuse sclerosis and periosteal new bone formation.

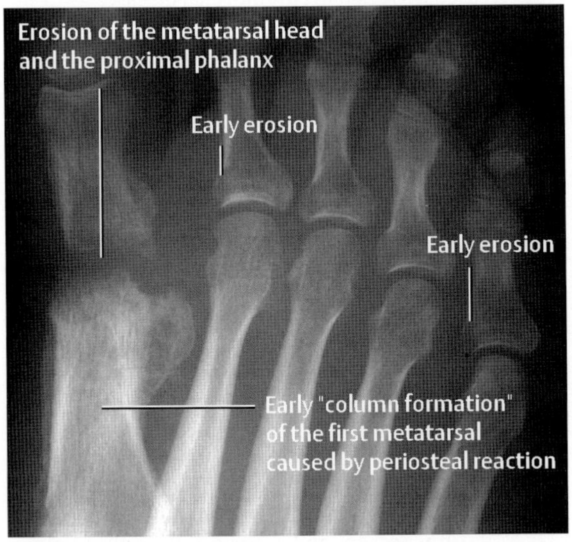

Fig. 9.**139** Female patient with diabetes mellitus.

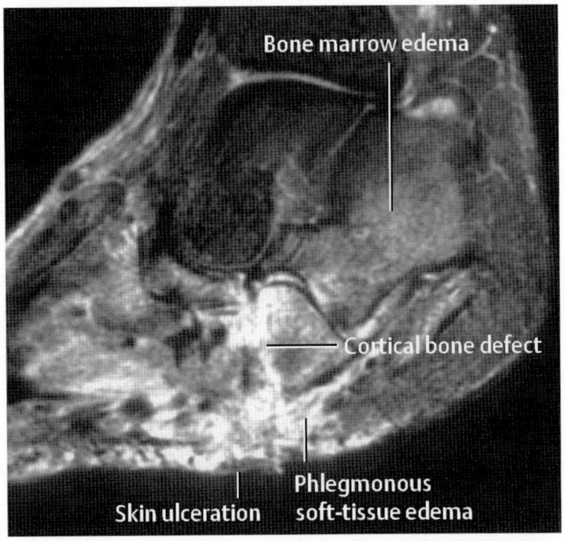

Fig. 9.**140** MRI STIR sequence: diabetic osteomyelitis of the foot, skin ulceration. The soft-tissue infection is confined to the lateral plantar compartment.

Crystal-induced Arthropathies and Periarthropathies

■ This is a heterogeneous group of joint diseases characterized by intra- or periarticular crystals deposited by different causative conditions. ■

The group includes:
- gout,
- calcium pyrophosphate dihydrate crystal deposition disease (CPDD, chondrocalcinosis),
- calcium hydroxyapatite crystal deposition disease,
- corticosteroid-induced crystal arthritis as an exogenous manifestation (Fig. 9.**141**).

Mixed types and overlapping of these conditions are by no means rare and make a clear separation difficult (Table 9.**12**).

PATH Crystal deposition in the joint or periarticular soft tissues can interact with the surrounding tissues in three ways:
- inflammatory reaction, clinically in the form of a synovitis,
- acceleration of degenerative destruction (caused by crystal shedding into the articular cavity),
- quiescence without evidence of bone production.

There are many different manifestations, and there is often marked discrepancy between the clinical symptoms and radiologic findings.

X-RAY Radiographs are the most important imaging modality. The evaluation should address:
- soft-tissue changes in the form of swelling or increased density (caused by tophi as seen in gout, effusion, and synovial changes) or in the form of calcifications (of cartilage, tendon, joint capsule, and possible pre-existing tophi),
- joint-space narrowing and osteophytes as signs of osteoarthritis,
- erosions or subchondral cysts, sometimes of considerable magnitude, caused by cartilage damage, synovitis, or pressure erosions (e.g., in tophaceous gout),
- destructive arthropathy as seen in the final stage.

DD The diagnosis is based primarily on the findings of radiography. The diagnosis can be confirmed with special laboratory tests if fluid can be aspirated from a joint effusion. The radiographic differential diagnosis can be **challenging**, since the findings overlap with other forms of arthritis and especially with osteoarthritis. In addition to 'thinking of the diagnosis', the typical distribution pattern and the characteristic constellation of the individual radiographic features endow each entity with a unique 'profile' (Table 9.**12**).

Gout (Gouty Arthritis)

■ Gouty arthritis is caused by the deposition of uric acid crystals. ■

PATH Uric acid is the end product of nucleic acid metabolism. Its increased synthesis or decreased renal excretion causes hyperuricemia.

Primary hyperuricemia:
- inborn abnormality of the nucleic acid metabolism (absent feedback inhibition) or renal excretion.

Secondary hyperuricemia:
- excess in exogenous nucleic acids (e.g., diet rich in nucleic acids) or endogenous nucleic acids (increased cell cycles as seen with myeloproliferative disorders, tumor regression during chemotherapy, etc.),
- decreased excretion in chronic renal disease.

If the concentration of uric acid exceeds the solubility value of 6.4 mg%, uric acid precipitates and is deposited as crystals, primarily in sites with low pH values (e.g., synovial fluid, tendon sheaths and bursae, subcutaneous tissue, and kidneys). This leads to crystal synovitis with damage to the articular cartilage by crystals precipitated along its surface.

In the late (chronic) stage of untreated gout, tophi develop. The tophus is formed when uric crystals precipitate in an acid environment and induce a chronic local inflammatory reaction. In the active phase, it is initially surrounded by very vascular granulation tissue and, in the static phase, by a fibrous connective tissue capsule. Macroscopically, its central mass looks like chalk (tophus = Latin: porous stone). The size of the tophi varies between a few millimeters and several centimeters. They are often found as clusters in either the soft tissues or bone.

CLINIC The onset of the disease typically occurs in the fifth decade, and men are affected 12 times more frequently than women. The preferred location of involvement is the first metatarsophalangeal joint; other preferential locations are listed in Fig. 9.**142**.

Stages of gout:
- Asymptomatic hyperuricemia.
- Acute gout: monoarticular pain attack (usually involving the first metatarsophalangeal articulation).
- Intercritical gout: symptom-free interval between acute gout attacks, lasting weeks to years. Later, the interval becomes shorter.
- Chronic gout: generally more than 10 years after the first gout attack. It is characterized by tophi, joint defects, and gout kidneys.

Therapy: Inhibiting the formation of uric acids (e.g., allopurinol).

Table 9.**12** Crystal-deposition arthropathies and periarthropathies: synopsis

Disease	Composition of crystals	Site	Predilection (target area)
Gout	Sodium urates	Articular and periarticular	First metatarsophalangeal articulation
Pyrophosphate dihydrate crystal deposition disease (CPDD)	Calcium pyrophosphate dihydrate (CPDD)	Fibrocartilage and hyaline cartilage, fiber-rich connective tissue, synovial lining	Knee, wrist
Hydroxyapatite crystal deposition disease (HADD)	Calcium hydroxyapatite	Periarticular tendons and bursae	Shoulder
Corticosteroid-induced crystal synovitis (Fig. 9.**141**)	Crystallized corticosteroids	Injection site	Injection site

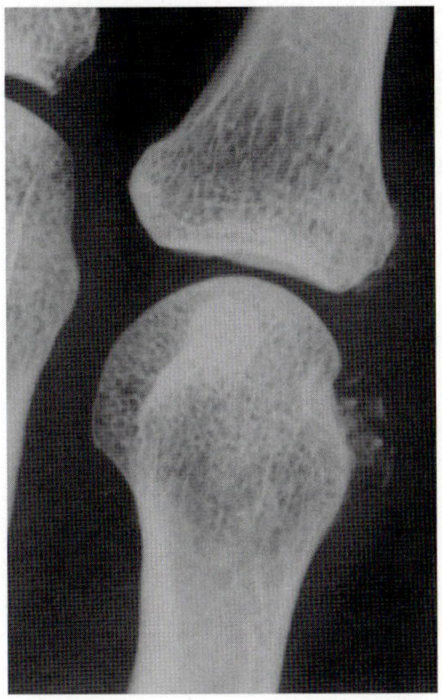

Fig. 9.**141** Corticosteroid-induced arthropathy (calcific deposits immediately after injection; complete resolution after 2 years).

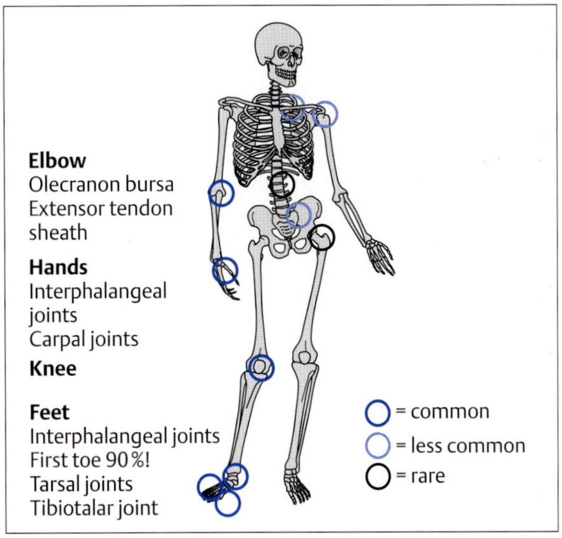

Fig. 9.**142** Distribution pattern of gouty arthritis.

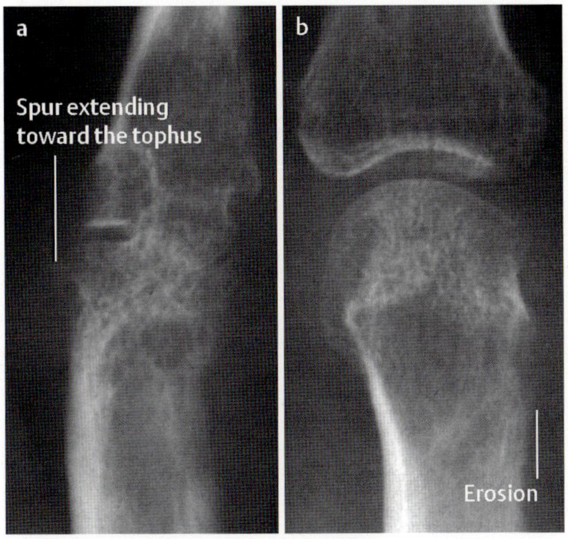

Fig. 9.**143** **a** Periarticular soft-tissue tophus with spur. Small periarticular tophi are also present. **b** Superficial erosive and proliferative changes.

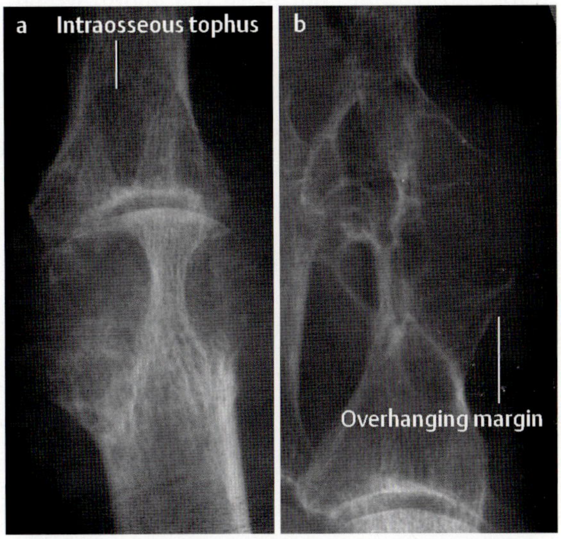

Fig. 9.**144** **a** Large periarticular osseous tophi. Concentric indentation of the metatarsal head. Notice the preserved joint space. **b** Large tophus with osseous destruction below the articular margin.

X-RAY In **acute** gout, the radiographic findings are either completely unremarkable or show nonspecific signs of acute arthritis (e.g., soft-tissue swelling) in locations targeted by gout.

In **chronic** gout, the detectable radiographic findings are all caused by tophi. Depending on the location, the findings can be grouped as:

Periarticular findings with secondary osseous involvement ('soft-tissue tophus'):

- Eccentric round-to-ovoid soft-tissue thickening (= matrix of the tophus). Occasionally, traces of calcific densities are visible.
- Tophus spur: spiculated periosteal reaction (Fig. 9.**143 a**).
- Erosive irregularities of the osseous surface (Fig. 9.**143 b**).

Osseous tophus ('medullary tophus'):

- Round or oval osteolytic area with a sharp border ('punched-out' appearance), often achieving considerable size (diameter exceeding 5 mm) with or without sclerotic border (depending on the activity). The osteolysis is usually subchondral and at the margin, but can also occur in the center of the bone (Fig. 9.**144 b**). Discrete radiolucencies in the spongiosa might precede the osteolytic foci.
- Subperiosteally growing tophi produce 'overhanging edges' (margins) due to periosteal elevation (Fig. 9.**144 b**).
- Subchondral osteolysis that extends into the joint, causing considerable mutilation (Fig. 9.**145**).

Osteoarthritic manifestation:

In longstanding gout, a crystal-induced osteoarthritis can develop and mark the gouty osseous changes.

SONO Sonographically, tophi appear as typical echogenic nodules with broad, indistinctly outlined, acoustic shadowing cast by the crystal in the center.

MRI If the diagnosis is unknown, MRI can be used to evaluate solitary large soft-tissue or bone tophi that can mimic tumors. If the diagnosis is known and resection of the tophus planned, MRI can be helpful in individual cases for visualizing the relationship of the tophus to surrounding anatomic structures.

Characteristic MRI findings correspond to the histology of the tophus:

- T2-weighted SE sequence (useful: frequency selected fat suppression): high signal intensity in the protein-rich matrix.
- T1-weighted SE sequence after administration of contrast medium: the surrounding granulation tissue exhibits intense enhancement (Fig. 9.**146**).
- Urate crystals by themselves have no signal and are not visualized within the protein mass because of their extremely small size.

DD Gout is a clinical diagnosis (typical pain attacks, hyperuricemia, crystals detected in the joint fluid). Occasionally, uricemia is not present at the time of the clinical examination.

The differential diagnosis of gout encompasses the entire spectrum of conditions that cause arthritis and osteoarthritis. However, some findings, if present, can be considered relatively specific for gout:

- typical first metatarsophalangeal articulation location,
- asymmetrical involvement,
- tendency to spread from medial to lateral (foot),
- absence of juxta-articular osteoporosis,
- partially intact articular surface and preserved joint space despite extensive osteolysis,
- osteolysis distant from the joint.

! The more an osteolysis in the articular end of a bone extends to the diaphysis, the more likely it represents tophaceous gout.
Any osteolytic focus exceeding 5 mm observed in a man is suspicious for gout.

More discriminating criteria for specific differential diagnostic questions are summarized in Table 9.**13**.

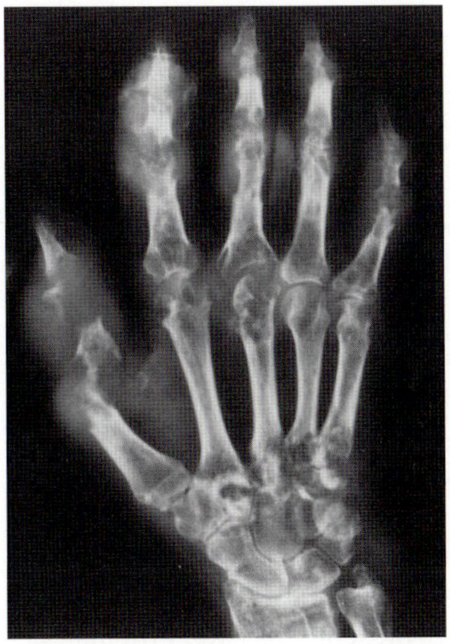

Fig. 9.**145** Mutilating gout.

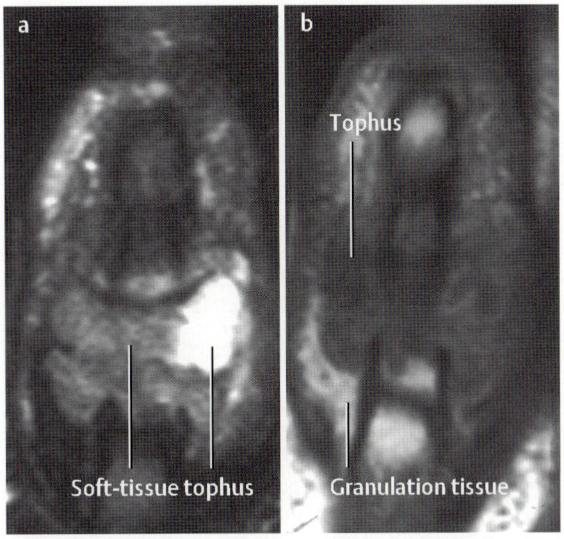

Fig. 9.**146** MRI of a large periarticular soft-tissue tophus at the middle finger.
a T2-weighted SE sequence with fat suppression: high signal intensity of the central matrix.
b T1-weighted SE sequence after administration of contrast medium: surrounding enhancing granulation tissue.

Table 9.**13** Differential diagnosis of gout

Differential diagnosis	Discriminating criteria
Gout with erosive changes	
Rheumatoid arthritis	Bilateral symmetric pattern (hands, feet), fusiform soft-tissue swelling, spread in the feet from lateral to medial, juxta-articular demineralization, early joint-space narrowing, rarely large (> 5 mm) and no osteolytic foci away from the joint
Psoriatic arthritis	Productive bone changes similar to those of gout, also mutilating joints No intraosseous tophus-like osteolysis
Erosive polyarthritis	Heberden and Bouchard nodes as well as occasional large subchondral cysts might mimic gout; symmetric involvement is indicative of osteoarthritis
Pigmented villonodular synovitis (PVNS)	Eccentric soft-tissue thickening and juxta-articular, also larger, osteolysis that might resemble gout, preferentially at the knee. In contrast to gout, no pain for a long time and late onset of symptoms (thus, no clinical arthritic signs)
Amyloid arthropathy	Soft-tissue thickening and erosive-cystic bone changes as seen in gout Only laboratory results, history, and histology help in the differentiation
Sarcoidosis	Cystic type can mimic gout, but sarcoidosis is painless
Solitary large soft-tissue tophus (rare)	
Bursitis, mesenchymal tumor	Differentiation only clinically, by MRI, by biopsy
Solitary large osseous tophus (rare)	
Intraosseous ganglion	Detection of fluid with MRI
Chondroblastoma	Strong tendency of the tumor to calcify
Giant-cell tumor	Detection of homogeneous soft-tissue tumor with MRI

Pyrophosphate Arthropathy

Synonym: Calcium pyrophosphate dihydrate crystal deposition disease (CPDD), chondrocalcinosis (often in reference to the radiologically evident cardinal sign of calcification), pseudogout (primarily used in the presence of gout-like pain attacks).

This is a crystal arthropathy characterized by the accumulation of calcium pyrophosphate dihydrate crystals, primarily in the fibrocartilage and synovial fluid.

PATH Etiology:
- **primary,** and often with familiar clustering,
- **secondary,** as a manifestation of metabolic or endocrine disorders (hyperparathyroidism, hypothyroidism, hemochromatosis, diabetes mellitus, and others).

Calcium pyrophosphate crystals are an intermediary metabolic product found in connective tissue. They characteristically accumulate in biochemically abnormal fibrocartilage, as found in disks and menisci, as well as in the superficial 'fibrocartilaginous' zone of the hyaline cartilage. They are also found in the synovial fluid of the joint and bursa and in fibrous connective tissue (joint capsule, tendon, or ligament).

CLINIC It occurs with increasing incidence after age 50 years and is a typical geriatric disease. Both genders are equally affected.

The crystalline deposits become symptomatic by inducing a synovitis, which can follow a variable course:
- chronic condition of variable intensity (commonest form),
- pseudogout (recurrent pain attacks, less severe than acute gout attacks, atypical location),
- asymptomatic (in about one-fifth of the cases, especially with calcification of the anulus fibrosis of the disk).

X-RAY Radiographs reveal periarticular calcifications and synovial swelling, and four different types of calcifications are described (Figs. 9.**148**, 9.**149**):
- Cartilaginous calcification: chondrocalcinosis in the true sense of the definition,
- Synovial calcification (rare special type of tophaceous pseudogout, characterized by large synovial calcification),
- Calcification of the joint capsule, ligaments, and tendons,
- Nonspecific soft-tissue calcium.

! Radiographic detection of fibrocartilage calcifications (e.g., menisci) is strong evidence of pyrophosphate arthropathy.

! Chondrocalcinosis with radiocarpal osteoarthritis change that is out of proportion to the rest of the hand is highly suggestive of CPDD.

Articular changes can also appear without visible calcium in the soft tissues. The classic signs of osteoarthritis must be observed amid the pattern typical for pyrophosphate arthropathy. Multiple subchondral cysts, some quite large and arranged in groups, can be present. Massive articular destruction is rare.

Other imaging modalities essentially play no role in further defining pyrophosphate arthropathy.

! To diagnose CPDD, the etiology of which is still unknown, it is important to search for typical radiographic signs in a systematic analysis with special attention directed to the distribution pattern (Fig. 9.**147**). Remember, 'what the first tarsometatarsal joint is for gout, the knee is for CPDD'.

DD
- **Osteoarthritis:** Since CPDD accelerates, or perhaps even causes, osteoarthritis, the differentiation from joint degeneration of other origin is often impossible.
- **Gout:** Notice the difference in the distribution pattern. Caution: Gout and chondrocalcinosis can be present at the same time.
- **Synovial soft-tissue calcifications of other origin,** e.g., synovial chondromatosis.

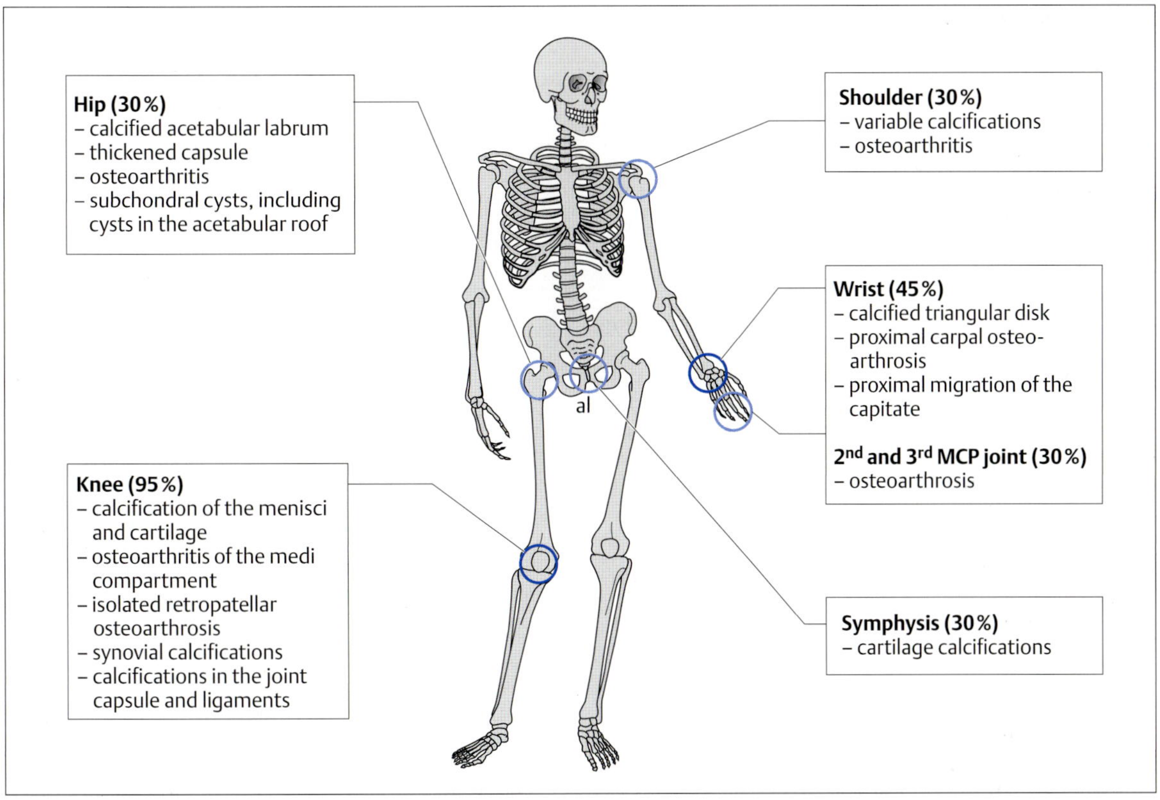

Fig. 9.**147** Typical pattern and distribution of calcium pyrophosphate dihydrate crystal deposition disease (CPDD): knees and wrists are preferentially – and bilaterally – involved, and, in contrast to gout, toes and fingers are not involved. The percentages stated in parentheses indicate the relative frequency of the involvement of the individual joints.

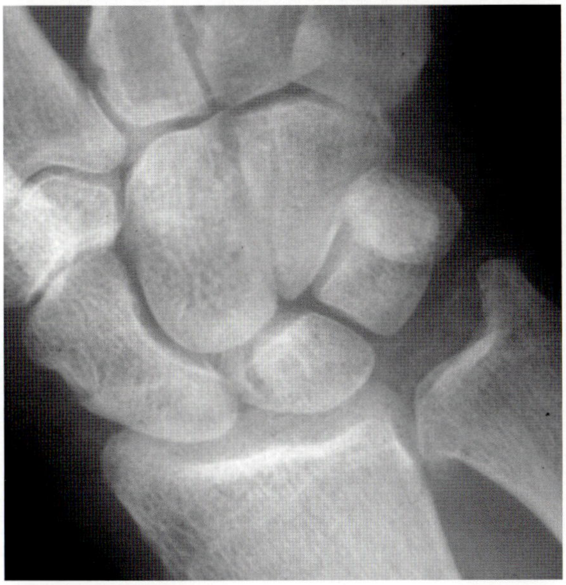

Fig. 9.**148** Chondrocalcinosis with calcification of the triangular fibrocartilage.

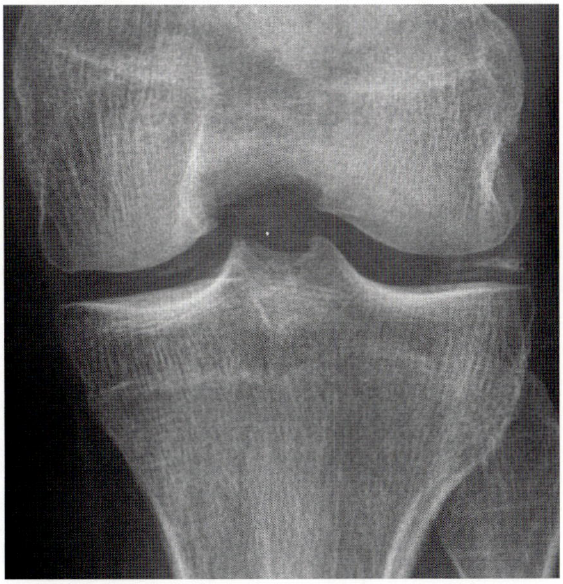

Fig. 9.**149** Nonspecific knee pain in a 41-year-old patient. Chondrocalcinosis with calcification in the menisci and hyaline articular cartilage.

Hydroxyapatite Disease

Synonyms: Calcifying tendinitis, peritendinitis, calcifying bursitis, periarthropathy.

■ This represents a primary periarticular calcification caused by deposits of hydroxyapatite crystals, which can induce painful inflammatory reactions. ■

PATH The deposition of chalk- or paste-like calcium may be related to age, trauma, or ischemia, but the exact cause is unknown. The needle-like, extremely small hydroxyapatite crystals are considered the most stable crystal type of alkaline calcium phosphate. The size of the calcific aggregates can fluctuate during the course of the disease process, and spontaneous resolution may occur.

CLINIC The condition occurs primarily in middle-aged and elderly patients, without gender preference. Patients usually have extreme pain in a single joint. The involved hand may also show erythema and swelling. Locations are:

1. shoulder and hip, at tendon insertions and bursae ('periarthropathy'),
2. elbow, at the triceps and collateral ligament insertions,
3. wrist, especially at the insertion of the flexor carpi ulnaris (pisiform bone and surrounding ligaments),
4. periarticular around the metacarpal, phalangeal, and interphalangeal joints.

Involvement of other locations, such as the greater trochanter, also occur.

X-RAY The cardinal findings are periarticular calcifications, which characteristically assume a hood-like configuration. The calcifications are dense, homogeneous, sometimes granular, and sharply demarcated (Fig. 9.**151**). Indistinct and milky-appearing calcifications are occasionally observed and are believed to have a higher spontaneous regression rate. Furthermore, indistinct calcification may be an indicator of acute symptoms.

! The 'Milwaukee shoulder' refers to destructive hydroxyapatite **arthropathy** and is often associated with a rotator cuff tear. Periarticular calcifications are usually absent.

SONO Calcium is detected on the basis of typical echogenic dome-like structures with acoustic shadowing (Fig. 9.**152**). Depending on the beam's angle of incidence and the reflectiveness of the calcium deposition, the sonographic findings can be of variable severity or even absent. Sonography might reveal calcium deposits that are radiographically obscured by overlying bone.

! Sonograms should always be correlated with the radiographs.

CT CT is the most sensitive method for the detection of calcium in the soft tissues.

MRI Calcifications generally have decreased signal intensity on both T1- and T2-weighted images. They may be surrounded by a halo of increased signal intensity on T2-weighted SE or STIR images if there is inflammatory edema within the affected tendons.

DD **Myositis ossificans:** The patient usually gives a history of trauma. In general, myositis ossificans does not directly affect tendon insertions and bursae as hydroxyapatite disease does.
Synovial sarcoma: The calcifications in this tumor are more spotty and scattered. Irregular osseous destruction may indicate the presence of a sarcoma.
Metastatic soft-tissue calcification seen in systemic imbalance of calcium pyrophosphate metabolism (e.g., renal osteodystrophy, chronic hemodialysis, vitamin D intoxication). Involvement of multiple sites and associated skeletal changes are the decisive criteria discriminating metastatic soft-tissue calcifications from the usually monoarticular hydroxyapatite disease.

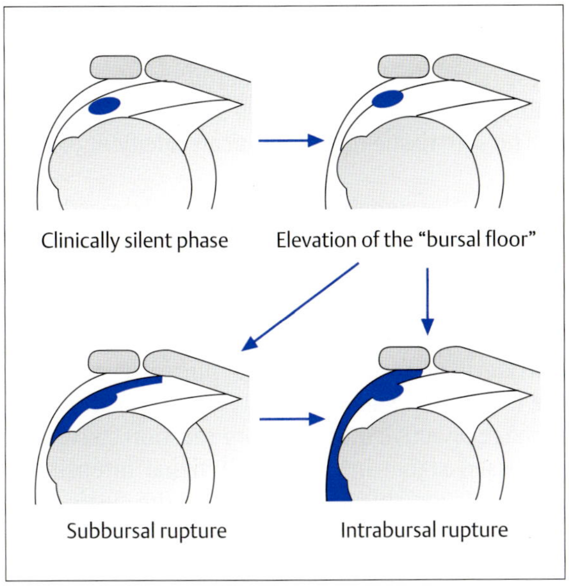

Fig. 9.**150** Phases of calcium hydroxyapatite crystal deposition at the shoulder (modified according to Moseley, 1969 and Resnick and Niwayama, 1995).

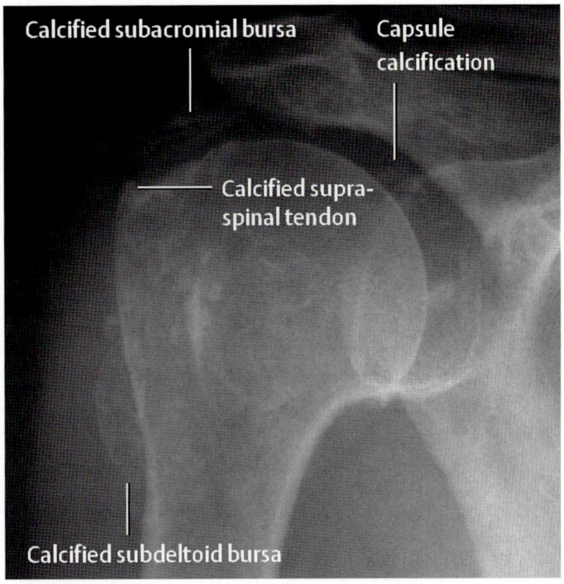

Fig. 9.**151** Calcium hydroxyapatite crystal deposition arthropathy of the shoulder.

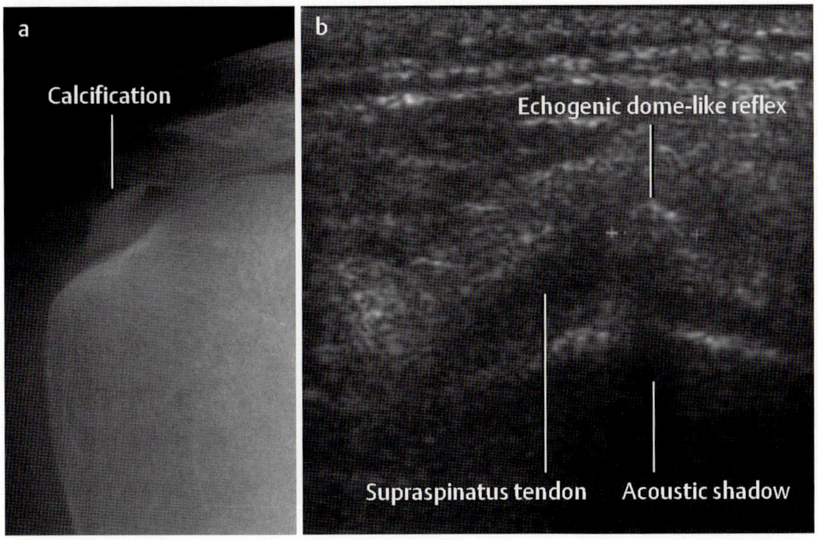

Fig. 9.**152** Radiograph (**a**) and corresponding sonogram (**b**) of supraspinatus calcific tendinitis with elevation of the bursal floor.

Arthropathy in Hemophilia

Synonym: Hemophilic hemarthrosis.

■ Hemophilia is an X-linked recessive hereditary hemorrhagic diathesis of differing severity with abnormal plasma clotting, usually due to a deficiency of factor VIII (Type A) or IX (Type B). ■

PATH Recurrent episodes of intra-articular and periarticular bleeding lead to inflammation and hypertrophy of the synovial membrane. Chemically induced toxic reactions and increased intra-articular and intramedullary pressure cause destruction of bone and cartilage.

At specific sites, such as the femoral head or talus, interosseous bleeding can result in osteonecrosis.

Additional muscular imbalance due to contractures increases the risk of spontaneous fractures.

CLINIC There are three main stages in hemophilia:

1. Intra-articular bleeding with restricted motion imposed by accompanying muscle spasms.
2. Subacute and chronic stage with chronic synovitis and joint destructions, muscular contractures, and atrophy,
3. Compartment syndrome or neurologic deficits as complications of the disease.

X-RAY The radiographic findings are:

- dense soft-tissue swelling caused by hematoma or synovial hemosiderin deposits (Fig. 9.**153**),
- regional or juxta-articular demineralization caused by the synovitis (leads to hyperemia),
- erosions, subchondral cysts,
- joint-space narrowing due to cartilage destruction, often accompanied by reactive subchondral sclerosis and osteophytes (Fig. 9.**154**),
- mutilating joint destruction (Fig. 9.**155**),
- in children: accelerated epiphyseal growth due to hyperemia.

Periosteal or interosseous hematoma may produce a **hemophilic pseudotumor.** Radiographically, these sharply demarcated radiolucencies appear bubbly and have trabeculae or septa.

The soft-tissue hematomas can calcify or ossify.

MRI The signal intensities of the hemarthrosis are variable and depend on the age of the blood. The signal intensity is usually low to moderate on both T1- and T2-weighted images, and may have confined areas of increased intensity. The hemosiderin deposits or synovial fibrosis is responsible for the low signal intensity, and subacute hemorrhage or active inflammatory reaction causes the increased signal intensity. The signal intensity of the cyst is variable and depends on the cystic composition.

DD

1. Other causes of a hemarthrosis include trauma, anticoagulation therapy, and myeloproliferative disorders. The changes are principally the same and are dominated by soft-tissue swelling.
2. Pigmented villonodular synovitis (PVNS) also has deposits of hemosiderin and other blood products, but is almost always monoarticular, whereas hemophilia is usually asymmetric and multilocular.
3. In childhood, juvenile chronic arthritis must also be considered.

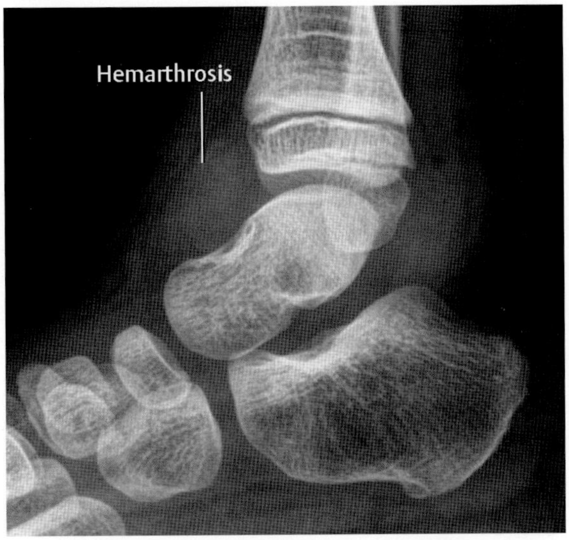

Fig. 9.**153** Dense hemarthrosis in a 7-year-old boy with hemophilia A.

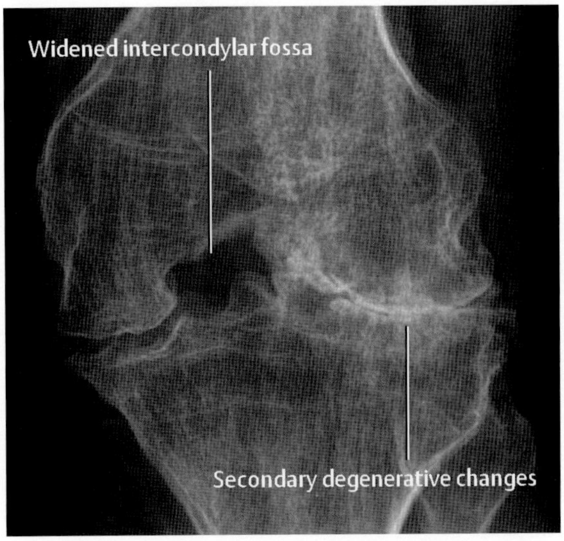

Fig. 9.**154** Advanced hemophilic arthropathy of the knee.

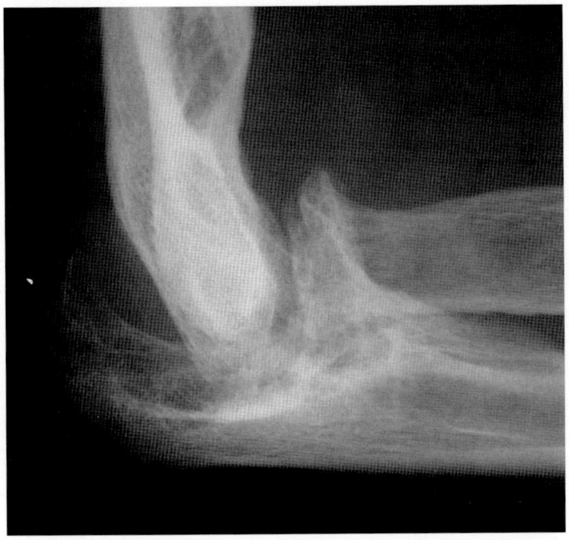

Fig. 9.**155** Mutilating arthropathy of the elbow in hemophilia A.

Tumors and Tumor-like Lesions of the Joints

Intraosseous Ganglion

Synonym: Subchondral synovial cyst.

■ The intraosseous ganglion is an osseous cystic lesion arising in the bone marrow space following intrusion of synovial fluid. ■

PATH The subchondral cyst has a fibrous wall and contains a gelatin-like material. The size of the cavity can vary considerably. The presumed traumatic pathogenesis differentiates the intraosseous ganglion from the degenerative detritic cyst. The defect can close off, and it is rare to detect a direct communication with the joint.

CLINIC Pain in the affected joint.
Age: The interosseous ganglion occurs in all age groups.
Location: The intraosseous ganglion prefers the joints of the long tubular bones.
Therapy: Excision with bone grafting.

X-RAY Conventional radiography shows the lesion to be a sharply demarcated singular radiolucency, generally with a thin sclerotic border measuring 0.2 – 7 cm (Figs. 9.**156**, 9.**157**). Septations can occur, but there are **no** intralesional calcifications. Individual lesions may be septated.

CT Because of the ability of CT to image structures without superimposing other structures, the break in the subchondral bone plate is more frequently visualized with CT than with conventional radiography (Fig. 9.**159**).

MRI The intraosseous ganglion has very high signal intensity on T2-weighted SE images (Fig. 9.**158**), usually equal to the intensity found in the joint effusion. With gadolinium, only the cyst wall shows rim-like enhancement. However, a few intraosseous ganglions also show homogeneous enhancement, especially those ganglions lacking a communication with the joint.

DD Benign, epiphyseally located tumors (e.g., chondroblastoma, osteoblastoma) can show similar radiographic features but often have calcifications and ossifications, which are **never** encountered in intraosseous ganglions. The osteoarthritic detritic cyst has similar features. Only the presence of osteoarthritis (joint-space narrowing, osteophytes, etc.) aids in differentiating the intraosseous ganglion from the detritic cyst.

Synovial Chondromatosis

Synonyms: Osteochondromatosis

■ A collection of cartilaginous or osseous bodies within the joint is referred to as synovial chondromatosis. It must be distinguished from synovial chondromas from osteoarthritis. ■

PATH Synovial metaplasia of unknown origin leads to the formation of tumor-like cartilage proliferations. These chondromas appear in large numbers and receive their nutrients from the synovial lining as long as they remain connected to it (in part stalk-like). Ultimately, they separate from the synovial lining and become **free** intra-articular bodies.

CLINIC Nonspecific articular pain, restricted motion, effusion.
Age: Any age group can be affected, esp. early adulthood.
Location: In general, monoarticular involvement, with knee, elbow, and shoulder most commonly affected. Other locations are possible.
Therapy: Surgical excision.

X-RAY **CT** Synovial chondromatosis is detectable only if the intra-articular bodies are calcified or ossified. The vast number of (free) joint bodies establishes the diagnosis. Osteoarthritic changes can result from mechanical irritation of the joint if the diagnosis is delayed (Fig. 9.**161**).

SONO An effusion is always detectable in sonographically accessible joints (e.g., knee, shoulder, hands, feet). Round foreign bodies of different echogenicity (depending on the degree of calcification) 'float' within the effusion.

MRI Multiple round bodies of low signal intensity are seen amidst the effusion of high signal intensity (T2-weighted SE image). They are confined to the joint. In general, MRI demonstrates the intra-articular loose bodies before conventional radiography does, since detectability with MRI is not contingent on lesion calcification or ossification.

DD Differentiation from synovial chondromatosis secondary to degenerative osteoarthritis is very difficult. Generally the loose intra-articular fragments from degenerative change will be fewer in number and larger. It also is the result of synovial metaplasia and essentially has identical findings, except that degeneratively caused synovial chondromas are fewer in number. The age of the patient and osteoarthritis found in other joints might help in the differentiation (Figs. 9.**160**, 9.**161**).

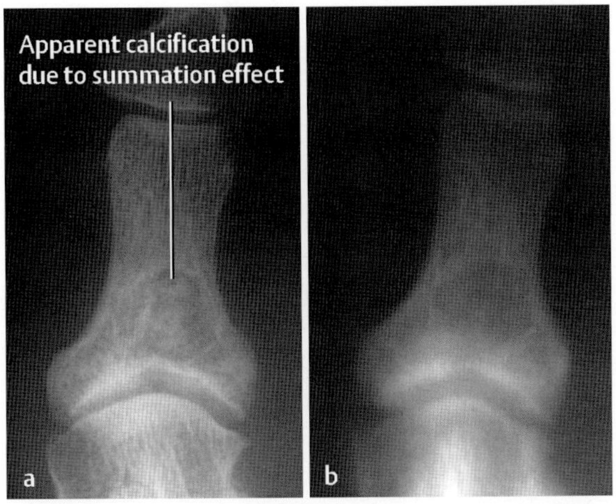

Fig. 9.**156** Intraosseous ganglion at the phalangeal base in a 60-year-old man. The PA radiograph (**a**) shows a calcific density projecting through the lesion. Conventional tomography (**b**) reveals this finding to represent a summation density without evidence of internal calcification of the ganglion.

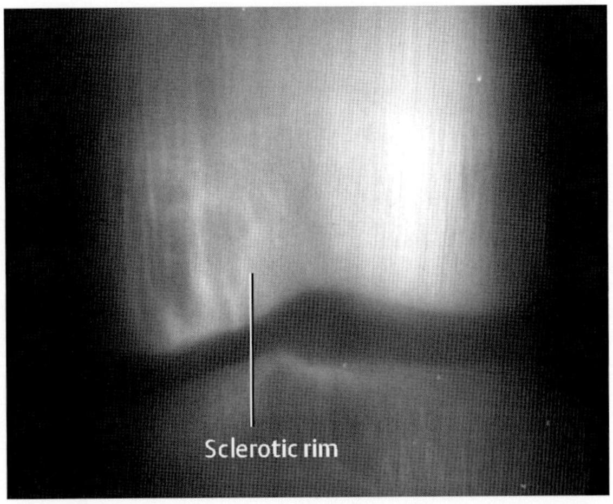

Fig. 9.**157** Conventional tomography of an intraosseous ganglion of the knee. A distinct radiolucency with a sclerotic rim is seen.

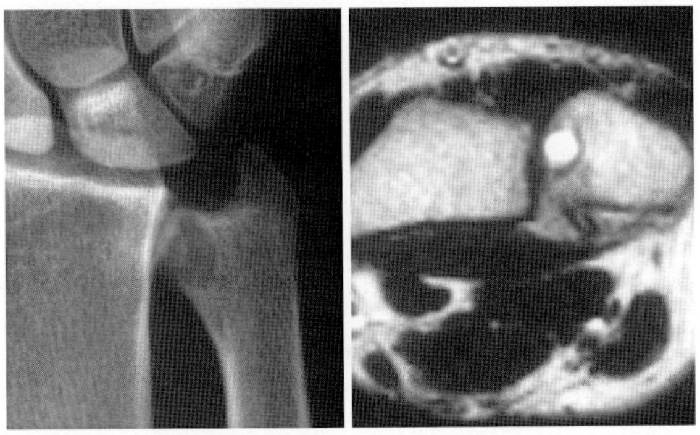

Fig. 9.**158** Intraosseous ganglion in the distal ulna and the corresponding MRI (high signal intensity on the T2-weighted SE sequence). In comparison to Fig. 9.**157**, the marked sclerosis is less pronounced.

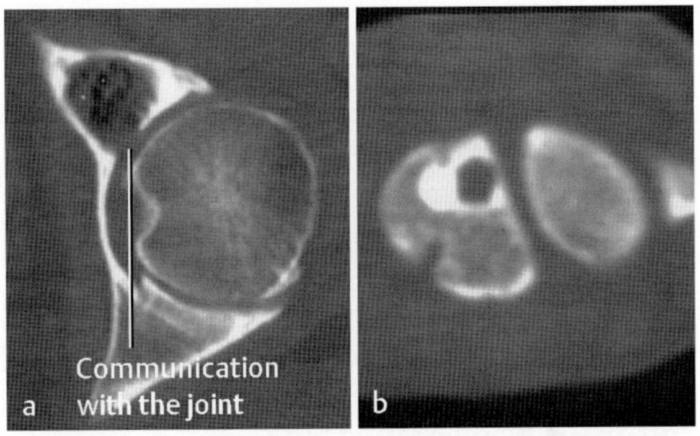

Fig. 9.**159** **a** Intraosseous ganglion of the hip. Notice the intralesional gas, which has reached the ganglion from the joint as part of joint degeneration (vacuum phenomenon). **b** Intraosseous ganglion in the lunate with marked marginal sclerosis. Both illustrations are axial CT sections.

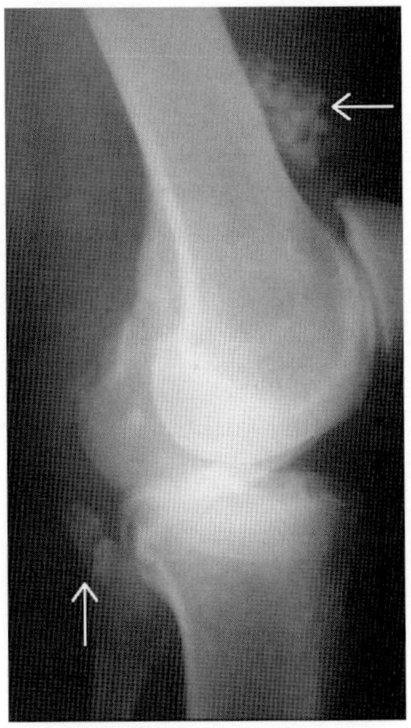

Fig. 9.**160** Synovial chondromatosis of an osteoarthritic knee in a 66-year-old man.

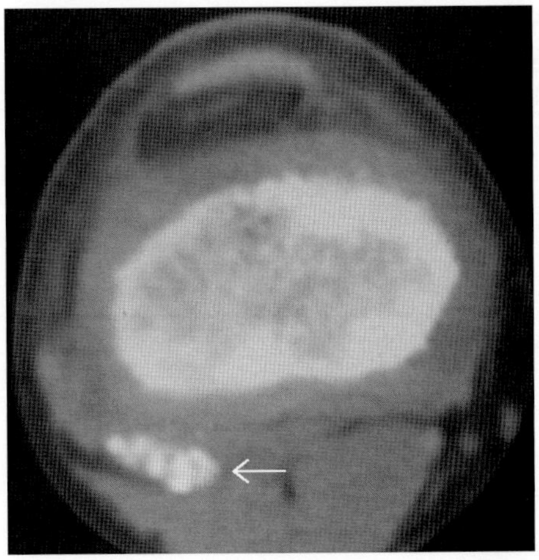

Fig. 9.**161** Synovial chondromatosis of the knee in an 8-year-old boy.

Pigmented Villonodular Synovitis (PVNS)

■ Pigmented villonodular synovitis is a benign proliferative disorder of the synovial lining arising in tendon sheaths, bursae, and joints. If located in a tendon sheath, it is also referred to as 'giant cell tumor of the tendon sheath'. ■

PATH PVNS is villous proliferation of the synovial lining containing hemosiderin that partially destroys bone.

PVNS is **not** an inflammatory process and is categorized as a tumor-like lesion because of its tumorous growth.

! PVNS (giant-cell tumors) of the tendon sheaths and bursae are included with the soft-tissue lesions (Fig. 9.**165**). The clinically conspicuous finding must be further evaluated radiographically to determine any osseous involvement.

CLINIC Recurrent pain and swelling of the affected joint, accompanied by restricted motion (possibly also intermittent joint locking) and serosanguineous or xanthochromatic joint effusion without preceding trauma.

Age: Adults in the third and fourth decade of life are primarily affected. It almost never occurs in children.

Therapy: Curettage. High recurrence rate.

X-RAY Two articular manifestations are distinguished:

Soft-tissue manifestation (60%–70%):

It is characterized by a soft-tissue swelling of extremely high density (hemosiderin). The joint space is normal in width, and the bone is not involved.

Osseous manifestation (30%–40%):

Multiple cyst-like radiolucencies of different sizes are located in the articular end of the bone. They are sharply demarcated and frequently surrounded by a sclerotic border (Figs. 9.**162**–9.**164**). **No** calcifications are seen within the lesion. The osseous lesions are invariably accompanied by soft-tissue swelling.

CT Soft-tissue tumors of an exceptionally high density are seen in the joint, usually with erosions in the articular ends of the bone (Fig. 9.**162**).

MRI The detection of hemosiderin is an important indicator of PVNS. The tumor typically has **low signal intensity** on T1-weighted **and** on T2-weighted SE images. If calcium can be excluded radiographically as causing the low signal intensities on the T2-weighted image, the intracapsular soft-tissue mass can be diagnosed as PVNS with a high degree of certainty. The tumor enhances (Fig. 9.**165**).

DD The radiographic features of pigmented villonodular synovitis are quite characteristic, and proposing a differential diagnosis is generally not warranted as long as more than one of the articulating bones are involved (Figs. 9.**163**, 9.**164**). A malignant synovial tumor must be considered in the presence of amorphous calcifications within a soft-tissue density and indistinctly outlined osseous erosions.

MRI easily distinguishes the intraosseous ganglion with its high signal intensity (high, fluid-equivalent signal) from PVNS.

Glossary

Synovial sarcoma (**synonym:** synovioma, Fig. 9.**166**): This tumor arises in the region of the synovial membrane, not only within the joints, but also in tendon sheaths and bursae (see also Soft-tissue Tumors, pages 200–202). In the joint, the malignant tumor is easily visualized as a soft-tissue mass with secondary bone destruction by MRI. A definitive diagnosis cannot be achieved by imaging, but the diagnosis can be suggested by virtue of the juxta-articular location and detectable calcifications (present in about one-third of cases).

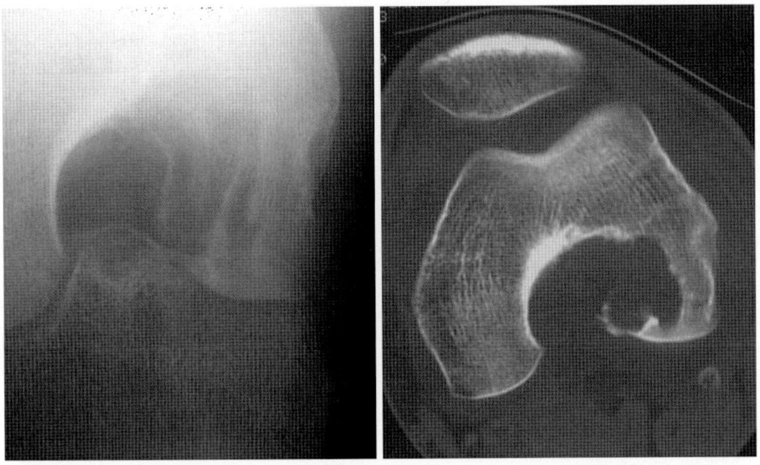

Fig. 9.**162** PVNS of the femoral condyle in an 18-year-old man.

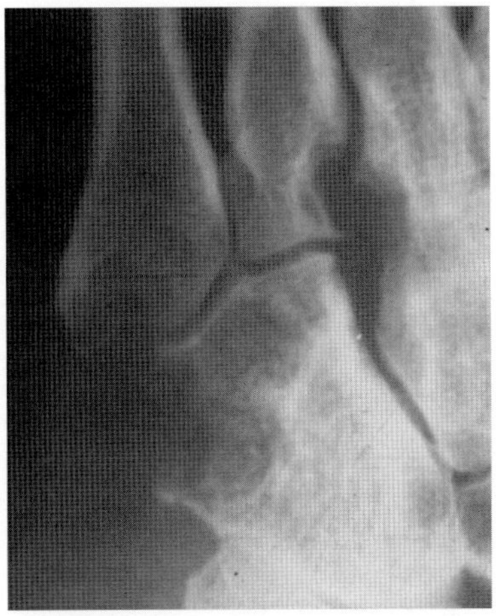

Fig. 9.**163** PVNS in the region of the Lisfranc joint line with several defects in the cuboid and adjacent metatarsals.

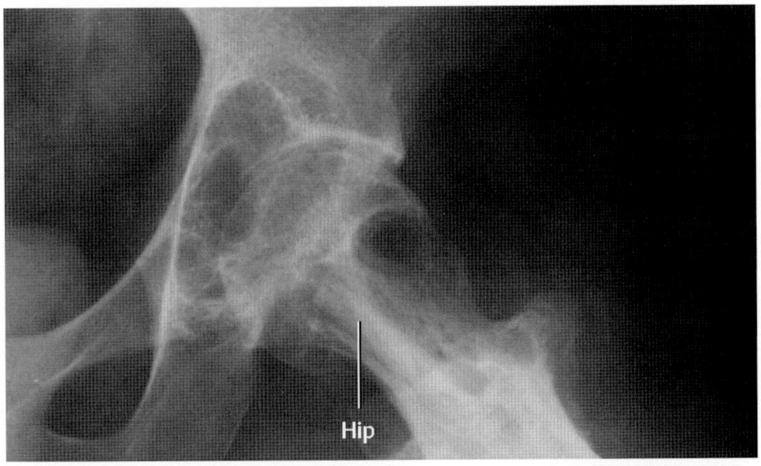

Fig. 9.**164** Recurrent PVNS of the hip in a 30-year-old man after resection of the femoral neck and rib graft. Notice that the disease crosses the joint.

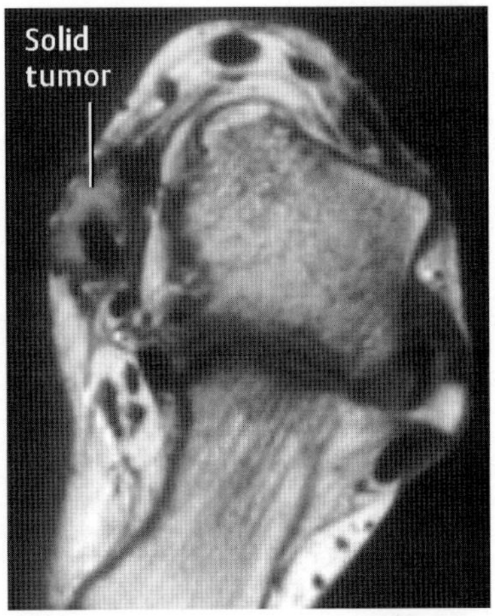

Fig. 9.**165** PVNS arising from the tendon sheath of the posterior tibialis muscle, T1-weighted SE image after administration of contrast.

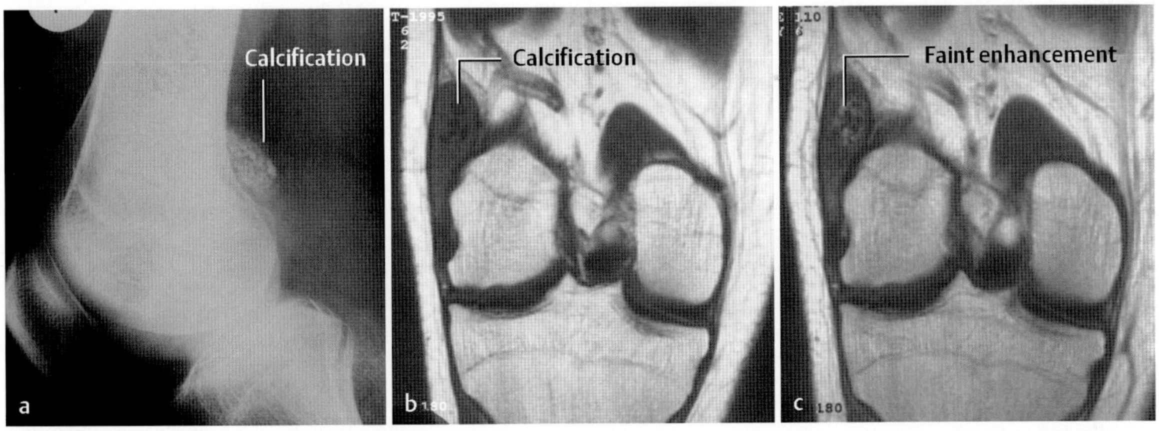

Fig. 9.**166** Synovial sarcoma of the knee. **a** The lateral radiograph shows calcification adjacent to and separate from the cortex. The T1-weighted MRI before (**b**) and after (**c**) administration of contrast medium shows a pocket-like extension of the joint capsule with calcifications and solid tissue (note enhancement).

Index

Page numbers in **bold type** refer to illustrations.

A

abscess
  Brodie's, *see* Brodie's abscess
  and post-traumatic osteomyelitis **149**
  soft-tissue 152, **153**
  and spondylodiskitis **337**
acetabulum
  fractures 58–61
    classification 58, **58, 59**
  roof arcs **59**
Achilles tendon
  erosive enthesopathy 349, **349**
  and Reiter syndrome **351**
achondrogenesis, *vs.* thanatophoric dysplasia 258
achondroplasia 258, **259**
  vs. thanatophoric dysplasia 258
acrocephalosyndactyly 274, **275**
acromegaly 254–255, **255**
acromioclavicular joints, renal osteodystrophy **249**
acromioclavicular separation 64, **64**
acute longitudinal radio-ulnar dislocation (ALRUD) 80
adamantinoma 180
adolescent kyphosis 328
Ahlbäck disease 224, 226, **227**
  vs. osteochondritis dissecans 226
Aitken's classification, fractures 14, **119**
Albers–Schönberg disease 270
algodystrophy 30
ALRUD, *see* acute longitudinal radio-ulnar dislocation
aluminum bone disease 250
amyloidosis 248, 254, **255**
Anderson and D'Alonzo classification, dens fractures 48, **49**
Andersson lesion 298, **349**
anemia 212–215
  aplastic 214, **215**
aneurysmal bone cyst, *vs.* osteoblastoma 160
angiography
  and bone tumors 157
  and pelvic injuries 56
  and soft-tissue tumors 200
angiomatosis, cystic 176
ankle 126, **127**
  fracture 120–125
    osteochondral 16, **17**
    typical findings **37**
    Weber type C 116
  ligamentous injuries 126, **127**
  rheumatoid arthritis 340
  stress views 126, **127**
ankylosing spondylitis 346–349
  diagnostic criteria 347
  differential diagnosis **359**
  juvenile onset 348
  vs. psoriatic arthropathy 353
  vs. Reiter syndrome 351
ankylosis 296, **297**
anterior cruciate ligament (ACL), tears 10
Apert syndrome 274, **275**
aplastic anemia 214, **215**
apophyseal variants 130
ARCO, staging 219
arteriovenous malformation 202
arthritis 294, **295,** 296
  bacterial 331, **332,** 334
  differential diagnosis 358, **359**
  echinococcal 334, **335**
  enteropathic, differential diagnosis **359**
  gouty 364
    distribution pattern **365**
  HIV-associated 331
  infectious 331, 332
    vs. osteoarthritis 314
    vs. pustulotic arthro-osteitis 288
  juvenile chronic 331
  Lyme 331
  vs. osteoarthritis 302
    signs **305**
  pathogenesis 304
  pathophysiology **303**
  psoriatic **305,** 352
    vs. Reiter syndrome 351
  reactive 350–351, **351**
    vs. ankylosing spondylitis 348
    differential diagnosis **359**
  rheumatoid, *see* rheumatoid arthritis
  septic, differential diagnosis **359**
  tuberculous **333,** 334
arthrography
  carpal derangement 92, **93**
  hip 104
  shoulder 66, **67**
  TFCC injuries 88, **89**
  trauma 6, **7**
arthro-osteitis, pustulotic 288–289, **289**
arthropathy
  corticosteroid-induced **365**
  crystal-induced 364–365
  enteropathic 354
  hemophilic 372, **373**
  neurogenic 360
  psoriatic 352–353, **353**
    vs. ankylosing spondylitis 348
  pyrophosphate 368
articular disease, HIV-associated 356
articular surfaces, fractures 16–18, **17, 18**
aseptic osteonecrosis 218
asphyxiating thoracic dysplasia 260, **261**
atlas
  fracture 48, **49**
  pediatric considerations 50
  rheumatoid arthritis **341**
avascular necrosis (AVN) 26, **27,** 248
  femoral head 218–223
    etiology 219
    vs. Legg–Calvé–Perthes disease 232
    staging 219
avascular osteonecrosis 218
avulsion fracture, anterior, spine 46
axis
  fracture 48, **49**
  pediatric considerations 50

B

bamboo spine 298
Bankart lesion 70, 72
Barlow maneuver 290
Barton fracture 84, **85**
basilar invagination 342, **343**
battered child syndrome 132–135
  diagnostic approach **135**
Bekhterev disease 346
Bennett fracture 96, **97**
birth trauma 134
bismuth poisoning 250
blade of grass radiolucency 276
block vertebra 298
Blount disease 224
blow-in fractures 42
blow-out fractures 42, **43**
Boeck disease 280
Böhler's tuberosity–joint angle 122, **125**
bone
  aluminum disease 250
  bruise, tibia **115**
  consolidation 24
  contusion, *vs.* reflex sympathetic dystrophy 30
  cyst, *see* bone cyst
  deformities 216
  infarct, *see* bone infarct
  infection 136–151
  ischemic 218–235
  island 182
    vs. osteoid osteoma 160
  marrow, *see* bone marrow

bone
plate, subchondral 292
loss 294, **295**
scan, *see* scintigraphy
spotted 270
bone cyst
aneurysmal 188, **188, 189**
vs. enchondroma 166
vs. giant cell tumor 170
vs. osteoblastoma 160
vs. simple 186
simple
vs. aneurysmal 188
juvenile 186, **186, 187**
bone growth
constitutional disorders 256–275
summary 257
normal 242, **243**
bone infarct 228, **229,** 230
definition 218
differential diagnosis 228, 230
vs. enchondroma 166
vs. fracture 22
vs. lipoma 177
bone marrow 212
degenerative changes, vertebral bodies 324
edema syndrome 230, **231,** 294
hyperplasia 212
and lipidosis 216
bone tumors
classification 154
imaging 157–158
primary 160–181
staging 157
Bouchard nodes 312, 314
bowing deformities 248
Bragard staging 226
breast carcinoma, metastasis **197**
Brodie's abscess 144, **144, 145**
vs. osteoid osteoma 160
brown tumor 244, **245**
vs. amyloidosis 254
vs. osteoblastoma 160
bucket-handle tear, meniscus 108, **109**
buckle fracture 14, **15**
bullhead sign, pustulotic arthro-osteitis **289**
burns 34
frostbites 34
bursitis, calcifying 370
burst fracture, spine 44, **45**
buttonhole deformity 96
button sequestrum 190, **191**

C

Caffey disease 282
calcaneus
insufficiency fracture **21**
lipoma **177**
calcification
intervertebral disks 346
ligamentous 318
soft-tissue **35**, 248, 284, **285**, 370
see also ossification
calcifying bursitis 370
calcifying tendinitis 370, **371**
calcinosis 284
idiopathic **285**
pseudotumorous **249**
calcitonin 242
calcium metabolism 242
calcium phosphate deposition disease (CPPD) 246
calcium pyrophosphate deposition disease (CPDD) 368, **369**
callus formation, and fracture healing 25, **25**
Campanacci osteofibrous dysplasia 180, **181**
carcinoma, *see* metastases; tumors
carpal bones 130
alignment 92
auxiliary lines
derangement 92–95
fractures 90, **91**
instability 92, 93, 94
osteoarthritis 314, **315**
carpometacarpal injuries 96, **97**
carpometacarpal joint, osteoarthritis 314, **315**
cartilage
articular 292
degenerative changes **309**
fragmentation **309**
hyaline articular 308
repair 310
cellulitis, phlegmonous 152, **153**
cement fracture, hip prosthesis 104, **105**
chance fracture, spine 44, **45**
Chaput tubercle **121**
Charcot joint 314, 360, **361**
Chassaignac injury 78, **79**
child abuse, *see* battered child syndrome
chloroma 208
chondral fractures 16–18
vs. osteochondral 18, **19**
chondroblastoma 166, **167**
vs. giant cell tumor 170
chondrocalcinosis 244, 368, **369**
chondrodysplasia
metaphyseal 264, **265**
punctata 260, **261**
chondroma 166
periosteal **167**
tendon sheath **201**
chondromatosis, synovial 374, **375**
chondromyxoid fibroma 168
chondrosarcoma 168, **169**
vs. chondroblastoma 166
vs. enchondroma 166
vs. osteosarcoma 162
chondrosis 316, 320–325
Chopart joint 124
chordoma 180, **181**
chronic venous stasis 286, **286**
circumscribed osteolytic foci 296
classifications
acetabular fractures 58, **58, 59**
Anderson and D'Alonzo, dens fracture 48, **49**
ankle fractures 120, **121**
arthritides 331
atlas fractures 48
avulsion fractures, intercondylar eminence 114, **115**
bone tumors 154
calcaneal fractures 122, **123**
carpal bone instability 93
Danis–Weber, ankle 120, **121**
dens fractures 48, **49**
dysostosis 274
femoral fracture
distal **101**
head 60, **61**
neck 98, **99**
forearm fractures, distal 84, **85**
hangman's fracture 46, **47**
Hawkins, talar neck fracture 122, **123**
hip dislocation 60
humeral fractures, distal 76, **77**
Le Fort fractures 42, **43**
ligamentous injuries, sacroiliac joints 56, **56**
Meyers and McKeever, intercondylar eminence fracture 114, **115**
Monteggia fractures, ulna 83
Moore, tibial plateau fracture 114, **115**
Neer, proximal humeral fractures **75**
osteogenesis imperfecta 267
osteomyelitis 137
osteoporosis 236
Palmer, TFCC injuries 88
pelvic injuries 54
Pipkin, femoral head fracture dislocation **61**
plafond fractures 116, **117**
pseudarthrosis 26
sacroiliac ligamentous injuries 56
skeletal lesions 156
spinal fractures 44
talar neck fractures 122, **123**
tibial fractures 114, **114, 115, 119**
Tile, pelvic injuries 54, **55,** 56
Tossy, acromioclavicular separation 64
ulnar fractures 83
Weber, ankle 120, **121**
WHO, soft-tissue tumors 200
clavicular fracture
vs. acromioclavicular separation 64
vs. sternoclavicular dislocation 62
clay shoveler's fracture, spine 44
cleidocranial dysplasia 262, **263**
coccyx, fractures 50
codfish vertebra 212, **237**
Codman tumor 166
collagenosis, mixed 356, **357**
collateral ligaments
grading of injuries **112**
tibiofibular 126, **127**
Colles' fracture 84, **85**
compartment syndrome 34
muscle necrosis **35**
soft-tissue calcification 34, **35**
compression fracture, spine 12, **12,** 44
computed tomography (CT)
arthrography, shoulder 70
avascular necrosis, femoral head 222, **223**
and bone tumors 157
degenerative spinal disease 326–327, **327**
and insufficiency fracture 22
joint diseases 293
myelography 322, **323,** 326

computed tomography (CT)
quantitative 240–241
trauma 4, 6, **7**
condyles, femoral, fracture 16, **17**
congenital hip dysplasia 290, **291**
connective tissue diseases
articular changes 354
inflammatory systemic 331
mixed 356
Conradi–Hünermann chondrodysplasia 260
cord remnant **329**
coronoid process, fractures 80
cortical desmoid 194, **195**
vs. osteosarcoma 162
corticosteroid therapy 252–253, **253**
and arthropathy **365**
joint changes 362
cotton-wool skull **275**
coxitis, *vs.* Legg–Calvé–Perthes disease 232
CPDD, *see* calcium pyrophosphate deposition disease
CPPD, *see* calcium phosphate deposition disease
craniocervical transition 48
cranium, *see* skull
crescent sign, distal humeral fracture **76**
CREST syndrome 355
CRMO, *see* osteomyelitis, chronic recurrent multifocal
Crohn disease 354
Crouzon disease 274, **275**
cruciate ligaments 110, **111**
CT, *see* computed tomography
cystic angiomatosis 176
cysts 202
detritic 302
vs. lipoma 177
meniscal 112, **113**
post-traumatic 28, **29**
subchondral 296, **297**
acetabular roof **305**
tibiofibular joint **313**
synovial 318, 322

D

dactylitis **213**
Danis–Weber classification 120, **121**
David Letterman sign 94, **95**
degenerative osteoarthritis, post-traumatic 28, **29**
Denis, three-column spine model 50, **50**
dens
fracture 48, **49**
rheumatoid arthritis **341**
densitometry, bone 240
de Quervain fracture dislocation 90, **91**
dermatomyositis 355–356
calcinosis **285**
desmoid 202
cortical 194, **195**
periosteal 194, **195**
desmoplastic fibroma 178
DEXA, *see* dual-energy X-ray absorptiometry
diabetic foot 362
diabetic osteoarthropathy **363**
diabetic osteomyelitis **363**
differential diagnoses 336
achondroplasia 258
acromioclavicular separation
vs. clavicular fracture 64
adamantinoma 180
Ahlbäck disease *vs.* osteochondritis dissecans 226
amyloidosis 254
anemia 214
ankylosing spondylitis 348
arthritis 358, **359**
asphyxiating thoracic dysplasia 260
battered child syndrome 134
bone cyst, aneurysmal 188
bone infarct 228, 230
bone marrow edema syndrome 230
Brodie abscess 144
chondroblastoma 166
chondrodysplasia punctata 260
chondrosarcoma 168
chordoma 180
chronic osteomyelitis, *vs.* fracture 22
cleidocranial dysplasia 262
crystal deposition arthropathy 364
dyschondrosteosis 260
enchondroma 166
eosinophilic granuloma 190
erosion 294, **295**
Ewing sarcoma 172
fibrous cortical defect 184
fibrous dysplasia 194
fractures 22
Gaucher disease *vs.* Niemann–Pick disease **217**
giant cell tumor 170
gout 366, 367
growth variants 130, **131**
hemangioma 176
hemarthrosis 372
hydroxyapatite disease 370
hyperparathyroidism 246
hypochondroplasia 262
hypophosphatemia 268
intraosseous ganglion 374
joint disease 294, 296
Legg–Calvé–Perthes disease 232
lipoma 177
lymphoma, malignant 210
metaphyseal chondrodysplasia 264
metastases 198
mucopolysaccharidosis 272
multiple epiphyseal dysplasia 262
myelofibrosis 216
myeloma 206
myositis ossificans 286, **287**
osteoblastoma 160
osteochondroma 164, 166
osteochondrosis dissecans 234
osteoid osteoma 160
osteomyelitis 142
osteopetrosis 270
osteosarcoma 162
Paget disease 278
patella, partite 100
periosteal reaction in children 282
plasmocytoma 206
psoriatic arthropathy 353
pustulotic arthro-osteitis 288–289
pyrophosphate arthropathy 368
reflex sympathetic dystrophy,
vs. arthritis 30
Reiter syndrome 351
rheumatoid arthritis 342
rickets, hereditary 268
sarcoidosis 280, 281
shoulder impingement syndrome 68
simple (juvenile) bone cyst 186
spondyloepimetaphyseal dysplasia 264
sternoclavicular dislocation
vs. clavicular fracture 62
synovial chondromatosis 374
systemic lupus erythematosus 355
thanatophoric dysplasia 258
toxic osteopathy 250
tuberculosis 150
ulnar elongation 86
diffuse idiopathic skeletal hyperostosis (DISH) 282, 328, **329**
vs. ankylosing spondylitis 348
complications 328
vs. pustulotic arthro-osteitis 289
digital luminescence radiography 4
DISH, *see* diffuse idiopathic skeletal hyperostosis
DISI, *see* dorsal intercalated segmental instability
diskitis 331
disks, *see* intervertebral disks
dislocation
ankle 12, **12**
anterior, spine 44, **45**, 46
atlantoaxial 48
carpal **95**
distal forearm 88, 89, **89**
facet joint 46, **47**
fingers 96
foot 124
hip 60
posterior, spine 46
sternoclavicular 62, **63**
disuse osteoporosis 28, **29**, 294
vs. reflex sympathetic dystrophy 30
dorsal intercalated segmental instability (DISI) 92
dual-energy X-ray absorptiometry (DEXA) 240, **241**
dyschondrosteosis 260, **261**
dysostosis 256, 274, **275**
multiplex 272, **273**
dysplasia
osteofibrous **181**
thanatophoric 258, **259**
dysraphism, spinal **361**
dystrophy
see also reflex sympathetic dystrophy

E

echinococcal arthritis 334, **335**
echinococcosis, skeletal 150
elbow
  dislocation 78
  mutilating arthropathy **373**
  pediatric **79**
  rheumatoid arthritis 340
  tennis 78, **79**
empyema, shoulder **333**
enchondroma 166, **167**
  vs. bone infarct 228
enchondromatosis 266, **267**
enthesopathy 306, **307,** 350
  erosive, Achilles tendon 349, **349**
eosinophilic granuloma 190, **191**
  vs. Ewing sarcoma 172
epicondylitis, radiographic findings 78, **79**
epidermoid 194
epiphyses
  cone shaped 128, **129**
  dysplasia, multiple 262
  fractures, tibia 116
  growth zone, development 128 – 131
epiphysiolysis
  distal tibia 118, **119**
  femoral head 100, **101**
  tibia 116
Erlenmeyer flask deformity **213,** 214
erosion 294, **295**
erysipelas 152
Ewing sarcoma 172, **172, 173**
  vs. eosinophilic granuloma 190
  vs. osteomyelitis 142, 143
  vs. osteosarcoma 162
exostosis
  cartilaginous 164
  cauliflower **164**
  multiple cartilaginous 266, **267**
extension fractures
  radiography 46
  spine 46

F

facet joint
  dislocation 46, **47**
  osteoarthritis 318, **319,** 326
  unilateral blocking 46
facial bones, fractures 40, **41,** 42
  classification 41
Fanconi anemia 274
fatigue fractures 20
Felty syndrome 342
femoral head
  avascular necrosis 218 – 223
    staging 219
  fracture dislocations 60, **61**
  osteonecrosis 224
  osteoporosis, idiopathic 232
femur
  fractures 98, **99,** 100
    distal, classification **101**
  French telephone deformity 258
  see also femoral head
fetal alcohol syndrome 260
fetal warfarin syndrome 260
fibroma 200
  chondromyxoid 168
  desmoplastic 178
  nonossifying 184, **184, 185**
fibromatosis 202
  congenital generalized 266
  mandible **203**
fibro-osteoplasia, secretory 244
fibro-ostitis 306, **307,** 348
fibro-ostosis 306, **307**
fibrosarcoma 178, **179**
fibrous cortical defect 184, **184, 185**
  vs. bone infarct 228
fibrous dysplasia 192 – 195
  vs. adamantoma 180
  vs. bone infarct 228
  vs. Brodie abscess 144
  ground glass appearance
    192, **193, 194**
  Pagetoid manifestation **194**
  polyostotic 266
  vs. simple bone cyst 186
fibula
  fracture, typical findings **37**
  head, fractures 116, **117**
fingers
  fractures and dislocations 96
  sausage-like **353**
fish mouth sign, osteoporotic fracture 52
flake fractures 2
flexion fractures
  radiography 46
  spine 44, 46
flipped meniscus sign 108
fluoroscopy, joint diseases 293
fluorosis 250, **251**
foot
  compartments **362**
  diabetic 362
  dislocation 124
forearm
  distal, dislocation 88
  fractures, pediatric age group 82
  proximal, fractures 80 – 83
foreign body reaction 28, **29**
Forestier disease 328
fractures
  acetabular 58 – 61
  ankle 120 – 125
  articular surfaces 16 – 18, **17, 18**
  in battered child syndrome **133, 135**
  Bennett 96, **97**
  calcaneal 122, **123, 125**
  carpal bones 90, **91**
  classifications and types 12 – 23
  clavicular 62, **63**
  complications after 26 – 31
  compression 12, **12**
  and cyst formation 28, **29**
  distal forearm, classifications 84, **85**
  distal radius, in children 86, **87**
  femoral head 60, **61**
  femur 98, **99,** 100
  fingers 96
  flake 2
  forearm
    distal 84 – 87
    pediatric age group 82
    proximal 80 – 83
  Galeazzi 82, **83**
  healing 24 – 26, **25**
    times 36
  insufficiency 12, **239**
  intertrochanteric 98, **99**
  Jones 124, **125**
  Maisonneuve 120, **121**
  malleolus, medial 118
  metastatic, signs 52, **53**
  metatarsal bones 124, **125**
  midfacial 42
  and MRI 8, **9,** 10
  olecranon 80
  osseous consolidation 24
  osteoporotic, signs 52, **53**
  patella 100 – 102
  pathologic 12, 22, **23**
  pediatric 14, **14, 15**
  pelvic 54 – 56
  pelvic rim 54
  pilon, tibia 116
  plafond, tibia 116
  reporting 36
  Rolando 96, **97**
  Salter–Harris type II, radius
    82, **83**
  signs 40
  spine, new *vs.* old **51,** 52
  stable *vs.* unstable 50
  stress 12, 18, 20
  subchondral, femoral head 222
  talar 122, **123**
  tibia, distal 118, **119**
  tibia and fibula 116, **117**
  trabecular 24
  traumatic 12
  treatment 24, 25
  types, important 12, **13**
  typical findings **37**
  vertebral, osteoporotic
    vs. metastatic 52, **53**
  Winterstein 96, **97**
Freiberg disease 226
French telephone deformity 258
frog leg view 100
frostbites 34
  osteolysis **35**
Frykman classification, distal forearm fractures 84, **85**
fungi, osseous infection 136

G

Galeazzi fracture 82, **83**
ganglion, intraosseous 374, **375**
ganglion cysts 202
  interosseous, *vs.* amyloidosis 254
gangliosidosis 272
gap healing 24
Garden classification, femoral neck fracture 98, **99**
Garré sclerotic nonpurulent osteomyelitis 150, **153**
Gaucher disease 216, **217**
geodes 296
giant cell reparative granuloma 194
giant cell tumor 170, **171**
  vs. aneurysmal bone cyst 188
  vs. chondroblastoma 166

giant cell tumor
vs. enchondroma 166
vs. simple bone cyst 186
glenohumeral joint, and shoulder dislocation 72
glenoid labrum 72
avulsed **73**
glenoid ligament, avulsion **69**
glenoid rim, fracture **71**
glomus tumor 176
glucocerebrosidosis 216
golfer's elbow **79**
Gorham–Stout disease 176
gout 364, 366
erosions 294
mutilating **367**
vs. pyrophosphate arthropathy 368
granulocytic sarcoma 208
granuloma, giant cell reparative 194
granulomatosis, Langerhans 190
greenstick fractures 14, **15**
forearm 82
ground glass appearance, fibrous dysplasia 192, **193, 194**
growing fracture 14
growth
disturbance, post-traumatic 28
pattern, bone lesions 156
variants, differential diagnosis 130, **131**

H

hair on end appearance, skull 214, **215**
hallux valgus 314, **315**
hand–foot syndrome 212
Hand–Schüller–Christian disease 190
hangman's fracture 46, **47**
Hawkins classification 122, **123**
healing, fractures 24–26, **25**
time 36
Heberden nodes 312, 314
hemangioendothelioma **176**
hemangioma 174–176, 202
hemangiopericytoma **201**
hemarthrosis **373**
hemophilic 372, **373**
hematologic disorders 204–217
hematoma, post-traumatic **29, 33**
hematopoiesis, extramedullary 214, **215**
hemochromatosis, *vs.* osteoarthritis 314
hemophilia
arthropathy 372, **373**
hemarthrosis 372
vs. juvenile rheumatoid arthritis 344
Hill–Sachs lesion 70, **71, 73**
hip
arthrography 104
bone marrow edema syndrome **231**
congenital dysplasia 290, **291**
dislocation 60
internal fixation 106, **107**
osteonecrosis 218–223
stages 219
post-surgical 102–107
prosthesis
bipolar 102, **103**
cemented 104, **105**
cement fracture 104, **105**
follow-up after 103
loosening 104
self-locking 104, **105**
total 102, **103,** 104
histiocytoma
benign fibrous 178, **178**
vs. fibrous cortical defect 184
malignant fibrous 178, **179**
histiocytosis X 190
HIV-associated arthritis 331, 356
Hodgkin disease 210, **211**
Honda sign, sacrum **21**
host response, bone tumors 156
H-shaped vertebra 212, 216
humerus
capitellum, normal position 76, **76**
fractures
classification **75, 77**
distal 76, **76, 77**
proximal 74, **74, 75**
shaft 74, **75**
head
osteonecrosis 224, **227**
segmental division 74, **74, 75**
Hutchinson/Chauffeur fracture **85**
hydroxyapatite disease 370, **371**
hyperostosis
acquired 289
condensans, clavicle 289, **289**
frontalis interna 282
hyperparathyroidism 244–247
bone loss symptoms 246
differential diagnosis 246
hypertrophic osteoarthropathy 282, **283**
hypochondroplasia 262
hypoparathyroidism 250, **251**
hypophosphatemia 268, **269**
hypophosphatemic rickets 244

I

impaction, subchondral 18, **18**
impingement syndrome, shoulder 65
impingement test, rotator cuff 66
infantile cortical hyperostosis 134, 282, **283**
infarct, in sickle cell anemia **215**
infection
after fracture 26
bone 136–151
soft-tissue 152, **153**
instability
carpal bones 92, 93, 94
distal radial fractures 84
dorsal intercalated segmental 92
pelvic fractures 54–57
shoulder 70–73
spine 50, **51,** 52
volar intercalated segmental 92
insufficiency fractures
defined 12, 20
and MRI 8
intercondylar eminence, avulsion fractures 114, **115**
interosseous ligaments, distal 126
intervertebral articulations
changes 318, **318, 319**
degeneration 326
intervertebral disks
calcification 346
degeneration 316, 320–325
diseases, imaging 326–327, **327**
herniation **323, 325**
osteochondrosis **324**
prolapse 316, 322, **323**
retromarginal 328
protrusion 316, 322, **325**
sequestered 316, **317**
intraosseous ganglion 374, **375**
involucrum 143
ischemic bone disease 218–235

J

Jefferson fracture, atlas 48, **49**
Jeune syndrome 260
joint disease
arthritis *vs.* osteoarthritis, overview 302–305
degenerative 308–330
terminology 310
hematologic 360
inflammatory 331–359
metabolic 360
neurogenic 360
pathologic–radiologic correlations 302
signs 293
tumors and lesions 374–377
joints 292–377
anatomy 292–293
capsule 292
injury 2, **3,** 8
mouse ears **353**
space narrowing 296, **297,** 302
synopsis 292–301
synovial, anatomy **292,** 292–293
Jones fracture 124, **125**
Judet, oblique views **55**
Judet and Letournel classification 58, **58, 59**
Jüngling disease 280
juvenile bone cyst 186, **187**
juvenile hematogenous osteomyelitis 138
juvenile kyphosis 328
juvenile rheumatoid arthritis 344–345, **345**
differential diagnosis **359**
juxta-articular osteoporosis 294, **295**

K

Kahler disease 204
Kaplan syndrome 342
Kienböck disease **27,** 224
kissing contusion, knee 110, **110**
knee
internal lesions 108–113
kissing contusion 110, **110**
ligaments 110, **111,** 112
pain, and MRI 8, 10
Köhler disease **129**
I 224
II 224, **225,** 226

Köhler's teardrop sign **58**
kyphosis 328

L

Langerhans granulomatosis 190
Lauenstein view 100
lead poisoning 250, **251**
Le Fort classification, fractures 42, **43**
Legg–Calvé–Perthes disease 224, 232, **233**
  vs. Meyer's dysplasia **131**
leiomyosarcoma **200**
Léri–Weill disease 260
Letterer–Siwe disease 190
Letterman sign 94, **95**
leukemia 208, **209**
  vs. myelofibrosis 216
ligaments
  injury 32
  sacroiliac 56, **56**
  spinal 318, **319**
  tibiofibular collateral 126, **127**
limbus vertebra 328
lipidosis 216
lipoma 177 – 179, 200 – 202
liposarcoma 202
  vs. lipoma 177
Lisfranc articulation 124
locking, facet joint 46, **47**
Looser zones 244, **245**, 248
lower extremity
  fracture, typical findings **37**
  trauma 98 – 127
  see also ankle; foot; knee; thigh; *specific bones*
luminescence radiography, digital 4
lunate bone
  avulsion **91**
  osteonecrosis 224, **225**
lunatomalacia 224
lunatotriquetral dissociation 94
lunotriquetral ligament 94
Lyme arthritis 331
lymphangioma 176, 202, **203**
lymphoma
  malignant 210, **211**
  vs. myelofibrosis 216

M

macroglobulinemia, Waldenström 206
Madelung deformity 260
magnetic resonance arthrography (MRA) 10
  carpal derangement 94, **95**
  shoulder **73**
  shoulder imaging 68, **69**
  wrist **91**
magnetic resonance imaging (MRI)
  and articular surface fractures 16
  avascular necrosis, femoral head 222, **223**
  and bone tumors 158
  degenerative spinal disease 326 – 327, **327**
  and insufficiency fracture 22
  joints 301, **301**
  malignancy signs, soft-tissue tumors 200
  trauma 8, **9**, 10
    indications 11
Maisonneuve fracture 120, **121**
malformation, arteriovenous 202
malignancy
  lymphoma 210, **211**
  soft-tissue, MRI signs 200
  see also tumors
malleolus, medial, fractures 118
Manaster rules, classifying skeletal lesions 156
mandible, fibromatosis **203**
mastocytosis 216, **217**
  vs. myelofibrosis 216
Matta acetabular roof arcs **59**
Mayfield staging, carpal instability 94
McCune–Albright syndrome 266
McKusick metaphyseal chondrodysplasia 264
Melone classification, distal forearm fractures 84
melorheostosis
  dripping candle wax appearance 282, **283**, 284
  radiographic signs 270, **271**
meniscus
  anatomy **109**
  degenerative changes 310
  lesions 108, **109**
  MRI signal alteration 108, **109**
  tears 10, 108, **109**
Menkes syndrome 134
metacarpal injuries 96, **97**
metastases **196 – 199**
  carcinoma **197, 199**
  and fracture, signs 52, **53**
  vs. myelofibrosis 216
  osteoblastic, *vs.* osteoid osteoma 160
  vs. Paget disease 278
  see also tumors
metatarsal bones
  fractures 122, 124, **125**
  osteonecrosis 224, **225**, 226
    staging 226
Meyer dysplasia, *vs.* Legg–Calvé–Perthes disease **131**, 232
Meyers and McKeever classification 114, **115**
Milwaukee shoulder 370
mineralization, ossification centers 130
mixed collagenosis 356, **357**
mixed connective tissue disorder (MCTD) 356
Monteggia fractures 82, **83**
  classification 83
  and elbow imaging 78
  and olecranon 80
Morquio's disease 264
MPS, *see* mucopolysaccharidosis
MRA, *see* magnetic resonance arthrography
MRI, *see* magnetic resonance imaging
mucolipidosis 272
mucopolysaccharidosis (MPS) 272, **273**
  type IV, *vs.* spondyloepimetaphyseal dysplasia 264
multiple cartilaginous exostosis 266, **267**
multiple enchondromatosis 266
multiple epiphyseal dysplasia 262, **263**
multiple myeloma 204
muscle injuries 32 – 35
  defined 2, **3**
muscle necrosis, compartment syndrome **35**
mutilation, joints 296, **297**
myelofibrosis 216, **217**
myelography 322, **323**
myeloma, differential diagnosis 206
myelopathy, and DISH 328
myositis ossificans 286
  enhancement **287**
  vs. hydroxyapatite disease 370
  post-traumatic 28, 34
  radiographic signs **287**
  zonal pattern **287**
myxoid liposarcoma **203**

N

nasal bones, fractures 42
navicular bone
  fracture **91**
  osteonecrosis 224, **225**
necrotic bone disease 218
Neer classification, proximal humeral fractures **75**
Neer projection, shoulder imaging 66, **67**, 70
neurogenic osteoarthropathy 360, **361**
newborn osteomyelitis 136, **137**, 138
Niemann–Pick disease 216, **217**
non-Hodgkin lymphoma 210, **211**
nonossifying fibroma 184, **184, 185**
  vs. aneurysmal bone cyst 188
nucleus pulposus 324, **324**

O

occipital condyles, fracture 48, **49**
occult fractures, and MRI 8, **9**
olecranon, fractures 80, **81**
Ollier disease 266
Ortolani maneuver 290
Osgood–Schlatter disease 116, **117**
ossification
  ligamentous 318
  soft-tissues 284, **285**
  see also parasyndesmophytes; spondylophytes; syndesmophytes
ossification centers 128 – 131
  distal humerus 76, **76**, 77
  secondary 124
  tibial tuberosity 116, **117**
osteitis
  condensans
    clavicle 289
    ilii 282, **283**
  deformans 276
  fibrosa cystica 244
  multiplex cystica 280
osteoarthritis 296
  vs. arthritis 302
  atrophic 310
  degenerative, post-traumatic 28, **29**
  degenerative signs **311**

osteoarthritis
erosive **305,** 310
facet joints 318, **319**
pathogenesis 302, 304
pathophysiology **303**
peripheral joints 308–312
vs. pyrophosphate arthropathy 368
osteoarthropathy
amyloid 254
diabetic **363**
distribution pattern **309**
hypertrophic 282, **283**
neurogenic 360
osteoblastic metastasis **197**
osteoblastoma 160, **161**
vs. Brodie abscess 144
osteochondral fractures 16–18
vs. chondral 18, **19**
osteochondritis dissecans 218, 234, **235**
vs. Ahlbäck disease 226
vs. normal variant 130, **131**
osteochondrodysplasia 256
osteochondroma 164–166
vs. myositis ossificans 286
osteochondromatosis 374
osteochondrosis 320–325
dissecans 234
intervertebral disks **325**
osteodystrophy, renal 248, **248, 249**
osteofibrous dysplasia 180, **181**
osteogenesis imperfecta **239,** 266, 267
vs. battered child syndrome **133,** 134
vs. hypophosphatemia 268
osteogenic sarcoma 162
osteoid osteoma 22, 160, **161**
osteolysis
after frostbite **35**
foci, circumscribed 296
massive 176
osteoma 182, **182, 183**
osteoid 22, 160, **161**
parosteal, *vs.* osteochondroma **165**
osteomalacia 242, 244, **244**
osteomyelitis 136–149
acute, diagnosis 143
vs. bone marrow edema syndrome 230
chronic 22
vs. osteoid osteoma 160
vs. osteosarcoma 162
chronic recurrent multifocal (CRMO) 144, **145,** 150
classification 137
complications 140, 142
vs. eosinophilic granuloma 190
healing 140
hematogenous
acute 136, 138–142
adult 138
chronic 142, **143**
vs. Ewing sarcoma 172
juvenile 138
juvenile hematogenous 138
plasma cellular 150
post-traumatic 146–149
vs. reflex sympathetic dystrophy 30
sclerotic nonpurulent, of Garré 150, **153**
and sickle cell anemia 212, 214, **215**
osteonecrosis 216, 218–227
definition 218
lunate bone **27,** 224, **225**
metatarsal heads, staging 226
vs. osteoarthritis 314
summary 224
osteopathia striata 270, 282
osteopathy 236–255
neurogenic 360
toxic 250, **251**
osteopenia 219, 230, 248
osteopetrosis 270, **271**
osteophyte **313**
formation 310
mixed 298
osteopoikilosis
epiphyseal bone islands 182, **183**
punctate sclerotic foci 270, **271**
osteoporosis 220, 236–241
circumscripta 276, **277**
classification 236
disuse 28, **29,** 294
vs. reflex sympathetic dystrophy 30
hand **239**
idiopathic, of femoral head 232
and insufficiency fracture **21**
postmenopausal **237,** 238
senile
cortical thinning **239**
fracture types 238
transient 230, 294
osteoporotic fracture, signs 52, **53**
osteosarcoma 162, **163**
vs. myositis ossificans 286
vs. osteoblastoma 160
vs. osteomyelitis 142
vs. simple bone cyst 186
vertebral metastasis **321**
osteosclerosis 270
vs. myelofibrosis 216

P

pachydermoperiostosis 282
Paget disease 276–279
complications 276
differential diagnosis 278
vs. hemangioma 176
vs. myelofibrosis 216
preferred sites **277**
Palmer classification, TFCC injuries 88
pancytopenia 274
Panner disease 224, 226
parasyndesmophytes 298
psoriatic arthropathy 352, **353**
Reiter syndrome 351
steer-horn **299**
patella
dislocation 100, 102
fractures 100–102
osteochondral fracture 16, **17**
partite 100, **101**
patellar tendon, tear 100, **101**
pathologic fractures 12
Pauwels classification, femoral neck fracture 98, **99**
pediatric age group
battered child syndrome 132–135
fractures
forearm 82
humerus, distal 76, **76**
radius, distal 86, **87**
growth disturbance, post-traumatic 28
leukemia 208, **209**
osteomyelitis
differential diagnosis 142
in newborns 136, **137,** 138
periosteal reaction, differential diagnosis 282
pseudosubluxation, C2/3, 50, **51**
toddler's fracture 14
trauma 128–135
spinal 50
tuberculosis 150
see also infantile; juvenile
pelvico-cleidocranial dysostosis 262
pelvis
disruption, classification 54
fracture lines **57**
injuries, Tile classification 54, **55,** 56
squared 258
trauma 54–61
pencil-in-cup mutilation **297**
periarthropathy 370
crystal-induced 364–365
periosteal desmoid 194, **195**
periosteal reaction 18, 20, **353**
lamellar 296, **297**
peritendinitis 370
peritumoral edema 158–159
phalanges, squared 214
phleboliths **201**
phlegmonous cellulitis 152, **153**
phosphate diabetes 244, **269**
phosphorus poisoning 250
Pierre–Marie–Bamberger disease 282
pigmented villonodular synovitis (PVNS) 296, 376, **377**
vs. amyloidosis 254
vs. hemarthrosis 372
vs. osteoarthritis of knee 312
Pipkin classification, femoral head fracture dislocation **61**
plafond fractures, classification 116, **117**
plasma cellular osteomyelitis 150
plasmacytoma 204–207, **207**
vs. amyloidosis 254
vs. giant cell tumor 170
vs. hemangioma 176
POEMS syndrome 206, **207**
poisoning, metal 250, **251**
Poland syndrome 274
polyarteritis nodosa 356
polyarthritis, chronic 338
polycythemia vera 216
polydactyly 274
polymyositis 355–356
differential diagnosis **359**
polyostotic fibrous dysplasia 266
Pott disease 334
Preiser disease 224, 226
progressive systemic scleroderma (PSS) 355
differential diagnosis **359**
pronator quadratus sign 86, **87**
prostatic carcinoma, metastasis **197**
pseudarthrosis 26, **27**

pseudo-Charcot joint 362
pseudocyst, subchondral 220
pseudodeficiency rickets 268
pseudoepiphyses 128
pseudohypoparathyroidism 250
pseudospondylolisthesis **329**
pseudosubluxation, C2/3, in children 50, **51**
pseudotumor, hemophilic 372
psoriatic arthritis, differential diagnosis **359**
psoriatic arthropathy 352–353, **353**
  vs. ankylosing spondylitis 348
psoriatic morning star **353**
PSS, *see* progressive systemic scleroderma
pustulotic arthro-osteitis 288–289, **289**
PVNS, *see* pigmented villonodular synovitis
pyknodysostosis 270
pyrophosphate arthropathy 368

R

radiography
  conventional
    and bone tumors 157
    and facial fractures 40
    spine 45
    trauma 2, 3–10
  digital luminescence 4, **5**
  follow-up after hip replacement 103
  fracture reporting 36
  hip, internal fixation 106, **107**
  peripheral joints 294, **295,** 296
  sacroiliac joints 298, 300
  spine 298
radius
  fractures
    head 80, **81**
    neck 80, **81**
  head, subluxation 78
  Salter–Harris type II fracture 82, **83**
Recklinghausen's disease of bone 244
reconversion, bone marrow 212
reduction anomalies 274, **275**
reflex sympathetic dystrophy (RSD) 30, **31**
  and juxta-articular osteoporosis 294
  see also bone marrow, edema syndrome
Regazzoni plate 102, **103**
Reiter syndrome 350–351, **351**
  vs. psoriatic arthropathy 353
renal osteodystrophy 248, **248, 249**
renal transplantation 248
resorption, bone, in hyperparathyroidism 246, **247**
retinacula, patellar 112, **113**
rhabdomyolysis 34, **35**
rheumatic fever 331
  vs. juvenile rheumatoid arthritis 344
rheumatoid arthritis 338–343
  vs. amyloidosis 254
  vs. ankylosing spondylitis 348
  criteria 339
  differential diagnosis **359**
  juvenile 344–345, **345**
  and osteolytic foci 296
  vs. Reiter syndrome 351
  seronegative 342
rickets 134, 242, **243**
  hereditary 268
  vs. hypophosphatemia 268
  vs. metaphyseal chondrodysplasia 264
  pseudodeficiency 268
  vitamin D-resistant 244
Rolando fracture 96, **97**
Romanus lesion 298, **299,** 346
roof arcs, acetabulum **59**
rotation, atlantoaxial 48
rotation fractures, spine 46, **47**
rotator cuff **65**
  lesion 65–66
  rupture 65
  shoulder joint, and MRI **9,** 10
Rubinstein–Taybi syndrome 274
Rüedi–Allgöwer classification 116, **117**
rugger jersey spine **249**

S

sacral ala view 54, **55**
sacroiliac joints
  ligamentous injuries, classification 56, **56**
  radiographic signs 298, 300
  subchondral resorption 246
sacroiliitis **335, 347,** 354
  Reiter syndrome **351**
  variegated picture 228, **299,** 346
sacrum
  butterfly view 54
  fractures 50
  insufficiency fracture **21**
Salmonella osteomyelitis **141**
Salter–Harris classification, fractures 14, **14, 15**
  type II, radius 82, **83, 87**
SAPHO syndrome 288
sarcoidosis 280–281, **281**
sarcoma
  granulocytic 208
  synovial 202, 376, **377**
scaphoid bone
  fat pad sign 90, **91**
  osteonecrosis 224, **225,** 226
scapholunate ligament **91,** 94
scaphopisocapitate alignment 86
Schachman metaphyseal chondrodysplasia 264
Scheuermann disease 328, **329**
Schmid metaphyseal chondrodysplasia 264
Schmorl's nodes 328
scintigraphy
  acute hematogenous osteomyelitis 138–140
  avascular necrosis of femoral head 220, **221**
  and bone tumors 157
  and insufficiency fractures 20, **20**
  joints 300
  metastases 196
  and trauma 10
scleroderma, calcinosis **285**
sclerosis, subchondral 296, **297**
  hip **219,** 220, **220**
sclerotic nonpurulent osteomyelitis 150, **153**
scoliosis 328
seat-belt injury 44
senile osteoporosis 28
sequestrum 143
  button 190, **191**
  in chronic osteomyelitis **149**
Sharp syndrome 354, 356, **357**
shear fractures, spine 46, **47,** 48
shepherd's crook deformity, fibrous dysplasia **194**
shiny corner sign 346
  spondylitis **299**
shoulder
  dislocation 70–73, **71**
  empyema **333**
  hydroxyapatite disease **371**
  impingement syndrome 65
  instability 70–73
  Milwaukee 370
shoulder girdle, trauma 62–74
sickle cell anemia 212, **213,** 214
skeletal dysplasia 256–271
skeletal echinococcosis 150
skier's thumb **97**
skull
  cloverleaf 258
  cotton-wool appearance **275, 277**
  fractures 38, **39**
  osteoma **183**
  plasmocytoma **205**
  trauma 38, **39**
SLE, *see* systemic lupus erythematosus
Smith fracture 84, **85**
soap bubble pattern, fibrous dysplasia 192
soft-tissue
  abscess 152, **153**
  calcification 248, 284, **285**
    compartment syndrome 34, **35**
  changes, trauma-induced 32–35
  infections 152, **153**
  involvement, bone lesions 156
  ossification 284, **285**
  swelling 294, **295**
  tumors 200–203
    classification 200
    follow-up 202
    glossary 202
    treatment strategies 159
sonography
  and bone tumors 157
  joints 300, **300,** 301
  quantitative 240
  shoulder imaging 66, **67**
  and soft-tissue infection 152, **153**
  trauma 8, **9**
spinal canal, stenosis 318, 326
spine
  bamboo appearance 298
  compression fracture 12, **12**
  degenerative changes 316–330, **321**

spine
degenerative disease, imaging 326–327, **327**
dysraphism, and osteoarthropathy **361**
fractures
classification 44
extension 46
flexion 44, 46
rotation 46, **47**
instability 50, **51,** 52
normal, nucleus pulposus **324**
radiographic signs 298
rheumatoid arthritis 340–342, **343**
rugger jersey appearance **249**
trauma 44–53, 48, **49**
see also vertebrae
spondylitis 331, 332, 354
ankylosing, *see* ankylosing spondylitis
anterior 298
bacterial, *vs.* ankylosing spondylitis 348
infectious 334–**337**
spondyloarthropathy
erosive **255**
juvenile, *vs.* rheumatoid arthritis 344
seronegative 331
spondylodiskitis **325,** 331, **337**
vs. amyloidosis 254
vs. ankylosing spondylitis 348
bacterial *vs.* tuberculous **337**
infectious 334–**337,** 336
tuberculous 334, **335**
spondyloepimetaphyseal dysplasia 264, **265**
spondylolisthesis **327**
spondylophytes 298, **299**
spondylosclerosis, hemispheric 321
spondylosis deformans, *vs.* ankylosing spondylitis 348
spotted bones 270
squared phalanges 214
staging
ARCO 219
avascular necrosis, femoral head 219
bone tumors 157, 159
Bragard 226
Legg–Calvé–Perthes disease 232
Mayfield, carpal instability 94
osteochondrosis dissecans 234, **235**
osteonecrosis
hip 219
metatarsal heads 226
Stecher view, carpal bone fractures 90, **91**
steer-horn parasyndesmophyte **299**
stenosis, spinal canal 318, 326
sternoclavicular dislocation 62, **63**
sternocostoclavicular hyperostosis 282
Still disease 344
Streptococcus pyogenes 152
stress fractures 12, **21, 23**
and MRI 8
stress reaction 18, **19**
stress views, ankle 126, **127**
subchondral cysts 296, **297**
hip 304, **305, 311**
tibiofibular joint **313**
subchondral impaction 18, **18**
subluxation
anterior, spine 44, **45,** 46
atlantoaxial 48
posterior, spine 46
radial head 78
see also pseudosubluxation
subscapularis tendon, MR arthrography **69**
Sudeck disease 30, 230, 294
sugar loaf sign 355
supraspinatus tendon, tear **67, 69**
swan-neck deformity 96
symphalangy 274
symphysis pubis, disruption 54, **55**
syndactyly 274, **275**
syndesmophytes 298, **299**
synovial chondromatosis 374, **375**
synovial cysts 318, 322, **323**
subchondral 374
synovial fluid 293
synovial joints, decompression **339**
synovialoma 376
synovial plicae 112, **113**
synovial sarcoma 376, **377**
syphilis 150
syringomyelia, and osteoarthropathy **361**
systemic lupus erythematosus (SLE) 355, **357**
differential diagnosis **359**

T

talar fractures 122, **123**
talomalleolar joint spaces, asymmetry 126
talus, necrosis 224
tarsal bones 130
anatomy **124**
fractures 122–125
teardrop fracture
extension 46
spine 44, **45**
teardrop sign
blow-out fractures 40, **43**
Köhler's **58**
temporal bone, fractures 38, 40, **41**
tendinitis, calcifying 370
supraspinatus **371**
tendon injuries 32, **33**
tendon ruptures, lower extremity 100
tennis elbow 78, **79**
Terry Thomas sign 94, **95**
TFCC, *see* triangular fibrocartilage complex
thalassemia 214
thanatophoric dysplasia 258, **259**
Thiemann disease 224
Thomas sign 94, **95**
thoraco-pelvic–phalangeal dysplasia 260
three-dimensional imaging 6, **7**
tibia
distal fractures, in growth period 118, **119**
and fibula, fractures 116, **117**
fractures 114
pilon fractures 116
plafond fractures 116
tibial plateau
fracture dislocations **115**
fractures 114, **114, 115**
tibial tuberosity, avulsion 116
tibiotalar joint, rheumatoid arthritis **343**
Tietze syndrome 289
Tillaux–Chaput tuberosity 120, **121**
toddler's fracture 14
tophus **365,** 366, **367**
torus fracture 14
Tossy classification, acromioclavicular separation 64
toxic osteopathy 250, **251**
trabecular fractures 24
trauma 2–135
in children 128–135
definitions 2, **3**
fractures
classifications 12–23
complications 27–31
healing 24–26
reporting of 36
types **37**
and imaging 2–10
practical suggestions 11
lower extremity 98–127
meniscus 108
musculoskeletal, imaging 2, 3–10
and osteomyelitis 146–149
pediatric age group 128–135
pelvis 54–61
radiography
conventional 4, **5**
digital 4
shoulder girdle 62–74
skull 38, **39**
and soft-tissue changes 32–35
spine 44–53
typical findings **37**
upper extremity 74–97
triangular fibrocartilage complex (TFCC) 8, 86
injuries 88, **89**
tuberculosis
vs. eosinophilic granuloma 190
skeletal 150, **151**
and spondylodiskitis 336
tuberculous arthritis **333,** 334
tuberculous spondylodiskitis 334, **335**
tuberosity, of Tillaux–Chaput 120
tuberosity–joint angle, Böhler 122, **125**
tumorlike lesions 154, 182–199
tumors 154
bone, primary 154–181
from bone marrow 172, **173**
bone-producing 160–163
cartilage-producing 164–171
from connective tissue 177–179
glomus 176
joints 374–377
matrix 156
primary, and metastases 196
soft-tissue 200–203
vs. soft-tissue abscess **153**
vascular 174–176
malignant 176
see also malignancy; metastases

U

ulna
- fracture, typical findings **37**
- variance 86, **87**

uncovertebral joints **318**
upper extremity
- trauma 74 – 97
- *see also* elbow; forearm; hand; wrist; *specific bones*

V

vacuum phenomenon **253,** 336
- sternoclavicular dislocation 62, **63**
- and vertebral fracture **51**

vascular tumors 174 – 176
- malignant 176

vertebrae, vertebral bodies
- in achondroplasia **259**
- block 298
- codfish **237**
- cod-shaped 212
- compression 198
- end plates, degenerative changes 316, 318
- facet joint osteoarthritis **318**
- H-shaped 212, 216
- ivory **197**
- limbus 328
- marrow changes 324
- in osteoporosis **237**
- pear-shaped deformity 264
- rounded **298**
- squared 298, **299**
- vertebra plana 190, **190**
- washed-out appearance **244**
- *see also* spine

VISI, *see* volar intercalated segmental instability
vitamin D overdose **253**
vitamin D-resistant rickets 268
volar intercalated segmental instability (VISI) 92
Volkmann triangle **37,** 120

W

Waldenström macroglobulinemia 206
Weber classification, ankle fractures 120, **121**
Winterstein fracture 96, **97**
wrist
- auxiliary lines
- magnetic resonance arthrography (MRA) **91**
- and MRI 8
- positioning 86, **86, 87**
- *see also* carpal bones; metacarpal injuries

X

X-ray absorptiometry, and osteoporosis 240 – 241

Z

Zellweger syndrome, *vs.* chondrodysplasia punctata 260
zygoma, fractures **41,** 42
zygomaticomaxillary complex (ZMC), fractures 42